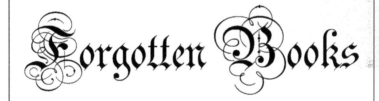

ISBN 978-1-397-31006-4
PIBN 11375127

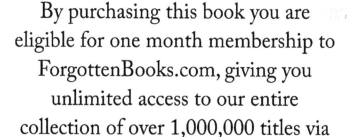

English
Français
Deutsche
Italiano
Español
Português

www.forgottenbooks.com

Mythology Photography **Fiction**
Fishing Christianity **Art** Cooking
Essays Buddhism Freemasonry
Medicine **Biology** Music **Ancient
Egypt** Evolution Carpentry Physics
Dance Geology **Mathematics** Fitness
Shakespeare **Folklore** Yoga Marketing
Confidence Immortality Biographies
Poetry **Psychology** Witchcraft
Electronics Chemistry History **Law**
Accounting **Philosophy** Anthropology
Alchemy Drama Quantum Mechanics
Atheism Sexual Health **Ancient History**
Entrepreneurship Languages Sport
Paleontology Needlework Islam
Metaphysics Investment Archaeology
Parenting Statistics Criminology
Motivational

JOURNAL

OF THE

American Veterinary Medical Association

FORMERLY

AMERICAN VETERINARY REVIEW

(Original Official Organ U. S. Vet. Med. Ass'n)

EDITED AND PUBLISHED FOR

The American Veterinary Medical Association

BY

PIERRE A. FISH, ITHACA, N. Y.

Index Volume LIII

NEW SERIES VOLUME VI

ITHACA, N. Y.

Published by the American Veterinary Medical Association

1918

List of Illustrations, Volume LIII, New Series, Vol. 6

Author's Index

Index to Volume LIII.   New Series Volume 6

JOURNAL

OF THE

American Veterinary Medical Association

Formerly American Veterinary Review

(Original Official Organ U. S. Vet. Med. Ass'n)

PIERRE A. FISH, Editor   ITHACA, N. Y.

Executive Board

—————, 1st District; W. HORACE HOSKINS, 2d District; J. R. MOHLER, 3d District; C. H. STANGE, 4th District; R. A. ARCHIBALD, 5th District; A. T. KINSLEY, Member at large.

Sub-Committee on Journal

J. R. MOHLER   R. A. ARCHIBALD

The American Veterinary Medical Association is not responsible for views or statements published in the JOURNAL, outside of its own authorized actions.
Reprints should be ordered in advance. A circular of prices will be sent upon application.

VOL. LIII., N. S. VOL. VI.   APRIL, 1918.   No. 1.

HORSEFLESH

Evidence indicates that from the time of the cavemen in northern Europe all of the larger domesticated animals, including the horse, were used for food purposes. Later the tribes of northern Europe sacrificed the horse, as the most noble animal, to their Gods and the ceremonies of sacrifice were accompanied with great feasts in which horseflesh was largely consumed. With the growth of Christianity the idolatrous custom of sacrifices was denounced and in the effort to abrogate pagan worship edicts were issued against the consumption of horseflesh, not apparently because of any inherent quality in the flesh, but for religious reasons. Christianity has apparently been responsible for prohibiting horseflesh for food along lines somewhat similar to the Arabic and Jewish prohibition against the use of pork. Sentiment has also been a factor. The horse, more than any other animal, perhaps, has been man's friend and servant. In war he has helped to win victories: in peace he has added to his owner's prosperity. Strong ties of affection have developed between horse and master.

With perhaps the exception of swine, all of the domesticated animals are more or less cleanly in their habits and are of use to man in other ways than yielding up their flesh for his consumption. The cow is the wet nurse of humanity. Without her milk the hu-

man population of the earth could not be sustained nor maintained, especially during the early years of infancy. In olden
times and in some areas still, the bovines do the work of the horse
in tilling the soil. The sheep provides us with material for our
clothing. All possess some qualities which are on a par with some
human attributes. Maternal affection, during the period of help-
lessness of the young, is strongly developed. The cow is docile and
unresisting; the gentleness of the lamb is proverbial—and yet we
eat them.

On sentimental grounds the only consistent course is vegetari-
anism. Protein and fat as well as carbohydrate may be obtained
from vegetable sources . Man is an omnivorous animal. Nature
has endowed him with a mouth and digestive apparatus which can
utilize either an animal or vegetable diet and a taste or appetite
for a mixed ration. There is also evidence that the more concentrated animal protein is more easily digested and assimilated resulting in more pronounced bodily vigor and stamina.

War has been responsible not only for much traditional glory
for the horse, but it has also brought him down to the inglorious
level of the other domesticated animals. The ban against the use
of horseflesh was undoubtedly imposed to break up pagan worship
rather than to any injurious dietetic effect or for any great respect
for the horse. The custom, once established, has been maintained.
During the French revolution and the Napoleonic campaigns, it
was necessary at times to use horseflesh to avoid starvation. During the Danish siege in 1807 it was utilized. To a vanquished people, sustenance is of more immediate importance than glory. The
pangs of hunger may overcome the pangs of conscience and religious scruples yield to the necessity of keeping alive the vital
spark. Although earlier records are not available, it would appear
that early in the nineteenth century some of the European countries
permitted the sale and use of horseflesh as a necessary or progressive measure.

A state of siege and the hardships of war, with accompanying
food restrictions, have apparently been responsible for a return to
the early practices of the consideration of the horse from a dietary
standpoint. From 1840 and 1850 some of the European countries
have sanctioned the public sale of horse meat. The practice has
grown, indicating that there has been a desire for it and this has
been still further emphasized by the fact that horse meat has been

supplied at a much lower rate than that of the other domesticated animals. Subject to the same careful veterinary inspection as for other food animals, there is little or no possibility of the communicability of disease to the human subject. With proper supervision and inspection there have been no more indications nor reports of dietary troubles than from other meats.

Horse meat has sometimes been substituted for beef without detection on the part of the consumer. In comparison the essential difference is that the fibers of horseflesh appear to contain a somewhat higher proportion of glycogen and the fat is of a somewhat softer consistency. Because of this it is claimed the flavor varies slightly from beef but the difference disappears when the fat is removed. The taste has also been stated to be slightly sweeter than ordinary meat. Such articles of food as oysters, lobster and liver contain glycogen and are highly prized. The claim has also been made that horse meat has a greater percentage of nourishment than beef, mutton or pork.

In America the use of horse meat has not attracted attention until recent years. Twenty years ago the government inspected horse carcasses for export to Denmark, but the trade from this country was not apparently kept up for more than three or four years. The present war and considerations of public welfare have brought the matter to the surface in a number of localities. The sale of horseflesh has been permitted in St. Louis; Cincinnati; New York; Portland, Oregon; and doubtless in a number of other places. Reports indicate that local consumption is on the increase and in some instances the supply has not been able to keep up with the demand.

The question is also an economic one. There are some millions of people here from foreign countries where horseflesh has been consumed and who would be glad to continue its use if available. There would at the outset, be a considerable demand for it here and the demand would increase. There is an export market for it among our allies and this market would undoubtedly grow. The head of one of the horsemen associations has stated that there are 4,000,000 horses in this country that might as well be eaten. If the dressed carcass would average from 400 to 500 lbs. there would be from 1,600,000,000 to 2,000,000,000 lbs. of meat available with a per capita quantity of 16 to 20 lbs. for a population of 100,000,000. Many horses are on ranges where the pasturage might be available for our other animals or where the soil might be utilized for the production of cereals. At this time waste is criminal. The world must be fed and edible food of all kinds should be utilized. Sentiment for the horse should be respected just as the sentiment of vegetarians is respected. There is no thought of compulsion in enforcing the eating of flesh of any kind, but where such an important source of food supply is available and it is clearly evident there is a demand for it, there should be no unnecessary delay in making it available. The horse can do his bit in the dietary of civilization as well as the other domesticated animals. Custom should not be allowed to stand as a barrier when necessity demands progress. The use of the horse for food is beyond the experimental stage. There is no more danger from eating this form of flesh than any other commonly used. The horse is proverbially clean in his habits. Compared with poultry and swine there is no discussion—yet we balk at the horse and swallow swine.   P. A. F.

EIGHT REASONS FOR EQUINE MEAT AS FOOD

First, horseflesh has not been eaten in the past in our country largely because we have been influenced by an unsound public sentiment and popular prejudice created by religious and other decrees of less enlightened nations than our own.

Second, horseflesh should be eaten because the flesh is rich and nutritious. The horse is one of the most cleanly animals by nature and spurns impure and unwholesome food. The food that hogs and ducks will consume, the horse rejects. The horse is almost immune from tuberculosis, while the cow, hog and chicken are very susceptible. The mare's milk is one of the richest animal food products known to science.

Third, horseflesh should be placed upon the market, because a large part of our population in the large cities have been afforded in their native countries access to this cheaper kind of meat, and thus helped in their struggle for a better existence.

Fourth, every humane society in the land should join heartily in this movement because it would help solve one of the most trying problems that daily concerns their splendid work. To punish by fine and imprisonment the man who works a hopelessly and incurably lame horse adds many hardships to the owner and many times makes his children go to bed hungry and weak. It is no solution of the man's misfortune to fine and imprison him, and break down the wife and mother at home with her children's need for food, clothing, perhaps medicine and a roof over their heads, thus adding another economic problem for civic and charitable bodies to solve.

Fifth, one of the principal forms of food consumed by the horse is oats. This food, so rich in nutritious elements and long prepared for human consumption in the form of breakfast food, is now so costly as to be almost beyond the reach of the working classes.

Sixth, many of the horses properly forced off the streets by humane agents are kept by their ignorant and impoverished owners for weeks with the hope of curing them, and large quantities of now the most expensive foods, oats and corn, are worse than wasted. The owner dreads the destruction of the animal because that means the payment of a fee for removal of the body, and in finding of some new employment to keep his family and himself.

Seventh, the sales marts of our cities are besieged for relief by owners in their desperation, and many times out of sympathy for these unfortunates permit the sale of these animals against their better judgment, and thus add to the horse's extended suffering. The temptation to traffic in these animals, to clandestinely move them from place to place, and to unload part of their burden on someone else less able to bear it, is a problem so difficult of solution by the humane societies that even the imposition of many thousands of dollars in fines annually (I have heard as high as $30,000 a year and imprisonment) does not rectify the wrong. Neither does it add to greater humaneness, which we hope and pray will come out of this terrible and terrifying war.

Eighth, every horse that might be sold for food consumes daily eight times as much by weight as would sustain a man. Every day he is fed impoverishes his owner when there is no remedy for his crippled legs or body. Such horses ofttimes eat, but waste as much again as would maintain a sound horse at work. There is waste of labor spent in the hopeless struggle trying to cure such horses, waste of food and medicine, which ought to be conserved.

W. H. H.

EUROPEAN CHRONICLES

Bois Jerome.

OXYUROSIS IN EQUINES.—Under this name the learned professor of Alfort, A. Raillet, proposes to study the series of troubles that are due to nematodes of the large intestines of equines and which belong to the genus *Oxyuris*.

Although these helminths, fed especially on the vegetable detritus of the large digestive organs, are scarcely parasites, and by some authors are considered as harmless, yet numerous and positive observations show that they are liable to promote various troubles, some of which have a direct relation to their evolution and others perhaps are related to some products of secretion which are manifestations of the physiological activity of parasites.

In opening his subject, Professor Raillet gives an historical discussion which begins with 1782, when Goeze was the first to describe and give an illustration of the oxyure of horses under the name of *Tricocephalus,* which in 1788 Schrank called the *T. equi,* and in 1803 was transformed by Zeder into *Mastigodes equi.* In the same year Rudolphi called it the *Oxyuris curvula* and in 1849 it was named *O. equi* by Em. Blanchard.

Later, and between the years 1859 and 1901, many articles were written by various authors, viz.: Rudolphi, Gurlt, Gribel, Jerke, Raillet, Probstmayer, Looss, Luistow, etc., until finally the type species of the genus was admitted as the *Oxyuris curvula* of Rudolphi, which is the *Tricocephalus equi* of Schrank, and must therefore take the name of *Oxyuris equi* of Schrank, whose distinctive characters are those given by Raillet, describing the male and female parasite with their varieties, that may be observed in different cases, especially calling attention to differences in the length of the tail in each sex.

Oxyuris equi lives in horses, donkeys, and mules. It has been found in zebras. It is in the diaphragmatic curvature of the large colon, where it is generally met with normally. It has been found in a duck. It is a cosmopolitan parasite and is found in all countries where there are equines and yet, although recognized as common parasites by veterinarians the statistics relating to them are not numerous. One is given in which a horse had evacuated 300 long tailed oxyuris and at the post mortem of which 30 more were found, 8 of which were males.

There are two other species of oxyuris, the *O. poculum* and the *O. tenuicauda,* both of which present only a zoological interest.

'Continuing his interesting article Raillet writes on the evolution of the parasites and of their pathogenic action telling the reader successively the opinions advanced by various writers from Hurtrel d'Arboval down to our day and relating the facts advanced by English, French and German observers, he summarized all in the symptomatology as consisting in local manifestations universally admitted and in general trouble insufficiently established.

The former consist first in a violent, unresisting, although intermittent pruritis, which is manifested by the animal rubbing the posterior part of the body against surrounding objects. The animal holds down his tail tightly, curves his vertebral column, pushes against the walls or sides of his stall and with force rubs against them, sometimes almost in a frenzy. In the anal region, almost always the perineum and often also at the base of the tail, crusty plates of various sizes, yellowish, greenish or of dirty grey color are seen adhering to the inflamed and sometimes excoriated skin. The skin of the perineum may also be scratched or inflamed. Frequently also the crusty scabs and the excoriations are found at the inferior portion of the root of the tail. The caudal appendix has the hairs altered, they are curly, torn and easily pulled out. Inflammation of the anus does not seem to be a common observation.

The general symptoms observed by many veterinarians are a noticeable loss of flesh, accompanied sometimes with anemia and perhaps cachexia. Colic has been observed but may, however, be due to other causes than the parasites.

While this is the summary of the observations of the various authors, the diagnosis of oxyurosis can be established without great difficulty—the pruritis of the perineal region and the depilation of the tail at its base, with the scabby oviparous collections on the perineum, all tell the story.

The presence of worms attached to the anus, certainly in the feces or if necessary a rectal exploration will be positive evidence of the condition.

The prophylaxis and treatment are then considered. The former is difficult. The treatment is easy. Tartar emetic, corrosive sublimate as Van Swieten solution, areca nut powder, thymol, followed by purgatives, etc., have their advocates. Raillet advises enemas of tepid soap water or acidulated with vinegar or with corrosive sublimate 1 per 2000 or a mucilaginous emulsion of thymol. These enemas must be large and repeated as often as necessary. The cutaneous lesions heal of themselves and disappear spontaneously or with antiseptic treatment.

The bibliography of the article of Prof. Raillet gives a long list of publications covering a space of years from 1782 to 1913 and offering to the inquirer a most complete collection of writings upon this subject which has been reviewed by the masterly article of the worthy professor of Alfort.

. 📧 📧 📧

VETERINARY DENTISTRY.—Notwithstanding the fact that American Veterinary Science is quite in its youth, when compared with that of old Europe, no one will ignore the many valuable contributions that have been given for the elevation and benefit of our profession and several names are already inscribed in the archives of good work performed. Among them, some will remain comparatively unknown; others will be remembered for years to come.

It is to Dr. House, I believe, that one of the most frequent, essential and important opportunities of surgical application is due. If today *veterinary dentistry* is a specialty, if it has the honor of a collegiate department, occupied by professors of eminent ability, it is due to the work started by Doctor House many years ago. I am under the impression that I am but one who can remember to have witnessed his ability, his dexterity and the success met with, although some failures may have occurred.

These remarks are suggested by a communication published in the *Bulletin de la Societe Centrale* of Paris in October, 1917. It is from the pen of a Belgian veterinarian, Professor Jos. Hamoir, actually doing service at the central infirmary of the Belgian army. The author is already well known by his writings, even in America, and the communication referred to is entitled: *Study on the Dental and Paradental Affections of the Horse.*

The subject has already been treated in the various classical works on surgery and therapeutic treatment, but Prof. Hamoir has had such extensive opportunities and been able to give so much attention to the patients observed that his article has been considered of such value that it was referred to the Commission on Recompense for the recognition it deserves.

The author first develops the importance of the problem of mastication, especially with horses the principal object of the article. As the function of mastication has for its essential organs, the molar teeth, it is of them that Hamoir speaks principally and divides the causes which disturb the mechanism of mastication and renders its functions insufficient, into *physiological* and *pathologi-cal*. These being related either, 1st, to a congenital fault in the opening of the jaws or a *reciprocal anomaly* in the molar surfaces; 2nd, of a congenital anomaly of structure of some molars; 3rd, of dental diseases, such as fractures, luxations, caries, etc.; 4th, of paradental affections, alveolitis or primitive or secondary alveolo-dental periostitis.

This long consideration is divided into two chapters.

In the first are treated, in succession: 1st, the *dental crisis*, which means the period from two to three and one-half years of age, on the average, during which successively takes place the change between the milk and adult molars; 2nd, the *dental irregularities*. With Belgian veterinarians, with exceptions, the name of *chiçots* is given to the sharp and cutting asperities that occur on some teeth. The word *chicotomy* is used to refer to the operation for the removal of those asperities; 3rd, *overgrown teeth*. These are called *surdents* and mean the condition of a sound molar grown above the general level of the dental arch to which it belongs; 4th, *dental caries;* 5th, *fractures;* 6th, *alveolar periostitis.*

In the second chapter, under the heading of *paralveolar affections,* are treated: 1st, the *sinusitis of dental origin,* and 2nd, the *osteomyelitis* of similar origin.

It is not possible for me to go into further consideration of this valuable paper. To have enumerated the various subdivisions and give a faint idea of what is in it, is all I can do. The causes, symptomatic manifestations, lesions with their progress and various localizations, results and treatment demanded to restore the dental apparatus to a proper condition, are points that the reader must look up for himself in the *Bulletin de la Societe Centrale.*

RENGUERA.—This is the name given, in Peru, to a paralytic sheep disease to which Mr. S. H. Gaizer, F.R.C.V.S., gives much consideration in Sir John M'Fadyean's journal.

After telling how he was requested to investigate the subject, the author gives the local geographic and climatic conditions of Peru, treats of the sheep-farming customs and comes to the history of the disease.

The word *Renguera* is probably derived from the Spanish word "rengna" meaning "injured in the back". The origin and spread of the disease is without reliable information. It has existed in Atocsaico, one of the largest farms in that country, for six years and also in neighboring farms. The number of animals affected varies and in some instances the losses have been such that sheep raising had to be abandoned.

The symptomatology is as follows: the disease occurs only in sheep. The symptoms commence in lambs from the age of 14 days old to that of 5 or 6 months. It is manifested by a partial loss of control of movements of the hind legs and quarters with a tendency to knuckling. At rest the animal stands with a wooden-horse attitude, so as to keep its balance. When forced to move, both hind legs move forward by jumps. If made to go faster there is a twisting of the hind legs around one another, followed by a fall, with the animal on its side, but often on its back with legs in the air. After a few moments the lamb recovers, rises again until another collapse occurs. With all that, the animal appears perfectly healthy and if left alone for a rest, after recovering from its exhaustion, he will move about apparently well.

There are acute and chronic cases. In bad cases in lambs a not uncommon symptom is observed, viz.: a slight up and down trembling of the head and more rarely of the whole body. The fore limbs then show loss of control.

The paralysis is always progressive from behind forward in fatal cases. When this occurs in young lambs, it usually comes within a week.

Apart from the nervous manifestations the affected animal is otherwise normal and all his functions are regular.

Perfect recovery has not been observed.

The post mortem lesions were, (1) increase in the peritoneal, pericardial and pleural fluids, which were frequently slightly tinged with hemoglobin; (2) a darker color of the liver in most cases; (3) slight but never marked increase in the coloring of the cranial and spinal meninges; (4) occasional catarrh of the small intestine in lambs; (5) not infrequently patchy endocarditis.

The possible nature of *renguera* and the attempts to transmit the disease with brain inoculation, with blood, cerebro-spinal fluid, peritoneal and pericardial fluid and by methods of feeding, did not prove successful in experiments.

An almost constant association of a micrococcus with the disease suggested a large number of inoculations which were made on hoggets and lambs, all of which are concisely recorded in Mr. Gaizer's article which is closed with the following conclusions:

"Renguera is a new and hitherto undescribed disease of lambs, occurring in the Peruvian Andes.

"Sheep only appear to be susceptible.

"Renguera belongs to the class of nervous diseases, to which louping-ill, scrapie and swing back in Britain and pataleta in South America belong.

"Renguera is distinguishable from louping-ill by its affecting lambs only and by there being no convulsions in any form of the disease. From scrapie it is distinguished by there being no symptom of skin irritation. No comparison can be made with swing back. It closely agrees with some of the descriptions of pataleta but not with others.

"Renguera is almost constantly associated with a micrococcus which can be grown from the fluids and tissues of the body, including, sometimes, the brain and spinal fluids; but in the absence of success in all attempts to transmit the disease either with the coccus or any of the fluids and tissues of the body, it is not possible yet to say if this coccus is the causative agent.

"Curative measures hold but little promise of success. Prevention may be found by further experimentation.

"The occurrence of the disease at an altitude where ticks do not exist should be of special interest as it shows that ticks are unnecessary for the propagation of at least one sheep disease of the nervous type."

ASPHYXIATING GASES ON HORSES.—If the noxious effects from these gases are well known in human medicine, from the numerous instances that have been observed and studied on the various battle-fields; where an obus (shell) loaded with chloroformiate of trichlorated methylen and chloropicrine was used, the results accompanying the explosion of such on horses and mules have not yet had much publicity in our periodicals. On that account, the observations reported by Veterinarian Francois and Doctor Nicolas are full of interest.

The former relates two observations. In one, which occurred on the front at Verdun, the teams of fifteen wagons delivering munitions to artillery battery positions had been exposed to the effects of asphyxiating gases and were in such condition that it was thought first an utter impossibility to bring them back to camp. One hundred and two horses were affected. Sixty-one were very sick, 33 less seriously and 8 were in such state that none were expected to recover. These horses were divided into three groups, separated, and isolated in the woods close by, in the shade and having quiet and free ventilation.

The second observation related to a smaller number of horses, thirty-four, which were also divided into three groups as in the first case, viz.: 18, 11 and 5 horses, according to their condition.

The description of the symptoms in the sickest of the animals is minutely described and concisely summarized by Dr. Nicolas as observed by him. Severe dyspnea, abortive cough similar to that observed in heaves or emphysema, rosy, spumey nasal discharge, loud respiration with mucous rales, dull cardiac sound, hypertensive pulse, small, cyanotic mucous membranes, lumbar reflex absent or reduced. Everything indicated difficulty in respiration due to the edema of the lungs, as characterized by the nasal discharge; edema which has been observed in men who died from intoxication by chlorine gas and in dogs experimentally intoxicated with it.

The progress of the trouble is, notwithstanding the severity of the attack, without alarming aspect. After seventy-two hours, three days, improvement was noticed in the animals that suffered most and in a few days *all* the horses of the two observations of Francois were able to resume their work, none showing afterwards any ill consequence of the intoxication.

According to Francois the condition, of the sick ones, was due to an attack of tracheo-bronchitis with possibly a slight extension of capillary bronchitis in the anterior portion of the pulmonary lobes.

The treatment indicated as a preventive is the use of a mask, simple in its construction and of sufficient solidity to be adapted to all kinds of bridles and not interfere with the bit, to be easily applied and permit the frequent application of compresses on the head. As a curative treatment, shady, airy and sheltered exposures seem to be essentially and almost the only indication.

In human medicine, says Nicolas, venesection early and free, injections of ether, cold rectal enemas, camphorated oil, strychnine and also inhalations of oxygen gas have their advocates.

So far the treatment resorted to in human medicine has not been applied to our animals.

▨ ▨ ▨

SUMMARY FROM RECENT PUBLICATIONS RECEIVED AND BIBLIOGRAPHIC NOTES.

Those marked "X" will be summarized. Those marked "O" will appear in abstracts.

VETERINARY RECORD—Dec. 8th. (O) Undiagnosed—Dec. 12th. Acute articular rheumatism in the horse—Tetanus—Dec. 25th—Undiagnosed—(O) Azoturia in forage poisoning—Two cases of tetanus—(O) Acute spreading disease of the alveolar periosteum in horses.

VETERINARY NEWS—(from Dec. 22 to Jan.) A few successful cases— Magnetic and electric forms of pressure on animals—(O) A few diseases affecting animals in Northern Rhodesia.

VETERINARY JOURNAL.—(December) Treatment of pneumonia by intra-tracheal injections—Poll evil—(O) Tubercular arthritis of cervical vertebrae in a mare—(O) Case of goitre in a dog—Rheumatism or what?—(O) Necrotic vaginitis in cattle—(O) Subcutaneous emphysema—Reminiscences of a remount officer in the U. S. Army—(X) Somme veterinary medical association —(O) Obituary of Prof. A. E. Mettam.

CLINICA VETERINARIA—(Nov.) Upon the experimental ictero-hemorrhagic spirochetosis of dogs—Second case of spirochetosis in white rat—Etiologic examination of the uterine secretion in the diagnosis of the diseases of the uterus—Trichina in Italy—(O) A case of pasteurellosis in man.

IL NUOVO ERCOLANI—(Nov. and Dec.) New researches upon the etiology and transmission of pulmonary pest—Judgment against two empirics gelderes.

REVUE DE PATHOLOGIE COMPARÉE—(O) Efficacious treatment of sarcoptic mange in horses—(O) Camphor in diseases of cardiac vessels.

REVUE GENERALE DE MED. VETER.—(X) On the operation for cartilaginous quittor.

RECUEIL DE MED. VETER.—(X) Pathogeny of goitre in horses—Horse chestnuts in the food of animals.

BULLETIN SOCIETE CENTRALE—(O) New center of sarcoptic mange in rabbits—Contagious stomatitis in the horse—(O) Rare localization of epizootic lymphangitis—(O) Intoxication with phenic acid followed by death— (X) Studies of digestive pathology—(X) Differential diagnosis between calculus and coprostasis of horses.

ANNALES DE L'INSTITUT PASTEUR—Bacteria of dusts. A. L.

—Dr. C. L. Norris, formerly at Wheeling, W. Va., has been transferred to Fort Worth, Texas.

—The daily press reports the arrest of Fritz Hagerman alias Charles Aisenbach at Susanville, California, who confessed that it was the common understanding that the plots of the Industrial Workers of the World to poison cattle and burn grain, farm houses and lumber mills were supported by German money.

SOME STUDIES OF THE TUBERCULIN TEST*

M. H. REYNOLDS
University and State Live Stock Sanitary Board, St. Paul, Minn.

I have recently had occasion to make a special study of tuberculin test records of herds that have been under continuous observation and tuberculin test for a number of years. The studies which I am presenting are taken from the work of several different men of the University and Live Stock Sanitary Board. It does not appear practical to try to give more than this general statement of credit because many of the individual cases represent the work of several men.

In most of the later cases used, the work was done by the author in the course of certain tuberculin test research studies that have been under way for several years. I appreciate very much the assistance I have had in these studies from the State Live Stock Sanitary Board, through Drs. Ward and Whitcomb.

There are several points which I wish to bring out in this discussion :

That a simultaneous or combination test is more accurate than either test alone, no difference which test we use.

That we should be slow to condemn any recognized test, especially on limited experience.

The desirability of simultaneous or some equivalent form of testing in the case of very bad herds, very valuable animals, or any conditions under which extreme accuracy is desirable.

The value of carefully made clinical observations and herd history.

That we too frequently overlook warnings in the form of low reactions.

That any tuberculin test should be considered as merely an aid in diagnosis and not the diagnosis.

The unwisdom of generosity in diagnosis with valuable animals.

That we must not condemn all cattle that show 106.0 on temperature test, or pass all that stay below 103.0, in other words, we have been looking too much at the top of the thermometer for our reactions.

*Presented at a joint session of the Minnesota and Wisconsin State Veterinary Associations, 1917.

Nothing that I may say should be taken as a condemnation of either recognized test. My experience and the experience of others show that they are all useful. Each has certain advantages and all three have faults.

The following cases have been selected as *types* and should be so considered. Such cases have occurred over and over in my experience.

To simplify these cases and focus attention on the particular point under consideration, I shall usually omit many details essential to a good test record. We shall assume that the management of details as to stable conditions, feed, water, temperature hours, etc., was intelligent and correct.

OVER-LOOKING WARNINGS. These cases will illustrate also the fact that we must not look at the top of the thermometer altogether for our reactions.

. CASE 1. A young Jersey cow was eighteen months old at the time of her first test in August, 1914. Her highest preliminary temperature was 102.2. Her post-injection temperatures were 102.5, 103.2, 102.0, 102.4, 103.0, 102.8.

This heifer was tested again in December, 1914. Her preliminary temperature was 102.0. The post-injection temperatures were 103.6, 102.2, 102.0, 101.8, 101.4, 102.8; diagnosis "doubtful".

She was omitted from the regular herd test in November, 1915, on account of pregnancy, usually a mistake, and so in this case. We do not now omit pregnant cows from a herd test, unless they are actually or about calving.

However, this cow was retested in January, 1916, and gave a clear temperature reaction as follows: High preliminary, 101.2. Second day temperatures, 104.2, 105.8, (watered) 103.4, 102.6, 102.4, 102.1. Autopsy of February 4, 1916, showed lymph glands enlarged and caseo-calcareous with a caseo-calcareous area in the lung substance, lesions evidently old. Such cases are not rare.

What does this case teach? Does it not plainly teach that such cases should not be omitted from herd test on account of pregnancy or any other ordinary cause? Does it not show a very plain warning in the test of August, 1914, repeated even more plainly in the test of December, 1914? This cow was in a valuable herd for two years after she may have been a spreader of tuberculosis. Those temperatures of August and December should have been taken more seriously.

CASE No. 2. A yearling Jersey heifer was tested in November, 1913. High preliminary temperature was 101.4. Post-injection temperatures, 102.0, 102.0, 102.0, 101.2, 102.0, 102.4. Diagnosis, non-tuberculous. She was retested in May, 1914, her temperatures running as follows: High preliminary, 101.4. Post-injection, 102.6, 103.0, 101.3, 101.4, 101.8, 101.0. Diagnosis "doubtful".

This heifer was tested again in December, 1914, and given a diagnosis of "non-tuberculous". Nothing significant appears in the record of this test.

In November, 1915, this cow was given simultaneous thermal and intradermal. She gave a typical reaction by both thermal and intradermal tests. Her skin reaction at 72 hours was marked "xxxx" (extreme) and was still very conspicuous at 120 hours. For years there had been an occasional reaction in this large and valuable herd. You all know that sort of history. Perhaps two reactions this year, no reactions next year, two reactions the year following, one the next, etc. This heifer may have given a warning in those three last post-temperatures in her November, 1913, test: 101.2, 102.0, 102.4, and later temperatures should have been taken. In her test as a two-year-old in May, 1914, she gave a very plain warning, which was also overlooked in that preliminary 101.4, and her two first post-injection temperatures of 102.6, and 103.0.

This case shows clearly what happens in a series of tests between the healthy non-reacting heifer and the tubercular cow and is worthy of rather critical study. Was she infected and on the border line between reaction and no reaction, when tested in November, 1913?

Do not these cases illustrate one of our faults, where we overlook tuberculous cattle and leave them in the herd as sources of subsequent loss and worry?

Take this next case of a very valuable shorthorn cow where such a warning was overlooked and very serious losses resulted.

CASE No. 3. A shorthorn cow, six years old, was tested in August, 1914. Her preliminary temperatures were 102.2, 103.6, 102.2. Her second day temperatures were 103.3, 102.4, 102.0, 102.1, 103.6, etc., intradermal reaction negative. These temperatures suggest that this cow had passed her maximum at the first morning temperature or was beginning to show reaction in the three last temperatures and that those first temperatures should have been seriously considered, in spite of the high preliminary temperatures.

This cow was given a diagnosis of non-tuberculous, and bought at a very long price. She failed rapidly during the fall, and by the last of October was very greatly emaciated, had a chronic cough, and was very feeble. Autopsy October 29, 1914, showed very extensive, generalized miliary tuberculosis of the lungs. The bronchial, mediastinal, and other glands were involved. The gland lesions were calcareous. The lung substance lesions were acute. Following her purchase, this cow was very closely associated in confined quarters, with a particularly valuable herd, previously tested, and supposed to be clean or practically so.

After this association with Case 3, the herd showed a serious number of reactions, and there followed serious losses. What was the trouble? Well, those first three and the last three post-injection temperatures should have been seriously considered, and purchase should have been refused. The veterinarian's advice not to purchase this cow would have saved a great deal of trouble and serious losses.

I consider this cow's test of August, 1914, as another illustration of a low reaction. It shows also the possibility of a positive reaction with the post temperatures actually lower than the high preliminary.

CASE 3A. The next case is very suggestive in several respects. It shows (a) plain warning overlooked, (b) conflict between thermal and intradermal, and (c) an error in judgment by the veterinarian who made the previous test in question. More weight should have been given to things other than temperatures.

In November, 1916, I tested 29 animals in a certain herd, by the simultaneous thermal and intradermal method. All passed quite clear, excepting three, Case 3A, and two other cows standing one on either side of her. Her morning, mid-day and late afternoon preliminary temperatures ranged from 101.2 to 101.7. Her second day temperatures at approximately two-hour intervals from 7 a. m. to 5 p. m., ranged 101.2, 103.9, 105.8, 104.5, 104.0, 102.9, 102.4. Third day temperatures were normal, maximum 101.7. On the first day there was promise of a very pronounced typical intradermal reaction but this practically disappeared during the second twenty-four hours. Diagnosis based solely on thermal test would ordinarily be tuberculosis and the diagnosis based solely on intradermal would ordinarily be "non-tuberculous". But on account of the fact that the two cows standing on either side of "3A" must evidently be held for retest, it was decided to mark her as "suspicious", put her in quarantine, and arrange for a future test, especially as we desired to continue our studies of this case.

The other two cows will be passed over by a statement that both, on their second day temperatures, gave a slight reaction, which was marked as "doubtful"; but on subsequent test in April, 1917, they both passed clearly negative by all three tests.

It was certainly interesting, however, to have the two cows standing closest to "3A" show this suggestive temperature disturbance, especially as "3A" had come from a notoriously tuberculous herd. Following this case a little farther I retested this cow in April, 1917, some five months later, giving all three tests, simultaneously. She was given this time a large dose of tuberculin and gave a clear, satisfactory thermal reaction. The intradermal test was again negative or practically so. At least there was no local reaction but what under ordinary circumstances in routine test work would be passed over as unimportant. However, she gave a very marked and positive reaction on the sensitized ophthalmic test. This cow was killed, and her report shows slight caseo-calcareous lesions in the anterior mediastinal glands. A careful examination was made of the other visceral and body lymph glands but no other macroscopical lesions could be found.

What lessons are taught by this case? She had been tested in September, 1915, by a very experienced and conscientious operator. Her three preliminary temperatures: morning, mid-day, and afternoon, were rather high: 103.3, 104.0, 102.2. She was given only 2 c.c. of tuberculin, although from a notoriously bad herd.

Her second day temperatures were: 102.0, 102.2, 103.2, 103.4, 103.4. This cow was one of four or five animals purchased not long before from a tuberculous herd. All the other animals in this particular purchase had reacted in the September, 1915, test and were condemned. This cow was considered as a little suspicious at the time but the operator did not feel justified in condemning her as "tuberculous" or "suspicious" and she was left in the herd, fortunately as it appears, without much harm, unless we assume that the two cows standing on either side of her when I first tested the herd, had become slightly infected by her and had recovered—a mere hypothesis. Here was a reaction where the second day temperatures did not go above 103.4, and were actually below the maximum preliminary temperature. For several years I have been getting more and more suspicious of a series of temperatures showing gradual rise to what would ordinarily be considered as at most only "doubtful", perhaps 103.0 or 103.2, when there is no obvious explanation in the way of feeding, thirst, high stable temperature, exercise, etc., to account for such range of temperatures.

LESSONS. The lessons from "3A" are obvious. A plain warning reaction overlooked; some tuberculous animals will react to one test and not to another; there are such things as low reactions (true in all our tests); an error of judgment in estimating known bad herd history, the value of a simultaneous test, and with her bad herd history, she should have had a larger than 2 c.c. dose of tuberculin. This cow could have been safely condemned as tuberculous in her 1915 test, just as well as in her test of April, 1917, and risk to the rest of the herd obviated.

Fearing that the cases which I have selected as typical or illustrating certain specific points, may mislead you as to my average results with either test, I shall say that you are not warranted in drawing any general conclusions from these following cases to the effect that the intradermal test: e. g., is unreliable, because I could easily recite a large number of studies where reverse conditions have held true, and where in case of conflict between intradermal and thermal or between the intradermal and ophthalmic, the intradermal subsequently proved to be the correct test.

The next few studies selected as typical of certain cases show especially *the value of the simultaneous or combined tests and clinical data.*

CASE 4. A pure-bred Galloway cow, six years old, was given simultaneous thermal and intradermal tests November, 1916. Her high preliminary was 101.4. Her post-injection temperatures were 101.5, 102.2, 103.4, 103.2, 102.2, 101.6. Her intradermal reaction was quite negative. Diagnosis "doubtful" about equivalent to "no test". Considered as probably non-tuberculous and left in the herd.

Considering the history of this herd which was good—practically clean for several years—a perfectly negative skin reaction, it was extremely probable that this heifer was non-tuberculous; that the intradermal test was correct, and this temperature curve, which, without the intradermal test, must have been considered as very suspicious, was due to causes other than ·tuberculin.

In this case a valuable young cow was saved to the herd by the use of the simultaneous test and personal knowledge of the herd history.

The next case shows the help of a simultaneous test, and the importance of clinical observation and experience.

CASE 5. A young Jersey bull, about eight months old at the time of his first test, in November, 1916. This young bull was given simultaneous thermal and intradermal tests. His high preliminary temperature was 103.0. His second day temperatures were 104.4, 104.8, 105.0, 105.2. This was a peculiar case and temperatures were continued on the third day, at 10 a. m., 105.4; 5 p. m.; 102.0. Intradermal results at twenty-four, forty-eight, seventy-two, and one hundred and twenty hours all quite negative.

Here apparently we have a temperature reaction, but a quite negative skin reaction. Close observation of the animal showed that there was something wrong with him that did not impress us as constitutional disturbance, associated with tuberculin reaction. It would be a little hard to define exactly what that was but the bull was depressed, respiration hurried. There was that abnormally long, evenly maintained high temperature, continual to the forenoon of the third day. He was subsequently retested several times at considerable intervals by thermal and intradermal methods and his tests were always quite negative. Subsequent autopsy was entirely negative. Here we have what might have been a very misleading temperature reaction, but with a perfectly negative intradermal and a clinical disturbance that did not suggest tuberculosis. We felt safe in considering this young bull as probably nontuberculous and his subsequent history gave a very strong probability that this was correct.

Our study was continued of the greater diagnostic value of the simultaneous test and the value of careful observations in connection with tests, taking certain selected cases from the G. R. herd. Seventy-eight animals were tested in December, 1915, by the simultaneous thermal and intradermal. The records of three animals are especially interesting.

CASE 6. Six-year-old cow "Shorthorn" showed the following second day temperatures: 101.4, 105.2, 105.0, 105.2, 105.0, 103.6. This cow had received the ordinary intradermal dose of tuberculin —three or four drops—at the proper time and on the second day showed this apparent temperature reaction. Her intradermal reaction was quite negative. Observation showed that she was distinctly tympanitic, and was in some distress during the second day of test. Retest by simultaneous temperature and intradermal was quite negative. Considering the practically clean record of this herd, and the completely negative skin reaction and clinical data, the reasonable presumption is that those second day temperatures had no diagnostic relation to the tuberculin test and that the intradermal negative reaction was the correct one.

CASE 7. Occurred in this same herd and test "Gilbert 3", sixteen-months-old heifer, showed for highest preliminary 101.6. Her second day temperatures were 101.0, 100.8, 102.2, 103.4, 103.4, 101.8. Her simultaneous intradermal test was completely negative and the heifer was very much in heat during the second day of test. Considering the practically clean herd, her history, clinical observations made during the test, negative skin reaction, and negative retests, it is extremely probable that her thermal reaction had no diagnostic connection with the injection and that the heifer was non-tuberculous. She was so considered and left in the herd. I think wisely so. Without the skin test and without the observations, what else could we have done, except to diagnose tuberculosis? .

CASE 8. Is another one from this same herd and test. Nelly 2 illustrates the same lesson and emphasizes the fact that these cases are not rare. During the second day her temperatures went up to 106.4. Her intradermal reaction was perfectly negative. This occurred in a practically clean herd, with a good history. Examination showed an acute mastitis. Such cases could just as easily occur in a tubercular herd and without the careful observation a non-tuberculous cow would be pronounced tuberculous with the embarrassment and losses which usually follow the killing of a non-tuberculous cow, diagnosed as tuberculous.

CASE 9. Illustrates the value of combination test and herd history and is a good example of what I call "vagaries of the tuberculin test". Here we have a very good thermal reaction during the preliminary temperatures before the animal had received any tuberculin; another reaction after the injection; and both in a case that was not tuberculosis at all. A valuable young Holstein bull, 9 months old, was under test for sale in September, 1916. He was given simultaneous thermal and intradermal tests. During the test he was watered at 8:30 a. m., and at 5 p. m. Preliminary temperatures, beginning in the morning, were 102.3, 103.3, 104.3,

104.0, 104.1. Temperatures the second day at about two-hour intervals from 6 a. m., to 9 p. m., were: 102.3, 102.9, 101.3, 102.1, 102.9, 104.2, 103.2. Note the drop in temperature from 102.9 to 101.3, the bull having been watered in this interval. Here we have a ¡very nice reaction beginning with the first temperature after watering: 101.3, 102.1, 102.9, 104.2, 103.2. But this young bull was passed and sold as sound with my approval because a very careful intradermal was completely negative; the animal was young, the weather was hot; this occurred in a practically clean herd. There was no constitutional disturbance.

Assuming that this bull was non-tuberculous, which is extremely probable, we have here a case that illustrates strange things which may occur in the course of a test and the necessity of taking many factors into careful consideration in making diagnosis in such a case. Under the circumstances we might have postponed the test when we found those high preliminary temperatures, but this could not very well be done on account of the necessity of immediate action. It was my duty to express an opinion, if I could, as to whether this bull was tubercular or not. Here we had a reaction curve, before injection, another reaction curve after injection and yet the animal probably not tuberculous.

Knowledge of the history of the herd, personal information concerning details of the test, the help of a simultaneous intradermal, etc., enabled us to complete a desirable sale, at once, and saved a valuable animal which might otherwise have been condemned as tuberculous.

In late years I have repeatedly included animals with high preliminary temperatures and animals in advanced pregnancy and have yet to regret this policy.

In 1914 I had a suggestive experience along this line. It was necessary to test a lot of young bulls under purchase at a point outside of the state. This was in July. The weather was hot, especially on the first day of test and the test could not be postponed. These were all young animals, eight or ten months old.

CASE No. 10 showed the following preliminary temperatures: 103.0, 102.8, 103.4. His second day temperatures ran quite normal for age and weather, the highest being 102.4.

CASE No. 11. Preliminary temperatures 102.8, 103.2, 103.4. Second day temperatures normal.

CASE No. 12. Preliminary temperatures 102.6, 103.9, 104.0. Second day temperatures normal.

CASE No. 13. Preliminary temperatures 104.9, 103.7, 104.0. Highest second day, 103.6.

CASE No. 14. Preliminary temperatures 104.6, 102.1, 103.4. Highest second day, 103.6.

These young bulls were given the temperature test, a simultaneous intradermal test and the skin test was in all cases absolutely negative, and were all approved for purchase and I think quite properly so. Their after-history so far as known, has been quite satisfactory.

If the temperatures are normal during the second day, as has been the case very often in my experience, I feel as safe in pronouncing the animal non-tuberculous and after several years of experience in testing everything in the herd (1), including heavily pregnant cows, I have never seen anything on careful observation to show me that this was unwise. There are good reasons for including such animals in the test. Our herd test is then complete. Someone does not have to go back to make retest. We are not leaving untested and possibly tuberculous animals for an indefinite period in the herd. On the other hand, if temperatures continue high through both days of test, and a double test is not used, the animals may be retested by the intradermal or perhaps preferably by the ophthalmic. I have seen much more harm from leaving untested animals in the herd than from including such animals in the test, which we are usually advised not to do.

CASE 16. Was clearly positive to the intradermal, but negative to a simultaneous thermal and subsequently negative at different times to all tests. We shall study this case at close range.

Here we have a case that has been quite unusual in my experience and one that caused considerable trouble. A valuable young bull was given simultaneous thermal and intradermal test in April, 1916. He was then about two years old, weighed 1500 pounds; dose 3 c.c. of Bureau tuberculin injected at 8:30 p. m. His highest preliminary temperature was 102.2. His post-injection temperatures, beginning at 6 a. m., and continuing at intervals of two hours, until 4 p. m., were as follows: 102.6, 103.0, 102.4, 101.2, 102.6, 101.2.

(1) Young calves are given intradermal or ophthalmic test.

The history of his intradermal test is the especially significant feature of this case in view of his negative thermal reaction. The intradermal injection was also given at 8:30 p. m., April 21st. April 24th, 5 p. m., approximately seventy hours after injection, the intradermal reaction was graded "xxxx" very marked, and typical. The diagnosis on thermal test was "healthy". The diagnosis on intradermal, considering the negative thermal reaction was given as "suspicious". Alone it must have been "tuberculous". This bull was subsequently tested several times by different methods, with negative results.

There is an interesting feature of his temperature chart in this April, 1916, test. With his highest preliminary temperature 102.2, his first three temperatures the second day were 102.6, 103.0, 102.4. Whether these should have been given more consideration or not, is a question.

I am convinced that we have all possible variations in extent of tuberculin reactions and that this applies to all three tests— from zero to extreme positive. If one animal may show a temperature disturbance running up to 106.0, or 107.0, and another animal in the same herd, with the same tuberculin and tuberculous, gives a maximum reaction of 103.2, I know of no reason for concluding that a third tuberculous animal in the same herd with the same tuberculin may not give maximum temperature reactions of 102.6, or 103.0, the high post-injection temperatures shown in this test by this young bull.

Continuing this young bull's history I find that he was retested October 13 and 14, 1916, some six months later. At that time he was approximately two and one-half years old, weighed 1625 pounds, was given 6.5 c.c. of Bureau tuberculin at 9 p. m. His highest preliminary temperature was 101.4. His post-injection temperatures began at 5:30 a. m., and continued at about two-hour intervals until 9 p. m., with a maximum of 102.

On account of his previous history, temperatures were taken on the third day, but were low normal.

Here we have an unusually careful thermal test with a very large dose of tuberculin and a negative reaction in a young animal.

I tested this bull again May 21st to 25th, 1917, by simultaneous intradermal and sensitized ophthalmic. Both tests were, so far as could be determined, by careful observation, negative.

Then what about that apparently typical intradermal reaction

in April, 1916, accompanied by those first three second-day temperatures, 102.6, 103.0, 102.4, the highest preliminary having been
102.2?

This animal was young. At the time of that first test in April,
1916, he had come six weeks before from another herd that had
been officially tested for several years and in which there had been
no known reactions in recent tests. Previous to coming into the
herd, he had been tested, when seven months old, in October, 1914,
and apparently gave a remarkable series of temperatures: preliminary, 102.3, 102.2, 102.3; after injection, 102.0, 102.1, 102.1,
102.1, 102.0. He was omitted for unknown reason from the herd
test in 1915. After purchase he was kept in a large open box stall
in a well ventilated room in which all the bulls and some young
stuff were kept, and in which there had been no recent reactions.
The previous late fall test in this herd showed three reactions in a
total of about one hundred tests; neither reaction was in the bull
stable.

The cows were in two different rooms and at some distance
from the bull room. There was no communication, except at time
of service, and the possible transfer of infection by attendants,
and there had been little recent tuberculosis in the herd. The chance
for infection, therefore, in the herd where he was tested was very
remote.

This bull came from a herd that had an unusually good history
and yet after about six weeks in the second clean or nearly clean
herd, he gave a very typical skin reaction with negative temperature reaction, and subsequent retests by all three methods were
negative.

What is your diagnosis? Usually a typical reaction by either
intradermal or ophthalmic means tuberculosis. I am not quite so
sure of a positive thermal. As to which test misses the most tuberculous cattle, that is another question.

If, then, this young bull was tuberculous in April, 1916, what
about the simultaneous temperature test, and what about his subsequent negative tests? This sort of thing puts the operator in a
peculiar predicament.

I suspect that he *was* tuberculous in April, 1916. I now suspect these three early morning temperatures constituted a low
temperature reaction, or at least a good warning. Possibly he was
very slightly and recently diseased; the virus may have been of

low virulence and he may have recovered and eliminated to such an extent that reaction is no longer possible. Or he may have been tuberculous in April, 1916, be still tuberculous, and fail to react now and react good and plenty a year from now—but I do not expect him to do so.

Continuing this study, we might take up a herd group where the several tuberculin tests have shown what I have called, for want of a better term, "their vagaries".

CASES 18-29. Last month I gave a special retest in a certain herd to 13 valuable animals. The test this time was by the simultaneous single ophthalmic and thermal, with special ophthalmic, 8 per cent tuberculin, for the ophthalmic work. These animals were retested because in my regular herd test of May 21st to 25th, 1917, by the simultaneous intradermal and sensitized ophthalmic, twelve animals had given "doubtful" or "suspicious" eye reactions. The other one had given a "suspicious" skin reaction with negative ophthalmic.

One of the twelve had given "doubtful" on both eye and skin reactions.

On the retest June 27th and 28th, 1917, by the thermal and ophthalmic, all 13 passed quite clear on temperature, seven gave apparently positive eye reactions, 1 suspicious eye, 2 doubtful eye, 3 negative eye test.

Eleven of these same animals had been in a general herd test November, 1916, and been given simultaneous thermal and intradermal tests. One young animal had intradermal only, and one calf, included in the two later tests, was not in fall test of 1916. These twelve animals passed clear at that time, unless we consider significant some very slight skin indurations about the size of a matchhead which we have always, in a thousand tests or more, considered unimportant. We get these in a very large percentage of presumably healthy animals and ignore them in diagnosis.

This situation occurs in a herd which we believed to be free from tuberculosis. This herd of 107 animals, including those under special study, in the fall test of 1916, had passed clear excepting one tuberculous cow.

This experience raises some rather serious questions. Was there so much tuberculosis in a herd which we had every reason to consider clean, or practically clean, after many tests? Did the thermal test fail us in so many cases? I have believed for some

time that there is an important number of tuberculous cattle that
will react to either test and not to another test, but have never believed and do not yet believe that there are so many as this experience would seem to indicate. Is it possible that an intradermal or
thermal injection given simultaneously with or a few hours before
the ophthalmic, can sensitize the eye of a healthy animal so as to
give a false ophthalmic reaction under ophthalmic test? I suspected for some time that this might be the explanation of such
experiences, but we had a very clear cut and positive trial to the
contrary in which the intradermal and sensitized ophthalmic test
in combination were given to thirty-two young cattle where the
circumstances are such that it is exceedingly improbable that any
were tuberculous. The intradermal was given four hours before
the first ophthalmic, yet all of the thirty-two passed one hundred
per cent clean by both tests, without any reasonable suspicion, so
that what might have been a pretty explanation of sensitization in
the non-tuberculous is spoiled.

SUMMARY. The points brought out in this summary have
each been illustrated several times in the cases selected as types
for illustrations.

It is quite apparent that some tubercular cattle will react to
one test and not to another.

A simultaneous or combination test is more accurate than
either of the same tests used alone.

Any of our tests may fail occasionally and we must be slow in
condemning.

A simultaneous or combination test is especially desirable, in
case of badly infected herds or very valuable animals, or in any
place where extreme accuracy is unusually important.

We often overlook plain warnings in the way of low reactions
and look too much at the top of the thermometer for our reactions.

Careful clinical observations and a knowledge of the herd history are very important in all cases of suspicious or apparently
positive reactions.

We should regard any tuberculin test as an *aid* to diagnosis
and not as *the* diagnosis.

We should realize more clearly the importance of mature judgment and clear, hard thinking in estimating reaction or absence of
reaction.

All of the tests, especialy the thermal, are liable to show peculiar results: e. g., Case No. 9, where we had a very good temperature curve before injection, another one after injection, and the animal concerned was probably not tuberculous.

We all know but we sometimes forget that we must not be generous with suspicious or doubtful reactions because animals are valuable.

It is not wise, as a rule, in ordinary stable herd work to exclude from test, on account of pregnancy or high preliminary temperature unless there is other obvious clinical reason. More harm will be done, as a rule, by omissions than by their inclusions.

GENITAL TUBERCULOSIS OF CATTLE*

W. L. WILLIAMS
Department of Obstetrics and Diseases of Breeding Cattle, New York State Veterinary College at Cornell University

Tuberculosis of the genitalia of cattle has generally been considered as rare and of scant scientific and economic importance. William Williams[1] states, "If the cow be in calf, abortion is apt to occur; if not pregnant, the condition called nymphomania is frequently present". Law[2] states, "The generative organs also occasionally suffer, in which case an early and rather persistent desire for the bull (nymphomania) * * * In cases of uterine tuberculosis, the nymphomania may be supplemented by a purulent discharge. * * * Genital tuberculosis in the bull is associated with nodular swelling of the testicle, epididymis, or cord, hydrocele, and exceptionally tubercle on the penis or in the prostatic sac". Friedberger und Fröhner[3] state that genital tuberculosis occurs rarely in both sexes and may invade any portion of the genital system. Hutyra und Marek[4] mention tuberculous epididymitis and orchitis, and assert that rarely the testis undergoes tuberculous abscessation, with a consequent fistula. They consider penial tuberculosis as extremely rare, and claim that when it occurs the

---

*Presented at the Tenth Annual Conference for Veterinarians, Ithaca, N. Y., Jan., 1918.

(1) Principles and Practice of Veterinary Medicine, 1875, p. 347.
(2) Veterinary Medicine, Vol. IV, 1902, pp. 448,449.
(3) Speciellen Pathologie und Therapie.
(4) Spezielle Pathologie und Therapie der Haustiere.

glans penis becomes studded over with tubercles. Quoting Hess, they regard uterine and tubal tuberculosis as rare and as causing sterility and nymphomania. Vulvo-vaginal tuberculosis is mentioned as a rare possibility.

Hoare[5] describes genital tuberculosis very briefly, without according it an important place. He admits the possibility of transmission by copulation, and mentions a single case of primary penial tuberculosis.

The general trend of veterinary literature concerning genital tuberculosis is in sharp contrast with my personal observations. The difference in view is possibly due to a variation in the direction of study. Veterinarians rarely look for genital tuberculosis, since ordinarily it does not affect the general well-being of the patient. Clinically, it is only when one concentrates his observations upon the diseases of the genital organs in connection with sterility that the recognition of genital tuberculosis becomes probable and its importance realized. The genitalia are not inspected frequently in the abattoir. They are not used as human food. When they are tuberculous, the lesions possess little or no importance in relation to the value of other tissues for food. Hence, much genital tuberculosis may pass unnoted.

The genital mucosa offers a highly vulnerable field for tuberculous invasion, but genital exposure to tuberculosis is rare as compared with exposure through contaminated food. That is, when open pulmonary tuberculosis exists, the patient is constantly contaminating mangers, food, and water by means of her sputum, so that companions are exposed daily and hourly. When genital tuberculosis exists, the exposure may be identical, because of the genital discharges contaminating food and water, but the special venereal exposure occurs only during the very brief period of copulation.

I have not observed tuberculous orchitis or epididymitis. There is no example of either in my pathologic collection of genitalia, and no specimen in the collection of any department of the college. The scattered records in veterinary literature of tuberculous orchitis and epididymitis do not serve as a very accurate basis for outlining the clinical symptoms. In a general way, it is stated that the epididymi and testes show painless enlargement and har-

---

(5) System of Veterinary Medicine.

dening. The demarcation between the epididymis and the testes gradually become clouded, and finally lost. Apparently the epididymis usually becomes involved first and the disease extends thence to the gland. The location of the tuberculous process is said to be usually in the parenchyma, having its basis in the mucosa of the epididymis and testis. In this manner the disease may be well advanced before peripheral inflammation or tuberculous extension involves the peritoneal coverings, to cause adhesions and hydrocele. Rarely, abscessation is said to ensue, resulting in a fistula.

The clinical diagnosis of tuberculous epididymitis and orchitis is difficult. The painless tumefaction of the testes is not characteristic of tuberculosis, but may ensue from various pyogenic infections. The peritoneal adhesions, hydrocele, and abscessation are quite as probable from other infections as from tuberculosis. Tuberculin offers, next to the excision of the testis and its examination, the best means for diagnosis. As is well known, tuberculin has its limitations, and may fail. If the patient responds to tuberculin, the evidence of tuberculous epididymitis or orchitis is not complete. Tuberculous lesions in other organs may cause the response to tuberculin, while the lesions in the epididymis and testis may be non-tuberculous. When but one testicle is involved, its removal and histo-biologic examination offers by far the most reliable means for diagnosis. If the disease has existed for some time, the removal of the testis is in no case of economic importance, because as a broad general rule chronic epididymitis or orchitis signifies incurable sterility of the involved gland. Hence its removal is no loss, but actually, as a rule, the best curative measure and the greatest available protection for the other testicle and for the breeding life of the bull.

The path of tuberculous invasion of the epididymis and testis has not been clearly learned. It is not primary. It does not seem to be secondary to penial infection. While I have observed several cases of primary penial tuberculosis, I have not noted subsequent tuberculous epididymitis or orchitis. It appears highly improbable that the tubercle bacilli would traverse the long urethra and vas deferens and reach the epididymis without leaving behind evidences of its passage in the form of penial or urethral tuberculosis. When wholly within the tubules of the epididymis or testis, as appears usually to be the case, the invasion is apparently not direct from the peritoneum. When the scrotal peritoneum is first involved, it would appear probable that the invasion had occurred from the peritoneal cavity through the open inguinal ring. Apparently most instances of tuberculous epididymitis and orchitis are referable to hematogenic sources and constitute a part of generalized tuberculosis.

The prognosis for the involved gland is hopeless. If only one gland is involved, it may be successfully removed, leaving the bull perfectly fertile. The difficulty is that, the tuberculous epididymitis or orchitis, being usually a secondary rather than a primary lesion, the basic lesion remains and probably unfits the bull for breeding except when mated with infected cows held under the Bang plan. Even in such cases, it needs be determined that the vas deferens, vesicula seminales, prostate gland, and penis are free, or the bull becomes a serious menace even to tuberculous cows, because when such parts are involved tubercle bacilli may be ejaculated with the semen from the sound testicle and induce primary genital (venereal) tuberculosis in the cow, which may promptly bring her breeding life to a close.

Tuberculosis of the vas deferens, seminal vesicle, and prostate is possible, but apparently too rare to be of great economic importance. Tuberculosis of the vesicula seminales or prostate would tend to interfere with urination. The diagnosis of tuberculosis of these parts would be based necessarily upon rectal palpation.

PENIAL TUBERCULOSIS. Penial tuberculosis is comparatively common in the bull. The corpus cavernosum, urethra, and urethral mucosa are not so frequently involved as the submucosa of the glans, prepuce, sheath, and the adjacent penial lymphatics.

Tuberculosis invades any organ far more readily when the protective epithelium is wounded. The anatomy of the copulatory apparatus of the bull and the mechanism of copulation render epithelial injuries more probable elsewhere than in the mucosa of the glans penis itself. The penis of the bull (and of ruminants generally) is very firm. The transverse diameter and the consistency of the penis are but slightly modified by erection. The protrusion of the penis during copulation is brought about almost wholly by the elimination of the sigmoid flexure (see Fig. 12), the accomplishment of which requires the relaxation or overcoming of the retractor penis muscle. When at rest, the penis lies within the prepuce, above the sheath. The mucosa of the sheath

of the bull is not commonly distinguished from that of the prepuce
in the adult, although they have a wholly different embryologic
history. The sheath exists as a distinct structure at the time of
birth; the prepuce does not. In the new-born ruminant and porcine male, the sheath constitutes a comparatively short infundibu-
lum, terminating at the bottom in the meatus urinarius (Fig. 1).

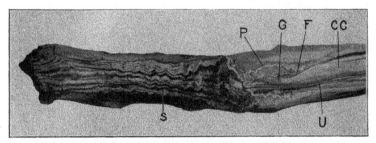

FIG. 1. Penis and sheath of bull calf, in sagittal section.
S, sheath; U, urethra; P, prepuce, not yet free from the glans; G, the interval
being occupied by soft embryonic tissue; F- fornix; CC, corpus cavernosum.

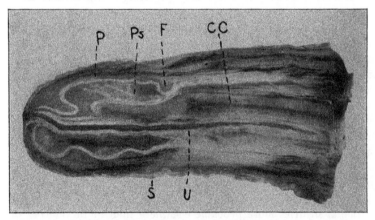

FIG. 2. Penis of bull calf with the sheath forcibly reflected over the glans.
Ps, preputial sac, occupied by embryonic tissue. Other letters same as in Fig. 1.

No part of the penis is exposed. At the time of birth, the two layers of mucosa, one of which is later to form the mucosa of the glans
penis and the other the mucous membrane of the prepuce, are firmly
adherent to each other, as shown in Figures 1 and 2. Later, when
sexual maturity approaches, the tissue between the two layers of
mucous membrane which serves to bind them together slowly gives

way, and the preputial sac finally becomes established. In the abattoir, one may observe every gradation of the development of the prepuce in veal calves. The gradations may be seen also in castrated males (Fig. 3). The prepuce may be totally absent, or there may be any degree of development, according to the degree of sexual development at the time of castration. The prepuce of the bull therefore represents that portion of the penial envelope

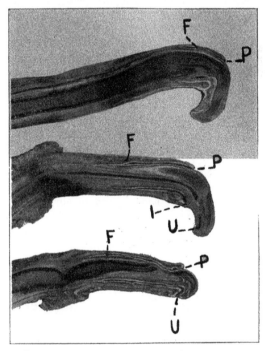

FIG. 3. Sagittal sections of penises of steers, showing gradations in the dehiscence of the prepuce from the glans.
P, prepuce; F, fornix; U, urethra; I, adhesive band on median raphe.

extending from the apex of the glans penis to the base when the penis is at rest. The sheath consists of that portion extending from the apex of the glans penis forward to the sheath opening.

The new-born ruminant or porcine male cannot protrude the penis, and if castrated early never becomes able to do so. The embryonic history is traceable in the anatomic characters of the two membranes. The preputial epithelium is very delicate and easily abraded; the epithelium of the sheath is coarser and offers higher resistance. The preputial mucosa is even and smooth; the sheath mucosa is thrown into wavy longitudinal rugae.

In coitus, the protrusion of the penis is effected by the momentary elimination of the sigmoid flexure (Fig. 12) which necessitates the elongation of the retractor muscle of the penis. When the glans is protruded beyond the prepuce and sheath, the prepuce and the sheath each becomes reflected upon the penis, to constitute its outer covering. For the moment, both preputial and sheath cavities cease to exist, and the mucosa of each, instead of lining their respective sacs, constitute the external covering of the penis. The reflection of these two membranes is made possible by the very loose areolar connective tissue lying between the mucous lining of the canal and the outer yellow elastic framework of the sheath derived from the abdominal tunic. The coital thrust of the bull is vigorous, or even violent. It is so violent that occasionally, as shown in Fig. 8, the prepuce is torn or ruptured. The abrasion or rupture is withdrawn at once, with the retraction of the penis, and there is carried along any infection which has entered the wound.

The superficial genital mucosa of the bull, as well as that of the ram and the boar, is further exposed to abrasions and consequent infection by the presence of the granules or nodules of the granular venereal disease—a chronic infection which is essentially universal. The granules or nodules frequently become inflamed, especially from excessive coitus, the epithelium at the summits of the granules becomes abraded, and hemorrhage ensues. It is not rare to see the granular venereal disease so severe that the parts bleed after each coitus, if the bull will copulate. Sometimes the pain is so great that he refuses to copulate; sometimes the swelling of the sheath is so great that the penis cannot be protruded—the bull has phimosis.

Therefore, in addition to the very delicate epithelium of the genital mucosa, the prepuce itself may be ruptured, or there may occur a multitude of minute abrasions at the summits of the granules regularly present. These abrasions offer special facility for invasion by pathogenic bacteria. If the cow is afflicted with tuberculous genital catarrh, any abrasions upon the penis, prepuce, or sheath of the bull existing or occurring at the time of copulation invites tuberculous infection. The entire group of such tuberculous infections may be classed as primary venereal or coital tuberculosis.

Primary tuberculosis of the male copulatory organs of the bull may involve any tissue or part contributing to the copulatory apparatus. The principal types I have observed are: (1) tuberculosis of the glans penis; (2) sheath tuberculosis; (3) preputial tuberculosis; (4) tuberculosis of the penial lymph glands.

1) *Tuberculosis of the glans penis* is not very rare. I have observed two cases clinically, and others in the abattoir. One clinical case was in a large Holstein herd bull. For some months he had been unable to copulate with small or medium-sized cows, but could do so successfully with large cows with commodious vulvae. Attempts at copulation were generally followed by a limited amount of hemorrhage. The glans penis was enlarged, especially at its apex. The surface was dark colored, congested, somewhat eroded, and suppurating slightly. Inability to copulate was apparently referable to the combination of four factors—the enlargement of the glans; the roughening of its surface, due chiefly to the destruction of the epithelium, thus hindering the introduction of the glans into the vulva; the pain; and the flaccidity of the diseased area. The penis was protruded readily. When the bull was confined upon the operating table, the penis could be pushed out of the sheath and prepuce by forcibly effacing the sigmoid flexure. When thus forced out and securely grasped so that the part could be readily inspected, it was seen that the apex of the glans for a distance of about three inches was much inflamed and enlarged, and bled readily upon touch. The diseased tip was dark livid, the epithelium largely destroyed, and the surface contaminated by purulent exudate. The appearances were strongly suggestive of tuberculosis. The diseased tip of the glans was amputated. The histologic appearances were those of tuberculous lesions, and stained smears showed tubercle bacilli. The operative wound progressed very favorably for a time, and the bull was promptly discharged from the clinic, apparently on the safe road to recovery.

The patient belonged to a breeder devoid of serious regard for the control of tuberculosis. It was understood that the disease was rampant in his herd and that he was more concerned about concealment than control. I was unable to follow the case. Apparently the patient, valued at about ten thousand dollars, had contracted the infection by copulating with a cow having genital tuberculosis. After becoming infected, he was evidently a very

serious menace to any cow free from genital tuberculosis with
which he might copulate. The venereal peril was limited chiefly
by the fact already related, that he could not copulate with most
cows and heifers, but only with those having commodious vulvae.
The attitude of the owner prevented any investigation of the herd
in an effort to learn whether any harm had come to cows from
copulation with this animal. So far as I have observed, he was

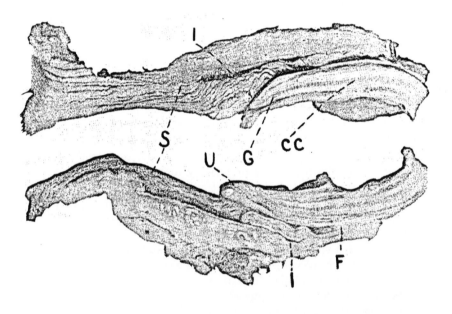

FIG. 4.   Tuberculosis of sheath and prepuce of bull.
S, sheath; U, urethra; G, glans; F, fornix; CC, corpus cavernosum, I,I, fissure
extending into tubercular mass.

one of the most dangerous bulls I have seen with genital tuberculosis, because in most cases copulation is more promptly and absolutely excluded and venereal transmission thereby avoided.

A very interesting abattoir specimen is illustrated in Fig. 8,
in which there has been a rupture of the prepuce and also tubercle
infection at the tip of the glans penis. I see no relation between
the two lesions.

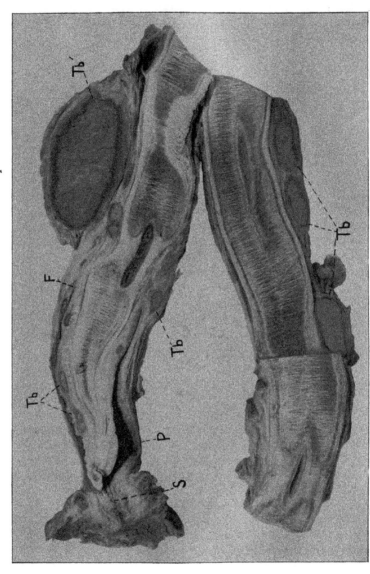

Fig. 5. Primary penial tuberculosis in bull. Sagittal section, with cross section and doubling S, sheath; P, prepuce (ventral side); Tb, tubercular masses; Tb', large abscess at base of glans. The dotted lines from Tb, at the left of the fornix, F, indicate tubercular masses in the submucosa of the glans

Tuberculosis of the submucosa of the glans is illustrated in Fig. 5. This specimen shows numerous tubercles in the submucosa. They were not recognizable clinically. The disease was brought to a crisis by the larger tuberculous abscesses in the prepuce and about the base of the glans, which rendered protrusion of the penis impossible.

(2) *Tuberculosis of the penial sheath* is presumably rare. I have but two well defined specimens in my collection. Both were obtained from the abattoir, and are without clinical history. One, Fig. 4, indicates that penial incarceration occurred early, rendering the animal impotent and causing him to be sent to the shambles. The other, Fig. 10, is a more complex case with rupture of the prepuce and tuberculosis of both glans and sheath. Clinically, the condition could not well have been differentiated, upon ordinary examination, from other infections of the sheath wall, especially actinomycosis. Among chronic infections, however, tuberculosis is far and away the most probable, and a provisional diagnosis of tuberculosis should be made. The tuberculin test may serve as an aid, but it is subject to severe limitations, since any reaction may be due to pre-existing tuberculous lesions in other parts of the body. If it is reasonably certain that the bull was tuberclefree prior to the development of the lesion, the test possesses great value. Exploratory incision through the external skin, and the removal of material for bacterial and inoculation studies, is of great diagnostic value.

So long as the bull can protrude the penis and copulate, he constitutes a serious menace. Since the infection is primary, the fundamental lesion is in the mucosa, and naturally open, and any tuberculous excretions occur within the sheath. The glans penis inevitably becomes contaminated, but not necessarily infected. In copulation, however, the surface contamination is carried into the vulva and vagina of the female. In protruding the penis also, as the reader will understand by studying Figures 6 and 7, until the swelling becomes too great for copulation to occur, the sheath mucosa is reflected and when the penis is fully protruded the tuberculous membrane itself constitutes the covering of the penial base and enters the vulva of the cow during coitus.

Accordingly it is essential that great care be exercised in handling inflammatory conditions of the sheath and, in making a diagnosis, that every available means be taken to eliminate the question of tuberculous infection. However, one must not incise the sheath deeply, for diagnostic or other reasons, lest the resultant cicatrix incarcerate the penis. If tuberculosis is diagnosed, the bull should be excluded from service, even to reacting cows, and promptly sent to slaughter.

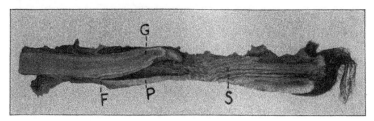

FIG. 6. Sagittal section of penis of bull, retracted within the prepuce.
F, fornix; G, glans; P, prepuce; S, sheath.

(3) ᐟ *Preputial tuberculosis* is apparently less common than tuberculosis of the glans or of the sheath. The preputial membrane, which is far more delicate than that of the sheath, is exposed during copulation to special injury at the base of the glans.

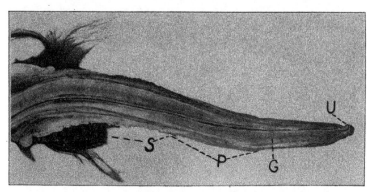

FIG. 7. Penis of bull, protruded from sheath and prepuce.
Lettering same as in Fig. 6.

At this point the epithelium of the glans becomes reflected, to constitute the lining epithelium of the preputial sac. At the moment of the copulatory thrust, the parietal, or outer preputial membrane, is suddenly and violently reversed, to constitute the covering of the penis from the base of the glans backwards for a distance approximately equal to the length of the glans itself. Further back, the sheath mucous membrane succeeds the prepuce as the mucous covering of the protruded penial body. The prepuce and the

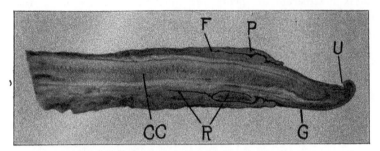

FIG. 8. Rupture of prepuce from coital violence.
CC, corpus cavernosum; F, fornix, P, prepuce; G, glans; U, urethra; R, coital rupture. At right end of the rupture the ruptured border of the prepuce is folded upon itself.

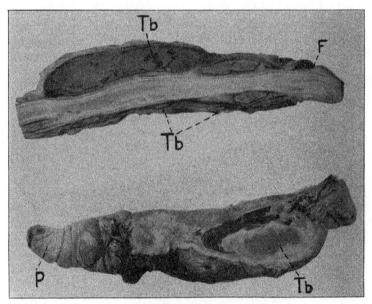

FIG. 9. Tuberculosis of the glans and penis.
P, prepuce; F, fornix; Tb, tubercular masses.

sheath mucosa become completely reversed. That end of the sheath mucosa which, while the penis was at rest, was situated most anteriorly now becomes most posterior. The mucosa of the sheath and of the prepuce become reversed in relation to each other. When the penis is at rest, the prepuce is behind the sheath, but when the penis is protruded the prepuce is in front of the reversed sheath mucosa. Accordingly the prepuce, at the point of its attachment to the base of the glans, is one of the most vulnerable points at which tuberculosis and other infections may effect an entrance. When infection occurs, it usually leaves scant trace in the epithelium of the glans, but involves chiefly the lymph glands of the submucosa.

As soon as infection occurs and inflammation is established, the loose areolar tissue between the prepuce and the external dartoid sheath becomes involved, adhesions occur, and the penis is incarcerated. By studying Figures 1, 2, 6, 7, 9, and 10, it will be

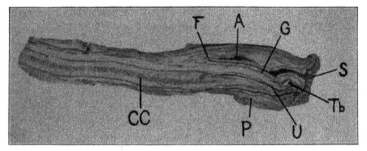

FIG. 10. Tuberculosis of glans and prepuce.
S, sheath; G, glans; P, prepuce; F, fornix; U, urethra; CC, corpus cavernosum; Tb, tubercle in tip of glans; A, tubercular abscess in prepuce.

seen that as soon as such inflammatory adhesions become established copulation is at an end, because the preputial wall cannot become reflected upon the body of the penis and the continuity of the outer with the inner layer at the base of the glans serves as an unyielding ligament, holding the penis firmly in its retracted position.

Clinically, the presence of the lesion is probably not observed until well established. That is, the infection probably occurs without attracting notice, and, if opportunity is granted, probably several copulations are made during the few succeeding days, without attracting attention. When the lesion has reached a certain development, a given copulation, especially with a heifer, irritates the lesion severely and sets aflame the established infection. Then the lesion is observed, and is naturally attributed to mechanical injury in the last copulation, which is only partly true. Then swelling in the preputial region becomes evident, incarceration of the penis follows quickly, and copulation cannot occur.

The diagnosis is fundamentally dependent upon symptoms essentially identical with those seen in sheath tuberculosis, except the lesion is located further backward, just anterior to the scrotum. It cannot be differentiated from other infections by an ordinary physical examination. Before an accurate diagnosis can be made, it is essential to include the tuberculin test and bacterial search. In a breeding sense, the lesion is not subject to cure.

(4) *Tuberculosis of the penial glands* is by far the most commonly observed type of genital tuberculosis in bulls and sends more valuable breeding sires to the shambles than any genital lesion, perhaps more than all other genital lesions combined. Apparently entering through a lesion, either recognizable or unrecognizable, of the glans, sheath, or prepuce, it may involve the lymph glands at any point from the margin of the sheath, along the prepuce, and up to and above the sigmoid flexure. Clinically, in opening the small peri-penial abscesses, I find them containing thick pus, the abscess walls dark, angry red, *without calcification.* The lymph glands lie chiefly along the sides of the penis. When involving the small glands outside the mucous membranes of the sheath and prepuce, the inflammatory adhesions soon prevent the reflection of these membranes upon the exterior of the penis, make its protrusion impossible, and exclude copulation. Swellings in the region, usually well defined and painless, are evident. Abscessation gradually develops, but the abscesses are small, their walls sclerotic, non-fluctuant, and without a tendency to "point" or break. The lesions are well illustrated in Figures 5, 9, 11 and 12.

Sometimes the sigmoid lymph glands are involved, while those of the sheath and prepuce are slightly or not at all affected. In such cases, as shown in Figures 11 and 12, the chief clinical phenomenon is inability to protrude the penis and copulate. The inflamed glands induce adhesions which inhibit the elimination of the sigmoid flexure. Palpation of the region enables the veterinarian readily to detect the enlarged glands.

The enlargement of the lymph glands of the sheath, prepuce, or sigmoid flexure constitutes strong evidence of primary venereal tuberculosis. Other infections may induce similar adenitis, but commonly the veterinarian is justified in diagnosing provisionally

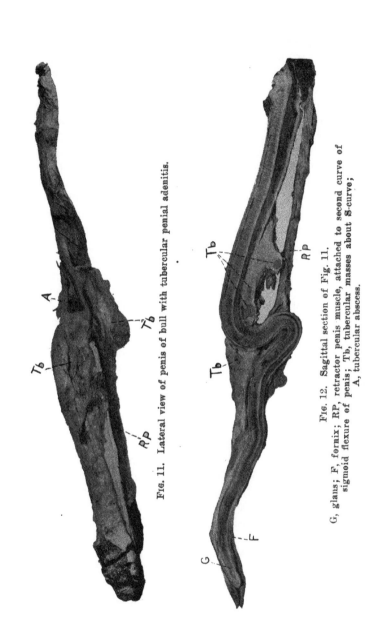

Fig. 11. Lateral view of penis of bull with tubercular penial adenitis.

Fig. 12. Sagittal section of Fig. 11.
G, glans; F, fornix; RP, retractor penis muscle, attached to second curve of sigmoid flexure of penis; Tb, tubercular masses about S-curve; A, tubercular abscess.

such lesions as tuberculosis. He may, should circumstances de-mand, search for bacterial or other evidence. On the whole, any chronic adenitis of these glands ruins the breeding value of the bull and dictates slaughter. A positive diagnosis is highly impor-tant, even when made post mortem. If it is tuberculosis—and that is the rule—there must be highly dangerous cows in the herd, the genitalia of which should be subjected to very rigid search for tu-berculosis. While a bull may become infected in copulating with a cow when the exterior of the vulva is contaminated with tubercle-bearing fecal excreta, this is improbable. The assumption should generally be that the infection has arisen from copulating with a female having tuberculous genital catarrh. Such an offender should be detected and eliminated. She is almost always incurably sterile. She constitutes a great peril to any breeding sire, and is one of the worst of "spreaders" of tuberculous infection.

TUBERCULOSIS OF THE FEMALE GENITALIA. Every part of the genital organs of the cow is subject to invasion. My collection con-tains examples of ovarian, tubal, uterine, cervical, and vaginal tuberculosis, and I have observed clinically vulvar tuberculosis.

(1) *Ovarian tuberculosis* is very rare, but is far more com-mon than orchitic tuberculosis. The ovary is more exposed to the infection than the testicle, especially in the presence of extensive peritoneal lesions. I have obtained but two good examples. One of these, Fig. 13, is highly interesting, because casual examination suggests that the avenue of invasion of the ovary was through the physiologic lesion, the crater of a ruptured ovisac. The dense in-vesting tunic of both the testis and the ovary appears to offer a highly effective barrier against tubercular invasion, with the im-portant difference that in the ovary there occur intervals (ovula-tion) when the tunic is ruptured and its continuity temporarily in abeyance. Viewed in this light, more ovarian than orchitic tu-berculosis might be expected. Apparently this is true. Neverthe-less, the ovary is highly resistant to the infection, as compared with other portions of the female genitalia. Frequently the uterus and oviducts are highly tuberculous, while the ovary remains nor-mal. Generally, when the oviducts are involved, the pavilion is adherent to the ovary, and the peritoneal side of the pavilion is studded over with tubercles, as shown in Figures 15, 16, and 17, but the adherent, encapsuled gland resists invasion.

Ovarian tuberculosis cannot, in my experience, be directly and positively diagnosed clinically. Clinical diagnosis is not highly important, since ovarian invasion rarely, if ever, occurs without tubal and uterine tuberculosis, each of which is open to reasonably safe clinical diagnosis. So far as I am aware, ovarian tuberculosis induces no clinical symptoms. There is a definite impression given in veterinary literature that ovarian tuberculosis causes sterility at times, but there is no evidence that it plays an essential rôle. So far as I have seen, it is the coexisting tubal and uterine tuberculosis which causes the sterility. Statements occur also (Hutyra

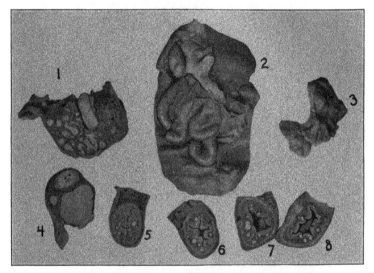

FIG. 13.   Tuberculosis of ovary, oviduct, and uterine walls.
1, section through oviduct, showing a mass of tubercles; 2, oviduct, enlarged and adherent, with adherent ovary shown at the upper left hand corner; 3, normal oviduct, for comparison; 4, ovary, showing above a tubercular mass, and below and to the right a corpus luteum; 5, 6, 7, 8, cross section of uterine horns, showing tubercles in submucosa.

and Marek, Law) that genital tuberculosis, either through the invasion of the ovaries or otherwise, induces nymphomania. No evidence is submitted upon the point. The power of tuberculosis of any portion of the genital tract to cause nymphomania is probably pure legend. A careful study of nymphomania shows it to be due to a definite type of cystic degeneration of the ovary, wholly devoid of any trace of relation to tuberculosis. Genital tuberculosis

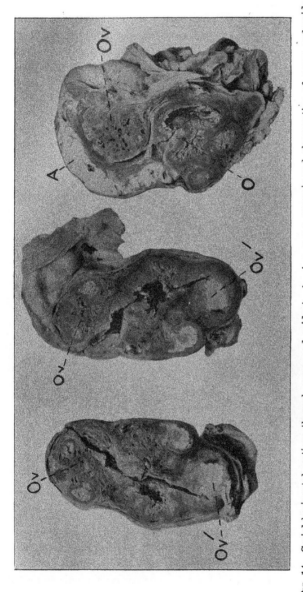

Fig. 14. Serial horizontal sections through ovary and oviduct, showing severe necrosis and abscessation of ovary and oviduct Ov', section through greatly enlarged, abscessed ovarian end of oviduct; O, ovary; A, parovarian adipose tissue

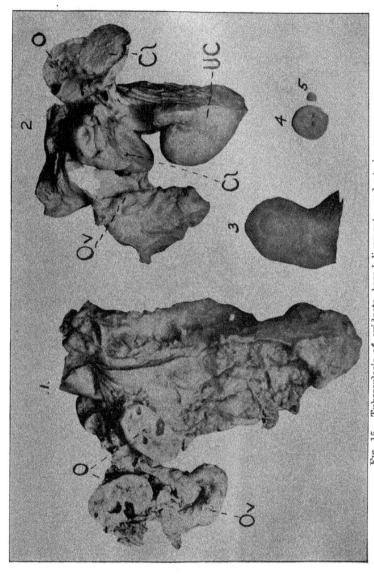

Fig. 15. Tuberculosis of oviducts, broad ligaments, and uterine cornu

O, ovary; Ov, oviduct; Cl, corpus luteum; UC, uterine cornu; 1, ovary (divided) oviduct and broad ligament; 2, ditto and uterine horn; 3, cross section of horn, showing faintly numerous tubercles in submucosa; 4, tubercular, and 5, normal oviduct, in cross section

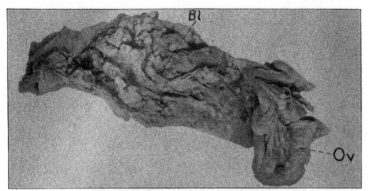

FIG. 16. Tuberculosis of broad ligament.
Bl, broad ligament; Ov, oviduct.

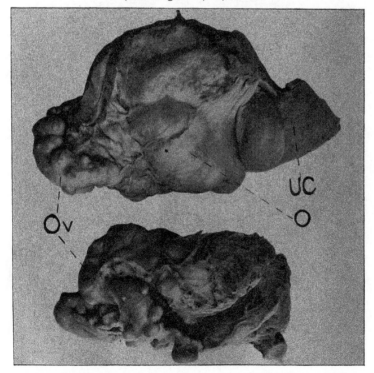

FIG. 17. Tuberculosis of ovary and oviduct, the oviducts being very nodular and
enlarged, the ovary adherent in the pavilion and broad ligament.
Ov, oviduct; O, ovary; UC, uterine cornu.

and the nymphomaniacal type of ovarian cyst may co-exist, but that is not evidence of either identity or relationship.

(2) *Tubal tuberculosis* is, next to uterine tuberculosis, the commonest type observed in the genitalia of cattle. In many specimens, the appearances suggest that the infection has invaded the oviducts centrifugally from the peritoneal cavity through the pavilion. In other instances of even severe uterine tuberculosis, the oviducts are free. Tuberculous oviducts are usually recognizable by rectal palpation. They become enlarged and very hard. Generally they are adherent and studded over with large tubercles. The tuberculous tubes vary in transverse diameter up to 0.5 inches or over. When much enlarged, they become elongated and thrown into folds lying in front of and lateral to the ovary, as shown in Figures 18 and 19. The disease may be confused with ordinary pyosalpinx or hydrosalpinx. In ordinary pyosalpinx there are two types. In the first and commonest, there is not much pus and the oviducts are not greatly enlarged, but are very firm and of even contour. In the second type of pyosalpinx, the pus is voluminous and the oviduct walls attenuated, giving a soft fluctuating tube, with thin, atonic walls. In hydrosalpinx, the oviduct is distended with lymph, firm and fluctuant. Tuberculous salpingitis is, in my experience, always nodular, the tubes very hard, adherent, and quite large.

Tuberculosis of the oviduct is almost, if not always bilateral, rendering the animal incurably sterile as well as a peril in a breeding or milk herd. The pus from tuberculous pyosalpinx escapes through the uterus and cervix to the vagina, to constitute a very serious menace to the bull.

(3) *Uterine tuberculosis* is the commonest type of genital tuberculosis in cattle. It is the most dangerous type of genital tuberculosis. The peril of uterine tuberculosis to other cattle is double. It is supremely dangerous to the bull when copulating with the affected animal. The discharges resulting from the tuberculous uterine catarrh soil the vulva, tail, thighs, and ultimately the udder, and contaminate milk. Thus the milk becomes intensely dangerous for calves, for other animals, and for man. In its peril to animal and human health, uterine tuberculosis vies with tuberculosis of any other organ. Uterine tuberculosis is quite variable, showing three somewhat separable types:

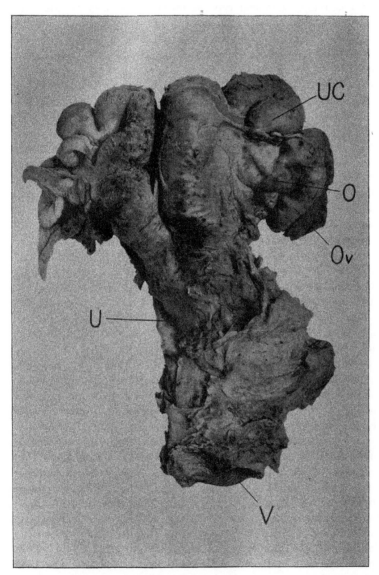

FIG. 18. Dorsal surface of tuberculous oviducts, uterus, and vagina, showing
extensive pelvic adhesions and adhesions of ovaries in pavilion
of oviduct and broad ligament.

O, ovary; UC, uterine cornu; Ov, oviduct; U, uterus; V, vagina.

(a) Peritoneal uterine tuberculosis with extensive pelvic adhesions, as shown in Fig. 18.

(b) Tuberculosis of the glandular structures of the uterine mucosa, as shown in Figures 21 and 22.

(c) Tuberculosis of the epithelial layer of the mucous membrane, as shown in Fig. 23.

No clear line of demarcation can be drawn between the three types, but in most cases one of the three groups of lesions predominates.

In uterine tuberculosis there is generally a persistent, obstinate uterine catarrh. In some cases the catarrhal discharge is inconspicuous. In some cases the tuberculous uterine catarrhal discharge is inconspicuous. Douching the uterus may reveal very little pus. In some cases of tuberculous uterine catarrh, uterine douches affect the catarrh favorably for a time, but permanent relief I have not observed. In cases where there have been apparently favorable results from douching, misleading the practitioner as to the nature of the malady, limited observation indicates that copulation sets the infection aflame. In other cases, such as Figures 21 and 22, the catarrh is profuse, but not generally fetid. Like tuberculosis of the oviducts, uterine tuberculosis is usually, if not always symmetrical, or bicornual. Generally the uterus contracts extensive pelvic adhesions. In many cases the peritoneum is so involved that ovaries, oviducts, uterus, and broad ligaments constitute a complex adherent mass, as in Fig. 18, where it is difficult, though generally possible, to identify the various parts by rectal palpation. Pelvic adhesions due to genital tuberculosis resemble strongly pelvic adhesions due to other infections. The adhesions due to tuberculosis are often accompanied by palpable tubercles. Their recognition aids materially in diagnosis. Non-tuberculous pelvic adhesions are frequently accompanied by sclerotic abscesses of an ovary, oviduct, uterine horn, or the three areas combined. Tuberculous pyosalpinx and pyometra, with necrosis of the uterine mucosa, as indicated in Figures 21 and 22, is common enough, but I have not observed extensive tuberculous abscesses involving the ovaries, oviducts, uterus, or broad ligaments. There is one important difference in the clinical history of tuberculous and non-tuberculous pelvic adhesions. The non-tuberculous adhesions are commonly preceded by acute metritis, largely with placentitis and retained fetal membranes. Tuberculous pelvic adhesions ordinarily arise independently of acute metritis.

The cow from which Figures 18 and 19 were taken was entered in our clinic for sterility. There was slight uterine catarrh (tuberculosis of the uterine mucosa) which abated under aseptic douches. The ovaries, oviducts, and uterus were normal by rectal

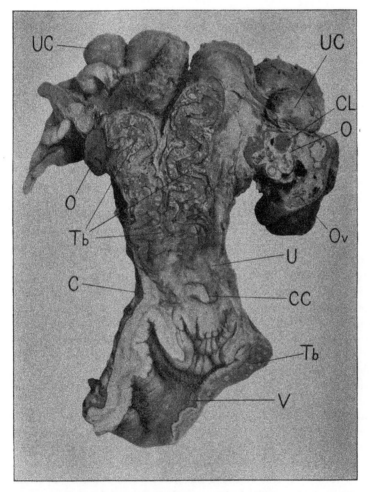

FIG. 19. Horizontal section of Fig. 18, showing tubercles, Tb, in uterine and vaginal walls. The right oviduct, Ov, is greatly enlarged, especially at its ovarian end, crossed by the line from O.

CL, corpus luteum in right ovary, O; C, cervix; CC, cervical canal. Other lettering same as in Fig. 18.

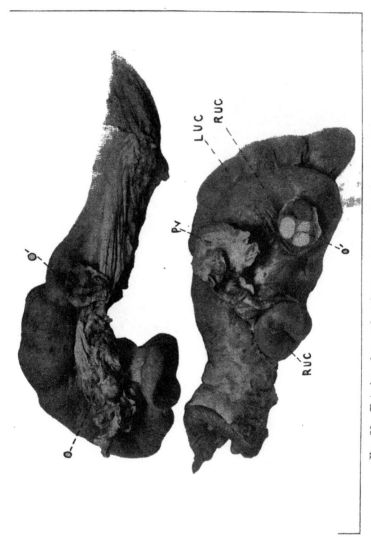

FIG. 20. Exterior of severely tubercular uterus without pelvic adhesions

⊙, divided right ovary in situ; ⊙', ⊙', excised portions of ovaries lying in uterine cornu; Pv, pavilion of right oviduct spread out and covering remnant of right ovary; RUC, RUC, right horn; LUC, left horn

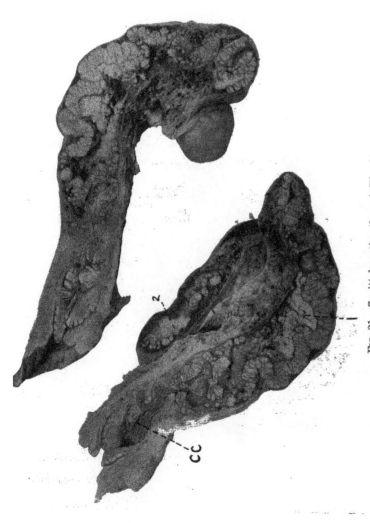

Fig. 21. Sagittal section through Fig. 20

tubercular pyometra, showing pus masses in cornual cavity; 2, pus masses in apex of cornu; CC, cervical canal. The corrugated uterine walls are everywhere thickly set with tubercles

palpation. She appeared so well that she was mated with a valuable herd sire. Soon afterward, she broke down, and upon re-examination genital tuberculosis was evident. When destroyed, extensive generalized tuberculosis was revealed. As she entered our clinic without a history, but upon the assumption of freedom from tuberculosis, no careful search was made in that direction. Apparently the disease reached its crisis at about the time of copulation, the patient gave way to the infection, and a diagnosis of genital tuberculosis became practicable. Fortunately the sire escaped, largely because the cow was douched just prior to copulation. The case illustrates vividly the insidious and subtle manner in which genital tuberculosis in the cow may develop and how the veterinarian needs be on his guard.

In some cases the tuberculous uterus remains to the end free from adhesions, as in Figures 20, 21, and 22. It is a significant fact that in my collection those uteri in which the mucosa is most extensively involved and which have undergone the maximum increase in size have suffered least from pelvic adhesions. Is this because in such cases as Figures 20 and 22 the infection of the uterine cavity has been primary (venereal) and in those cases with extensive adhesions, as in Fig. 18, the infection has invaded the tract by continuity from the general peritoneum? The freedom of the oviducts in Fig. 20 appears to emphasize this suggestion.

When the uterus is enlarged and sclerotic and comparatively free from adhesions, the tuberculous character is difficult of clinical recognition. One may meet with similar sclerotic hypertrophy in actinomycosis (primary genital) and in chronic purulent sclerotic metritis with destruction of the uterine mucosa. In such cases, however, the outlook for the breeding life of the patient is hopeless and an accurate clinical diagnosis is not imperative. In some cases of uterine tuberculosis, the masses of tubercles are so voluminous that they throw the uterine walls into great transverse folds which may be palpated per rectum. When such folds are present, they have a distinct diagnostic value. Usually in chronic abscessation of the uterus due to ordinary pyogenic bacteria or to actinomycosis, while the uterus is enlarged and hard, it is very irregular in outline. At one point there may be little or no enlargement. In actinomycosis and in pyogenic abscessation of the genitalia, some one part usually forms a great abscess or abscesses quite overshadowing other lesions, but in tuberculosis there is a

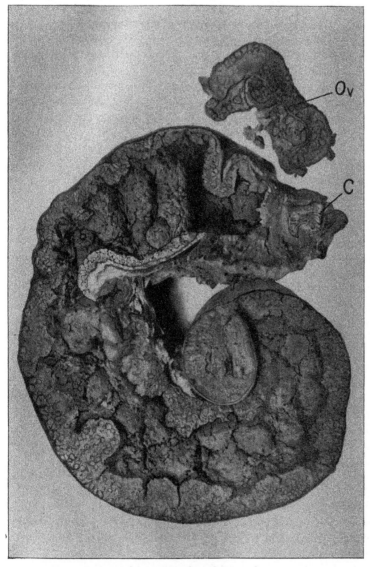

FIG. 22. Advanced tubo-uterine tuberculosis, with necrosis of mucosa
and pyometra.
Ov, oviduct, greatly enlarged and consisting of a mass of tubercles;
C, cervical canal.

strong tendency to symmetrical enlargement. The two horns are approximately alike in volume, form, and consistence. This is important to remember in making a diagnosis. In one cow of great breeding value, a reactor to tuberculin, which had not calved for two years and had long suffered from an abundant, fetid, highly repulsive genital discharge, I found one uterine horn much enlarged, three or four inches in its transverse diameter, and irregular in its contour. The other horn was approximately normal. The findings by palpation, in conjunction with her reaction to tuberculin, led me to diagnose uterine tuberculosis. The autopsy revealed, instead, a macerating fetus, the bones of which caused the irregular bulging of the cornu. Had I recognized the fact that in uterine tuberculosis the enlargement of the horns is usually symmetrical and that the pus from the tuberculous uterus is not usually fetid, the error would probably have been avoided. In those cases of uterine tuberculosis where only the superficial mucous layer is involved, as in Fig. 23, the diagnosis by ordinary clinical examination fails. The ovaries, oviducts, and uterus are normal to palpation, the uterine catarrh is insignificant, and no outstanding clinical evidences of genital tuberculosis are present.

The outstanding elements in the differentiation of utero-tubal tuberculosis are the pelvic adhesions, the tubercles in the genital peritoneum, the symmetrical enlargement of the uterus, and the obstinate uterine catarrh. No one of them warrants a positive diagnosis. If the patient reacts to tuberculin, the probability of genital tuberculosis is increased. No data are at hand regarding bacterial search of the genital discharges. Such search would probably aid materially in diagnosis. A negative tuberculin test is not conclusive evidence that genital tuberculosis is not present. The very valuable herd bull from which Fig. 5 was made quite certainly contracted the infection from a cow which had successfully passed several tuberculin tests, in spite of severe utero-tubal and general tuberculosis, with tuberculous uterine catarrh. While in many cases, such as delineated in Fig. 18, quite an accurate physical diagnosis of genital tuberculosis may be made, not all cases may be detected. The important point is that utero-tubal tuberculosis may almost always be tentatively diagnosed by rectal palpation and the veterinarian and owner placed on guard. So long as the symptoms named are present, the tentative diagnosis of utero-tubal tuberculosis is not only justified, but obligatory, from the sanitary standpoint. When uterine catarrh is present, copulation is contraindicated by every consideration of hygiene. Fertilization cannot occur; coitus aggravates the catarrh and imperils the bull. The retention in a dairy of a cow with obstinate uterine catarrh is unjustified by every consideration of health and decency. The af-

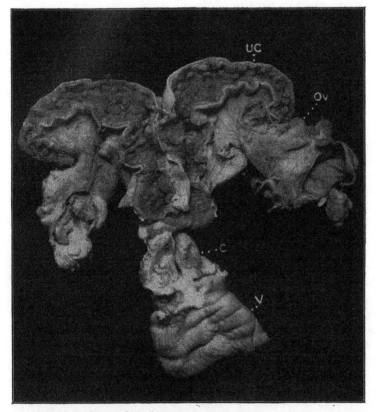

FIG. 23. Miliary tuberculosis of the superficial uterine mucosa of a virgin heifer.

V, vagina; C, cervix; UC, uterine cornu; Ov, oviduct. The uterine horns are laid open to show the numerous small tubercles upon the mucous surface.

flicted animal is unfit to associate with others in such a manner that their food may become contaminated with the genital discharges.

A tentative diagnosis of utero-tubal tuberculosis works no serious injury. If the cow recovers, the recovery automatically corrects the diagnosis; if she fails to recover, she is worthless for breeding or dairying, and fit only for slaughter, whether the infection be tuberculous or otherwise.

(4) *Tuberculosis of the cervix* is presumably rare. I have but one specimen (Figures 24 and 25) derived from the abattoir, and hence without a clinical history. In this case, the uterus and oviducts are also involved. The illustrations suggest the probable clinical features. The greatly swollen, hard, smooth lips of the cervix are apparent, and could not well be missed by an expert ex-

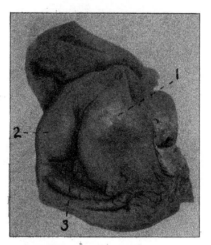

FIG. 24. Tuberculosis of the vaginal portion of the cervix.

1, greatly enlarged tubercular lip of os uteri externum; 2, a second, lesser tubercular tumefaction of lip; 3, mucous folds of the first annular cervical fold. Between it and 1 is the os uteri externum.

amining the genitalia clinically. While uterine catarrh was evidently present in this animal, it presumably had nothing to do with the cervical lesion. The lesion was apparently closed and caused no discharge. The surgeon, meeting with such condition, would logically incise the tumor, laying bare the nature of the lesion. I have repeatedly opened cysts in these parts. In so doing, I always draw the cervix back into the vulva before operating, so that the field is freely open to view and the contents which may be released are readily seen. If purulent, they at once raise the question of tuberculosis, which, once raised, should not be dismissed until the diagnosis has been made perfectly clear. On no account should a cow be permitted to copulate when a cervical lesion exists, unless it is clearly shown to be non-tuberculous. Even harmless-appearing cysts should not be passed over carelessly. Like vulvar cysts, discussed below, they may be tuberculous. The cervical lesion, when open, is evidently extremely dangerous.

(5) *Vaginal tuberculosis* is apparently very rare. Fig. 19 illustrates the only specimen in my collection. It was not recog-

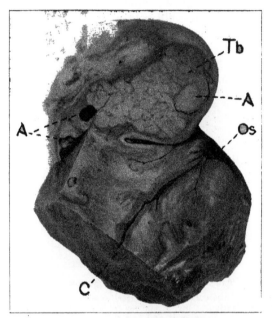

FIG. 25. Sagittal section of Fig. 24.
Os, os uteri externum; C, cervical canal; Tb, tubercles in lip of os uteri; A, A, tubercular abscesses.

nized clinically, although I examined the patient several times. However, I did not search for vaginal tuberculosis. Possibly it was of recent origin.

It is important for the veterinarian, in dealing instrumentally with diseases of the genitalia, to bear in mind that he may, by the use of the uterine forceps, implant the infection in the cervix, or in the vagina at its point of continuity with the cervix. He may re-infect these parts, through instrumental lesion, with the discharges from the patient's uterus. If careless in his methods, he may carry the infection from a tuberculous cow to a healthy one. Under reasonable precautions, the danger is quite negligible. Fig. 19 shows that in this case the tuberculous lesions are within the vaginal wall and closed. If open, the lesion would have the same danger as that of the cervix.

(6) *Vulvar tuberculosis* has occurred twice in my practice, each time readily diagnosed, though in one case the nature of the lesion was at first misleading. In this case, at the first examination,

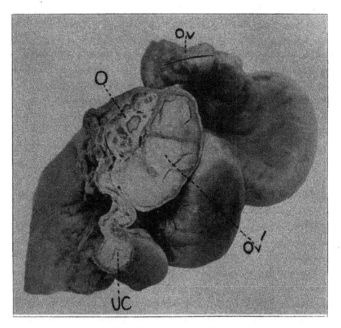

FIG. 26. Uterus of Figs. 24 and 25.
O, bisected ovary; Ov, greatly enlarged and very nodular oviduct; Ov', cystic ovarian end of oviduct; UC, cross section of horn.

a cyst one inch in diameter lay in the vulvar lip and was incised just at the labial margin, and a small amount of sero-purulent content escaped. Prior to my next examination, the patient had reacted to the tuberculin test, and when I next examined her, the lesion presented the typical characters of a tuberculous ulcer. My second case was more readily diagnosed. The vulvar lip, which was swollen and sclerotic, presented an old fistulous opening, from which small volumes of thick pus could be pressed out. Centripetally, a

tuberculous gland, two to three inches in diameter, lay alongside
the vagina. In addition, both supramammary glands were greatly
enlarged, and at each internal inguinal ring glands three inches in
diameter were palpable. Autopsy showed severe generalized tuberculosis.

Vulvar tuberculosis is evidently a *very* dangerous type for the
bull. In my second case, the cow had been bred to the herd bull,
valued at more than ten thousand dollars, but a few days before my
examination. Fortunately he escaped infection.

Having regard for the facts set forth, it seems remarkable
veterinary writers have given so little attention to the subject of
genital tuberculosis in cattle. The failure to give the subject due
consideration is apparently due to two circumstances: (1) the
average veterinary practitioner fails to diagnose the disease in
either sex; (2) in the abattoir, the genitalia are not ordinarily inspected.

In the bull, the preponderant types disable the patient for
coition and he must be sent to the shambles, regardless of the nature of the disease. He is impotent, and ceases to be of value as a
sire. The fact that a highly dangerous cow lurks somewhere in
the herd is not recognized. The cow with utero-tubal tuberculosis
is sterile, and beyond that fact the practitioner fails to go.

Careful study must make it apparent that genital tuberculosis is not rare and that it offers one of the most, if not the most
dangerous train of lesions observed in any form of tuberculosis.
Most types of genital tuberculosis in the bull are highly dangerous
to cows with which he may copulate, so long as he is capable of
copulation, but the bull often becomes quickly incapacitated sexually and the special venereal dangers are placed in abeyance.

The cow with genital tuberculosis, be it tubal, uterine, cervical,
vaginal, or vulvar, is intensely dangerous. I have seen more valuable breeding bulls sent to the shambles from serving such cows than
for any other cause, or for all other causes combined. The genital
discharges from open lesions find their way inevitably along the
tail, thighs, and escutcheon over the udder to the teats. There it
is taken with the milk when a calf sucks, or the milk is contaminated
as it is drawn, and finally consumed by calves or people.

The control of these dangers evidently depends chiefly upon
the more general and accurate diagnosis of genital lesions in both
sexes and the more general adoption of efficient sex hygiene in

breeding cattle. The lesions are to be detected through two chief agencies—dairy inspection and inspection of the genitalia¹ in connection with sterility. At present, dairy inspection fails utterly in most cases in relation to genital disorders. Repeatedly I find, in regularly inspected herds, and even in certified dairies, cows with quarts or gallons of fetid pus in the uterine cavity, large volumes of which are pressed out from time to time while the cows are lying down. Advancement in this field is one of the most urgently needed reforms in dairy inspection. The greatest weapon for the control of the danger lies in the more general inspection of the genitalia of cattle, as a safeguard against sterility and abortion. It is becoming more and more apparent that a careful physical examination of the genitalia of cows, prior to breeding, is a wise precaution of distinct scientific and economic importance. It is beginning to dawn upon some progressive breeders of pedigreed cattle that, before permitting the herd sire to serve a cow, her genitalia should be subjected to a careful inspection and that she should not be bred until it is determined, so far as possible, that she is sound. A study of the problem indicates further that the breeder should take far greater care in the sex hygiene of the bull. If penial injuries and infections are to be averted, having first ascertained that the genital organs of the cow are healthy, the external genitalia of both cow and bull should be carefully washed before permitting copulation. It is highly important, in the prevention of penial lesions, which may serve as infection avenues, that the crusts of pus in the vulvar tuft of hairs of the cow be removed by washing. Otherwise, these crusts of pus may be caught and forced into the vulvar opening, to abrade the penial mucosa. After copulation, the penis, prepuce, and sheath of the bull should again be carefully and efficiently douched. These precautions go hand in hand with those designed to control sterility and abortion.

—Dr. William F. Biles has been transferred from College Park, Md., to Louisville, Ky., to take charge of hog cholera educational and demonstrational work in that city, vice Dr. Hanawalt, deceased.

—Dr. W. M. Balmer has removed from Boston, Mass., to Wilmington, N. C., in charge of federal meat inspection at that place.

CANINE COCCIDIOSIS, WITH A NOTE REGARDING OTHER PROTOZOAN PARASITES FROM THE DOG*

MAURICE C. HALL, Ph.D., D.V.M., and MEYER WIGDOR, M.A.
Research Laboratory, Parke, Davis and Company, Detroit, Mich.

In a recent paper, Hall (1917) reported the occurrence of a coccidian in dogs in Detroit and stated that its size precluded the idea that it was *Diplospora bigemina*, so far as available literature showed. An examination of Stiles's (1892) original paper and of the measurements given by Fantham (1916) leads us to the conclusion that this coccidian at Detroit is *D. bigemina*. In the first 200 dogs examined here, this parasite was found in 15, or 7.5 per cent, a frequency that warrants some study of this organism and which suggests that it is probably much commoner in American dogs than our present lack of information would suggest. Another thing which warrants consideration of this protozoan is the fact that it is reported as one of the species occurring in man. In 1915, Wenyon reported a coccidian (*Eimeria Coccidium*) from soldiers on the Gallipoli Peninsula, and the same year Woodcock reported *Isospora*, a generic name sometimes used in place of *Diplospora*, from soldiers in the same locality. (The available literature states that *Diplospora* develops 2 spores each containing 4 sporozoites, while *Isospora* develops 2 spores each containing a variable number of sporozoites.) Castellani (1917) says that coccidiosis in man is comparatively common in the Balkans and notes a number of cases, stating, in comment, that treatment was unsatisfactory. Inasmuch as our soldiers may yet fight on any of the battle fronts surrounding the Central Powers, the diseases to which they may be exposed deserve especial consideration at this time. Moreover, the disease in the dog has received very little study.

In the case of dog No. 127, a heavily infected animal, this coccidian showed a marked tendency to occur in adherent groups in the feces. We use the method of examining the feces described by Hall (1917) and in spite of the use of the mechanical agitator, coccidia were commonly found in clusters of two to twelve in the feces of this animal. We regard this as perhaps due to an adhesive character of the oocyst wall or to a particularly mucilaginous quality of this dog's feces.

*Read before the Southeastern Michigan Veterinary Medical Association, Jan. 9, 1918.

Stiles (1892) notes that this species occurs in dogs and cats and in the polecat, *Putorius putorius*. Railliet and Lucet (1891) have reported these as different varieties, *Coccidium bigeminum canis, C. bigeminum cati*, and *C. bigeminum putorii*. Weidman (1915) has reported another variety, *C. bigeminum canivelocis*, from swift foxes in the western United States. Stiles notes that the coccidia from the intestine of the dog which have been referred by various authors to *Coccidium perforans*, the form from the rabbit intestine (regarded by some workers as identical with *Eimeria stiedae*), are probably *C. bigeminum*. Recently Guillebeau (1916) has reported *Eimeria stiedae*, the coccidian commonly found in the liver of rabbits, from the liver of dogs, but in his review of this paper (Guillebeau, 1917), Railliet concludes that the organisms described are not coccidia, but blastomycetes. Railliet does not regard the hepatic organisms described by Lienaux, Clark, Marcone, or Olt as coccidia, and notes that forms described by Perroncito are trichosome eggs. He believes that *Diplospora bigemina*

Fig. 1. *Diplospora bigemina*. Oocyst with the two spores, each containing four sporozoites and a residual body. Highly magnified.

from the mucosa and submucosa of the intestinal villi is the only coccidian known from the dog, and that while hepatic coccidia may occur in the dog, no case of the sort has been established. In passing we note the following editorial from the *Pacific Medical Journal* of July, 1916:

"COCCIDIOSIS. This disease, said to be more or less prevalent in San Joaquin Valley of California, is produced by a protozoan or psorosperm. The parasite is found in the excreta of dogs, hogs, and in the intestine and liver of rabbits and in bones of the human family. Some forty cases are known. Most of them originated in the San Joaquin Valley. The mortality is 100 per cent. The most recent case occurred in Los Angeles County Hospital."

There appears to be some misunderstanding or error involved here.

Most of the material we have examined falls within the range of measurements given by Hall (1917), the oocysts measuring 36 to 40 μ long by 28 to 32 μ wide. Fantham (1916) gives a range of 22 to 40 μ by 19 to 28 μ. These forms have 2 spores, each spore measuring 10 to 20 μ in diameter (Fantham gives a range of 10 to 18 μ), and each spore contains 4 sporozoites, each 12 μ long by 4 μ wide, and a residual body (Fig. 1). In one animal, Dog No. 223, we found a smaller strain of coccidia, the oocysts measuring 20 by 18 μ in diameter, the spores 12 by 11 μ in diameter, and the sporozoites being 10 μ long and 3 μ wide. The distinction in size between the coccidia in this animal and the other coccidia was quite marked and naturally raises the question whether this should be regarded as a strain, a variety, or a species. It is possible that there are several species of *Diplospora* in the dog, characterized by considerable differences in size, or there may be one species developing various strains under certain determining conditions. This is not a matter on which we care to pass judgment, but it is a question which apparently deserves investigation. If we understand the figures given by Stiles and other writers, the oocysts from European dogs are about 10 μ in diameter, the small ones at this point are about 20 μ in diameter, while the large ones here and the forms reported by Weidman (1915) from the western swift fox, examined in the Philadelphia Zoological Garden, attain a diameter of 40 μ.

Some incidental attempts to culture our coccidian material gave the following results: Coccidia of the larger strain, in feces from dog No. 127, were kept in a 10 per cent solution of potassium bichromate, as advocated by Cole and Hadley (1910), at room temperatures. The culture was not examined until the ninth day, at which time most of the oocysts had spores containing sporozoites. A second bichromate culture was made up of coccidia-infested feces of dog No. 210 and kept at a temperature of 23° to 29°C. During the first 24 hours the oocyst material divided to form the two sporoblasts. During the next 24 hours, the spores formed and the sporozoite development went on to the production of two to four cells to a spore. During the third day, sporozoites were present in almost all oocysts. Under such favorable conditions, then, feces containing this coccidian would probably be infective for other susceptible animals by the fourth day. A third culture from the feces of this same dog, No. 210, was made at the same time as the one just noted, but was made with tap water. At the same temperatures as the preceding culture, this culture with water showed no apparent change the first 24 hours. During the next 24 hours some cell division was observed in the oocysts. The subsequent development proceeded very slowly and the early stages of sporozoite development were not noted until the eighth day. On the fourteenth day several oocysts were found showing developed sporozoites. A fourth culture was made with the smaller strain of coccidia, the infected feces of dog No. 223 being cultured in 10 per cent potassium bichromate at temperatures of 20° to 23°C. During the first 24 hours, cell division had proceeded to the point where there were 2 well-defined sporoblasts. During the second 24 hours, development proceeded to the formation of 4 well-defined sporozoites. This material was fed to dog No. 173, which it failed to infect, but this dog seemed to have acquired immunity to cocci-diosis. It appears, then, that feces of dogs infected with *Diplospora bigemina* may become infective for susceptible animals under very favorable conditions in 48 hours, probably, and under unfavorable conditions may remain uninfective for two weeks or longer. It is unlikely that conditions in nature very often approach the favorable conditions afforded by the use of potassium bichromate solution and the maintenance of the temperature noted, and consequently the development period in nature probably is a matter of weeks rather than days as a rule.

To ascertain the length of time required for the coccidia to develop from the infecting sporozoites in the dog to the appearance of oocysts in the feces, the following experiments were performed:

Dog No. 216, under treatment with Fowler's solution, was given a heavy concentration of sporozoites about 1 hour after receiving Fowler's solution. The dog vomited about 15 minutes later, probably losing some of the coccidian material in this way. Fecal examinations for the following 13 days were negative. Dog No. 219, having shown no coccidia on a single fecal examination, was fed a heavy infestation of sporozoites from the feces of dog No. 127. The feces showed no coccidia the next 3 days; the fourth day was Sunday and the feces were not examined; the fifth day oocysts were found in the feces, the cycle from sporozoite to oocysts in the feces requiring at least 4, possibly 5, days. Dog No. 130, having shown no coccidia on a single fecal examination, was fed a half dram of a bichromate culture of feces containing coccidia. No coccidia were found in the feces the next two days and no feces were passed the third day. On the fourth day, oocysts appeared in the feces, among them an oocyst containing 2 spores, which suggests that the oocyst in the 1-celled stage, as ordinarily found in the feces, was present on the third day. The post mortem examination of this dog on the fifth day after feeding the coccidia showed numerous coccidia in various stages of development in the intestinal wall. Dog No. 173 was given a half dram of culture containing coccidia in bichromate solution. Fecal examinations through the following 10 days were negative. The feces were not examined the eleventh day, but on the twelfth day they were examined and oocysts found. The developmental period from the ingestion of sporozoites, therefore, appears to require from 4 days, possibly as little as 3 days, to 11 or 12 days. A culture of coccidia in potassium bichromate was fed to a rat, but fecal examinations were still negative at the end of 19 days, and the examinations were abandoned with the presumption established that rats are probably not capable of infection with D. bigemina under ordinary circumstances.

Although the treatment of coccidiosis is generally unsatisfactory at present, it has been noted by investigators that infestations are commonly self-limited; after the host is infested, the coccidian reproduces by schizogony for a time, spreading the infestation more widely in the host, but after a time the parasitic elements undergo the sexual transformation leading to the formation of oocysts intended for the dissemination of the infection to other host animals, the schizogonous cycle comes to an end, and the infestation terminates. We had occasion to observe this for D. bigemina in the case of dog No. 173. As noted above, feeding of infective material led to the infestation of this dog and the appearance of oocysts in the feces on the twelfth day. Oocysts were numerous in the feces of this dog for a little over a week. On the tenth day of oocyst occurrence in the feces there was a marked falling off of their number and very few were found the next two days. No oocysts were found thereafter, so the infestation required 12 days before oocysts appeared in the feces and lasted only another 12 days so far as the presence of oocysts showed infestation. Fecal examinations for the next 61 days showed no oocysts, in spite of attempts at re-infestation.

Crawley (1912) states in regard to the self-limitation of coccidiosis: "Apparently, however, no immunity is produced, and another attack of the disease may result from a fresh infection from without.'' An experiment along this line was carried out in connection with the self-limitation of infection of dog No. 173. After this dog had been infested by feeding, had shown the infestation for 12 days, and had then been apparently free from infestation for 14 days, the animal was given 2 mils of material from the same infective culture of *D. bigemina* that had previously infected it. No oocysts were found in the feces during the next 18 days. Nineteen days after this attempt to infect the dog, the animal was given 3 mils of a heavy concentration of coccidian material obtained from this animal while it was showing an abundance of coccidian material in the feces. No oocysts were found in the feces during the next 16 days. Seventeen days after this second attempt, the animal was given 4 mils of a culture of the small strain of coccidia found in dog No. 223. No oocysts were found in the feces during the next 11 days, at which time the dog was killed. This dog had shown no sign of coccidiosis after having been fed 3 cultures at intervals of 11, 28 and 47 days previous to death. The animal had been susceptible to coccidiosis when first given infective material after being found negative. In all other cases where we fed the same coccidian material to dogs, we infected the animals without difficulty, except in the case of dog No. 216, which could not be infected with oocysts from infected feces of this dog (No. 173). In this case (No. 173) we failed to infect the dog with the same strain that had originally infected it, with the coccidia taken from the dog's own feces, and with a totally different strain, morphologically distinguishable and from a different animal. The obvious explanation that occurs to us is that this dog had developed an immunity to *D. bigemina*. Other explanations may be figured out, but they seem less plausible than this, and we submit that this is apparently a case of acquired immunity to coccidiosis. The apparent immunity to the small strain is evidence, though not conclusive, that this and the larger form are only different strains of a single species.

As regards the pathological significance of *D. bigemina,* we have but little information, but the following notes may serve some purpose: Dog No. 130 presented a clinical picture of distemper and died of pneumonia, probably due in part to distemper and partly to an accident in drenching. The small intestine showed diffuse hemorrhagic points, most pronounced in the ileum, especially the lower ileum near the valve. Scrapings of the mucosa showed the coccidia to be most abundant in the ileum, less so in the jejunum and least so in the duodenum. These findings of increasing numbers of coccidia with increasing severity of lesions may be correlated, but in the absence of sections indicating the relation of the coccidia to the hemorrhage, we do not care to hazard a definite opinion. Dog No. 173 showed numerous fine petechiae in the intestinal mucosa, and these were especially numerous in the Peyer's patches, giving these a uniformly dark appearance. No sections were made and this dog had shown no oocysts in the feces for 45 days. Dog No. 127 showed innumerable pinpoint petechiae in the ileum, but it would be unsafe to draw conclusions based on this one dog, as the animal figured in other experiments. The intestine of dog No. 223 was macroscopically normal except for the presence of hook-worm petechiae. Other dogs that had coccidiosis were used in experiments that complicate the post mortem findings and leave the effect of the coccidiosis uncertain. However, we may note that Weidman (1915) found what he regards as a variety of *D. bigemina* in hemorrhagic, ulcerative enteritis in the swift fox, raising the question as to the possible etiological relationship. In view of the fact that coccidia are destructive to epithelial tissue and that some species fairly closely related to *D. bigemina* are known to be highly pathological, it would seem reasonable to suppose that *D. bigemina* might be distinctly pathological at times, though the apparent good health and lack of post mortem lesions in other dogs makes it certain that it often does no visible damage.

A few clinical observations may be noted in this connection. As regards the presence of febrile conditions, we find the following: Dog No. 173 showed a preliminary temperature of 101.5° before the feeding of coccidia to the animal. During the next ten days, in which no oocysts were found in the feces, the animal's temperature was as follows, no temperature being taken on the fourth day: 101.7°, 101.0°, 100.3°, 101.2°, 102.4°, 103.0°, 101.1°, 101.6°, 99.8°. This shows a slight rise in temperature on the sixth and seventh days. No temperature was taken on the eleventh day. On the twelfth day oocysts were found in the feces and were abundant for the next 7 days. This period was marked by a steady rise in temperature as follows: 100.0°, 101.0°, 101.2°, 101.4°, 101.8°, 102.0° (no temperature taken the eighteenth day after feeding), 102.4°. The following days there was a marked falling off in the number of oocysts in the feces and a simultaneous drop in temperature as follows: 101.5°, 100.8°, 101.0°. Oocysts then disappeared from the feces, the temperatures persisting within the limits of normal temperatures as follows: 100.3°, 100.0°, 101.9°, 101.0°, 100.0°, 100.8°, 100.4°. Dog No. 219 showed a preliminary temperature of 102.0°. This animal had distemper and a pronounced goitre, conditions which complicated the clinical picture of coccidiosis. After feeding the coccidia and while no oocysts were found in the feces, the animal's temperature dropped and then rose as follows: 101.0°, 101.8°, 103.4° (no temperature taken the fourth day after the feeding). The next day oocysts were found in the feces and again the temperature dropped and rose as follows: 101.0°, 102.4°, 102.8°, 102.7°, falling the next day to 101.6°. Three days later the oocysts were very scarce in the feces and the temperature fell to 100.0°. The animal was put on anthelmintic treatment at this time, introducing another complication, but no more oocysts were found in the feces and the temperature remained under 100.0°. Dog No. 130 apparently got some of the drench containing coccidia into its lungs. No preliminaary temperature was taken. The day after the animal was given the coccidia, the temperature was 104.0°, the next day 103.2°, the next day 101.0°. During this time there were no oocysts in the feces. The following day, oocysts appeared in the feces and the temperature rose again to 102.4°, the animal dying of pneumonia the following day. Post mortem examination showed areas of red hepatization in all the lobes of the lungs.

A consideration of the temperatures given suggests that there is a slight elevation of temperature during the period that oocysts are found in the feces, but it would be unsafe to generalize from so few cases. A consideration of the temperatures of a number of dogs not infested experimentally, but found infested on fecal examination, shows the following temperatures for periods when oocysts were present in the feces (some feces were only examined on one day for oocysts): Dog No. 66—101.3°, 101.5°, 101.4°, 101.0°, 101.5°, 102.5°, 98.8°, 95.0°, followed by death (case complicated by pneumonic condition of left median lobe and by administration of coal-tar preparation); No. 112—101.9°, 101.0°, 102.0°, 101.4°, 101.0°; No. 119—102.2°; No. 127—102.5°; No. 129 —101.5°; No. 139—101.3°; No. 167—101.2°; No. 168—101.6°. Taking the figures given by Malkmus (1912) as the normal for the dog, 99.5° to 102.2°, we are impelled to the conclusion that intestinal coccidiosis in dogs, due to the presence of *Diplospora bigemina*, is an afebrile condition.

In the experiment dogs which were given some attention with reference to the presence of coccidia, diarrhea was noted as follows: Dog No. 173 developed a diarrhea on the sixth day after oocysts appeared in the feces, and had a bloody diarrhea on the last day in which oocysts appeared in the feces. Dog No. 219 developed a diarrhea on the second day after oocysts appeared in the feces; the following day there was much gas in the feces; the following day there were blood and gas in the diarrheal feces, the blood persisting in the diarrheal feces over the period in which oocysts were found and while the experiment remained uncomplicated by other factors. Dog No. 130 developed a diarrhea on the first day that oocysts appeared in the feces. Inasmuch as diarrhea is a prominent symptom of coccidiosis in man, cattle, rabbits and birds, and is a logical sequel of the coccidian injury to the intestinal mucosa, we are of the opinion that the diarrheas observed may reasonably be associated with the coccidiosis as perhaps its most prominent symptom. It is a point that deserves further investigation, but it may be tentatively accepted as in accord with the probabilities. In the case of this species which undergoes much of its development in the submucosa, there appears to be no diarrhea while only the developmental stages in the submucosa are present, but the passage through the mucosa of the oocysts gives rise to injury resulting in the production of diarrhea. Light infestations may not show diarrhea; the organism is present, but no clinical picture of coccidiosis is presented.

For some reason, the protozoan parasites of dogs in this country have received very little attention and there is little known on the subject. It is possible that such parasites are as scarce as the scanty literature would suggest, but there is no evidence that such parasites have been looked for. The following list of protozoan parasites recorded from North and Central America is made up to a considerable extent of records of experimental infestations. The list covers only references readily available and is not intended as an exhaustive compilation.

Entameba venaticum was described from dogs in the Canal Zone by Darling (1915). This protozoan was found in the colon on post mortem examination and appears to be pathological.

Trypanosoma hippicum, described by Darling in 1910 from

solipeds in the Canal Zone, has been inoculated into dogs at the same locality, according to the same author (Darling, 1913).

Trypanosoma equiperdum was reported by Mohler (1911) at Washington in a dog imported from France to this country after inoculation with the trypanosome of dourine for comparison with American strains, and American dogs were inoculated with this French strain.

Trypanosoma evansi, the cause of surra, is reported from an experimentally infected dog by Mohler, Eichhorn and Buck (1913) at Washington.

Babesia canis, the cause of canine piroplasmosis or malignant protozoan jaundice, has been reported from dogs in Porto Rico.

Spirochaeta sp., an organism merely noted as "a spirochaete", is said by Gray (1913) to have been found in infective venereal granuloma of the dog in the United States by Beebe and Ewing of Cornell.

Treponema pallidum, the organism of syphilis, has been successfully inoculated in dogs by Bertarelli, and dogs may have been, and very likely have been, inoculated with this organism in the study of experimental syphilis in this country.

PROTOZOAN (?). Foster (1912) reports what he regards as an undetermined protozoan as the cause of protozoic stomatitis or sore mouth of dogs in the South. Of the mouth lesions, he says:

"Microscopic examination of sections made through these lesions, stained by Jenner's method, reveals a protozoic infection of the mucous glands, which is associated with streptococcic infection. The infecting organisms are found in the glands themselves and also in the ducts near the surface. Experiments thus far do not permit me to classify the protozoa in its proper place. * * * I find it to be actively motile, possessing a movement indicative of bipolar flagellae, although I have not as yet stained any. It reproduces by simple fission, will grow on simple media, and presents chromatin granules. Stained from pure culture, it frequently appears as crescent-shaped on account of its movement. * * * In shape it resembles a grain of barley. Injected into the mucous membrane of a healthy subject it will produce the disease, from which it may be again obtained. It is non-sporulating."

Leishmania americana, or *Leishmania tropica americana*, the organism causing the American variety of Oriental sore, is not definitely reported from dogs in North America, so far as we are aware. However, Oriental sore has been reported from man in Panama by Darling (1911) and the disease and its parasite has been found in dogs in South America by Pedrosa, according to Lavern (1916). Lavern states:

"The cases of natural infection of dogs by *Leishmania americana* are very rare. In 1912, Pedrosa observed, in northern Brazil, two dogs that had ulcerations of the nasal mucosa. One of the dogs * * * was in bad condition; he had cutaneous ulcerations beside the lesion of the left nostril; smears made from scrapings from the nasal ulcer showed numerous Leishman bodies identical with those from the human subject. The master of the other dog had an ulcer of the foot that was diagnosed as leishmaniosis, and he made the dog lick his ulcer; the animal thereby became directly infected * * *; the diagnosis rested on the macroscopic appearance of the ulceration, and the history of the case."

Rangelia vitalii was described by Carini and Maciel, in 1914, from the blood of dogs in Brazil. It is said to resemble *Leishmania*, but lacks a visible centrosome. It causes a disease known as nambiuva, bleeding ear, yellow fever of dogs, or blood plague, characterized by icterus and cutaneous and internal hemorrhage. It has not yet been reported from North or Central America, so far as we are aware.

Neuroryctes hydrophobiae, is the name applied to the supposed protozoan organism causing rabies. However, the etiological agent in rabies is commonly regarded as not yet established. The well known Negri bodies are regarded as diagnostic of rabies, but their identity with, or relation to, the cause of rabies is still debated. Owing to the laxity in our treatment of dogs, rabies is rather common in the United States.

SUMMARY. *Diplospora bigemina* has been found in 7.5 per cent of 200 dogs examined at Detroit. The occurrence of this coccidian in man in other countries gives it considerable importance and it may be found to occur in man in this country. The coccidian is reported from the western swift fox, indicating that it may occur in the West, the home of the fox, or may occur in the East, where the foxes examined were living in a zoological garden.

Under favorable temperature conditions, oocysts in 10 per cent potassium bichromate solution appear to develop infective sporozoites in two days, but under less favorable conditions, probably more nearly those found in nature, this may require two weeks or

longer. From the feeding of oocysts containing infective sporozoites to the appearance of oocysts in the feces of the dogs fed, a
period of as little as 3 or 4 days to as much as 11 or 12 days may
elapse. Infections are self-limited. In one animal oocysts were
present in the feces for 12 days; subsequent attempts to infect this
animal failed and there was apparently an acquired immunity to
coccidiosis.

With infestations naturally acquired, dogs often show a practically normal digestive tract post mortem, but with heavy infestations, usually the result of feeding coccidia experimentally, hemorrhagic conditions have been found that may be related to the presence of the coccidia. The disease is afebrile, though experiments
suggest that there is a slight elevation of temperature during the
time that oocysts are found in the feces. Diarrhea, at times with
the presence of gas or blood in the feces, appears to be, and probably is, a symptom of canine coccidiosis.

The following protozoa have been recorded in dogs in North
and Central Ameerica: *Entameba venaticum, Babesia canis, Diplospora bigemina, Spirochaeta sp., Neuroryctes hydrophobiae* and
an undetermined form regarded as protozoan.

The following protozoa have been reported in experimental
infestation in dogs in North and Central America: *Trypanosoma
hippicum, Trypanosoma equiperdum,* and *Trypanosoma evansi.*

Treponema pallidum, an organism only too common in man
in this country, has been inoculated in dogs by Bertarelli, *Leishmania americana* has been found in man in Panama and in dogs in
Brazil,, and *Rangelia vitalii* has been reported from dogs in Brazil.
Any or all of these forms might be found in dogs in this country,
but we find no existing records.

CASTELLANI, A. 1917. Notes on tropical diseases met with in the Balcanic and
    Adriatic Zones. *Jour. Trop. M. and Hyg.,* Vol. 20 (17), Sept. 1, pp.
    198-202.

COLE, LEON J., and PHILIP B. HADLEY. 1910. Blackhead in turkeys: A study
    in avian coccidiosis. *R. I. Exp. Sta. Bull. 141,* pp. 137-271, 11 pls.

CRAWLEY, HOWARD. 1912. The protozoan parasites of domesticated animals.
    Bu. Anim. Indust. Circ. 194, pp. 465-498, pls. 37-42, figs. 63-75.

DARLING, S. T. 1911. Oriental sore in Panama. *Arch. Int. Med.,* Vol. 7, May,
    pp. 581-597, 6 figs.
    1913. The immunization of large animals to a pathogenic trypanosome

(*Trypanosoma hippicum* (Darling)) by means of an avirulent strain. J. *Exp. Med., Vol.* 17, (5), pp. 582-586.

1915. Entamebic dysentery in the dog. *Proc. Med. Ass., Isthmian Canal Zone,* Vol. 6, (1), pp. 60-62.

FANTHAM, H. B. 1916. Protozoa. In *The Animal Parasites of Man,* London, pp. 25-210, 119 figs.

FOSTER, ALLAN A. 1912. Protozoic stomatitis, or sore mouth of dogs. *Kans. City Vet. Coll. Quart., Bull. 36,* June, pp. 872-874.

GRAY. HENRY. 1913. Venereal diseases in the dog, rabbit, hare and fowl. *In* Hoare's A System of Veterinary Medicine, Chicago, Vol. I, pp. 366-371.

GUILLEBEAU, A. 1916. Parasitic occurrence of *Eimeria stiedae* in the liver of the dog. (*Schweitz. Arch. Tierheilk.*), Vol. 58, (11), pp. 596-602, 6 figs. (Not seen.)

1917. Idem. *Rec. d. Méd. Vét.,* Vol. 93, (1-2), pp. 71-73.

HALL, MAURICE C. 1917. Apparatus for use in examining feces for evidences of parasitism. *Jour. Lab. and Clin. Med.,* Vol. 2, (5), FEB., pp. 347-353, 3 figs.

1917. Parasites of the dog in Michigan. *Jour. A. V. M. A.,* n.s. Vol. 4, (3), June, pp. 383-396.

LAVERAN, A. 1916. American leishmaniosis of the skin and mucous membranes. *New Orleans M. and Surg. Jour.,* Vol. 68, (9), March, pp. 582-606.

MALKMUS, BERNARD. 1912. Clinical diagnosis of the internal diseases of domestic animals. Chicago, 259 pp., 57 figs.

MOHLER, JOHN R., ADOLPH EICHHORN, and JOHN M. BUCK. 1913. The diagnosis of dourine by complement fixation. *Jour. Agric. Research,* Vol. 1, (2), Nov. 10, pp. 99-107.

RAILLIET, ALCIDE and ADRIEN LUCET. 1891. Note sur quelques éspeces de coccidies encore peu étudiées. *Bull. Soc. zool. de France,* Vol. 16, (9-10), Nov.-Dec., pp. 246-250. (Not seen.)

STILES, CHARLES W. 1892. Notes on parasites. II. *Jour. Comp. Med. and Vet. Arch.,* Vol. 13, (9), Sept., pp. 517-526, figs. 1-7.

WEIDMAN, FRED. D. 1915. *Coccidium bigeminum* Stiles in Swift foxes (Habitat Western U. S.). *Jour. Comp. Path. and Therap.,* Vol. 28, (4), Dec. 31, pp. 320-323, 3 figs.

—Dr. R. A. Gregory has removed from Forest City, Ark., to DeWitt, Ark.

—Dr. H. F. Lienhardt, formerly at Wayne, Pa., is now located at Manhattan, Kans.

—Dr. J. M. Jehle, formerly at Des Moines, has charge of hog cholera control work in five counties with headquarters at Grinnell, Ia.

AN APPEAL FOR EQUINE MEAT AS A FOOD*

W. Horace Hoskins, D.V.S., New York, N. Y.

When conferences are being held as to the amount of whale meat that can be secured to meet meatless days, and these inhabitants of the deep live wholly a cannibal life; when shark meat is quoted at 20c a pound and their meat was once despised and their source of sustenance like that of a whale; why should anyone shudder at the consumption of equine flesh, when it lives only on the richest cereal grains and the most succulent grasses of the plains and mountains of the west, where the air and sunshine are the purest and the valleys and hills are watered by the freshest and least-soiled water of our land?

Why should we send men down to the perils of the deep to secure whales when on our western plains we have upwards of two millions of horses, with their rich and nutritious flesh, ready for the slaughtering pens?

Why should we seek shark meat at 20c a pound when clean and wholesome equine steaks can be placed upon our tables at 15c per pound?

Are we not guilty of serious neglect and almost criminal indifference to the well-being of millions of our people in the great cities who have had access to this meat in their own lands and are denied it in our own country? What is our answer to the daily story of many weeks of fifty deaths a day in our great metropolis from pneumonia, and almost a like number from tuberculosis that are contributed to largely by an insufficient amount of animal food because of an actual scarcity, and the inevitable high prices resulting and the relative low wage?

How are we to answer future generations if the little children of our day are denied a sufficient quantity of milk for their proper sustenance and growth, because of the high price and dangers of contamination; and, at the same time deny their mothers sufficient animal food while they foster, conceive and suckle these babies that are to be our future men and women; when right at our doors in these meatless and wheatless days is a vast, untouched source of animal food, rich, clean, wholesome, free from tuberculo-

---

*Presented at the meeting of the Veterinary Medical Association of New Jersey, January, 1918.

sis and the using up of which would afford hundreds of thousands of acres of land ready for the tilling to lessen our wheatless days?

Why should we have to cry out in our land for this relief and tell the story that follows in so graphic a manner and to plead for legislation, national, state and municipal, to reestablish federal and to establish state and municipal equine meat inspection and give immediate relief?

When Germany from month to month carefully figures the dimensions and weight of her dogs as a part of her available food supply!

When her women will visit the interned camps of American prisoners, and offer to prostitute their bodies for a cake of soap, because of the scarcity of fat!

When every ounce of equine fat is conserved for food, and not a pound of her horseflesh but what is given out with the same exactions as any other kind of animal food!

When her highest skilled veterinarians are commandeered to save every hoof possible in the exhaustion of her own horses and only those taken in battle afford any contribution to her depleted supply at the battle front! When agriculture has forced her to make beasts of burden of her women, to cultivate her fields and maintain her crops. We in America stand aghast at our great animal food shortage, and because of our past prodigality and wastefulness in our beef supply, seem dazed and perplexed when right at our doors stands ready for sustenance and our economic helpfulness, one of the richest, cleanest, most nutritious sources of animal food in the world.

Worse than wasteful, we are nearing the line of criminal negligence, for we cannot dodge the responsibility of the unparalleled losses from pneumonia and tuberculosis stalking over our land just now; so largely contributed to by an insufficient animal diet for our people, because of the high price of beef, mutton and pork, and the relative low wage of those who daily work.

We recall with seeming surprise and astonishment that our soldiers in the Civil War subsisted many weeks and months on horseflesh, maintaining their strength and courage.

We forget the siege of Paris, when for six months her people were sustained and saved by horseflesh, her chief animal food.

We are unmindful of the fact, that the American Indian preferred the meat of horses to that of buffalo, that they followed to the death, when Uncle Sam had no condemned horses for their sustenance.

Almost immune to tuberculosis and the condemnations of carcasses from this disease on the killing floor would be of no moment, while 9% of the hogs, killed under federal inspection, are sent to the rendering tank as unfit and unsafe for food, because of generalized tuberculosis. Upwards of three to five per cent of our beef cattle go the same way, from the same cause, and yet this is the white man's as well as the red man's plague in every period of American history.

The only disease that gives us any serious consideration as to the wholesomeness of equine meat, is that of glanders, yet this disease is so rare in man that a recognized case in our land is of sufficient interest to have the story graphically told by the associated press in every paper in our land.

Stranger than fiction is the fact that a large per cent of the condemnation of Uncle Sam's horses in the army and on the Indian country borders, was for glanders and yet the Indians ate these carcasses uncooked and our records show no prevalence of glanders in the death records of these early occupants of our land.

Equally interesting is the fact that cooking the meat to the usual temperature of a broiled steak, makes innocuous this meat so far as any danger of transmission is concerned.

Again we know as a recognized scientific truth that the muscle fibre is resistant to any contamination of this form of disease.

Meatless days, wheatless days, are serious charges against even so wasteful and prodigal a nation as ours has been.

Hides, horns, and hoofs, that brought easy wealth and pelf, as the flesh rotted and the bones bleached on our western and southern plains, as we lived in a fool's paradise, and indulged in "Mulberry Seller's dreams", that there would ever be a day of reckoning.

The question is up to us now with a fearful force. Shall we let two millions of horses, fed on the richest grasses of our fertile plains, producing the richest foods, of the safest and most wholesome kind, grown in the open mountain range air, free from the dangers of contamination of domesticity, and enriched in its nutrition by its muscular activity as it roams over the unfenced lands, gathering its rich succulent grasses from non-infested pastures, or shall we accept the dangers of the other than beech nut fed hogs, or the products of contaminated pens, stables, barn yards and chicken roosts and then boast of our intelligence and keen perception?

Shall we continue to encourage every moral wrong, that has kept pace with the economic wrongs of our land, and allow millions of pounds of wholesome food go to waste, deny to the animal food raisers of the west these grasses for sheep and cattle, or deny to our own people and lift our pleas to God for more plentiful and abundant crops, when these horses are roaming over thousands of acres that ought to be tilled and growing grains to save the lives, of millions of our brothers and sisters in the war torn, war crazed, poverty stricken, hungry and cold allied countries?

Shall we continue to condone every moral wrong back of which is an economic one?

———◆———

THE CLASSIFICATION OF INFLAMMATIONS

SAMUEL HOWARD BURNETT, Ithaca, N. Y.

Of course the matter of most vital concern to a veterinarian is to be able to recognize the nature of pathological conditions on meeting them. It is also a matter of a good deal of importance that he express himself in describing his experiences so other members of the profession can get a clear understanding of his meaning. A confused use of terms is usually an indication of a lack of clearness of concept. The use of ambiguous and poorly defined terms accounts for part of the haziness of some of the descriptions encountered. An idea must not only be clear and distinct, but be expressed clearly.

This difficulty is especially apparent in regard to inflammation. Inflammation is a large subject. Parts of it are difficult; but the entire subject is made unnecessarily so by the confused use of terms. It is sometimes surprising to find how much less difficult and less confusing is the study of actual cases and specimens than what has been written about them.

The following simple classification of inflammations is offered in the hope that it may be of help. I believe no one will find it difficult to use. The terms are not new. They have been in use a long time. The arrangement is somewhat simplified. An attempt has been made to make the meaning of the terms clear.

For convenience of description and reference, inflammations are separated into a few groups.. It is in the main an artificial classification. The same fundamental processes are present or may be present in each group and in each individual case of each group. Intermediate forms between the different groups occur. It is not the purpose of this article to discuss the meaning of the several varieties of inflammation. It should be kept in mind, however, that inflammation is merely a local reaction. It is the local expression, as it were, of the interaction between the cause and the vital forces present in the body. A study of the expression of the interaction of these is of great value. It helps to an understanding of the disease. A classification of the reactions makes it easier to grasp the meaning of the conditions found.

In general, inflammations are named according to the predominant or more important process present. There are exceptions to this. Certain injuries and the resulting reactions are well enough known to have names of their own rather than classified names. Some of these are according to the character of the injury (wound, laceration), some according to the cause (sunburn, frost-bite), or the character of the reaction (abscess, ulcer). When different processes are present in about equal degree, a combination of names is used: as a degenerative and exudative or a fibrino-purulent inflammation.

The following schema presents the commonly occurring forms of inflammation:

GROUP 1. EXUDATIVE—
   fibrinous
   hemorrhagic
   serous
   purulent
   catarrhal
     desquamative
     serous
     mucous
     purulent

GROUP 2. PARENCHYMATOUS

GROUP 3. NECROTIC—
   suppurative
   ulcerative
   diphtheritic
   caseous
   gangrenous

GROUP 4. PROLIFERATIVE—
   simple
   granulative
   chronic productive

Some inflammations are named according to the cause, as *glanders pneumonia, tubercular mastitis, actinomycotic glossitis.* It gives needed information to add a term giving more definitely the character of the lesion, as *caseous tubercular lymph-adenitis* or *productive tubercular omentitis.*

GROUP 1. Exudative inflammations are those in which the predominant feature is exudation. The more important other processes present are degeneration, active hyperemia and proliferation. Degeneration of the vascular endothelial cells makes exudation of fluid possible. There may be degeneration of other cells due to the direct action of the cause of the inflammation or it may be a secondary effect. The coagulation of an exudate may deprive cells of their supply of nourishment. Again cells may be injured by substances produced by disintegration. Active hyperemia precedes exudation. With exudation the hyperemia is lessened. An abundant exudate presses on the capillaries and usually produces a local anemia in the midst of the exudate. With absorption of the exudate and proliferation of new tissue, hyperemia extends toward the central part of the area. Hyperemia persists at the edge of the area containing the exudate. Proliferation of connective tissue occurs in all cases where there is a considerable amount of exudate. The presence of fibroblasts and young blood vessels indicates that at that place the resisting and healing forces of the body are overcoming the cause of the injury. When there is a considerable amount of fibrinous exudate healing is by the formation of granulation tissue. A mistake sometimes made is to call such a stage of a severe fibrinous inflammation a chronic productive inflammation.

When the principal feature in the inflamed area is fibrin, it is called a *fibrinous* inflammation; when fluid containing but little fibrin, a *serous;* when leucocytes, a *purulent;* and when red corpuscles, a *hemorrhagic* inflammation. A fluid poor in fibrin is not necessarily a serous exudate. There must be other processes present indicating an inflammation. Serous exudate and edema are not synonymous terms. When there is an exudate from a membrane in which are desquamated cells it is known as a *catarrh.* It is named according to the character of the exudate; as a *serous, mucous* or *purulent* catarrh or *catarrhal* inflammation. When the desquamated cells are present in large numbers, it is known as a *desquamative catarrh* or *catarrhal* inflammation. In a desquamative catarrhal inflammation there is often proliferation of the cells that are cast off.

GROUP 2. Parenchymatous inflammations are those in which

degeneration or necrosis of the functional cells is the predominant process. The supporting tissue, being more resistant, suffers less damage. This form of reaction is found in glands (liver, kidneys, pancreas, salivary glands, thyroid glands, mammary glands and ovaries), in skeletal muscle and in cardiac muscle. In very severe forms, there may be necrosis, e. g., *acute yellow atrophy of the liver.* The supporting tissue is not extensively involved in the necrosis. The more common kinds of degeneration found are cloudy swelling, granular, fatty and lipoid degenerations. Sometimes there is a marked degeneration of the functional cells and an abundant exudate in the supporting (interstitial) tissue. Such a condition is sometimes called a *diffuse* inflammation (*acute diffuse nephritis.*)

GROUP 3. Necrotic inflammations are those in which the most important process is necrosis which affects both the functional and the supporting tissue. All the kinds of necrosis occur—coagulation, liquefaction, caseation and gangrene. A *suppurative* inflammation is one in which there is suppuration. A *diphtheritic* inflammation is one in which there is wide spread coagulation necrosis. Inflammations with focal or nodular coagulation necrosis are not called diphtheritic, simply necrotic. A *caseous* inflammation is one in which the necrotic area or areas is caseous. It occurs as one or more restricted areas. An inflammation with wide spread gangrene is known as a *gangrenous* inflammation. An *ulcerative* inflammation is characterized by the presence of one or more ulcers. A form of ulcerative in which the defect remains and is without suppuration is sometimes called an *erosive* inflammation.

GROUP 4. Proliferative inflammations are those in which proliferation of tissue is, from the beginning or nearly so, the predominant process. They may be divided into three sub-groups, partly according to the kind of cells that react and partly according to the character of the reaction. In proliferative inflammations, the causes are not severe enough to produce much death or degeneration of tissue; but rather serve to stimulate proliferation. Endothelial cells proliferate readily and rapidly, as do lymphadenoid cells.

In the first sub-group (simple proliferative), blood vessels and connective tissue do not proliferate to any extent.. In most cases of acute inflammation, proliferation is not the predominating process. It is sometimes important enough or sufficiently characteristic to deserve recognition in the name, though proliferative is generally not a part of the name. They are usually classed as varieties of exudative inflammations. *Glomerulo-nephritis*, some cases of *acute splenitis* and *lymph-adenitis*, and *desquamative catarrhal pneumonia* are examples.

The second sub-group comprises inflammations in which rapid production of connective tissue and blood vessels (granulation tissue) is the predominant process. The formation of excessive granulation tissue ("proud flesh") is an extreme case. An interesting example of this sub-group is diffuse, i. e., wide-spread *productive tubercular omentitis* in cattle, in which the omentum is covered with young tissue, mostly connective tissue well supplied with blood vessels.

The third sub-group consists of the inflammations in which the slow formation of connective tissue is, from the first or nearly so, the most conspicuous process. The inciting cause is comparatively mild and exerts a long continued action. This variety is called *chronic productive* inflammation. Other tissue than connective tissue may take part in the proliferation; but to a lesser extent, as in *chronic hypertropic gastritis*.

—Six counties in southeast Texas have voted to take up systematic tick-eradication work. They are Galveston, Jefferson, Harris, Tyler, Houston, and Montgomery. Five other counties, Brazoria, Hardin, Jasper, Angelina, and Newton, are to vote soon on tick eradication. The progress so far made in southeast Texas is regarded as very encouraging, because headquarters for the work in this section were established at Houston as recently as October, 1916. In the 24 counties in southeast Texas, 485 dipping vats are available for use; 52 of them were constructed in January of this year.

—Clifton D. Lowe, D.V.M. Ohio State University, 1910, has just been appointed to the position of Southern Field Representative of the American Aberdeen-Angus Breeders' Association, with headquarters at Knoxville, Tenn. The territory assigned includes the Southwest as well as the Southeast. Dr. Lowe has specialized in animal husbandry subjects for several years.

—Dr. Fred W. Graves has removed from Hillsboro to Wingate, Ind.

THE CLEANING AND DISINFECTION OF LIVE STOCK CARS*

S. F. MUSSELMAN, State Veterinarian, Frankfort, Ky.

When asked by the secretary of your committee on sanitary science and police to present a paper at this meeting on the cleaning and disinfection of live stock cars, I gladly accepted and welcomed the opportunity to present this important subject to which entirely too little attention has been paid by sanitarians because of their failure to compare the cost with the results.

There is not a subject on your program, which if generally adopted, would be of more importance to the live stock industry of the nation or of greater value in its protection and conservation. During the present crisis when it is brought home to us daily that there is a world shortage of beef, pork and mutton, that we must increase these supplies and that the United States has practically the world to feed, it behooves each of us, particularly those engaged in live stock sanitation, to use every possible means at our command to aid in the protection and production of live stock.

During our recent campaign against foot-and-mouth disease we were taught many very valuable lessons in the control and eradication of disease, and had we profited by them to the extent that we should have, there would be no world shortage of beef, pork and mutton, but on account of the inconvenience to a few individuals I fear we have allowed ourselves to drift back into "the same old rut". It was clearly demonstrated that even so serious a disease could be controlled and eradicated by the enforcement of certain measures—among others, and by no means the least important, was the cleaning and disinfection of all live stock cars, without which I doubt if success would have followed our efforts. February 17, 1915, the Bureau of Animal Industry issued order No. 233 requiring that all live stock cars within the United States be cleaned and disinfected. At about the same time practically every state issued similar orders applying to both inter- and intra-state shipments. These orders had a far reaching effect not only in the eradication of foot-and-mouth disease, but to them is credited a marked decrease in losses from other communicable diseases.

*Presented at the 54th Annual Meeting of the American Veterinary Medical Association, Section on Sanitary Science and Police, Kansas City, Mo., August, 1917.

In Kentucky we were so favorably impressed with the effect of these orders that we decided to make some investigations, which proved to us that our saving from hog cholera, alone, would amount to a half million dollars for the year. This result was good and sufficient reason for us to make our order permanent.

Much to our surprise, the Bureau believing that foot-and-mouth disease was under control, and without giving sufficient consideration to the general results following the enforcement of order No. 233, issued order No. 239, effective July 15, 1915, revoking order No. 233. This action on the part of the Bureau was closely followed by similar action in many states, thus practically compelling all others to do likewise.

A great deal of pressure was brought to bear upon us and many requests were made that we rescind our order, but before doing so and realizing that it was practically impossible to continue this alone, I sent the following letter to the Bureau of Animal Industry and the live stock sanitary official in every state:

"February 2, 1916.

Dear Doctor:

In view of the fact that quarantine orders issued by the Bureau of Animal Industry and the different states requiring the cleaning and disinfection of all railway cars handling live stock moving inter-state during the foot-and-mouth disease quarantine of 1914-15, losses from contagious and infectious diseases among the live stock of Kentucky were materially decreased, and I presume similar conditions existed in your state, the State Live Stock Sanitary Board of Kentucky adopted similar regulations to be effective permanently. This regulation has caused the railroad companies to charge $2.50 per single deck car and $4.00 per double deck car, and this charge is the cause of considerable complaint and is objected to by shippers and commission men, and I am almost daily in receipt of requests to modify this regulation, but owing to the great benefits derived from its enforcement, no modification has been made.

Is it not your opinion that such a regulation adopted by all the states would cause the railroads to maintain disinfecting stations where all cars could be cleaned and disinfected and would materially assist in the work of controlling contagious and infectious diseases among live stock? As hog cholera is more widely prevalent than any other live stock disease, the above mentioned regulation would certainly assist very materially in the control of this disease.

If you approve this regulation will you not attempt to secure its adoption by your Board? If other states do not join us in this matter, I fear we will be forced to modify our regulations.

Please let me have an expression from you as soon as is convenient.

Very truly yours,
(Signed) S. F. MUSSELMAN,
State Veterinarian."

In due time the Bureau replied stating that the "Federal requirements could not be enforced by the Bureau in respect to cars used in shipments, which are intra-state, only". Considering the importance of the question I felt that all states should have replied promptly, but to my great disappointment only twenty-six states replied within sixty days and none since. All of these approved such a regulation. Some called attention to the fact that they had had similar regulations in force, but were compelled to rescind them. Twenty of the twenty-six objected to the prevailing charges that the shippers must pay. Ten of the twenty-six stated that they would gladly cooperate in the enforcement of such a regulation if all states would adopt it, but that they could not "go it alone". Mind you, Kentucky was at that time "going it alone", but because of our failure to get immediate support from our surrounding states, we, like all others, were compelled to modify. Eight of these twenty-six states estimated the saving in other live stock diseases, due to the cleaning and disinfecting of live stock cars, amounted to sums ranging from one-quarter of a million to a million dollars. If it is worth that much to eight states what would it be worth to forty-eight?

What are the objections to the cleaning and disinfecting of live stock cars? After many inquiries I have been unable to find but one objection—that is, to the unreasonable charge made in 1915, namely $2.50 for a single deck car and $4.00 for a double deck car. These charges we know are exorbitant, and there is no doubt that they had a great deal to do with the revocation of the cleaning and disinfecting order.

Kentucky has only one public stock yard, at which federal inspection is maintained, and the management of those yards had good reason to object to this order because they were losing shipments, that under normal conditions would be consigned to them. On account of this charge of $2.50 and $4.00, they were being diverted to other yards. For instance, many shipments from Tennessee are made to the Kentucky yards, and when shippers would

drive their live stock to the railroad stations for loading, the agent
would add $2.50 or $4.00 to the freight bill, if consigned to Kentucky. This of course would meet with the shippers' objection,
and the agent would promptly reply that they would not have to
pay this if shipments were consigned to other yards. In many instances the stock was loaded in the car ready to go, but on account
of this extra charge the shipper would bill his stock to some other
point. Was that a cleaned and disinfected car or not?

If we could have secured the cooperation of the railroads at
that time to the extent that they would have made a reasonable
charge, there would have been no trouble in making such an order
permanent, as shippers will not object to a reasonable charge, if
it will in any way benefit them. When the shipper bills his stock,
he is required to sign a contract binding him in many ways, but
the railroad only agrees to rent him a car and transport the car to
destination, if on their line, or to place where the connecting carrier will receive and carry it to or toward its destination. In a
conversation with a railroad employee, who is in charge of the live
stock department, I asked what kind of a car they furnished. He
stated a clean car; I then asked what he meant by a clean car. He
promptly replied that a clean car was one that had not been detained
in quarantine because of handling diseased stock. I then asked
what about the litter and manure contained in the cars. He replied that they would remove that if the shipper wanted it, but
they didn't often want it because they (the shippers) would then
have to bed the car. Who usually beds a car? "Of course they
could do it themselves, or we'll do it for $1.50 a car."

The railroads are compelled by law to furnish clean passenger
cars, and I believe they should also be required to furnish clean
live stock cars. How much better would it look to see on a live
stock contract these words: "The carrier hereby agrees to furnish
for the transportation of said live stock a car, that has been cleaned
and disinfected under proper supervision since last used in the
transportation of live stock, for which an additional charge of
$1.00 is made"?

Let us see if we cannot fix a reasonable charge. According to
the report of a statistician in the United States Department of
Agriculture there are 1,075,000 carloads of live stock shipped annually between points in the United States. At $2.50 per single
deck car and $4.00 per double deck car, estimating that 20% are

double deck cars, it is found that the annual cost to the shippers would amount to $3,010,000. The railroads were taking advantage and were making enormous profits, as was shown in more than one instance. It was proven to the Inter-State Commerce Commission that cars could be cleaned and disinfected at a cost, that would not exceed $1.00 per car. The charge at Indianapolis was $1.00 per single deck and $2.00 per double deck car. One of the big trunk lines running into Chicago was required on one occasion to show the actual cost of cleaning and disinfecting a car. Their representative at that hearing stated that it cost 20c a deck to clean them, 15c to disinfect, and 10c for sanding—a total of 45c, which we can by a few figures show to be about the actual cost.

During the early part of 1915, cresol compound, which was then in general use, could be purchased in any quantity for $1.00 per gallon. About six gallons of the disinfectant solution are required for each car. A solution containing 3% of cresol would necessitate 24 ounces, or less than 20c worth of disinfectant for each single deck car. Estimating that two men could clean and disinfect fifteen cars in one day and were being paid $2.00 per day, each, for their labor, we see that for $7.00 ($4.00 for labor and $3.00 for disinfectant) fifteen cars could have been cleaned and disinfected in one day, making the total cost per car of 45½ cents. These facts were known by many shippers, and of course this extra charge made the work unpopular, yet the live stock industry was profiting. We estimated our saving from hog cholera at a half million dollars, and seven other states reported saving a like sum, which means that eight states alone saved in live stock, principally hogs, $4,000,000, at a cost to all states of $3,010,000.

Let us go farther and compare the cost at present prices to the probable saving. Practically all chemicals have advanced in price from 50% to 100%, yet we can purchase cresol compound, or its equivalent, in quantities of ten gallons or more, for considerably less than $2.00 per gallon. The cost of labor has also advanced and we will allow it an advance of 50%. Allowing $2.00 per gallon for disinfectant, $3.00 a day, each, for labor, using the same two men, who have not improved any by experience but are still disinfecting fifteen cars per day, we find that cars can be cleaned and disinfected for 80c per car. It is reasonable to believe that the men used for this purpose would, with experience, improve and that by working systematically, even without the railroad providing regular disinfecting stations along its lines, more than double the amount of cars could be cleaned and disinfected in a day and considerably less disinfectant solution needed, which must in time greatly reduce this cost. Allowing the railroads a reasonable profit for this work, to say nothing of that accruing from the saving in the hauling of tons and tons of filth in these cars and the price for which great quantities of it can be sold for fertilizer purposes, there would be little, if any, objection to paying $1.00 for a single deck car and $1.50 for a double deck car. Assuming that there are 25,000 more car loads of live stock shipped between points in the United States, annually, than when the previous estimate was made and that 20% are double deck cars, we find that the cost to the shippers would be $1,210,000. Modern equipment and trained men will greatly reduce this cost. If Kentucky and seven other states saved by the cleaning and disinfecting of all live stock cars $4,000,000 worth of live stock in one year, it is not unreasonable to estimate the annual saving to each of the forty-eight states at $100,000. According to this estimate, which I consider very conservative, it will cost $1,210,000 to save $4,800,000. This fact certainly deserves our consideration.

The object in cleaning and disinfecting all live stock cars is to remove or destroy all infectious material contained therein, thus eliminating a very common means of disseminating live stock diseases.

I will not go into detail and describe the process of cleaning and disinfecting a car, as I presume you all are familiar with it, but I will give you an example of how the work was often done in 1915 and which no doubt had something to do with the charges of $2.50 for a single deck car and $4.00 for a double deck car. Four cars on a siding at an out-of-the-way station were held for cleaning and disinfecting before being loaded for intra-state shipments. The railroad called for supervision. An inspector was sent, the railroad furnishing his transportation, which would have amounted to $5.00 if a ticket had been purchased. The inspector found two section hands waiting with a hoe, shovel, broom, one three-gallon bucket, whitewash brush, one gallon can cresol compound, and about one bushel of lime. These men went to work scraping out the litter and manure into a pile alongside the car. A few shingles were secured from a nearby house for cleaning out the cracks and crevices and ledges outside where the hoe and shovel would not reach. The car was swept and then washed with the broom, and water that had to be carried in the one bucket from a well about two hundred feet from the car. This took some time, of course, as quite a number of trips were necessary. After the washing was completed, the same bucket was used for the disinfectant solution. Four ounces of cresol compound and about two pounds of lime were added to each gallon of water and spread over all surfaces, and as nearly as possible into all cracks and crevices with a whitewash brush, which you know required more time. The remainder of the lime was spread over the piles of litter and manure after sprinkling them with the disinfectant solution. Cleaning and disinfecting these four cars required practically all day at an expense to the railroad of $3.00 for labor, $1.00 for disinfectant, 20c for lime, and the inspector's transportation valued at $5.00—a total of $9.20 for four single deck cars. Thousands of cars were cleaned and disinfected under similar circumstances and at similar cost, which would, of course, increase the average.

Instructions for cleaning and disinfecting cars are contained in paragraph 1, section 5, of Bureau of Animal Industry order No. 245:

"Remove all litter and manure from all portions of the car, including the ledges and framework outside; clean the interior and exterior of the cars; and saturate the entire interior surface, include inner surfaces of the car doors, with a permitted disinfectant."

A great deal is said here in a very few words, and there is no reason for its misinterpretation.

If all states and the Bureau would get together and issue a uniform regulation requiring all cars used in the transportation of live stock between points in the United States, or in their respective states, to be cleaned and disinfected after unloading and before being again used for the transportation of live stock, I am sure the railroads would cooperate and provide regular stations along its lines equipped with modern appliances and trained men where cars could be cleaned and disinfected under the supervision of state or federal inspectors in a very short time and at little cost.

Because of the decrease in livestock diseases, as a result of such a regulation, both the live stock industry and the railroads will profit thereby to the extent that there will be a larger production of live stock, hence an increase in the number of shipments.

Believing that the results obtained will more than justify the means, I request that you all give this subject earnest consideration and see if you cannot agree that the cleaning and disinfection of all cars used in the transportation of live stock between points in the United States will be of great aid in the prevention of live stock diseases and help materially in reducing the high cost of living.

———◆———

DISCUSSION

DR. TORRANCE: It has always been a surprise to us in Canada that the United States has not appeared to be aware of the vast importance of this subject, "The Disinfection of Live Stock, Cars and Yards". When the foot-and-mouth disease broke out in the United States we were informed that the Chicago Stock Yards were being cleaned and disinfected for the first time in forty years. That outbreak appeared to have required the disinfection of places which had never been disinfected before, and apparently you are at the present time slipping back into the old rut.

In Canada we have been fully convinced of the benefit of this work for a great many years. My predecessor, Dr. Rutherford, introduced the system of car cleaning and supervision of stock yards, which has been in existence now for over eleven years, and I do not think anyone in Canada would be willing to go back to the old system. We have a staff connected with my branch which supervises all this work. We have traveling inspectors, one for the east and one for the west, and all the points where quarantine is going on, and see that our local inspectors are properly supervising the work at every distributing point on the railroad. At each railroad center we have a paid inspector employed by the department to see that the cars are properly cleansed and disinfected, and when he is satisfied that this work has been well done, he puts a card on the car door certifying to that effect. Shippers of live stock have a right to refuse a car which does not bear that card, and we find that it is very seldom necessary, as the railroads have got into the routine of always returning stock cars to the cleaning stations after they have been used.

When a car reaches a cleaning station the first thing is to remove all the litter, clean it out as carefully as possible, sweep it, and then it is scrubbed with a broom and water from a hose. After the thorough washing, the disinfecting takes place. The disinfectant is one approved by the department, is mixed under the supervision of our inspector, and applied by means of a spray pump, so that every crevice is thoroughly saturated. We always insist upon the disinfectant being mixed with lime water. Not only is lime a pretty good disinfectant in itself, but the use of lime enables the workman to see that every part is being reached. If you are using a colorless fluid it is difficult to tell whether you have covered all the parts of the car.

Our railways are required to keep all the stock yards clean and disinfected, and traveling inspectors are always on their heels. If they find a stock yard anywhere that is not in a normal condition, they are immediately required to clean this stock yard, or it is closed to traffic. Whitewash is applied in these yards at least once a year, and if necessary, oftener. We maintain such a constant supervision over them that it is usual to notice, in traveling through Canada, that all the stock yards you come to look nice and white and clean.

We are thoroughly convinced of the benefit of this system, and when the railroads a short time ago decided that it was time to make the shipper pay for this, the public did not object. The railroads had been paying for it before. Now the shippers are paying for the cleaning and disinfecting of the cars and in spite of that there is no demand to have it done away with. We are quite satisfied that we are getting full value for the money that is spent in this work in the protection of our live stock.

I might say incidentally that hog cholera infection in Canada is a very small issue with us, confined to a few localities, and the loss from it is trivial. You can say the same with regard to glanders and we fancy that our losses from both of these diseases have been reduced to a minimum, in consequence to a large extent of this system of disinfecting stock cars and yards. I am glad that a professional speaker has brought the attention of the association to this subject. It is a very important one in the conservation of live stock, and its value to the country can hardly be overestimated.

DR. L. E. NORTHRUP: After four years' experience in cleaning and disinfecting railway cars, auto trucks and farm wagons at the public stock yards in Indiana, I would endorse Dr. Musselman's paper in its entirety.

Dr. Musselman states that twenty-six states replying to his letter objected to the price charged for this work, and they should have objected. Over in Indiana we are cleaning 150 cars per day at a charge of $1.00 per single and $2.00 for a double deck, and the contractor is doing this work well and making a lot of money. The cost of the work per car, however, depends a great deal on the condition of the weather. In the Winter season with a heavy pile of frozen litter it will take a man three hours to thaw and remove, while in warm weather it takes one man only about twenty-five or thirty minutes to do this.

Indiana keeps two veterinarians and one layman to placard these cars as they come in. After being cleaned and approved, a release card is then placed on the car signed by the Inspector.

In regard to Kentucky going it alone, we have been at this work since 1913; not only cars, but we now have a great number of auto trucks, which, not like the railroad cars, never leave private property or go on to property where live stock is kept. These trucks run continually over the highway, and some of them are great double deck auto trucks, which necessitates our keeping a man to see that they are properly cleaned as soon as unloaded, under the General Law of Indiana, Act of 1913, Chapter 135. This is a good law and other states should have a similar one, putting all markets on a uniform basis.

The Doctor asks, ''What are the objections?'' Our impression is that the real objection to the cleaning and disinfecting of stock cars is the payment of the service fee.

It is a debatable question as to who should pay this fee. At first one might say that the railroads should do this or pay for it the same as a passenger coach, but we found that these cars were shipped over many lines and possibly rented, the company making delivery only getting a short haul, while in the case of the passenger coaches, they are owned by the railway company using them and are used only between terminal points.

Indianapolis is losing some interstate business from Illinois and Ohio because of assessing the $1.00 charge for cleaning against the shipper, as per tariffs allowed by the Interstate Commerce Commission, since Ohio and Illinois do not have such general cleaning laws. We believe, however, that this loss is small compared to the benefit.

The cleaning and disinfecting of cars certainly prolongs the life of the equipment, consequently the railway companies should be and are willing to pay for the same. You know that on intrastate business the charge is paid by the railroad, the public service commission having suspended the tariffs. They are now awaiting a decision. Should it be decided against the shipper, the railway companies will lose some more of this business, until all adjoining states pass similar laws.

I can hardly see how Dr. Musselman figures that all the gain he mentions came from the car cleaning alone. We believe, and the results after the general clean up from foot-and-mouth disease proves, that the cleaning and disinfecting of the small pens, chutes and scales along the railroad lines where hogs and other live stock are loaded, exchanged, unloaded for feeding in the country, and where farmers drive in and out with farm wagons, is of much greater importance than the cleaning and disinfecting of cars in which slaughter stock is shipped to market.

I will say, however, that the cleaning and disinfecting of cars belongs to the equipment, the railway equipment, and the railroad companies should pay for that—there is no question about that. In Indiana we find that they are willing to pay for it.

Dr. James Fleming: Looking at this matter from the viewpoint of the large market center it seems that the live stock shippers, railroad companies and other agencies opposed a uniform regulation governing cleaning and disinfection of all live stock cars, because (1) shippers contend that it was the duty of the railroads to furnish clean and disinfected cars without additional expense, (2) the railroads attempting to and succeeding in assessing the costs against the shippers and (3) the contention between the final and initial carrier as to which company is responsible.

The problem is to prevent animals from contracting disease while in course of transportation. We may resolve the problem into four elements: railroad cars, public stock yards, country loading points, roads and trails. In case of hog cholera, the country roads are an important factor. Where the disease exists, the roads and local stock pens are reasonably sure to be infected, and the infection is readily picked up by hogs while being driven along the roads or held even a short time in the pens.

Glanders and shipping fever of horses are perhaps more frequently communicated by the instrumentality of stock yards, with their mangers, feed troughs and watering places, than the cars. The opportunity for communication of mange, contagious abortion and tuberculosis, is not greater in cars than stock yards. The end to be attained, therefore, requires not only disinfection of cars, but also the country loading place, and, more essentially, the public stock yards, be maintained reasonably free from infection, by frequent cleaning and disinfection. Diseases we have always with us, such as shipping fever, contagious abortion and hog cholera, would be materially reduced, and in case any exotic disease gained entrance to the country its spread would be slower. The official machinery necessary for the enforcement of efficient cleaning and disinfection would aid in the early discovery of such disease.

The charge of $2.50 and $4.00 for cleaning and disinfecting cars seems to be exorbitant. I once supervised the job of cleaning and disinfecting twenty-five double deck sheep cars at Chicago. Some of the cars contained manure to a depth of fifteen inches, which was so hard packed that picks had to be used to loosen it up. A gang of twelve men worked continuously nearly forty-eight hours on this job. How many tons of manure and bedding were thrown out would be a guess. But it is safe to say that the hauling of the weight removed from a point in Montana to Chicago, at regular live stock rates, would have cost the road more than the cost of removing same. This is an extreme case, the point is that it does not cost the railroad any more to remove the old bedding and manure than it does to haul same back to new loading point, but in case of two or more roads being concerned in the haul, the receiving line passes the empty car with the old bedding to the initial carrier, shifting the responsibility as far as cost of cleaning and disinfection is concerned to the originating line, although it may have a very short haul. Naturally the initial carriers oppose cleaning and disinfection, unless at rates that an ordinary section gang, without special facilities, could make a profit for the road. If the cost of cleaning and disinfection could be equitably distributed among the lines sharing the haul, a large part of the opposition by railroads would be eliminated, and as the essayist says: "the public would stand for a reasonable charge for cleaning and disinfection, if shown that the protection is real."

There are specific instances where the cleaning and disinfection of cars prior to loading seem superfluous, as hogs being shipped for slaughter to a large market where the pens are always infected; fat cattle being shipped where it is known they will be slaughtered within a few hours before they could possibly develop any disease from exposure in the cars. This is a railroad argument against universal cleaning and disinfection of live stock cars and must be answered before results can be had.

These statements are made, not to minimize the necessity for cleaning and disinfection of stock cars each time used for the purpose of carrying live stock, but to point out that the freeing of the lines of transportation from infection will involve also the frequent cleaning and disinfection of public stock yards, in a more effectual manner than is now practiced and also a more stringent enforcement of the state laws against driving infected animals along public highways or over commons. Will the states cooperate to the extent necessary to achieve the latter object to a reasonable degree? Will the public submit to the restrictions necessary, and will they pay a reasonable charge for the cleaning and disinfection of cars, perhaps an increased yardage charge? Is the time ripe for this forward move? For we readily admit that it would be a forward move toward the effectual control of communicable diseases.

As has been pointed out, the removal of bedding and manure immediately after the unloading of live stock saves the railroads vast tonnage on the empty haul, in that way paying for the cost of its removal, at least. Considering this factor, we see no reason why the roads should be entitled to a profit on the cleaning of the cars. The cost to the shipper could be much lower than is charged, even than the actual cost of cleaning and disinfection, and yet be an economical proposition to the roads.

With full cooperation of the states and federal government, it is to be hoped not only that the cleaning and disinfection of cars can be accomplished but that the other avenues of infection, yards and highways, may be effectually controlled, thus answering the possible contention of the roads that infection is not prevented by the disinfection of cars alone.

DR. MUSSELMAN: The reason I did not take up the cleaning and disinfecting of yards was because it was a departure from the subject, but it, of course, is of material importance and should be taken up later. I was of the impression, and am yet, that the cleaning and disinfection of cars can be governed or can be arrived at earlier than the disinfection of stock yards. It doubtless is a subject of sufficient importance to have all sanitarians interested and state live stock sanitary boards should have a conference, or in some way adopt uniform regulations requiring that all stock yards be cleaned between hauls.

VETERINARY EDUCATION IN NEW YORK STATE*

THOS. B. ROGERS, D.V.S., Woodbury, N. J.

I have been requested to answer Dr. Gannett's paper as a representative of the New York American Veterinary School.

I wish to impress upon you at the outset that I make no attack whatever upon Dr. Gannett. Indeed, it is in my opinion a matter for gratification that a young and successful man should be willing to take time that he might well utilize to better pecuniary advantage in order to make the very strong plea that he has made on behalf of his Alma Mater. If a man does not always look with affection upon the country of his birth, the home of his childhood and the halls of his Alma Mater, there is something lacking in his moral and mental make-up.

Listening tonight to Dr. Gannett's address and having been privileged to hear him read it at the last meeting of this association, my mind automatically went back to a statement to be found in one of Macaulay's essays. Macaulay quotes Plutarch to the effect that Lysias, one of the most celebrated of the Athenian orators, was requested by a defendant to prepare for him a plea to be offered before an Athenian tribunal. The defendant finally took back the plea with the statement that the first time he read it he deemed it excellent; at the second reading he liked it less, and finally, after reading the paper a number of times, he came to the conclusion that it was no defense at all. Lysias said, ''But you forget that the judges will hear it but once.''

I do not hesitate to apply the story to Dr. Gannett's paper. At first hearing it was calculated alike to impress and convince, but carrying its matter into the quiet of the study, dissecting it paragraph by paragraph, I am driven to the conviction that while the good doctor has furnished us with an excellent example of special pleading, his eulogy of Cornell University and his disparagement of the New York American Veterinary College alike must fail their purpose. The inductions that he forms from his premises are in great part irrefutable, but he has fallen into an error quite common to humanity in starting his discourse with premises that are in the main erroneous.

*Read at the February meeting of the Veterinary Medical Association of New York City.

Let us dissect his argument and we find that:

Dr. Gannett advances a number of minor propositions and then grouping them into the far reaching major premise that there is no reason for the further continuation of the New York American Veterinary School—asks us to consent to its absorption by Cornell.

The principal minor premises are:

A. There is not room for two veterinary schools in the State of New York.

B. The Cornell school has ushered from its portals many distinguished alumni.

C. There is a progressive diminution of the number of veterinary practitioners in Greater New York.

D. The New York American School has not lived up to its opportunities.

E. Opportunity for the acquirement of veterinary education is greater in Ithaca than in New York City.

PROPOSITION 1. New York cannot support two veterinary schools. This proposition shows most conclusively that the attitude of the Cornell school is purely rural.

The Veterinary Department of Cornell, the New York American Veterinary School, should draw on the entire continents of North and South America for their students. The fact that the State gives support to an institution does not limit the scope of the school, indeed, if the work done is good work, students will gravitate to the institution alike from the continents and the islands of the sea, the teaching staff will have a cosmopolitan reputation, will be free of the guild the world over. If, however, two schools cannot be allowed to exist then it seems to me that Cornell should step down gracefully and ask for absorption into the older historic institution, the New York American Veterinary School. The contention that the lion of Ithaca and lamb of New York shall lie down together with the "lamb" inside will not, I am assured, be admitted by any alumus of the New York American Veterinary School. However, the facts, as they seem to me, point to the necessity for the continued existence of both schools, one should supplement the other. The country school of Ithaca offers the advantage of instruction in cattle pathology, and practical obstetrics, in the hygiene of milk on the farm, in the study of cattle feeds and cattle feeding. In New York the student has access to a wealth of

clinical material in horse, dog and cat practice, in ring judging of
horses and dogs, in scientific shoeing, in quarantine and abattoir
work, and in milk and meat inspection, diagnosis of equine lameness and in examination for soundness under practical men.   Indeed, I am convinced that if the Ithacan could spend one session
in New York and the New Yorker a session in Ithaca both would
be the better for the arrangement.   Lastly, a great city offers opportunities for extra collegiate education, the whirl of Broadway,
the commerce of the river fronts, the parks, monuments, and public buildings, the strangers within the city gates, the melting pot of
the ghetto, are educational factors of the highest importance; the
veterinarian at his best must be a citizen of the world; if his outlook has been confined to Jones cross roads and a country college,
he is handicapped in the race of life.   To paraphrase Tennyson,
better fifty years of New York City than a cycle of Ithaca or any
other country town.

PROPOSITION 2.   The Cornell school has ushered from its portals many distinguished alumni.   We admit this, but call Dr. Gannett's attention to the undoubted fact that men equally celebrated,
equally accomplished, equally devoted to the welfare of the veterinary profession, have passed from the portals of every veterinary
school on the American continent, good, bad or indifferent, rendering credit alike to themselves and their Alma Mater.   It is almost
useless to consume your time with furnishing examples.   But, in
our audience tonight I see several gentlemen whose careers would
reflect credit on any veterinary institution in the world.   Berns,
Hoskins, Ellis, Gill, Cochran, Smith, compare favorably with the
best from any school, anywhere at any time.   As evidence I call
your attention to what follows:

The history of the class of 1902 of the American Veterinary
College is briefly as follows: Of a graduating class of 52 members,
44 made good, and of these 44 about half of the number assumed
and maintained distinguished places in their profession.

Again—here is a little list of early alumni of the New York
American Veterinary School, most of them from the earlier classes,
many of them two-session empirics like myself and Dean Hoskins:

W. L. Zuill '80—Professor of Veterinary Surgery, Veterinary
Department, University of Pennsylvania.

W. H. Rose '80—Pioneer B. A. I. worker, still active.

C. W. Crowley '76—Distinguished practitioner of St. Louis,
Missouri.

. A. Holcombe '76—Professor, State Veterinarian, B. A. I.

. H. Wray '78—B. A. I., Rep. Great Britain.

W C. Corlies '76—Humane Society worker.

S. S. Field '78—One of New York's best known practitioners.

C. Curtice '79—Investigator, B. A. I. worker, Parasitologist.

J. C. Meyer '76—Distinguished practitioner of Cincinnati, Ohio.

G. H. Roberts '88—Indianapolis Veterinary College.

M. R. Trumbower '86—Ex-State Veterinarian, Illinois, Veterinary Sanitary Control work.

W. G. Hollingworth '84—State Veterinary Medicine.

M. E. Knowles '84—Now Major Knowles, State Veterinarian, Montana.

G. H. Berns '79—Successful practitioner. Surgeon.

D. W. Cochran '80—Successful practitioner. Surgeon.

· J. W. Scheibler '85—State Veterinarian, Tennessee. Successful practitioner.

L. H. Howard '82—State Cattle Commissioner, Massachusetts.

G. H. Davison '90—Breeder. Agriculturist.

R. W. Ellis '89—Journalist. Successful practitioner.

H. D. Gill '84—Now Major Gill, N. A. V. C. Biological.

R. R. Bell '88—Journalist. Instructor. Successful practitioner.

PROPOSITION 3. "There is from year to year a progressive dimunition in the number of veterinary practitioners in Greater New York." Why this should be a reason for the wiping out of the New York American Veterinary School is utterly beyond our ken. In the language of the music hall ditty, "The flowers that bloom in the spring, tra, la, la, have nothing to do with the case." And it would be quite as reasonable for Dr. Gannett to attribute loss of members in the Presbyterian Communion, the increase of measles among children, or the increased cost of living to the ill doing of the New York American Veterinary College, as to cite the dimunition in the number of veterinary practitioners as a reason for abolishing the school. I would, however, desire to allay Dr. Gannett's fears about the state of his chosen profession. For while there is no doubt that the veterinarians of Greater New York have had their sources of income decreased through the advent of the automobile and motor truck, it is refreshing to know that there are large districts in the south and southwest which are crying for veterinary service, and I am assured if Dr. Gannett feels that his professional position and income have been rendered insecure in the City of New York through the general use of motor power, that there are many prosperous communities in the south and southwest that need veterinary service and would welcome him in their midst, rewarding him in such measure as would be satisfactory to him, and we know his service would be satisfactory to them.

It is idle to waste time on this proposition—it was probably injected into the discussion through inadvertence.

PROPOSITION 4. The New York American Veterinary Schools have not lived up to their opportunities.

Dr. Gannett undertakes, not unkindly, to disparage the school of Liautard in that it was not willing in its march through the times to lengthen the period of study or generally to conform with what seemed to be the modern requirements for the admission into the practice of veterinary medicine. As an old pupil of Dr. Liautard I wish to bear evidence to the very thorough course of instruction that was given in the old American Veterinary College by Professor Liautard and his staff, and when we consider that his work was purely a labor of love, that he received no financial return, the expenses coming largely from the pockets of the professors, instead of gravitating to the professorial pockets as at Cornell, it is quite remarkable that such men as Alexander Stein, James Robertson, Roscoe R. Bell, Alfred Large and their colleagues should toil patiently year after year in rendering this most unselfish service. No one realized better than Dr. Liautard, who was, we may remark in passing, the most accomplished all-around veterinarian that this continent has known, no one, we say, knew better than he that it was impossible to give as good a veterinary education in two sessions of five months as was desirable, and he must often have contrasted the requirements of his Alma Mater with those of the American school over which for so many years he presided with dignity and ability.

Liautard, however, did know that the great need of this country at the time when the American Veterinary College opened its doors in 1875, was practitioners of veterinary medicine possessed of at least an elementary knowledge of the principles of their profession. I entered the American Veterinary College in the session of 1877 and at that time the only qualified practitioner of veterinary medicine in the State of New Jersey was my preceptor, Dr.

James C. Corlies, of Newark, who received his diploma in 1876. At that time there was but one qualified veterinarian in the City of Philadelphia, Dr. J. W. Gadsden, an alumnus of the London School. And it was certainly wise and politic on the part of Alexander Liautard that he contented himself with accomplishing the attainable rather than wasting his time in vain regrets that it was not possible at that time in this great country to furnish a veterinary education as good as that obtainable in Alfort or Berlin. Wisdom was justified of its children. The young men passing into the profession during those early years reflected credit alike on themselves and their Alma Mater, The American Veterinary College. In one respect, the Liautard school was, in my opinion, ahead of its time in that it devoted its attention to teaching the principles of medicine, not insisting upon requirements, through the process of memorizing of a large number of facts in anatomy, physiology, chemistry, therapeutics, obstetrics, and hygiene, facts as readily forgotten as learned—and an experience of more than ten years as a veterinary examiner has made it clear to me that if more time were devoted to the teaching of principles and less time to work in the laboratory, the end results would be better.

PROPOSITION 5. Cornell offers greater opportunities for a complete education than does New York.

I cannot answer this better than by calling your attention to the fact that a portion of the medical curriculum of Cornell University is perforce given in New York City, and also to a clipping from a Philadelphia paper of recent date calling attention to the fact that the bulk of the senior class in engineering of Cornell are to take their final studies and obtain practical experience in the Harlan plant of the Bethlehem Steel Company, in Wilmington, Delaware.

Cornell has all the advantages and disadvantages of the fresh water college and this remark applies to every part of the curriculum.

I think that you will admit this contention falls flat and won't waste time on it, other than to say that a really good education does not consist in the acquisition of Regents counts, but in the attainment of such knowledge of our work as best fits us for our walk in life—our environment.

I somewhat fear that to Dr. Gannett, Regents counts are synonymous with education.

Alas! not so! The mind that best accumulates the results of this Buddhist prayer wheel of education is akin to a phonographic disk, purely receptive, thought free, receiving the written or spoken word, engraving it on the tablets of the memory, and pouring it out when "someone pulls the string," *verbatim et literatim,* this and no more.

SHIPYARD IS OPENED TO CORNELL SENIORS

Students Will Get Practical Training in the Harlan Plant, Wilmington, Del.

WILMINGTON, DEL., January 26.—Forty students of Cornell University, representing the bulk of the senior class in engineering of the university, will arrive in this city February 4, to continue their final studies and obtain practical work at their professions at the Harlan plant of the Bethlehem Shipbuilding Corporation.

This war measure, decided upon by Jacob G. Schurman, president of the University, and the management of the Harlan plant in this city, is an innovation, and the precedent thus established, if it works out successfully, will, it is predicted, be followed by other colleges and universities throughout the country.

The students during their last few months of practical study and work combined at the Harlan plant will be paid for their services.

The students will receive lectures on two evenings each week. The best men in the shipbuilding business that this country affords will be brought here for that purpose by the Harlan management. These lectures will be open to foremen of the Harlan plant and other shipbuilding plants in this section.

There will be no practical work during the day time, the students being under the supervision of Prof. Robertson Matthews, in charge of heat-power engineering at Cornell University. There will be classes for them between 5 and 6 o'clock on certain afternoons, these lectures being given in the drafting room of the plant.

The men will be divided into two classes—hull construction and engine construction. They will return to Ithaca about June 1 for the graduation exercises and receive their diplomas. It is hoped by the promoters of the plan that some of them will remain with the shipyards of this vicinity, Hog Island, Chester, Camden and the Harlan and Pusey & Jones plants of this city.

Because of the limited number of places they can fill the men will not displace any of the "old timers" now employed at the shipyards here. The local shipyards expect when the weather "breaks" to be able to inaugurate added departments and increase the present production, so that there will be plenty of opportunity for some of the men to place themselves here.

PROPOSITION 6. Prof. John W. Adams, of the Veterinary

Department of the University of Pennsylvania, stated that *"no great veterinary school is possible in a large city."*

The only thing that could induce us to treat this remarkable pronunciamento seriously would be the death of its sponsor and as Dr. Adams is happily very much alive we feel justified in calling attention to what follows:*

Let us assume the method of the Gazetteer:

"The London Veterinary School is situated in an unimportant but ancient borough occupying the major portion of the counties of Surrey and Middlesex and slopping over into Kent. London was in existence in Roman times but has not grown fast of late. Its principal industries are the manufacture of fog horns, London porter, and public sentiment. It sends one member to Parliament and many to the court of Quarter Sessions."

"The Berlin Veterinary School is situated in the German village of Berlin. Population in 1914 about 1400; in 1917 much less both in number and girth." "Alfort, in the environs of Paris, offers another evidence of Dr. Adams' acumen as 'Paris has no manufactures of importance, its male population spending most of its time seated along country roads termed Boulevards. Their occupation is the leisurely consumption of syrups and light wines and the criticism of female beauty'."

"Dublin, the home of the school of that name, is an Irish town of about 1600 inhabitants. Its important manufactures are revolutions and Dublin stout."

"Edinburgh and Glasgow owe their fame solely to the veterinary and medical schools there established, the towns having grown up around the schools. Industries are the vending of oatmeal, red herring and shorter catechisms, the former being the favorite food, the latter the preferred literature of the students. These students coming from a race distinguished by its reckless extravagance do not as a rule stay in Scotland if they can help it, preferring to prey and pray elsewhere."

"Calcutta, Melbourne and Bombay, situated as they are in

---

*At the March meeting of this association, Dr. Rogers made the following statement in writing regarding Dr. Gannett's quotation of Dr. Adams: "I called Dr. Adams up and put the question to him. As nearly as I recollect this is his answer:" "I did say that a well rounded veterinary education could not be acquired in a large city, but also pointed out that it was equally unattainable in a small town, in other words, a country town offered advantages in cattle practice, etc., while the great principles on which medicine depend could only be taught in a large city." (From the secretary of the association.)

British dependencies, are quiet burgs of little activity, especially in the hot season. Productions—half castes, gold dust, road dust, Asiatic cholera and funerals of the aboriginal inhabitants.''

We could carry this line of argument further but submit that we have demonstrated a *reductio ad absurdum.*

CONCLUSION. In closing, I desire to say a few words on the ethical and sentimental side of this question.

When our great country was struggling for its freedom, for conditions assuring the unhampered right to ''life, liberty and pursuit of happiness'' that great Frenchman, Lafayette, visited us and aided us with his sword and council. When the oppressed immigrant from king ridden Europe approaches our shores he is welcomed by Bartholdi's Statute of Liberty enlightening the world, a fitting gift from the great French Republic, to the Republic of the West.

Today, gentlemen, our boys are fighting shoulder to shoulder with their brethren of the French Republic to insure unhampered freedom and the right to live our lives in safety, comfort and happiness, and they will fight on, Frenchmen, Englishmen and American, until right is fully established and might dispossessed of its hideous power for evil.

There are men who would tell us that Republics are ungrateful, that legislative bodies are venal, that to gain political ends we must sell ourselves to politics, must ''creep and intrude and climb into the fold'' where the pastures of legislative appropriations blossom. I do not believe it. Upward progress under such conditions is impossible and we are rising year by year to a higher social and political morality.

I do believe that the legislators of Greater New York, of this Empire City, will go to Albany determined that the work done by the Frenchman Liautard shall still bear more and better fruit, and that the great library you have lately formally opened will find a fitting home in the noble buildings of a school of veterinary medicine, that appropriations sufficient to maintain and perpetuate the school will be freely given and that New York City will insist upon the legislature of your great State providing for the New York American Veterinary College in such wise as to be satisfactory alike to urban and suburban pride and patriotism.

Lastly, gentlemen, I submit that I have shown that Dr. Gannett's premises are from the standpoint of logic, false premises, and consequently that the inductions therefrom are false. Q. E. D.

CLINICAL AND CASE REPORTS

EMPYEMA OF THE CHEST AND GANGRENOUS NECROSIS OF LUNGS*

(Treated by Surgical Operation and Application of Ordinary Drainage Methods.)

D. D. LeFevre, Newark, N. Y.

So far as the writer has been able to learn empyema of the chest is considered by all veterinarians as an extremely fatal disease and our text books treat of it in a despairing manner.

During the past Spring the writer came in contact with such a case. It presented the earmarks of one of the worst forms and apparently was likely to turn into a case of rigor mortis.

Thorough drainage methods were then applied and immediate improvement, convalescence, and rapid permanent recovery followed.

To me, the case seemed of considerable importance and I believe that further experimenting along the same line should be undertaken by those who have the opportunity, therefore I present the following case report:

A careful record of the patient's pulse, respiration and temperature was kept throughout her entire illness, but for the sake of brevity a discussion of the treatment administered on many of the days will be omitted, and in this paper there is discussed those things that transpired on certain dates, which seem to have a particular bearing on the case.

March 3rd, 1917. Gray mare, 6 years old. Weight 1400 pounds. Arrived in Newark from Buffalo. During the next few days she suffered a mild attack of influenza, apparently recovering in about ten days. She was used on a coal wagon, working one-half day, delivering small orders, loaded light. The work was gradually increased until she was drawing full loads all day. I think she slightly worked beyond her strength for several days before she was taken sick.

March 30th. Worked hard all day in windy, cold, drizzly rain. At night she refused food and I was called. Her pulse was 60; respirations, 25; and temperature, 106. She was placed in a separate building in a large roomy box stall, with large air space.

*Read at the 10th Annual Conference for Veterinarians, Ithaca, N. Y., January, 1918.

It was supposed that she was threatened with pneumonia, or a relapse of influenza, or both, and treated accordingly.

March 31st. Pleurisy was diagnosed and appropriate treatment given. Arecolin, the best agent for aborting pleurisy, was not given. I presume that with most of you arecolin has become your regular treatment in cases of acute laminitis, and that you know it can be relied upon to abort acute pleurisy in from three to four days, the same as it does laminitis. Arecolin was not given. During early part of sickness the animal did not have my personal attention but the attention of another veterinarian.

April 2nd. Pulse, 70; respirations, 36; temperature, 104. The evening before, the animal received a good turpentine sweat, applied with canvas and a felt sweat jacket, using about one gallon of turpentine. Apparently some benefit was received.

April 4th. Pulse, 80; respirations, 24; temperature, 106. The patient had a hard chill, and without orders the owner administered two one-half pint doses of whiskey. During the next few days various medicines were tried without any apparent benefit.

April 7th. Pulse, 66; respirations, 22; temperature, 103.3. In the forenoon, shortly after this record was taken, the patient had another chill and that evening her record was, pulse, 100; respirations, 24; temperature, 104.

April 8th. Pulse, 84; respirations, 20; temperature, 102.5. She appeared to be growing worse quite rapidly. The chest was found to contain a considerable amount of fluid. She ate sparingly, and stood constantly in one place, head down and ears drooping, haggard countenance. Pulse had to be taken by auscultation, if moved slightly, pulse was considerably quickened, so that from, now on I was very careful not to disturb the animal until her record had been obtained. A large doughy swelling had appeared between her front legs. It had gradually extended up on the pectoral muscles, and backward under and along the sides of the chest, behind the front legs.

April 9th. Pulse, 95; respirations, 20; temperature, 102.5. Patient certainly is in bad shape and unless something is done for immediate relief, she cannot be expected to live more than two or three days. She reels or staggers as if about to fall, when she is forced to move; refuses food, and by percussion the chest is found to be at least one-half or two-thirds full of liquid.

April 10th. Pulse, 90; respirations, 19; temperature, 102.
After buckling two girts or surcingles tightly around the body of
the patient, for the purpose of obviating shock, the patient was
tapped on the right side of the chest, probably between the seventh
and eighth ribs. The swelling on the side of the chest was so great
that it was impossible to trace, or even with certainty distinguish,
the difference in feeling of the rib or intercostal space. A small
opening was made through the skin with a knife, choosing a place
low down and behind the front leg far enough to be out of the way
of its movement. The trocar was then passed slowly in, and after
some manoeuvering it finally entered the chest cavity. As directed
in books, at first a rubber tube was placed on the canula for the
purpose of leading the fluid into a pail, but as the canula frequently
became blocked and the tube interfered and finally becoming
blocked with coagulated serum, it was finally dispensed with and
the fluid allowed to flow directly from the canula into the pail.
When the canula became blocked it was first crowded one way and
then another, sometimes drawing out or pushing in a little, or the
stilet again passed, until the outward flow of liquid was again established. Sometimes a gurgling noise was heard in the canula,
showing that air was passing from the outside into the chest. At
such times the thumb, was used to immediately close the canula,
until the flow of liquid could be reestablished. In this manner
thirty or thirty-five quarts of liquid were drawn off. The patient
showed immediate relief, and by evening and for the next two or
three days, she showed a marked improvement. Her record that
evening was, pulse, 72; respirations, 20; temperature, 101.2.

April 15th. Five days later, her pulse, 80; respirations, 23;
temperature, 104. Patient declines all food and is apparently
gradually growing worse. It was found that the chest was again
nearly filled with liquid, therefore she was again tapped. The
fluid was somewhat thicker than before and seemed quite turbid.
More trouble was experienced with the canula becoming blocked
than the first time she was tapped. After drawing off about 15
quarts of the liquid, the operation had to be discontinued because
we could not get any more liquid, although percussion sounds indicated there was plenty of liquid left in the patient's chest. During the next few days no apparent improvement could be noticed,
but by giving larger doses of fluid extract of gentian we managed
to stimulate her appetite enough to get her to eat sparingly, and

in the meantime the attending veterinarian was doing some thinking. The client being a next door neighbor and valued friend, the veterinarian made up his mind that if this horse had to die, it was not going to die with a chest full of pus. Text books and current literature were carefully examined and about all that could be found was that if a patient reached the stage that this patient was in nothing more could be done, and no hope should be entertained. In short, it was that if the liquid in the chest would not come out through whatever sized canula the individual operator chose to select, that ended it, the patient must die. So a trip to Rochester was made and a large sized trocar secured, also a new injection pump, together with proper appliances and tubing so as to fasten the pump to the canula. Returning home armed with these various appliances, I remember that the attending veterinarian again felt quite confident.

April 19th. Pulse, 92; respirations, 18; temperature, 102.8. The patient was no better, and something had to be done. She was growing weaker and poorer every day. So the large sized trocar was then passed into the horse's chest. A quart or two of liquid, fetid pus oozed out. The pump was then applied and by vigorous efforts a small amount of pus was secured but the valves or piston of the pump seemed to leak, at least we could not get suction enough to extract a material amount of pus, so a spray pump much larger and stronger was hitched to the canula coupling apparatus, and a still more vigorous pumping procedure carried on with no better success at securing pus, and yet by percussion sounds both sides of the chest seemed to be about two-thirds full of some kind of liquid.

A small, thin trocar was then passed high up on the left or other side of the chest so as to confirm the diagnosis of liquid of any kind being in the chest. Upon removing the stilet a strong flow of quite clear liquid was obtained, and allowed to flow until the canula became blocked. Not wishing to run any chances of getting the other side of the chest infected, the canula was then immediately withdrawn. Probably one gallon of liquid was drawn from the left side of the chest.

Upon going back to the right side of the horse, pus was noticed to be oozing out of the hole made by the large sized trocar. A probe pointed bistoury was passed in and the hole was enlarged, up and down. The handle of the bistoury was now introduced and turned so as to spread the tissue apart, and pus began to flow quite freely. The pus was grayish, flocculent, and very fetid. After a while the hole became blocked, and the probe pointed bistoury was again introduced and the hole was considerably enlarged, so as to freely admit the passage of two fingers into the hole. The outward borders of the two adjacent ribs could be felt but the swelling on the sides of the chest was so thick that the fingers were not long enough to reach into the chest.

A long, stout dressing forceps was now entered and then opened or spread and turned crosswise in the hole. Traction was now exerted outwardly and thus the hole was opened quite widely. Immediately there was a free and abundant escape of pus and partly decomposed fragments of coagulated serum, which were highly fetid. Altogether that day, there were obtained one and one-half tobacco pailfuls of pus, estimated at probably thirty or thirty-five quarts. The job was then discontinued for the day, but pus continued to drip from the wound.

April 20th. Pulse, 86; respirations, 24; temperature, 102.8. In the morning the patient showed some improvement, but not so much as was expected. No surgical interference was attempted, the patient was allowed to rest, and the veterinarian did some more thinking as to the best line of procedure.

It was believed that when the operator quit work on the patient the day before, that the hole became blocked or plugged with some kind of tissue, whether living or dead tissue the operator did not know, and the operator was just a little bit worried about the taking of a pair of heavy stout dressing forceps and grabbing hold of various kinds of ornaments on the inside of a horse's chest and by force dragging them to the outside. He thought he would perhaps get hold of a piece of living lung and rupture it and get a bad hemorrhage and perhaps he had some other thoughts. However, it was finally concluded that if the patient was to be saved, thorough and permanent drainage must be established.

In the afternoon her pulse was 90; respirations, 22; and temperature, 103.4. The wound had ceased to drip and was closed by increased swelling. The hole was again enlarged, the dressing forceps were introduced and a procedure of exploring around by feeling in different directions was followed; by reaching forward and toward the median line, the impacts of the heart beats could plainly be felt on the rounding curve of the long dressing forceps. Above it was thought that the lung could be felt floating. By a spreading manipulation of the hole, sudden gushes of liquid were liberated. This liquid was much thinner than the day before. By percussion it was found that the liquid extended to nearly the same height on both sides of the chest, but it was at a much lower level than formerly. Either the partition between the two halves of the lungs had become ruptured or the liquid from the left side had seeped through the partition into the right side.

The manipulation of the hole in the chest was continued and after a time some dead tissue was noticed to protrude outwardly through it. The forceps were then closed on whatever tissue was between its jaws. Another forceps was used to spread the hole and by a process of manipulation, a strip of partially decomposed lung tissue, eight inches in length and varying from two and one-half to four inches in width was drawn out. Pus now gushed out freely. Several more small pieces of lung tissue were extracted at various times when they presented themselves in evidence by blocking the hole.

Some three or four quarts more than a tobacco pailful, probably at least 25 quarts of pus, were drawn from the horse this day, and after the pus ceased to flow a couple of quarts of warm creolin solution were injected into the chest cavity and coaxed out again.

April 21st. Pulse, 58; respirations, 18; temperature, 102.6. She ate and drank freely, was brighter, and moved around in her stall quite freely. The chest was again flushed out with warm creolin solution, and so as to establish permanent drainage, a hole was made, slightly superiorly and further forward, between the sixth and seventh ribs. A piece of drainage cloth was now grasped by the dressing forceps and carried in through the lower hole, and then upwards. Another dressing forceps was now passed in through the upper hole and with it the operator grasped hold of the drainage cloth that was being held with the lower forceps. The lower forceps were now loosened and drawn out, the upper forceps were drawn out, dragging the drainage cloth with it, which completed the operation of passing the drainage cloth around the seventh rib. A toggle stick four inches long and the size of a lead pencil was now tied fast to each end of the cloth and the patient was left for the day.

During the next two or three days, as the patient seemed to be eating freely and doing well, she was observed but not interfered with. There was a considerable discharge from the wound, part of it drizzling down the back of the front leg and the patient seemed to delight in licking up this discharge. She also licked the wound and occasionally bit at the seton or drainage cloth. In this she was not interfered with, as we recognized the value of auto-therapy. We also appreciated the advantage of having the toggle stick in the ends of the drainage cloth, for if the ends were tied together, there would be danger of getting her teeth caught fast in the cloth and perhaps injuring herself. It was noticed that the swelling on the breast and sides of chest was decreasing.

April 24th. Pulse, 76; respirations, 18; temperature, 104.5. When the patient was standing up, the wound was noticed not to drain freely, but when she lay down pressure was brought to bear on the ribs so that they were slightly sprung apart and the wound was somewhat opened, and some pus flowed out forming a puddle on the bedding. The patient also had a nasal discharge. The seton was removed, the hole was rimmed out and several quarts of pus escaped, a new seton was put in place, and two or three quarts of creolin solution were injected into the chest. The operator with a syringe injected it in different directions, so as to wash or rinse off the upper parts of the inside of the chest. In the meantime, the holes were kept plugged with cotton, so as to retain most of the creolin solution within the chest for several minutes. The animal coughed, blew her nose, began licking her lips and champing her jaws. The attendant remarked that the injected material appeared to flow from the mouth and nose, and this seemed to be the case.

The only explanation the writer can offer is that the lower border of the lung had sloughed off and on the 20th I had drawn it out through the opening in her side and that some of the bronchial tubes still remained open. The creolin solution passed through these tubes into the trachea and on into the mouth and nose. The patient was observed for a few moments and as no ill effect could be noticed the washing out was continued to completion, but the holes were never again plugged.

May 2nd. Pulse, 52; respirations, 24; temperature, 102.6. Patient was eating heartily. She was gaining in flesh. When led out on the halter she acted bright and walked strong and freely. The wound was discharging freely; the drainage cloth was changed; the hole was rimmed out and the chest washed out.

May 9th. Pulse, 46; respirations, 16; temperature, 102.6. The drainage cloth was changed; hole was rimmed out; the chest was washed out. When she was led out on the halter, she tried to kick and play.

May 20th. Pulse, 46; respirations, 16; temperature, 101.8. Drainage cloth was changed and chest washed out. She was still in a thrifty condition.

May 25th. Pulse, 44; respirations, 16; temperature, 101.5. The seton was changed, hole opened up, and chest washed out. She was turned out to pasture on a steep side hill, with a shed to run under during nights and stormy weather.

June 5th. Visited patient in the pasture lot; she appeared thrifty, ran and played with the other horses. The wound was discharging some. She had a slight cough. It was noticed that when she coughed the air was expelled through the hole past the seton in her side. The flesh had now grown so that it fitted closely around the seton or drainage cloth. We could not see that any air was sucked back through the hole into the chest after coughing, and it is wondered if the animal will not by this method be able to expel the air that is in the pleural cavity, and so by degrees get the lung again inflated to its normal capacity, if it is now or has been collapsed, or partly collapsed.

June 20th. The patient was thrifty; the seton was removed, and she was discharged.

In August she was placed at light work on the farm; the work was gradually increased until she was doing as much plowing and dragging as any horse on the farm. All the fall she has drawn to market great loads of two and three tons of cabbage and other produce. She is at the present time thrifty and doing well, and her present owner considers her the equal of any horse on his farm.

———◆———

A CASE OF NECK PUNCTURE

———

CAPT. J. H. GOULD, V.C., Division Veterinarian, 88th Division

———

A bamboo puncture extending through the skin of the left side of the neck through the muscles, ligamentum nuchae, to the skin on the right side of the neck. As the direction was slightly upward, the opening on the left side was enlarged and good drainage obtained. The parts affected became swelled and edematous. Cleansed the wound thoroughly and injected tincture of iodine.

Put on cold fomentations. Swelling continued to increase. In-jected fifty per cent Turkish oil three times daily and used fomen-tation of ten per cent Turkish oil and the swelling decreased until the parts were about normal. Healing seemed slow, as is often the case in deep punctures, so injected mixture of four ounces tincture of iodine, twelve ounces As-trin-gal, and water to make a quart.

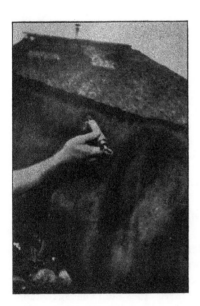 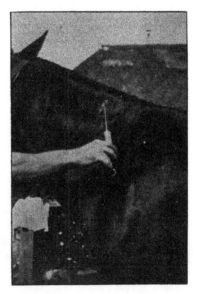

Injected three times daily for four days, then as discharge lessened, twice daily. Later once daily. After the fourteenth day very little discharge of a clear liquid came from the wound, so it was syringed out every two or three days with tincture of iodine, As-trin-gal mixture. Wound entirely closed in six weeks.

———◆———

COLD ABSCESS AND SERO-FIBRINOUS TUMOR

CAPT. J. H. GOULD, V. C., Division Veterinarian, 88th Division

The following pictures indicate the size of the growths and the parts affected:

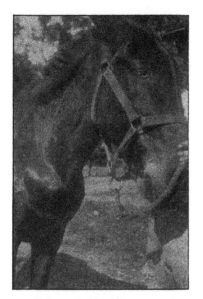
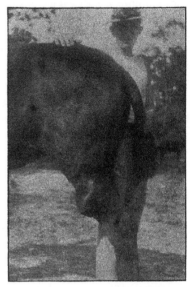

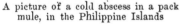

A picture of a cold abscess in a pack mule, in the Philippine Islands

A sero-fibrous tumor in the same mule. Probably caused by a severe bruise.

ABSTRACTS FROM RECENT LITERATURE

MORPHINE IN COLIC.—The method has been recommended by Messrs. Teppaz and Duprechou and referred to in the Society Centrale sometime ago. It relates to the administration of the alkaloid in intravenous injections.

If the classical treatment of colic, due to intestinal congestion or acute gastro-intestinal indigestion, applied at the beginning of the manifestations, is not followed by relief an hour afterward, or if the symptoms are very violent at the start they make in the jugular an injection of a solution of 0.25ct of hydrochloride of morphine, the regular dose in ampoules.

The effect is instantaneous, all bad symptoms subside.

The injection quickly quiets the pain. It is a simple treatment, easily applied and far superior to the administration per mouth of the tincture of opium.

However, if the intravenous injection of morphine presents advantages as to rapidity in the action of the narcotic effects, it does not offer a noticeable superiority over the subcutaneous injection. Morphine is only to be recommended against the manifestation of pain. Its inconveniences are not to be overlooked. Its paralyzing action on the intestines contraindicates it in cases of intestinal obstruction and its action on the blood vessels contraindicates its use in cases of intestinal congestion. A. L.

DEMODECTIC MANGE OF THE HORSE WITH CONTAGION TO MAN. G. Urbain, a Belgian Veterinarian. *Bull. Soc. Centrale.*—While visiting a farm to attend a cow, his attention was called to a horse which was very thin and had on the body numerous hairless patches on the head, neck and trunk. He made a diagnosis of sarcoptic mange which is common in the country where he practices. A young man on the farm had numerous spots in the forehead, cheeks and neck from which he took some of the secretions of the patches. Examining the material obtained from both horse and man, he found the demodex in it. The young man had been free from any skin trouble until he took charge of the mangy horse. The cutaneous lesions resembled those of chronic eczema. The hair came off in patches. There was no itching. Washing with arsenical solutions brought an easy recovery.

Cases of demodex in horses are not so very rare but the fact recorded above is not sufficient to prove the contagion even with the observation of folliculitis, replied Prof. Raillet. A. L.

CHOREA IN THE COW. W. R. Davis, M.R.C.V.S. *Veterinary News.*—The author has seen several cases which he thought resembled chorea in human beings and he records one of the cases as follows: He was called to attend a cow, 7 years old, Shorthorn, and found her standing and to all appearances very stiff. The breathing was quick, and the animal was sweating profusely. Every few minutes the eyes would be violently closed, causing a sort of grimace and a shake of the head, then the eyes would open widely again. There were twitchings in various parts of the body. On moving, each limb was violently flexed as if affected with stringhalt. Taken in a box stall, she lay down, with the eyes spasmodically shutting and opening; the body and limbs convulsively twitching. Feces and urine were normal. Pulse strong and full. Temperature 103°. The cow was six months in calf. Chloral and bromide of potassium were prescribed. Gradual recovery.

A. L.

TECHNIC FOR BLOOD EXAMINATION. (Abstracted from Marek's Clinical Diagnosis of Diseases of Animals, etc.)

COAGULABILITY. Place drop on cover glass, keep in moist chamber and observe progress of coagulation every minute by stirring with fine wire.

DETERMINATION OF HEMOGLOBIN WITH THE GOWER'S SAHLI HEMOGLOBINOMETER. Fill capillary pipette quickly up to 20 c. mm. mark with blood. Wipe carefully the point of pipette. Empty contents by blowing into graduated tube, into which a small amount of distilled water has been added. It is then thoroughly mixed with the water contained in the tube, and then is diluted by adding gradually water until the color corresponds with that contained in the picrocarmin tube, comparing it in proper. light before a white background. The scale indicates the hemoglobin contents.

COUNTING OF RED BLOOD CORPUSCLES. Draw blood without exerting pressure; wipe off first drop; the next one is carefully drawn up into pipette up to 0.5 mark. Without removing from the mouth the mixing pipette, its point is wiped quickly with finger or gauze and immediately following the diluting fluid is drawn up. This is either 0.9% Na Cl solution or Hayem's fluid (Hydrarg. bichl. 0.5 Natr. sulphuricum 5. Natr. chloratum 1 Aqua dest. 200). The fluid is drawn into the pipette, while this is gently rolled, at first rapidly, then slower until it reaches the mark 101. Then the point of the pipette is closed with the finger and shaken for two to three minutes to obtain uniform mixture of blood. Then the contents of the capillary tube is blown out. From the remaining fluid the counting chamber is filled, which should be used only when thoroughly clean. One drop is placed into the chamber, thereupon the cover glass is allowed to drop on the same, the contact surface should show Newton's color. The counting chamber should be completely filled to avoid air bubbles. Allow the slide to rest for two to three minutes allowing for settling of corpuscles.

The counting is undertaken under high magnification and the red blood corpuscles are counted by sliding the slide to the right; 20 squares are counted in a row, and the same way in the following rows. In all, at least 200 squares should be counted. In each square all red corpuscles are counted inside of the square and also those which cut the left and upper border, those on the two other borders are counted to the second row of squares.

The formula for establishing the number of red blood corpuscles per c.mm. is $N = 4000 \times Z \times V$. N. represents the number per c.mm., Z. the average number of corpuscles per square (obtained from the sum of the total count by dividing it with the number of counted squares), and V. represents the degree of the dilution.

COUNTING OF WHITE BLOOD CORPUSCLES. The principle for counting white blood corpuscles is the same as for the red corpuscles, only that a diluting fluid is used, which renders the red corpuscles transparent and also which stains the nucleus of the white corpuscles. The blood is diluted only 1:10 (on account of the corresponding small numbers of white corpuscles), and therefore a special pipette is used with a mark 11 on the end of the ampule. Turk-Burkers counting chamber is better suited for counting white corpuscles on account of the larger squares it contains. A 1% acetic acid solution is best adapted as diluting fluid with or without the addition of a 1% aqueous solution of gentian or methyl oroletts solution, which renders the red corpuscles transparent and the addition of the stain colors the nuclei of the white corpuscles.

The blood is drawn into the pipette up to mark 1 and then the diluting fluid to mark 11, and the further technic and counting is carried out the same as with red corpuscles.

EXAMINATION OF STAINED BLOOD SMEARS. Careful preparation of blood smears with the aid of a cover glass (in usual manner). Drying in air, fixation in absolute methyl alcohol three-fifths minute. Staining by Giemsa or other methods.

A. EICHHORN.

———◆———

CLINICAL CASES. J. Bouwmann, Deutch Veterinarian. *Veterinary News.* 1st. TORSION UTERI IN MARE.—In this, the author relates a number of cases and makes remarks about the colic which is caused by it and makes further remarks on the treatment of the torsion in the cow. The first case was one of right uterine torsion which terminated fatally after several hours of manipulation. A post mortem showed hyperemia of the peritoneum, in the bowels, mesentery and uterus.

The author follows this by remarks on six other cases where colic was present, only one of which was followed by death.

2nd. UNILATERAL PARALYSIS OF THE FACIAL NERVE IN A CALF DUE TO TUBERCULOSIS.—The calf was one year old. When examined there was much salivation and mastication was slowly performed. He was very emaciated. The right ear was hanging down, the right upper eyelid drooping, the eye ball had an oblique position and was retracted. The right pupil was as large as the left. The right nostril did not move, the right part of the upper lip was lower than the left. The skin of the head was sensitive to pin pricks. When the cornea was touched the eyelids did not close but when the head was not fixed, the calf reacted by head movements and by going sideways, showing that the cornea was sensitive. The calf did not grasp the food with his tongue. There was a purulent discharge from the right nostril. The calf was unable to back and moved as if he were tipsy. At the post mortem there was found tuberculosis of the pre-bronchial lymph glands and in the mesentery. The base of the brain had a compact mass of tubercles. In the first and second cervical vertebrae tubercles were also found. **A. L.**

THE SOLVENT ACTION OF ANTISEPTICS ON NECROTIC TISSUE. Herbert D. Taylor and J. Harold Austin. *The Journal of Experimental Medicine,* Vol. XXVII, No. 1, January, 1918.—Considerable stress may be placed on the relatively great solvent action of Dakin's hypochlorite solution as contrasted with the more recent and more stable chloramines of Dakin. The hypochlorite being such a good solvent of necrotic tissue, plasma clot and leukocytes, has preference over the chloramines in the treatment of infected wounds. The solvent action is due primarily to the hypochlorite content. This action is aided by the alkalinity of the solution. It seems probable that the greater instability of the hypochlorite solution, when compared with that of the chloramines, may be related to its greater solvent action. None of the solutions show a solvent action on blood clot when prepared in a reaction available for clinical use. **HAYDEN.**

HYDROBROMIDE OF ARECOLINE IN COLIC. Capt. C. E. W. Bryan, A.V.C. *Veterinary Journal.*—Arecoline is quite extensively used in the treatment of colic. The author has resorted to it in about 400 cases and for him, the hydrobromide is the salt which fulfilled all the requirements. The only occasions when he does not resort to it are in very mild cases, in those where the pulse is very weak and there is debility, in cases of acute tympanitis and in cases of diarrhea and exhaustion.

Generally one dose is sufficient. 2 gr. doses are used. In many cases, however, he has given a second and even a third dose; but in these cases he gives only one grain and that never until three hours have elapsed without effect from the first dose. The advantages claimed are: 1st, rapidity of action and therefore of result. If the animal has already a strangulated bowel, it kills it quicker. 2nd, rapid purgation. 3rd, no nausea or disturbance of appetite. 4th, all effects of the drug disappear after four hours. 5th, small bulk to carry, especially when one is on the march.

Percentage of deaths small and every fatal case proved to be one of strangulated bowel.   A. L.

FIBRO-MYOMA IN THE ABDOMEN OF A RETRIEVER. G. Gair, M.R.C.V.S. *Veterinary Journal.*—An eight-year-old retriever was losing condition and the abdomen grew larger. By examination a large firm mass could be detected in the abdomen. A rapid growth tumor was diagnosed and the prognosis being unfavorable the dog was destroyed. The tumor found at the autopsy weighed 13 lbs. It was situated among the intestines and adhering. On section it had a pink color and cotton ball appearance giving the characteristic picture of fibro-myoma. Its nature was made out by a microscopic examination.   A. L.

—The next meeting of the Kentucky Veterinary Medical Association will be held at Shelbyville, Ky., July 10 and 11.

Dr. Edward J. McLaughlin is now at College Park, Md., assisting in the demonstrational and educational work on hog cholera.

—The force of veterinary inspectors of the Bureau of Animal Industry employed upon educational and demonstrational work in connection with hog cholera at Springfield, Ill., has been increased by the addition of Dr. Matthew J. Huggins from Lincoln, Neb., and Dr. Frederick C. Jones from Columbus, Ohio.

—The Oklahoma State Board of Veterinary Examiners will meet at the State House, Oklahoma City, Okla., May 1st, 2nd and 3rd, 1918. All applicants for registration to practice veterinary medicine in the State of Oklahoma must appear for examination not later than 4 p. m. of the first day of the meeting.

—Dr. J. O. F. Price has removed from Lu Verne to Algona, Ia.

ARMY VETERINARY SERVICE

REGULATIONS GOVERNING VOLUNTARY ENLISTMENT IN THE ENLISTED RESERVE CORPS OF THE MEDICAL DEPARTMENT

Section 151 (b), Selective Service Regulations, provides for voluntary enlistment in the enlisted reserve corps of the Medical Department of the army as follows:

"Section 151 (b). Under such regulations as the Surgeon General may prescribe and upon receiving permission from the Surgeon General to do so, any medical student, hospital interne, dentist, dental student, veterinarian, or veterinary student may enlist in the enlisted reserve corps of the Medical Department, and thereafter upon presentation by the registrant to his Local Board of a certificate of a Commissioned Officer of the Medical Department of the Army that he has been so enlisted, such certificate shall be filed with the Questionnaire and the registrant shall be placed in Class V on the ground that he is in the military service of the United States. There is no other ground upon which such persons (as such) may be placed in a deferred classification."

The object of this provision is to enable the military authorities to place the above mentioned class of registrants in the military service where their experience and training can be utilized to best advantage.

For the purpose of obtaining better qualified officers in the Medical Department, it is the intention of the Surgeon General, if conditions permit, to allow medical, dental, and veterinary students to complete the course for a professional degree; and to allow hospital internes one year of practical training in a hospital. For this reason these men, after enlistment in the enlisted reserve corps, will be left on inactive duty until the desired training has been obtained; provided, however, that they make satisfactory progress, and that the conditions for obtaining such training are adequate. They may, however, be called to active duty at any time, if the need for their services is sufficiently urgent.

Since graduated dentists and veterinarians have already received a training adequate for the purposes of the Army, it will not be the policy of the Surgeon General to leave them on inactive duty; but they will be called to active duty as soon after enlistment as their services can be utilized in the enlisted force of the

Medical Department. Where practicable, they will be assigned to duty in the line of their professional work.

For the purpose of attaining these ends, the Surgeon General prescribes the following regulations:

1. Permission to enlist in the enlisted reserve corps of the Medical Department will be granted in the case of medical, dental, and veterinary students, hospital internes, dentists, and veterinarians, only to students in, and to graduates of, well-recognized schools.

2. The term "student" in these regulations shall mean a bona fide member of one of the regular classes in the regular course for the professional degree, in a well-recognized school. Such bona fide membership should be attested by an affidavit from the dean of the school, or from his authorized agent, duly executed before a notary.

> Note A: In the case of Medical Schools the "regular course" is understood to mean the usual four-year course leading to the degree of M. D. "Special", "premedical", graduate, and "post-graduate" students in medical schools, and persons studying medical subjects outside of schools which are legally authorized to confer the degree of doctor of medicine, will not be considered "medical students" within the meaning of these regulations.

> Note B: A medical school which offers only part of the regular course for the degree of M. D. may be recognized; provided the school is maintained for this purpose, and the equipment and teaching are equal to the standard of well-recognized medical schools; and provided the students of said school are acceptable for advancement in other well-recognized medical schools, which give a complete course for the degree of M. D. This provision refers particularly to the medical schools of universities which offer only the first two years of the regular medical course.

> Note C: In those medical schools which require for the degree of M. D. a fifth year, spent in hospital or laboratory, the member of the fifth class shall be regarded as "hospital-internes", within the meaning of these regulations, and not as "medical students".

> Note D: Restrictions corresponding to those for medical schools and medical students in Note A shall apply in the case of dental schools and veterinary schools, and in the case of dental students and veterinary students.

3. A "bona fide" student, within the meaning of these regulations, is one who has been duly registered by the school as a member of his class at the beginning of the school term; who has fulfilled the requirements of the school for admission to said class; who has been in attendance since the beginning of the school term, in accordance with the requirements of the school; and has satisfactorily done the work of his class to date. Unless a student has fulfilled all of these requirements, the dean should not issue to him the affidavit mentioned in Section 2.

4. In the case of a hospital interne, a dentist, or a veterinarian, who is a graduate from a well-recognized school, the fact of graduation from said school must be established by an affidavit from the dean of the school or his authorized agent, duly executed before a notary; which affidavit shall give the full name of the graduate, the name and location of the school, and the year in which the degree was conferred.

5. The term "hospital interne", within the meaning of these regulations, shall indicate a graduate from an approved medical school, or a student in the senior class of such school, who has received an official appointment in a hospital or medical school, which appointment involves either the care of hospital patients, or such advanced scientific study as will fit him for special scientific medical work in the Army.

6. Permission for "hospital internes" to enlist in the enlisted reserve corps of the Medical Department will be granted only when the conditions, in the opinion of the Surgeon General, are satisfactory for the purpose of training medical officers for the Army, and only to such number of internes in an approved institution as the Surgeon General may determine. Such permission will be further dependent upon the time of such appointment as interne, its duration, the character of the work, and the opportunities for training afforded the interne.

7. The Surgeon General will not recognize interneships in hospitals, sanitoriums or other institutions conducted for profit; or in small private hospitals (50 beds or less) ; or new interneships in any hospital, if established or added since May 18, 1917, to those previously existing, unless such new interneships are necessitated by and are proportional to an increase in the bed capacity of said hospital.

8. The approved period of interne service shall not exceed one year; it may begin, under suitable arrangements, any time within the last four months of the medical-school course; it must begin otherwise as soon as practicable after graduation; it must be completed within sixteen months from the last day of the month in which graduation occurs; and, if there is an interval of more than one month between the time of graduation and the beginning of the recognized interneship, the time must be spent in a way that will, in the opinion of the Surgeon General, improve the training of the graduate for army purposes. This intervening time, even if spent in a recognized hospital position, will not necessarily be counted as part of the year of interne service that may be allowed.

9. Permission for voluntary enlistment in the enlisted reserve corps of the Medical Department is hereby granted by the Surgeon General to medical students, dental students, and veterinary students in well-recognized schools (as defined in Section 1), provided they present to the recruiting officer affidavits that they are bona fide students in said schools (as required by Section 2); and recruiting officers are authorized to accept for enlistment in the enlisted reserve corps of the Medical Department those students who fulfill these requirements, and to enlist them, if acceptable under orders and regulations governing enlistments for the United States Army.

10. Permission for voluntary enlistment in the enlisted reserve corps of the Medical Department is hereby granted by the Surgeon General to dentists and to veterinarians who establish, to the satisfaction of the recruiting officer, in accordance with the requirements of Section 4, the fact of graduation from a well-recognized school; and recruiting officers are hereby authorized to accept for enlistment in the enlisted reserve corps of the Medical Department those dentists and veterinarians who fulfill these requirements, and to enlist them, if acceptable under orders and regulations governing enlistments for the United States Army.

11. All others, including "hospital internes", who may be eligible for voluntary enlistment in the enlisted reserve corps of the Medical Department under Selective Service Regulations, Section 151 (b), and by these regulations, must receive permission individually from the Surgeon General.

By direction of the Surgeon General.

AN EFFORT TO RETURN THE VETERINARY SERVICE
TO THE QUARTERMASTER CORPS OF THE ARMY

In a bill, H. R. 9867, introduced in Congress, the following paragraph was included:

So much of section sixteen of the Act making further and more effectual provision for the national defense, and for other purposes, approved June third, nineteen hundred and sixteen, as provides that the Veterinary Corps as therein constituted shall be a part of the Medical Department of the Army, is hereby amended so as to make the Veterinary Corps a part of the Quartermaster Corps of the Army; and, further, so as to authorize appointments of reserve veterinarians in the Veterinary Corps upon the recommendation of the Quartermaster General of the Army. Provided, That all appropriations made for the purchase of veterinary supplies and the hire of veterinary surgeons shall be available for the purpose for which made, and shall hereafter be disbursed through the Quartermaster Corps.

We understand this measure was not passed, on the point of order that it was new legislation included in a bill for appropriations. Army veterinarians were formerly in the Quartermaster Corps and there seems to be evidence that the combination was not a happy one. What bearing the reference in the bill, to all appropriations for the purchase of veterinary supplies and *hire* of veterinary surgeons, has upon rank for veterinarians is not clear. In the past, we believe the Quartermaster has not been particularly sympathetic toward rank nor generally appreciative of the work of the profession. Veterinarians have fought for many years for the recognition which has now come to them and any suggestion of retrogression should be promptly and earnestly counteracted. The association of the Veterinary Corps with the Medical Corps gives it recognition as a profession. The relations have been pleasant and there is a closer and more sympathetic relationship between human and veterinary medicine than the "hire" of the latter in a Quartermaster Corps. The present association with the Medical Corps unmistakably stands for greater efficiency for the veterinarians and efficiency in all branches is just what is needed to win in this war. Veterinary service among our allies has demonstrated its efficiency. We should profit by the experience of others. The fact that an effort has been made to disrupt the present satisfactory conditions of the veterinarians may indicate that further attempts are to be made. The profession should heed the warning and be on the alert to oppose any action that offers a suggestion of retrogression.   P. A. F.

Captain John H. Gould, Veterinary Corps, Division Veterinarian, 88th Division, United States Army, now stationed at Camp Dodge, has taken the examination given by the Surgeon General's office for the grade of Major.

Captain Gould is a native of Minnesota, born in Martin County, on the Minnesota-Iowa border, January 22, 1877. He was educated in high school, and then served in the war with Spain in the Twelfth Minnesota Infantry. Later, he was graduated from Ames as a doctor of veterinary medicine in June, 1902.

After practicing at Jackson, Minnesota, a few months, and being admitted to practice in both Minnesota and Iowa, he was ex-

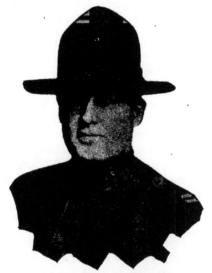

CAPTAIN JOHN H. GOULD

amined for veterinarian in the army, and was assigned to the Eleventh Cavalry. After two months' service at Fort Snelling, he joined his regiment in the Philippine Islands, returning to the United States in March, 1904.

He was stationed at Presidio, Fort Riley, and Fort Des Moines. He made an excellent record. He participated in the inaugural of President Roosevelt in March, 1905.

Ordered again to Fort Des Moines in October, 1905, he was again with his regiment, the Eleventh Cavalry. He took the regular medical course at Drake, and was graduated in June, 1907.

From June, 1907, he served at Forts Ethan Allen, Vermont; Oglethorpe, Georgia; ten months on the Texas border; in the Colorado strike zone; and again to the Philippine Islands in June, 1915. His service and special duties took him all over the islands, and into China and Japan.

He was returned to the United States in November, 1917, and assigned to Camp Dodge, becoming a captain shortly thereafter, and being examined for his majority.

Captain Gould is a member of the American Veterinary Medical Association (1902), and of many clubs and associations, medical, military, civic, fraternal, etc., including the Des Moines Chamber of Commerce.

———◆———

—Lieutenant H. E. Van Der Veen has been recently transferred from meat inspection duty at Chicago, Ill., to unit work at Camp Sherman, Chillicothe, Ohio, under the supervision of Major Knowles, Division Veterinarian. The mortality from infectious diseases in horses has been very much reduced in this camp.

—Captain R. A. Greenwood, by order of the War Department, has been transferred from Camp Sevier, S. C., to Camp Meade, Admiral, Md.

—Dr. J. M. Twitchell, formerly at the Auxiliary Remount Depot at Camp Funston, Kansas, has been stationed at Camp Greenleaf.

—Major C. E. Cotton is stationed at Chicago, Ill., as General Veterinary Inspector for eight central states. Inspection of sanitation and hygienic conditions of railroad yards and feeding stations and stables from which purchasing boards buy public animals and the veterinary affairs in the Division Camps are among his duties.

—Dr. Bert J. Cady, Berkeley, Calif., has received a commission as Second Lieutenant and ordered to report for duty at Camp Fremont, Palo Alto, Calif.

—Dr. Columbus W. Tittle, formerly of Davis, Okla., has been commissioned Second Lieutenant, V.R.C., and is stationed with the 304th Cavalry, Camp Stanley, San Antonio, Texas.

—Dr. C. M. Haring, of the University of California, commissioned as Second Lieutenant, is stationed at Camp Greenleaf, Fort Oglethorpe, Ga.

—Lieutenant George E. Butin, formerly of Bellevue, Neb., is stationed at Camp Doniphan, Okla., 128th Machine Gun Battalion.

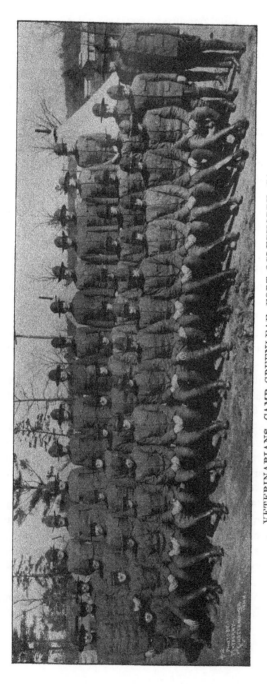

VETERINARIANS, CAMP GREENLEAF, FORT OGLETHORPE, GA.

Top row—left to right—Boyer, Summerville, Brown, O. W., Hughes, Coffeen, DeBoy, Smallbone, Twitchell, Rundle, Patterson, McCormick, March.

Middle row—Onley, Haring, Detwiler, Jansen, Moore, Kunnecke, Grace, Campbell, Cholvin, Campbell, Gieter, Maguire, F. X., Jensen, W. D., Muldoon, McGuire, Hunter, Adams, Dodsworth, Lacroix, Mackie.

Front row—Brown, Kneup, Harris, Fish, Brotheridge, Ackerman, Moye, Jones, Stifler, Hardenbergh, Udall, Meyers, Claris, Brown, Bailey.

—The Medical Officers' Training Camp at Fort Oglethorpe is divided into seven battalions, the seventh of which includes the veterinarians and psychologists. Company 27 (veterinarians) recently won the banner, after the Saturday inspection, for the best company after the second week of its organization. Among the competitors were companies of physicians which had been organized since last June. The banner is red and has inscribed upon it: "Do it Now," "Do it Well," "Smile, Damn You, Smile."

—Second Lieutenant M. W. Kreuziger has been transferred from Camp Lawrence J. Hearn, Palm City. Calif., to the 83rd Reg., F. A., Camp Fremont, Palo Alto, Calif.

—Lieutenant Charles C. Dobson, formerly at Muncie, Ind., is now at the Headquarters of the 76th Infantry Brigade, Camp Shelby, Miss.

—Captain Charles H. Jewell, of Camp Lee, Va., for many years in the Army service, received a commission as Major in the National Army, February 19.

ASSOCIATION MEETINGS

ALABAMA VETERINARY MEDICAL ASSOCIATION

The Alabama Veterinary Medical Association held its eleventh annual meeting at Auburn, Ala., March 1 and 2, 1918, at the College of Veterinary Medicine.

The first paper on the program was given by Dr. H. C. Wilson, Federal Veterinarian in charge of hog cholera work in Alabama. He discussed the use of serum and virus and gave the principal points that should be observed by veterinarians who administer them. Also the care and handling of the hogs. This brought out much discussion on the subject of immunity and the amount of serum and virus to use. It seemed to be the concensus of opinion that larger doses of serum and virus should be given in order to insure safe immunity.

A. R. Gissendanner, senior veterinary student, read a paper on Shoeing Draft Horses in the South. J. R. Sullivan, another senior veterinary student, read a paper on Shoeing the Light Horse in the South. These papers brought out a general discussion on the methods that were in common use and their defects. The great importance of having better educated farriers and veterinarians who have practical knowledge of horse shoeing, for use both in the army and in commercial life, was emphasized. J. H. Fussell, another senior veterinary student, read a paper on Removing One-half or One-quarter of the Cow's Udder. He gave the indications, precautions and successive steps in the operation.

The next subject was one that proved to be a live wire. "Why Should All Stock Cars, Stock Yards and Pens Be Regularly and Effectively Disinfected Under Official Supervision?" This was given by Dr. C. W. Ferguson. The results of the handling of a great many army horses and the movement of cattle, hogs, sheep, and other animals in infected cars, yards, etc., shows the absolute necessity for some supervision. The Army veterinarians present discussed the question from their standpoint and all seemed to agree that it was a positive necessity.

The value of studying poisonous plants was next brought out by Dr. M. W. Williams. All veterinarians present seemed to think that as a rule they did not receive sufficient instruction along that line while in college and many of them claimed that what they wanted to know was to recognize these poisonous plants as well as to know the poisonous principles, symptoms produced and treatment.

The next subject, "Impaction of the Rumen", was treated by Dr. J. S. Andrade. His method of handling this condition was to start the treatment with solutions of barium chloride, tartar emetic and then follow with repeated doses of caffein in the form of coffee. He reports a case where no action of the rumen was produced under two to three days and good recovery ensued.

The roaring operation in mules was next discussed by Dr. M. F. Jackson. This brought out considerable discussion and some seemed to think that there was a difference between the spasms of the larynx and laryngeal hemiplegia. This difference was not clearly defined.

Accredited herds was the next subject on the program but the veterinarian who was to discuss it was not present. Hence a general discussion of the subject was led by Dr. C. A. Cary and Dr. W. D. Staples. The general plan of the Government was brought out and every one present seemed to think that while a new thing it was a good one.

Reports of cases next came up, being discussed by several veterinarians. Dr. I. S. McAdory reported the removal of a large melanotic sarcoma from the shoulder of a mule, which weighed about six or eight pounds. It was removed successfully without loss of the animal. He also reported a cese in a cow that showed two punctures of the rumen which extended into the spleen, producing abscesses that extended apparently through the blood vessels to the liver and then to the lungs. No enlargement of the lymph glands was present. Dr. J. M. Luke next led a discussion on the treatment of azoturia with chloral hydrate, lobeline sulphate, etc. Dr. J. S. Cook reported a case of femoral hernia which apparently had two abdominal openings. He said as fast as he put the intestines into one opening they came out the other. He finally succeeded in stitching up the opening; and the animal (a one-year-old filly) recovered. This hernia was of one month's standing when he operated. He also reported a case that was apparently a choker or roarer. The animal died when it was cast for operation and post mortem revealed a forked clothes pin, five to six inches long, in the left guttural pouch. Dr. W. D. Staples reported the removal of a piece of wire that resembled a ladies' hat pin from the base of the tongue of a horse, the animal having gone without eating for several days. He also reported that nearly all disinfectants, weak or strong, were generally very irritating to a uterus that had been everted. He then brought up the question of the use of the stomach tube and most of those who discussed the subject seemed to think that a small single tube was better than a double tube and that passing it through the nasal passage was better than passing it through the mouth.

Lieutenant F. R. Harsh, of Camp Sevier, S. C., gave the method of handling influenza, pneumonia, etc., at the Remount Station. He seemed to think that vaccination or use of bacterins and medication had done very little good but that most cases recovered with fresh air in open corrals with protection from cold rains and cold winds. The death rate, as reported by him of all animals that were sick, was 4.8%. The animals were turned out in the corral and especially all that were able to move around. They could get at water and feed when they wanted it and inhaled plenty of fresh air. He thought influenza by itself was a mild disease but when complicated with septicemia or by *Bacillus equi septicus* it became very serious. He also stated that he had considerable trouble with scratches and grease but had obtained the best results by using white lotion.

Dr. G. A. Roberts discussed the subject of parasites, and especially the hook worm and nodular disease. He seemed to think that these parasites were responsible for the death of a great many cattle and sheep in the South. He also seemed to think that prevention by changing cattle to non-infected pastures in the spring and early summer months was the best line of treatment.

On the night of March 1 the Veterinary Medical Association of the College entertained the State Association at a ''War Banquet''. This was one where they were short on food and long on talk. There was a flow of language and a feast of reason, minus logic. The chief feature of the banquet was the Service List presented by the students, giving the names and rank of the veterinarians who are graduates of the Alabama Polytechnic Institute and in the U. S. Army. While the banquet was one of the very best some speakers that have been nearly always present were missed.

On the morning of the 2nd of March one of the belated speakers came in. It is necessary to mention this because there is only one of his kind. We refer to Dr. W. L. Stroup, universally known as ''Country'' Stroup of Corinth, Mississippi, who has an original, unique and effective method of collecting debts. According to him it is the only sure method on earth. We cannot reproduce his method here because it would spoil its effect to give it in cold type. There is only one man who can tell about it and that is Stroup himself. Just before the clinic he gave this to all present in his unique style and language. The clinic was well attended and more cases were presented than could be taken care of. Dr. Geo. R. White was chief operator. He spayed a cat and a cow, caponized a chicken, castrated a mule and a cryptorchid horse. Dr. W. D. Staples inspected and made diagnoses of a case of obscure lameness and a case of chronic indigestion. Dr. W. L. Stroup made a diagnosis of an eye trouble, corneitis due to traumatism. A deep seated abscess of the shoulder was inspected and Dr. R. I. Kearley advised delaying the operation. Two collie bitches were spayed by one of the veterinarians present. A case of fistulous withers with a Merillat tube in it was exhibited and a case of a mule where two water bags had been removed was also exhibited. There were several minor cases of lameness.

The next annual meeting occurs at Birmingham, Ala., on February 20th to 22nd, 1919, in connection with the third annual meeting of the Southeastern States Veterinary Medical Association. Dr. A. H. French of Birmingham was elected president of the Alabama Veterinary Medical Association for the ensuing year.

C. A. CARY, Secretary.

ANNUAL MEETING OF THE CENTRAL CANADA VETERINARY ASSOCIATION

When the fifteenth annual meeting of the Central Canada Veterinary Association opened in St. Andrews Hall, Ottawa, Ont., on February 6th last, Dr. George Hilton, president of the society, read the following message from Dr. F. Torrance, Veterinary Director General and honorary president of the association:

"Regret absence prevents my attending meeting; for success of which present my best wishes."

The wishes of the honorary president, as expressed in his telegram from Toronto, were realized. "The best attended and altogether most successful meeting we have ever held," a member put it when the last business was done.

There were afternoon and evening sessions and in order to promote good fellowship as well as vary the usual literary diet, a very successful little dinner was held at The Plaza at which nearly fifty members sat down. Over the coffee and cigars Mr. Gordon Rogers, of the Health of Animals Branch, entertained with several well chosen recitations and his humorous and witty sallies at the expense of the veterinary profession provoked much merriment. Altogether the dinner, which was the first held, proved such an enjoyable affair that it has undoubtedly come to stay.

That the members fully appreciated their responsibilities and anticipated a large attendance was evidenced by the very able papers presented for discussion. At the afternoon session Dr. Higginson, of Hawkesbury, gave an excellent address on "Parturition and Some of Its Problems" and the lively discussion thereon more than repaid the Doctor for the time and trouble taken. Dr. Bellamy, of Alexandria, read a paper entitled "Differentiating the Intestinal Disorders of the Horse", the subject being handled in a masterly manner and bearing all the earmarks of a careful and studious practitioner. Drs. James, of Ottawa, and McMaster, of Cornwall, also gave many useful pointers in their remarks on "The Examination of Horses for Soundness" and "The Treatment of Serous Sacs of the Shoulder". Professor E. A. A. Grange, Principal of the Ontario Veterinary College, Toronto, gave an interesting address at the afternoon session and entered whole heartedly into the discussions of the various subjects presented.

Dr. Fowler, of Toronto, who kindly consented to be with us, entertained the members with reminiscences of strange cases met with during his surgical career and exhibited specimens including rudimentary teeth taken from dentigerous cysts of the testicles. He also gave some very valuable hints to the practitioners present. Dr. Charles H. Higgins, Ottawa, Canadian representative of the Lederle Laboratories, gave a talk on "Bacterial Vaccines, Sera, etc.", which was much appreciated by all. Dr. S. Hadwen, Pathologist of the Health of Animals Branch, Ottawa, spoke on "Miscellaneous Diseases of Animals Including Poisonous Plants" illustrated by lantern slides. This was such a popular as well as illuminating talk that Dr. Hadwen was unanimously elected an honorary member of the Association then and there. Another notable contribution, illustrated, "Contagious Abortion of Cattle", was made by Dr. J. C. Reid, of the Biological Laboratory, Ottawa. An interesting display feature at the meeting was an exhibit of pathological specimens of animal diseases prepared by Dr. J. A. Allen, also of the Biological Laboratory.

Five new members were initiated into the good graces of the association, namely, Dr. A. A. Etienne, Montreal; Professor Albert Dauth, Laval University, Montreal; Professor N. E. McEwen, McDonald College, Ste. Anne de Bellevue, Que.; Dr. R. H. Foster, Renfrew, Ont.; and Dr. George D. Ackland, Newboro, Ont.

The following officers were elected: Dr. F. Torrance, honorary president; Dr. George Hilton, president; Dr. N. M. Bellamy, vice president; Dr. A. B. Wickware, secretary-treasurer; and the following executive slate: Drs. A. A. Etienne, L. Mulligan, J. B. Hollingsworth, W. C. Young, A. R. Metcalfe, J. Langevin, P. E. Pallister and C. H. Higgins.

Those in attendance were: Professor Albert Dauth, Professor N. E. McEwen, Professor E. A. A. Grange, Dr. W. G. R. Fowler, Toronto; Drs. P. W. O'Hara, Manotick; W. Nichols, Kingston; A. A. Etienne, Montreal; W. C. Young, Almonte; J. M. Bourdeau, Embrun; D. DeMoulin, Lancaster; H. S. Perley, Hanover, New Hampshire, U. S. A.; R. H. Foster, Renfrew; George Ackland, Newboro; W. L. Caron, J. Langevin and A. H. Younghusband, Hull; J. A. Allen, O. Hall, S. Hadwen, H. Laframboise, P. E. Pallister, F. H. S. Lowery, L. Mulligan, A. E. Moore, Robert Barnes, H. E. Marshall, Capt. B. L. Wickware, M.D., C.A.M.C., D. B. Kennedy, W. H. Marriott, A. B. Wickware, A. H. Harris, J. B. Hollingsworth, H. D. Sparks, A. E. James and Dr. A. E. Cameron, of the Entomological Branch, Ottawa; W. C. McGuire and J. D. McMaster, Cornwall; J. A. Bean, Winchester; A. R. Metcalfe, Vankleek Hill; A. C. Morrison, Chesterville; and J. Beaudette, Martintown.

The weather was very inclement, the mercury registering around 20° below zero, accompanied by a snow storm and many were unable to get to Ottawa due to delayed trains and the impassable nature of the country roads. However, the meeting was the best ever held with a record attendance of nearly fifty, and from all indications the association and veterinary profession of Central Canada is coming into its own. The outlook for next year is very bright and with an unprecedented spirit of optimism prevailing we anticipate enrolling many new members and sending your journal an eye-opener as regards a wide-awake veterinary association.

A. B. WICKWARE, Secretary.

VETERINARY INSPECTORS' ASSOCIATION

The regular meeting of the Veterinary Inspectors' Association was held in the Club Rooms of the B. A. I. in the Drovers Bank Building, Chicago, February 8, 1918, at 8 o'clock, P. M. The wives of the veterinarians were invited and many were present. Dr. J. B. Johnson, president of the association, welcomed the ladies. The orchestra of the B. A. I. was present, and, led by Dr. P. A. Franzmann, rendered a number of excellent selections. A number of solos were also given by friends of some of the association members, after which Dr. W. S. Sadler, surgeon, psychologist, author, lecturer, and Director of the Chicago Physiological Therapeutic Institute, was introduced, and presented his lecture on "Long Heads, Round Heads or What Is the Matter with Germany,"

Dr. Sadler immediately plunged into his subject, and endeavored to answer the question, "Why Did We Go to War with Germany?" From his own viewpoint, he stated: "Nine million blue-eyed, Nordic, long headed Germans have dominated 62,000,000 round headed and mixed type Alpine Germans, and taught them for the past forty years that they are more than ordinary men and are the especially selected people to rule and dominate the world."

He further stated that on the same territory where the great contending forces are fighting for supremacy today, the decisive battles of the world have been fought for untold centuries. The doctrine the German people are following is that might is right, and not that right is might. Their one thought is domination and rule; regardless of how they get there. This ideal of domination is built upon rigorous family discipline, and so severe is this training that many German children commit suicide rather than be subjected to the severe discipline of home. For this cause the percentage of suicides among children in Germany is greater than in any other country of the world.

He presented the civic and social conditions in Germany as follows: "The 10% of Nordic stock in Germany which includes the ruling and intellectual classes have turned traitor to civilization and, desiring to master the world, have poisoned the simple minds of the stupid round-headed Alpines, taught them the religion of valor, trained them for forty years in military psychology and developed in them a passionate devotion to the god of might, which makes them a menace to civilization."

Dr. Sadler then set forth twenty-five reasons why Germany must be beaten, chief among which are:

"Because Germany has become an international outlaw—an outcast among the civilized nations of the earth.

"Because Germany has mistaught and deceived a whole people; they are insane with Prussian poison and drunk with the delusion of world power.

"Because Germany's ambitions are wicked, her plans are unholy and her methods barbarous—because she has sinned against all mankind.

"Because they worship tyranny, reverence oppression, exalt hate, extol cruelty, practice dissimulation, and are obsessed with an insane national egotism.

"Because the nations of the earth can never dwell together in peace and unity and go about the pursuit of happiness unarmed without a victory over military Germany—the apostle of frightfulness on land and a ruthless pirate on the high seas.

"Because the world can no longer continue half democratic and half autocratic. After this great war it will eventually be either all democratic or all autocratic.

"Because of the unspeakable cruelties to women and children, the barbarous and immoral practices of the German soldiers, the crucifixion of Canadian officers and because of the terrible and frightful manner in which these war-mad Huns have conducted the whole war.

"Because civilization hangs in the balance. Human liberty and freedom is the goal for which we are fighting, and the world will not afford a safe abiding place for peaceful and liberty-loving men, if Germany wins this war.

"Because Germany has gone into moral bankruptcy, because she is spiritually insolvent, and the time has come for the civilized nations of the earth to sit as a solemn court of judgment to appoint a receiver either to reorganize or wind up the career of this brutal Germanic mighty establishment."

The Veterinary Inspectors' Association of the B. A. I. was organized in 1907 in the Chicago local laboratory by Drs. H. D. Paxson and L. Enos Day, the purpose of which was to discuss subjects pertaining to the work of the veterinarian in the Bureau of Animal Industry. The association meets on the second Friday of each month and is the oldest and perhaps the best attended of any association of its kind. The association at the present time maintains a library of about 300 volumes, covering the various branches of the meat inspection industry, also on building construction, and sanitary engineering.

H. B. RAFFENSPERGER, Resident State Secretary of Illinois.

———◆———

SOUTHWESTERN VETERINARY MEDICAL ASSOCIATION

The second annual meeting of the Southwestern Veterinary Medical Association was held at Benton Harbor, Mich.. February 21st.

Dr. Chas. S. McGuire, Dean of the Grand Rapids Veterinary College, cited interesting facts and statistics as to the present live stock conditions in the state and the effect of war on the live stock population of this country.

Dr. H. L. Grossman, of the B. A. I., read a very interesting paper on the relative value of different foods for hog feeding, touching also on the splendid work being carried on by the B. A. I. in the control of hog cholera.

Mr. W. R. Harper, Secretary of the State Live Stock Sanitary Commission, favored the members with a nice talk, pointing out the ways in which each veterinarian could be of real help to the Commission in carrying out their work.

Dr. Dunphy, State Veterinarian, told the members a great many very interesting facts, among which included a movement which is now on foot in this state to open up our present veterinary law in order to let down the bars to undesirables.

Mr. Harry Lurkin, County Agent, talked on cooperation among veterinarians and county agents, and the producing of little pigs that would be immune to hog cholera.

A schedule of prices was adopted by the members to meet the present conditions.

Each member pledged himself to exert his greatest efforts in his particular territory to the conservation of live stock and to cooperate with county agents, members of the B. A. I. and S. L. S. S. Commission, thereby doing his bit to help win the war.

Dinner was served at the Hotel Benton.

The following officers were elected: President, Dr. L. A. Hosbein, Coloma, Mich.; 1st vice president, Dr. H. P. Heinlan, Dowogiac; 2nd vice president, Dr. John Neville, Decatur; 3rd vice president, Dr. E. L. Kreiger, Benton Harbor; secretary-treasurer, Dr. E. C. Goodrich, St. Joseph.

E. C. Goodrich, Secretary-Treasurer.

THE DOMINION VETERINARY MEAT INSPECTORS' ASSOCIATION OF CANADA

The regular meeting of the Dominion Veterinary Meat Inspectors' Association of Canada was held on February 16th, 1918, in Occident Hall, Toronto. Although the weather was very inclement there was a good attendance and a lively discussion of the subjects presented augured well for the enthusiasm of its members. The executive committee presented a draft of the revised Constitution and By-Laws. This was dwelt with very carefully, each item being gone over separately and thoroughly. When completed it was decided to forward a copy to the Montreal Branch for their perusal and criticism.

Nominations were then received for the various offices and executive and some keen contests are looked for, judging from the names of the various nominees who had evidently been selected with due consideration as to their adaptibility for the office. The election will take place at the annual meeting on March 16th, 1918.

The secretary was instructed to invite Dr. Torrance to meet the association in Toronto at some date in the not too distant future to discuss various topics pertaining to the service.

During the month the members of the association and their ladies were entertained by President Dr. Bone at a progressive euchre, dance and musical evening. A very large attendance recorded the hearty appreciation of all and though the weather was extremely cold everyone reported a real enjoyable evening.

We have to thank Dr. Bone for his courtesy and goodheartedness and also for starting a course that might well be followed up and which would bring a more sociable and social feeling among all in the service.   T. E. H. FISHER, Secretary.

VETERINARY ASSOCIATION OF MANITOBA

The annual meeting of the Veterinary Association of Manitoba was held on Wednesday and Thursday, February 20th and 21st, at Winnipeg.

The proceedings commenced with the business session, at 2 P. M.

The meeting was presided over by Dr. H. N. Thompson, Virden, and there was a good attendance of members.

The financial statement showed the association to be in a flourishing condition.

The following were elected officers for 1918: President, Dr. W. J. Hinman, Winnipeg; vice president, Dr. J. A. Swanson, Manitou; secretary-treasurer and registrar, Dr. C. D. McGilvray, Winnipeg; council, Drs. W. J. Hinman, C. D. McGilvray, W. A. Shoults and J. B. Still, Winnipeg; Dr. H. Bradshaw, Portage-la-Prairie; Dr. A. G. Husband, Belmont; and Dr. J. A. Swanson, Manitou; examining board, Drs. W. J. Hinman, C. D. McGilvray, and W. A. Shoults, Winnipeg; auditors, Drs. Chas. Little and S. T. Martin; committee on veterinary education, Dr. R. A. McIntosh, Morden; Dr. M. B. Rombough, Winnipeg; Dr. H. N. Thompson, Virden; and Dr. J. A. Leadbeater, Brandon; committee on Constitution and By-Laws, Dr. W. A. Dunbar, Winnipeg; Dr. J. A. Munn, Carman; Dr. W. H. T. Lee, Minto; and Dr. S. A. Coxe, Brandon; program committee, Dr. W. A. Hilliard, Winnipeg; Dr. A. G. Husband, Belmont; Dr. C. A. Mack, Gilbert Plains; and Dr. S. T. Martin, Winnipeg.

The formation of an advisory board for the Dominion, on veterinary education, was discussed, and it was decided that this matter should be taken up with the other associations in Canada, to formulate some joint action.

A contribution of fifty dollars was made to the Salmon Memorial Fund, which is being raised by the American Veterinary Medical Association, for the purpose of commemorating the life-work of Dr. D. E. Salmon.

A discussion also took place in connection with amending the by-laws with regard to improving the method of electing the executive.

The evening session was specially well attended, and a number of instructive addresses were given.

Dr. Higgins, of Ottawa, dealt with Pertinent Features of Immunology, making special reference to blackleg in cattle, anthrax, contagious abortion and other animal diseases.

Dr. S. E. Hadwen, of the Health of Animals Branch, Ottawa, discussed Investigations in Swamp Fever of Horses.

Dr. W. A. Shoults, of Winnipeg, dealt with Laminitis of Horses, and illustrated his remarks by the use of diagrams.

Dr. H. N. Thompson, Virden, dealt with Operative Treatment of Poll Evil in horses.

Dr. C. A. Mack, of Gilbert Plains, presented a paper on Hemorrhagic Septicemia.

On the following day, Thursday, February 21st, a series of lectures and practical demonstrations were given at the Manitoba Agricultural College.

Dr. C. D. McGilvray, of Winnipeg, dealt with Tuberculosis of Cattle and the various methods of diagnosing the disease, interpreting test results, and the approved methods of suppressing this disease of cattle. Two reacting cattle were slaughtered and a careful post mortem made by Dr. J. G. Macdonald. The result of the examination confirmed the correctness of the tuberculin test as a diagnostic for the detection of tuberculosis.

The Operative Technique for Sterility in Cows was also demonstrated by Dr. C. D. McGilvray, and a post mortem examination of the animal confirmed the diagnosis as to the ovaries being the seat of the trouble.

Dr. S. Hadwen gave an illustrated address on investigational work conducted by him on Parasitic Anaphylaxis.

Drs. Shoults and McGilvray gave a practical demonstration on the clinical examination of horses, which elicited much discussion among the members.

The members present expressed themselves as being highly pleased with the meeting, and were unanimous in their expression that it was one of the best meetings of the association which had ever been held.

A vote of thanks was unanimously passed expressing the thanks of the association for the efforts put forth by the secretary-treasurer in making the meeting a profitable one for the members.

A vote of thanks was also tendered to G. W. Wood, Director of Animal Husbandry at the Manitoba Agricultural College, for the interest taken by him in making the meeting a success.

C. D. McGilvray, Secretary-Treasurer and Registrar.

SOUTHEASTERN MICHIGAN VETERINARY MEDICAL ASSOCIATION

The regular quarterly meeting of the association was held at the Griswold Hotel, Detroit, January 9, 1918, with about twenty members and visitors present.

Dr. H. E. States, Director of the Dairy and Food Department of the Detroit Board of Health, delivered an address on Municipal Milk Inspection. He gave the history of dairy inspection in Detroit and told how conditions affecting the milk supply had been gradually improved until Detroit had one of the best city milk supplies in the United States.

A paper entitled "Canine Coccidiosis, with a Note Regarding Other Protozoan Parasites from the Dog", by Dr. Maurice C. Hall and Meyer Wigdor, was presented by the senior author. Out of quite a large series of dogs examined in Detroit, the authors had found about 7½% to be affected with coccidiosis.

Dr. E. P. Schaffter, in charge of the local branch of the B. A. I., read a very interesting paper on "A Few Items on the Progress of Meat Inspection". Dr. Schaffter called attention to recent important changes in the meat inspection regulations, and explained the reasons for such changes.

The secretary read a communication from Dr. J. H. Blattenburg, chairman of the American Veterinary Relief Fund Committee, asking that one-half hour be devoted to securing subscriptions to the fund. It was decided to appropriate the sum of $20.00 from our treasury. in addition to the individual contributions from the members. Dr. E. E. Patterson started the ball rolling with a subscription of $25.00. Altogether our members have contributed over $150.00 to the fund.

Dr. F. J. Emmor, of Detroit, was admitted to membership, bringing our roll up to thirty-two.

A committee was appointed to draw up resolutions on the death of Dr. Melvin. Committee: Drs. S. Brenton, E. P. Schaffter and Maurice C. Hall. The resolutions were read as follows:

The Southeastern Michigan Veterinary Medical Association hereby expresses its deep regret for the loss sustained by the veterinary profession in general and the Bureau of Animal Industry in particular, in the death of

DR. A. D. MELVIN

the late head of the Bureau of Animal Industry. In his death veterinary medicine has lost an able and fair-minded executive, with a deep appreciation of the scientific and practical phases of the work he has so long and ably directed.

More than this, there has gone from us a friendly, kindly and true man, a personal loss no less great than the loss of an able veterinarian.

We recall his great services to the profession and to the live stock industry, and express to the Bureau of Animal Industry our sympathy for so great a loss, and we tender to his family our expression of deep sympathy.

The last number on the program was the question box. This brought out some good discussion of several very interesting bovine cases.

The subjects of papers promised for the next meeting were announced by the secretary. The meeting will be held the afternoon and evening of April 11, 1918.

H. Preston Hoskins, Secretary-Treasurer.

MICHIGAN MILK AND DAIRY INSPECTORS' ASSOCIATION

There was very much of a veterinary atmosphere about the annual meeting of the Michigan Milk and Dairy Inspectors' Association, held at Saginaw, February 6, 1918. Dr. H. E. States, Director of the Dairy and Food Department of the Detroit Board of Health, presided.

Dr. Ward Giltner, of the Michigan Agricultural College, delivered an address on the subject of contagious abortion. He dwelt especially upon the relationship between the abortion bacillus and the milk and udder of the cow. Dr. Giltner stated that there was nothing to be feared, from the standpoint of pathogenicity of *B. abortus* for human beings. He reported that he and his colleagues had recently completed some tests on this point, in which they had consumed daily large quantities of milk containing millions of abortion bacilli, with no apparent ill effects.

Mr. H. H. Halladay, President of the Michigan State Live Stock Sanitary Commission, addressed the meeting on the subject of "Regulations and Compensations Paid for Diseased Animals".

A paper on "Milk Transportation" was read by Mr. F. W. Fabian, of the Michigan Agricultural College. This paper gave the results of some experiments conducted by the author, with a view to determining the relative importance of certain factors in milk transportation on the bacterial content.

Dr. H. Preston Hoskins, of the Parke, Davis and Company Research Laboratories, read a paper entitled "Stable Disinfection". The author stated some of the fundamentals underlying disinfection, and pointed out the relationship existing between intelligent disinfection, animal health and clean milk.

The subject of "Tuberculosis Eradication as Carried Out by the U. S. Bureau of Animal Industry and the Michigan State Live stock Sanitary Commission, Cooperating with the Breeders of Pure-bred Cattle", was very ably presented by Dr. T. S. Rich, of the Bureau of Animal Industry.

Dr. William DeKleine, Health Commissioner of Flint, spoke on "Milk and Health". "City Milk Plant Operation" was discussed by Mr. E. O. Krehl, of Detroit, and "The Work of the Recent Milk Commission", by Mr. N. P. Hull, of Lansing.

Dr. J. R. Wardle, of Mt. Clemens, Chief Veterinarian of the Detroit Creamery Company, read a very interesting paper entitled, "Practical Production of Certified Milk". He told in detail of the methods employed in the production of certified milk. The milk from the dairy supervised by Dr. Wardle scored the highest number of points in competition at the Panama-Pacific Exposition.

The meeting closed with the transaction of some routine business. Dr. States was reelected president of the association.

H. P. H.

COMMUNICATION

SENTIMENT VS. HEALTH

Feb. 5, 1918.

Mr. Horace Hoskins.

Dear Sir—I saw in the *Spokesman Review* a suggestion you made in reference to fighting the scarcity of meat, by substituting beef by horse meat. I want to say in regard to it that if we can't win out in this war without the eating of horseflesh, we had better be whipped by the Germans. If you will leave it to the boys who are fighting I will be safe in saying that nine-tenths of them will feel as I do. Horse meat was never given us to eat, and I for one won't eat it if I know what I am eating, and I know that thousands, yes millions, are of the same mind. I regard a horse as next to human, and at times I think the animal superior to some in good common sense. A man who will advocate the like has a very weak spot somewhere where his brains should be.

I am engaged in the horse and cattle business, and I would no more think of eating one of my horses or a piece of one, any more than eating a piece of you, for I fear you are anyway half Hun, for that's quite similar to what they are doing, and saying.

Now you have heard what I have to say, or rather a small part of what I have to say, and I know there are many of my same opinion.

Respectfully yours,

Ray E. Libby, Twisp, Wash.

Feb. 14, 1918.

Mr. Ray Libby,

Twisp, Washington.

Dear Sir—Glad to have your views and note your comments on equine meat consumption.

Have you or I the right to say what others should eat in these meatless, wheatless and milkless days?

Have you or I the right to deny access to horseflesh for food to millions of our people, who have been privileged to buy it in the countries from which they have come?

Have you or I the right to contribute to the fifty to one hundred deaths a day in this great city from pneumonia and a like number from tuberculosis, largely contributed to by an insufficient meat diet, and a dangerous milk supply? Because of the high cost of beef, mutton and pork and the diseased dairy herds. Remembering that equines are almost immune from tuberculosis.

Have you a right to say that these animals, clean, wholesome and nutritious, for which by the tens of thousands, there is no future in the commercial world? Shall they continue to consume the grasses of the plains and deny the same to sheep and cattle for more rapid maturity?

Will you deny to the struggling wage earner for an existence, not a competence in old age, these thousands of acres, that should be growing grains, to help feed the 23% of underfed children in New York City, not to speak of the starving millions abroad?

Have you or I a right to inject our personal opinion in these matters, when the World is crying for food and we have it to give, when every acre of forage should be conserved to save human lives at home and abroad?

Respectfully yours,
(Signed) W. HORACE HOSKINS.

NECROLOGY

ROYAL B. KOONTZ

Dr. Royal B. Koontz died from tuberculosis, March 8, at the age of thirty-two years, at the home of his father near Stoyestown, Pa. He was a graduate of the veterinary college of the University of Pennsylvania in the Class of 1911. For a time he practiced with Dr. Prothero of Johnstown and later established a practice for himself at Barnesboro, Pa.

Dr. Koontz leaves a wife and three daughters.

JOHN T. CUNNINGHAM

Dr. John T. Cunningham died at Providence, R. I., September, 1917.

—Dr. Eugene Ferron has been employed as veterinarian and assistant manager of the cattle ranches of the Cauca Valley Agricultural Co. since August, 1916, at Palmira and in other parts of the Cauca Valley, Colombia, South America.

MISCELLANEOUS

—Veterinary Inspector E. B. Parker has been transferred from Colgate to Marietta, Okla.

—Dr. L. W. Burwell has removed from Clarendon, Ark., to Gahanna, Ohio.

—Dr. H. W. Witmer has removed from Bradentown to Ft. Pierce, Fla.

—Dr. D. E. Wright of Reno, Nevada, has removed to Colfax, Calif.

—Dr. Frank Bowne has removed from Paris Crossing to Pimento, Ind.

—Dr. M. E. Gleason, formerly at Fowlerton, Texas, has removed to San Antonio.

—Doctor and Mrs. H. Preston Hoskins of Detroit, Mich., announce the arrival of a daughter, Lois Margaret, March 4th.

—Dr. G. B. Munger, veterinary inspector on the meat inspection and hog cholera control forces of the Bureau of Animal Industry in Indianapolis, has been transferred to the hog cholera control force of Dr. James McDonald, Springfielld, Ill.

—The Illinois State Civil Service Commission will hold an examination, April 20, for Assistant State Veterinarian. The duties involve the sanitary control of live stock and making differential diagnosis under the direction of the Chief Veterinarian. Graduation from a veterinary college of recognized standing, and license to practice in Illinois and experience as a veterinarian required. Salary $8.00 a day when working.

—Lieut. H. L. Anderson, formerly of Thornton, Ia., is stationed with the 307th Cavalry, Del Rio, Texas.

—Lieut. Fred W. Graves, formerly of Hillsboro, Ind., is with the 326th Field Artillery, Camp Zachary Taylor, Louisville, Ky.

—Lieut. M. H. Gandy, formerly of Shreveport, La., is with the 309th Cavalry, Fort Sam Houston, Texas.

—Dr. Walter J. Taylor, formerly of California, who went to the Canal Zone, Panama, in 1916, to investigate anthrax outbreaks, has recently been put in charge of a new division which has for its purpose the management of cattle handling, plantations, dairy, hog and poultry farms.

—Dr. J. O. Wilson, formerly at Portal, N. D., has removed to Pierre, S. D.

—Dr. Klee, a nephew of Professor Bang, and formerly an assistant in the Clinical Department of the Veterinary School at Copenhagen, Denmark, is spending a short time in America visiting a few of the veterinary colleges. Dr. Klee is on his way to Lima, Peru, where he has a position with a veterinary live stock association.

—Press reports state that 240 government horses consigned to Covington, Ky., had died of suspected poisoning. Analyses of the stomachs indicated that belladonna and croton oil had been administered in some form.

—Dr. W. G. Bailey has removed from San Francisco to Vallejo, Calif.

—Dr. D. E. Sisk has removed from Mahomet to Gibson City, Ill.

—Dr. Adam A. Husman, formerly at Chicago, has been transferred to Memphis, Tenn.

—Dr. J. G. Murphey has removed from Oakland to Stockton, Calif.

—Dr. C. Ross has removed from New York City to Woodhaven, Queens Co., N. Y.

—Dr. G. P. Rebold has been transferred from Stockton to virus-serum inspection work at Oakland, Calif.

—Dr. Daniel Mattrocce, formerly of Merced, has accepted a position as veterinarian with Miller & Lux, Incorporated, at Los Banos, Calif.

—Dr. Lauderdale of the U. S. Department of Agriculture, is stationed in Laurens County, Ga., to assist in treating hog cholera.

—Lieut. John I. Handley, formerly of East Lansing, Mich., is at Headquarters 41st Division, Camp Hill, Newport News, Va.

—Dr. C. J. Cook has removed from Omaha, Neb., to Fort Keogh, Mont.

—FEED CARDS FOR HORSES. The City of Copenhagen has begun issuing feed cards for its horses. The number of horses in the city is estimated at 10,370. The cards allow for a large-size horse 3 kilos (6.61 pounds) of oats per day (instead of the unofficial 4 kilos which has heretofore existed). In addition to this, other feed, such as molasses and blood mixtures, may be used to the extent of 2 kilos per horse.

· —INCREASE IN MEAT ANIMALS. A statement given out by the U. S. Food Administration based upon compilations by the Department of Agriculture, shows that the total number of cattle in the United States on January 1, 1918, was greater by 1,247,000 head than on January 1, 1917. The number of hogs increased 3,781,000. The number of sheep and lambs was 1,284,000 more than at the beginning of 1917. This shows a total increase of 6,312,000 meat animals.

DUMB HEROES

There is a D.S.O. for the colonel,
　A Military Cross for the sub,
A medal or two when we all get
　　through,
　And a bottle of wine with our grub.

There's a stripe of gold for the
　　wounded,
　A rest by the bright seashore;
And a service is read as we bury our
　　dead—
　Then our country has one hero more.

But what of our poor dumb heroes
　That are sent without choice to the
　　fight,
That strain at the load on the shell-
　　swept road,
　As they take up the rations at
　　night?

They are shelling on Hell Fire corner,
　Their shrapnel fast burst in the
　　square,
And their bullets drum as the trans-
　　ports come
　With the food for the soldiers there.

They halt till the shelling is over,
　They rush through the line of the
　　fire;
The glaring light in the dead of night
　And the terrible sights in the mire.

It's the daily work of the horses,
　And they answer the spur and rein
With quickened breath mid the toll of
　　death,
　Through the mud and the holes and
　　the rain.

There's a fresh healed wound in the
　　chestnut;
　On the black mare's neck there's a
　　mark;
The brown mule's new mate won't
　　keep the same gait
　As the one killed last night in the
　　dark.

But they walk with the spirit of
　　heroes,
　They care not for medal or cross,
But for duty alone into peril unknown
　They go, never counting their loss.

There's a swift, painless death for the
　　hopeless,
　With a grave in a shell hole or field;
There's a hospital base for the cas-
　　ualty case,
　And a vet for those easily healed.

But there's never a shadow of glory,
　A cheer or a speech in their praise,
While patient and true they carry us
　　through
　With the limbers in shot-riven ways.

So here's to the Dumb Heroes of
　　Britain,
　Who serve her as nobly and true
As the best of her sons, mid the roar
　　of the guns,
　And the best of her boys on the
　　blue.

They are shell-shocked, they're bruised
　　and they're broken,
　They're wounded and torn as they
　　fall;
Yet they're true and brave to the very
　　grave,
　And they're heroes, one and all.

　　T. A. GIRLING, Veterinary Officer, C.A.V.C., France.

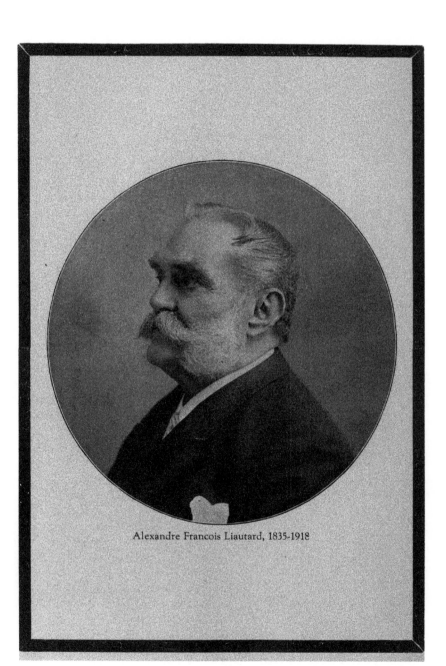

Alexandre Francois Liautard, 1835-1918

JOURNAL
OF THE
American Veterinary Medical Association
Formerly American Veterinary Review
(Original Official Organ U. S. Vet. Med. Ass'n)

PIERRE A. FISH, Editor   **ITHACA, N. Y.**

Executive Board
GEORGE HILTON, 1st District; W. HORACE HOSKINS, 2d District; J. R. MOHLER, 3d District; C. H. STANGE, 4th District; R. A. ARCHIBALD, 5th District; A. T. KINSLEY, Member at large.

Sub-Committee on Journal
J. R. MOHLER   R. A. ARCHIBALD

The American Veterinary Medical Association is not responsible for views or statements published in the JOURNAL, outside of its own authorized actions.
Reprints should be ordered in advance. A circular of prices will be sent upon application.

VOL. LIII., N. S. VOL. VI.   MAY, 1918.   NO. 2.

Communications relating to membership and matters pertaining to the American Veterinary Medical Association should be addressed to Acting Secretary L. Enos Day, 1827 S. Wabash Ave., Chicago, Ill. Matters pertaining to the Journal should be sent to Ithaca, N. Y.

CENTRALIZATION

The lack of centralized authority has been responsible for serious delay in certain branches. A system with division of authority means a consequent and deleterious division of responsibility. There is perhaps an undemocratic flavor to the idea of concentrating authority but it has the advantage of locating the responsibility promptly and speeding results.

The recent history of the railroad transportation is an apt illustration. The highly trained specialists of the railroad world who gave their services to the government accomplished more marvels than American railroads had ever accomplished before. In spite of all their efforts their work failed when the emergency arose because they were lacking in coordination. There was a lack in perspective, an inability to utilize all of the railroads as a single system. The lack of centralized authority was seen and admitted by the railroad men themselves and this authority was their solution of the problem. Since the Secretary of the Treasury has assumed the directorship of the railways there has been improvement. The arrangement has been bad for some of the roads, but it has improved transportation.

The airplane industry has not met expectations and centralized authority is demanded for this branch of the service. The allied armies have fought more or less independently for three years or over. There has been evidence of lack of coordination. There has doubtless been pride in the size and organization of a great national army and an unreadiness to place it under the supreme command of a General of another nationality. In opposition there has been an enemy highly organized and with authority very much centralized. The enemy, more favorably situated as to geographical position, has been able to swing armies from one front to another with the hope of conquering its opponents singly. The fighting has now centered upon the western front; the supreme test has begun and in the emergency the authority has been centralized in General Foch as Generalissimo. America is second to none in her pride and support of her Army—much of it still in the making. By brigading her troops with the gallant French and British defenders of civilization, she has waived selfish ambition of a great national army as a separate entity, when for the common good greater effectiveness may result. There has, throughout the war, been unity of purpose. With more complete unity of action, there is more promise of success.

If centralization of authority is desirable or essential in carrying out great projects in the Service, it follows that it is applicable as well to subordinate branches, each in its sphere. The veterinary corps has not been overburdened with authority. Its past history is over, but in its reorganization and future plans, centralization of authority is the goal to keep in mind. Healthy, normal soldiers belong to their commanding general; when sick, wounded and disabled they belong to the Surgeon General. Each is supreme in his own department. The Army animals belong to the Quartermaster's department; when sick or disabled they should belong to the veterinary department and veterinarians should have full authority over them until they are again fit for service. Our veterinary war history is in the making. It is wise to utilize the best features of veterinary service as shown in other armies and profit by the experience of others. Authority locates responsibility. Efficiency is the standard of success. This standard may make or break leaders but it must be maintained. An open page lies before our veterinary corps. The history written thereon will determine its future. We venture the prediction, when all is said and done, that it will compare favorably with that of others.

P. A. F.

■ ■ ■

GRADING COLLEGES

Although several months intervene before the Philadelphia meeting, it seems to the writer that there are a few problems that might well be considered and perhaps discussed in our JOURNAL prior to the August meeting.

The first problem in mind is the college situation. While the writer has never taken the college problem as seriously to heart as some of our members, believing, as he does, that such matters with a little assistance will eventually adjust themselves; at the same time it is fully realized that we have reached a point which is daily becoming more acute, where the veterinary colleges of North America, both State and private, must be so classified that prospective students who desire to take up the study of veterinary science will have some sort of a guide to aid them in choosing the particular institution from which to obtain instruction. Under existing conditions the prospective student has no means of definitely ascertaining which are accredited institutions and which are not. He usually applies to the most available college irrespective of its standing only to find when it is perhaps too late and to his sorrow that his chosen *alma mater* has a questionable standing, if any, with the profession he is entering.

Young men have come to the writer after graduation from unrecognized colleges seeking to obtain membership in the American Veterinary Medical Association and other recognition and have stated that they entered such institutions without knowledge and with no means of obtaining information which would in any way enlighten them as to their character and standing. They naturally assumed that as long as such colleges were operating under government sanction by state charter that everything was as it should be.

It is quite obvious that there can be no greater handicap for the recent graduate than to discover when he goes out into the world to follow his chosen profession that his credentials for which he labored so hard are not recognized by the existing authorities on veterinary education, the American Veterinary Medical Association and the United States Bureau of Animal Industry.

That there is an element of injustice in all this, that should be remedied if possible, goes without saying. The big problem confronting us is to determine wherein lies the remedy. Having in mind that suggestions might be asked for from men who are interested in this problem through the medium of our JOURNAL is what prompted the idea to broach the subject at this time.

In order to start the ball rolling in this direction the following suggestion is offered: that all colleges on this continent be scored by the committee on intelligence and education of the A. V. M. A. and depending upon the score obtained each college be placed in class A, B, or C, depending upon their facilities and qualifications to give instruction.

This plan has been and is being followed out by the Association of American Medical Colleges and that it has been successful is attested by the fact that the Surgeon General has decreed that only medical men who are graduates of class A or B colleges, as classified by the Association of American Medical Colleges, can obtain entry into the United States Service. Graduates of class C colleges cannot enter the medical corps as officers and boards of examiners of many states will not permit them to take state board examinations for entrance into private practice.

Let us adopt then as soon as may be practical some system of classifying our veterinary educational institutions which will at least be definite and mean something to the prospective student.

R. A. A.

EUROPEAN CHRONICLES

Bois Jerome.

RABIES IN GUINEA PIGS.—Probably this heading will be a surprise to some of our readers, who may ask what interest rabies of guinea pigs will offer. My excuse is the interest the subject may present from the point of view of comparative pathology and the value to those who experiment on the disease with these little animals. At any rate this contribution to the study of rabies in guinea pigs is in the *Annales de l'Institut Pasteur* and is signed by Prof. P. Remlinger, which is sufficient to indicate that the subject is interesting. It is to be regretted that its length does not allow an entire translation. I will give only extracts from it.

The clinical physionomy of rabies in guinea pigs is far from uniform. In the animal inoculated with street virus the furious form is most frequently observed. All the intermediate forms exist from the most violent to the most attenuated. After this statement, Doctor Remlinger gives a description of the various forms observed. First the furious form, then a more attenuated, the dyspneic, the pseudo-septicemic, the spasmodic, those in which the disease assumes such severity that like a shock death occurs generally between 24 and 36 hours or even in a shorter time, and before it has been possible to ascertain and fix the form of rabies that caused it. There are also the paralytic forms among which is that caused exclusively by fixed virus.

In a second portion of his article, the author presents a very interesting examination of the many factors that are liable to modify, in guinea pigs, the symptomatology of rabies and also its duration and progressive advance.

Among the principal factors is first considered the influence of the number of passages of the virus for the study of which, experiments were carried out with three viruses, in the second is the influence of the mode of inoculation and in the third that of the seat of inoculation and finally that of other foreign factors.

Following this important demonstration, the importance of which is principally from the point of view of experimentation, a minute comparison is made of the disease in guinea pigs and rabbits, and finally the article closes with the following résumé and conclusions:

"In opposition to rabies with fixed virus—always of a paralytic type—rabies with street virus has, in guinea pigs a most varied physionomy. The furious form is the most frequently observed, but all the intermediate forms exist. At times there is no agitation, the dominating symptom is dyspnea and the symptomatology is such that it resembles one of the numerous epizootic pulmonary affections of guinea pigs. The dyspnea may of itself be little marked and the analogy is then more like that of septicemia than a broncho-pneumonia.

"The spasmodic form, which is particularly observed after inoculation in the anterior chamber and nasal instillations, is very special. It is essentially characterized by a violent reaction, both objective and subjective, (prurit) at the point of inoculation, by pharyngeal rhonchus, spasms and convulsions. It has a great analogy with the form of rabies most common in man.

"The duration of declared rabies may, in guinea pigs, be very short. While the preceding forms, which run their course ordinarily in 24 to 48 hours, there is a form lightning like (foudroyante), the duration of which is so short that the disease escapes observation and death seems to occur suddenly. Hence in experiments on rabies, all pigs that die without symptoms can be considered as suspicious. Corpuscles of Negri should be looked for and the bulb be used for passage.

"The paralytic type is manifested under two forms, the relaxed and that with contracture or pseudo-tetani. Both may assume an ascending progress in their development and attain the syndrome of Landry, so frequent during rapid manifestations.

"A certain number of factors are likely to exercise influence upon the symptomatology of the disease. In passing from guinea pig to guinea pig, street virus becomes more active than from rabbit to rabbit. It may happen that after 8 or 10 passages, it kills in a fixed manner in 5 to 7 days. The first inoculations, starting from the dog, may give a paralytic form. After 2 to 4 passages the furious form, in its most severe aspect, may be observed. The severity of the symptoms diminishes afterwards. There are dyspnea, pseudo-septicemia forms, which towards the 20th passage, give rise to a paralytic form, which lasts to the end.

"The mode of inoculation, in the case of intramuscular or subcutaneous injections, the seat of inoculation, the age of the animal, the dose of injected virus, etc., have also their effect on the symptoms presented. If with the intracranial and intraocular injections, all the forms of rabies may be noticed, those in the muscles of the thigh or the soles of the feet give almost exclusively the pseudo-tetanic form. The analogy with tetanus is completed by the fact that in case of subcutaneous or intramuscular inoculations, paralysis almost always began at the inoculated region.

"Paralytic rabies is observed, especially in the street virus, in young animals and with a large dose of virus; while in adult age and with weak doses furious rabies prevails. In the experimental rabies of guinea pigs there is no splanchnic type comparable to the splanchnic type of tetanus.

"Guinea pigs are sensibly more susceptible to rabid virus

than rabbits. The period of inoculation is shorter and a smaller dose of virus or attenuated virus, harmless for the rabbit, causes the disease. There is then a great advantage which counterbalances in part the shortness of the disease and the variability of the clinical type. This must not be ignored in investigating rabies.''

SYNCHISIS SCINTILLANS IN HORSES.—Well known in man, this affection of the eye is almost entirely unknown in our domestic animals, except for two cases that have been clinically observed in Berlin, one in a horse, the other in a pigeon.

Veterinary Major Brock-Rousseau has observed one case lately and recorded it in the *Revue de Pathologie Comparée*.

It was in an aged gray mare. Both eyes had the aspect of a glass paper weight in which a quantity of small glittering bodies are fixed in the paste. The aqueous humor was filled with similar bodies, constantly in motion, and having the appearance of containing a quantity of golden dust in the cavities of the eye. Both organs of sight were alike and nothing else appeared which could explain such a condition.

As the affection has not been described in veterinary literature, says the writer, few facts are related by him.

It is said that about 1828 the discovery of scintillans synchisis was made by a physician, Doctor Parfait Davidson. In 1849 a German oculist noticed in sections made on several eyes, that cholesterin was present and that there had been preceding choroiditis. In 1876, besides the cholesterin, two new forms of crystals were discovered in eyes where the condition of scintillans had been observed, these were tyrosin and some phosphatic salts. In 1890 the anatomical changes were attributed by Gallannaerts to the choroid only—and finally Panas in feeding rabbits with naphthalin obtained an experimental scintillans synchisis, composed of crystals of sulfate and carbonate of lime without traces of cholesterin.

With this history we are brought to the definition of today, viz.: a rare form of softening of the vitreous humor, characterized by the presence of numerous (paillettes) broken crystals of cholesterin, floating in the interior and glittering as flakes of gold.

Examination with the ophthalmoscope is peculiar. When it is made with lenses of 18 or 20 dioptrics, if one gradually takes away the lens so as to bring it to the point of the various layers of the eye, he sees, after dilatation of the pupil, moving flecks of tyrosin recognized by their brilliant color and agglomerated masses of cholesterin with, sometimes, phosphatic agglomerations in the form of little balls covered with many dots. All these crystals may sometimes be observed by the naked eye and when they move they appear like gold dust. After dilatation of the pupil the vitreous humor has a very peculiar aspect, that of a brilliant kaleidoscope. With such conditions the sight is of course greatly impaired and often completely lost. There are cases where it remains almost normal and it is only accidentally that the oculist with the ophthalmoscope discovers the true condition of the eye.

The pathology of the disease is yet the subject of discussion and its etiology is in doubt. Old age, sex, some dyscrasia, syphilis, hepatic diseases seem to favor the genesis of the affection. In veterinary medicine all of these have only a secondary interest.

GOITER IN HORSES.—The pathology of the thyroid adenoma or goiter of horses is one which the previous articles of Prof. G. Petit of Alfort to which I have alluded in previous chronicles and to which I made reference under the title of epithelial tumors of the thyroid gland, has been the subject of another communication of valuable interest in the *Recueil* of Alfort.

Recalling the classification of the epithelial tumors, which he presented and which he divided into benignant (adenomas or goiters) and which can exceptionally be transformed into cancers, and the malignants, cancers proper or epitheliomas of various kinds. Prof. Petit, having treated of the latter in previous articles, says that he will complete the consideration of the subject by discussing now the pathology and evolution of the thyroidian adenoma or goiter, which, being synonymous in man, cannot be different in comparative pathology.

It will be understood that the study has for its object the sporadic, sometimes large and well characterized but more frequently encapsulated, invisible and not the endemic goiter which is so frequent in man at some climacteric, and has not been observed in equines.

In relation to the etiology, Petit says it is quite difficult to solve the question as like cancer, which at times follow it, both of these tumors result from the epithelial proliferation, independent of any characterized inflammation.

With the study of the pathogenesis various points are established.

For a long time it has been believed .that goiter was due to the proliferation of the cells which line the thyroidian vesicles. This was an error, as the adenoma comes from the multiplication of the epithelial vesicles which remain between the vesicles and exist at the embryonic stage. Plates showing this condition of the thyroid in the embryo are shown. It is probable that the adenoma is the manifestation or process of a glandular renovation. Adenomatous cells have no pigment, a fact which contributes to the whitish aspect of the small adenomas.

The growth of the adenoma takes place by a characteristic and well defined nodular arrangement, or by extension or diffused infiltration with indefinite areas. These two processes are illustrated by excellent plates.

In the massive or trabecular adenoma the tendency to neo-vesiculation is not indicated. For the cystic and the pseudo-cystic transformation the process is also different. In these the neovesicles are small microscopic cysts, which have a tendency to enlarge and mingle so as to form cavities more or less irregular and wide.

Although the thyroidian adenoma represents a precancerous condition it does not necessarily follow that it must degenerate as such ; yet cancer may be said to make its appearance more often in a gland having undergone the adenomatous transformation than in a normal gland.

The article of Prof. Petit closes with a schematic table of the three types of thyroidian adenomas with their cystic and pseudo-cystic form, viz.: the fundamental or initial, the diffused and their derivatives.

CARTILAGINOUS QUITTOR.—I am writing upon this subject as Professor Sendrail, Veterinary Major, gives a good article in Panisset's *Revue* in relation to the operation.

After a long critique of nearly all that has been written on it, with familiar objections on some of the methods of operation and a fair acknowledgement of the advantages the Professor gives a description of modifications that have withstood the test of a long and wide experience.

These modifications consist, above all, in limiting the parietal injury to the wall so as to retain for the foot a normal resistance and preserve its integral function.

Before the operation the foot is prepared by a normal paring and the application of an ordinary shoe. This is done standing.

The wall is thinned following a half circle extending 6 to 8 centimeters in length and 4 in height with its anterior boundary quite far from the extremity of the cartilage and posteriorly about two centimeters from the heel. This thinning occupies nearly half the height of the quarter and must be made very thin immediately below the coronary band.

The cartilage is exposed by a straight incision along the inferior border of the coronary band, joining both ends of the incision and embracing a piece of the podophyllous tissue about one centimeter wide. The external face of the cartilage is isolated from the skin with a double sage knife introduced under the coronary band and moved forward and backward as in the classical method. With a curette knife of Volkmann the ablation of the cartilage is made quite easily.

The ablation of the anterior portion of the cartilage is the delicate step of the operation and demands careful use of the instrument.

The lateral ligament of the joint can then be saved from injury. The operation is complicated only in cases of ossified cartilage. Although the necrosed portion of the cartilage may sometimes appear as the only diseased structure, Sendrail recommends the ablation of the entire cartilaginous plate.

An ordinary dressing, moderately compressed, is applied and held in place by rolling bands and is renewed according to indications.

The results obtained by this mode of operation in several hundred cases have proved very satisfactory but they nevertheless required from four to six weeks of rest.

A NEW VETERINARY MEDICAL ASSOCIATION.—If the report from a professional journal from America is correct and "more than 800 veterinarians have already been assigned to duty in the American Army" and probably a number of them will come to France, the news published in the veterinary papers of England will prove of interest to them.

Visiting and joining a veterinary association in time of war at the center of hostilities and mingling with confréres of similar aims and speaking the same language, will no doubt prove a great boon for our American confréres and present an opportunity they will accept with great pleasure.

I have already communicated with Professor F. Hobday, Veterinary Major, who is one of the officers of the association, and I hope to be able soon to give our American friends his reply to my inquiries if application for membership would be favorably entertained by the "Somme Veterinary Association" directors.

From the *Veterinary Journal* of England the following is given as notice of the organization:

At the suggestion that a Veterinary Medical Association be started at a centre "somewhere in France", as likely to be beneficial to the veterinary officers stationed in the neighborhood; the outcome was that the society should be called the "Somme Veterinary Medical Association"; that meetings should be held each fortnight, and a regular board of officers appointed and qualifications for membership adopted.

When the reply to my inquiries from Vice President Veterinary Major Hobday is at hand, I will communicate it to our friends in America.

SUMMARY FROM RECENT PUBLICATIONS RECEIVED AND BIBLIOGRAPHIC NOTES.

Those marked "X" will be summarized. Those marked "O" will appear in abstracts.

VETERINARY REVIEW OF EDINBURG. The first number of volume two has been published lately. It is a fine issue of 138 pages and like its predecessors presents to its readers concise abstracts, reports, reviews, notes on books, and bibliography of great value. There is in the number a review by Doctor Wm. Osler of Oxford University, a well known scientist, who wrote for the *Veterinary Review* on the *Essai de Bibliographie Hippique* which is published in Paris, and again on the *Birth of Modern Surgery*, a valuable addition to the subject, in which the great work of Lister in surgery is fully considered and credited. Among the reviews of this number, our friends in America will be pleased to read of the works of Professor Williams on Obstetrics, Doctor DeVine on Bovine Tuberculosis, and Kilbourn on the Pasteurization of Milk.

(X) MALADIES DU PORC (Diseases of Swine) by Prof. Moussu (Asselin and Houzeau, Paris). This text will facilitate the work of the veterinary practitioner and the breeder. It will receive consideration later.

JOURNAL OF COMPARATIVE PATHOLOGY AND THERAPEUTICS. Early history of veterinary literature (continued)—Bracken poisoning in cattle—Treat.

ment of red water by intravenous injections of tartar emetic—(X) Contagious abortion in mares and joint ill in foals—Etiology and serum
treatment.

VETERINARY JOURNAL, January, 1918. Distomatosis—Liver rot and flukes in
sheep and cattle—Diphtheric vaginitis of cattle—(O) Delayed fracture
of the humerus—(O) Radial paralysis in cows—(O) Adenoma of the
alopecia—A note on jhooling in camels.
February. Report on Ixodic lymphangitis—(O) Adenoma of the kidneys—Bacterial pyelonephritis in a cow—Aspergillus in birds, man and
cow—(O) An experience.

VETERINARY RECORD. Uterine torsion in cows, mares and cats—Malignant
edema—Tetanus—Bloody urine—Morphine in dog practice—(X) Filariasis of the withers in horses.

VETERINARY NEWS. Bloody urine—(O) Interesting cases.

IL NUOVO ERCOLANI. On the naso-fronto-maxillary resection in dogs.

LA CLINICA VETERINARIA. Bacteriologic researches on the typhoid affections
of horses—On the value of the method of Wulffi in the diagnosis of anthrax—(O) A case of puerperal mania—Tincture of iodine in the treatment of wounds.

REVUE DE PATHOLOGIE COMPARÉE. Epizootic abortion of bovines.

REVUE GENERAL DE MEDECINE VETERINAIRE. Life and work of A. Chauveau—
Treatment of lymphangitis in horses—(O) Old fistula treated by polyvalent serum.   A. L.

—KILLING HORSES. A new equipment for killing condemned
horses with illuminating gas has been installed in the Denver city
pound. A small air-tight stall is connected with the city gas main.
While the horse is munching his oats or hay from a manger in one
side of the stall the gas enters from a pipe directly underneath.
The animal gently and peacefully subsides into insensibility.—*The
Popular Science Monthly.*

—A force of federal inspectors engaged upon the eradication
of dourine, with headquarters at Albuquerque, New Mexico, have
been assigned as follows: Drs. Joseph L. Flanigan, Vernon A.
Dennis, Ben H. Steigleder, Guy E. Abrams, John J. Staab and
Gardiner B. Jones.

—According to an order issued by the Secretary of Agriculture,
the Federal quarantine against sheep scabies was lifted on April
15, 1918, from 136 counties in Texas with an area of 118,033 square
miles. This order is deemed to be of special interest at this time
because of the demand for mutton and wool.

STUDIES IN FORAGE POISONING*

Robert Graham, A. L. Brueckner and R. L. Pontius
Laboratory of Animal Pathology, Kentucky Agricultural Experiment Station
Lexington, Ky.

The sporadic appearance of forage poisoning in Kentucky has afforded opportunity to project a series of experimental studies upon feeds which were proved to contain the causative factor of the disease. Numerous suspected feeds in sporadic outbreaks of forage poisoning have been fed to experimental horses with negative results; in fact, difficulty has been experienced in establishing the feed responsible for the disease in certain outbreaks which have come to our attention. Attempts to isolate the causative factor from positive feeds (feeds which in ingestion experiments produced the disease) have in many instances resulted negatively.

During the course of experimental studies veterinary practitioners and stockmen of wide experience have been consulted and the prevailing impression regarding the etiology of forage poisoning seemed to associate this disease with moldy or inferior feedstuffs. In one instance positive feed was not visibly contaminated with molds, and certain molds isolated from supposedly poisonous feeds after being propagated in the laboratory were supplied to animals in feeding experiments with negative results.

The possibility of more than one cause of forage poisoning, or that a clinical disease resembling forage poisoning may be induced by more than one etiologic agent, is not disregarded nor is it claimed that the type of forage poisoning observed in Kentucky is necessarily the same intoxication occurring sporadically in the various states. Experimental data available at this time, however, indicate that the type of forage poisoning in horses and mules caused by the ingestion of an oat hay and an ensilage in remote outbreaks in Kentucky are closely related if not identical with a sporadic and clinical forage poisoning observed by Professor H. P. Rusk and Dr. H. S. Grindley* of the University of Illinois occurring on the McLean farm at Ottawa, Illinois.

*Presented at the 54th Annual Meeting of the American Veterinary Medical Association, Section on Sanitary Science and Police, Kansas City, Mo., August, 1917.

*Unpublished report.

In this paper are given a few preliminary experiments, with photographs, extracted from bulletins Nos. 207-208 of the Kentucky Experiment Station. The results of these studies corroborate in a measure the theory advanced by the late Dr. Leonard A. Pearson, wherein he mentioned the clinical analogy of forage poisoning in animals to meat poisoning in man. Infections of this type in man arising from extracellular toxin producing organisms are amenable to serum prophylactic treatment as pointed out by Kempner and Wasserman. The serological treatment of forage poisoning is thus suggested as the result of the apparent relation of serum immune to *B. botulinus* in protecting against a microorganism resembling *B. botulinus* isolated at the Kentucky Station from three feeds obtained from natural outbreaks of the disease. Serum immune to the strains isolated from the feeds proved equally efficacious in protecting small animals against a fatal *B. botulinus* infection as well as an artificial infection arising from the homologous strains.

Following a natural outbreak of forage poisoning in horses an oat hay was secured that possessed the property of producing clinical forage poisoning subsequently to ingestion. (See Figs. 1, 2 and 3.) The oat forage was moved to the Experiment Station where the threshed grain separated from the straw, as well as the straw independently, proved capable of producing clinical forage poisoning in horse and mule stock subsequently to ingestion. Water in which the grain and straw were immersed proved likewise infective to horses subsequent to drinking. Chicken feces obtained from the oat straw after threshing, disguised in wholesome feed of a horse, resulted in the disease, while chicken feces from remote sources, disguised in wholesome feed of horses, was not productive of the disease. Chickens, rabbits, guinea pigs, swine, sheep and goats freely consumed the poisonous oat grain without noticeable effect.

Contaminated feed may apparently retain its infective quality for several months in that two barrels of the oat hay in question were reserved for approximately two years and upon allowing horses to drink water in which the oat hay was immersed clinical forage poisoning resulted.

In 1916 Drs. Buckley and Shippen** brought out the patho-

** Jour. Amer. Vet. Med. Ass'n, 1917, 50, New Series 3, No. 7, pp. 809-816.

genic nature of *B. botulinus* to horses, and noted a clinical and anatomic resemblance of *B. botulinus* intoxication artificially induced in horses to sporadic forage poisoning. The pathogenic character of *B. botulinus* for horses as pointed out by Buckley and Shippen

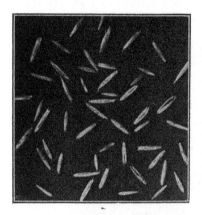
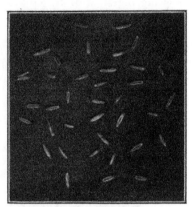
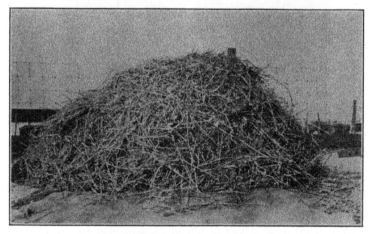

Figs. 1, 2 and 3, Bulletin 207, Kentucky Experiment Station
Griffith Oat Hay and Threshed Grain

was observed by the writers following the ingestion of 2 c.c. broth culture *B. botulinus**** disguised in wholesome feed and as the result of injecting 0.1 c.c. subcutaneously. The intoxication observed

*B. botulinus strain (N. B. S.) from Dr. Buckley, Washington, D. C.

following artificial infection with *B. botulinus* presented in some experimental horses symptoms and gross anatomic lesions resembling those found in forage poisoning. It was also reported by Buckley and Shippen that chickens were not noticeably affected following ingestion of *B. botulinus* broth culture in feed, yet the feces from chickens fed *B. botulinus* proved capable of inducing

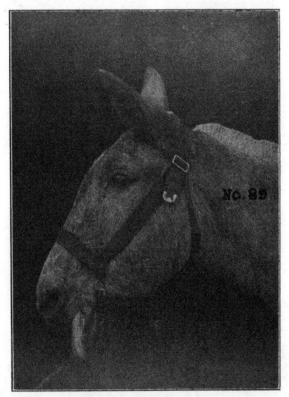

Fig. 4, Bulletin 207, Kentucky Experiment Station

fatal intoxication when fed to horses accompanied by the clinical features of forage poisoning.

Corroborating the infective property of chicken excreta following the ingestion of broth cultures of *B. botulinus* disguised in feed mule No. 89 was fed 95 grams of the chicken feces naturally voided. The feces were ground and thoroughly mixed in wholesome feed and given to the mule on December 21st. The ration of this animal then consisted of wholesome feed and water. The animal appeared normal until the morning of December 26th, at

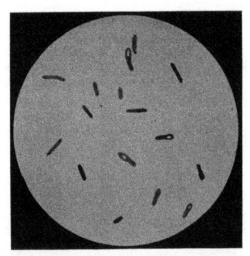

Fig. 8, Bulletin 207, Ky. Exp. Sta.

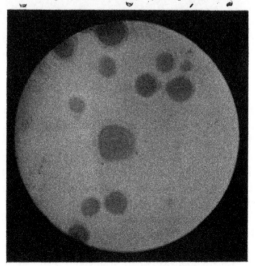

Fig. 9, Bulletin 207, Ky. Exp. Sta.

which time there was observed a marked muscular weakness, pharyngeal paralysis and restlessness; the tongue was paralyzed and pendulous. Fig. 4 was made at 10 a. m. on December 26th and at 3 p. m. the animal became permanently decumbent, followed by death on December 27th.

From the internal organs of horses fatally .afflicted from drinking the poisonous oat hay water previously mentioned numerous plantings were made in different cultural media under conditions favorable to the development of *B. botulinus*. Samples of the oat water direct from the barrel were also cultured and placed under similar favorable conditions. From the cecum contents of experimental horse No. 91 fatally afflicted from drinking the oat water, a Gram positive, anaerobic, sporulating, rod-shaped organism, 0.8 to 1 micron wide and 2½ to 6 microns long, was isolated.

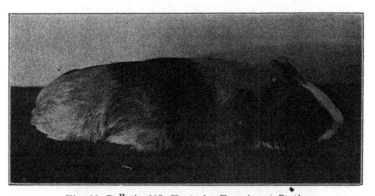

Fig. 10, Bulletin 207, Kentucky Experiment Station

This organism resembled *B. botulinus* as to morphological and cultural characters and it was administered to small animals.

A healthy guinea pig received per os 0.2 c.c. broth culture of the anaerobic bacillus isolated from the cecum of horse No. 91 on February 14, 1917. Fig. 10 represents the prostrate condition of this pig at 11 a. m. February 15th, 24 hours after being infected. Death occurred at 7 a. m. February 16th.

Experimental horse No. 94 was allowed to ingest with wholesome feed 4 c.c. broth culture of the anaerobic organism isolated from the cecum of horse No. 91 on February 14, 1917. The animal remained apparently healthy until February 19th, at which time there was manifest paresis of the pharynx and a marked general weakness. The plate for Fig. 11 was made on February 19th and the following morning the animal was permanently decumbent.

After remaining in a moribund condition for three days death followed on February 23rd, nine days after feeding the culture.

Postmortem examination of horse No. 94 revealed hemorrhagic lesions in the outer wall of the small intestine and on the inner wall numerous punctate hemorrhages and highly injected areas were found. The gross findings at autopsy in other horses similarly infected involved congestion of the lungs, areas of hyperemia, congestion and hemorrhage in the mucous and serous membranes. In the connective and supporting tissue of the body gelatinous infil-

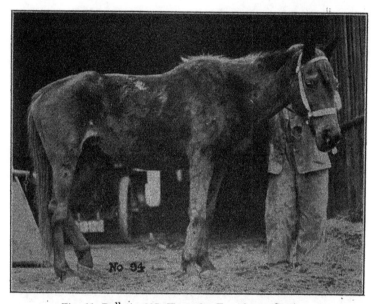

Fig. 11, Bulletin 207, Kentucky Experiment Station

tration was frequently observed. Gross changes were very slight or not discernible in other animals artificially infected.

From the cecum of horse No. 94 an anaerobic bacillus resembling the organism used to infect this animal (originally isolated from cecum of horse No. 91) was regained. 0.5 c.c. of the organism in broth given per os to guinea pig shown in Fig. 14 resulted in intoxication and death in 25 hours.

The fatal effect of *B. botulinus* as pointed out by Drs. Buckley and Shippen and the resemblance of artificially induced *B. botulinus* intoxication in horses to clinical forage poisoning prompted

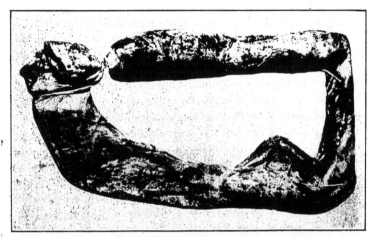

Fig. 12, Bulletin 207, Kentucky Experiment Station

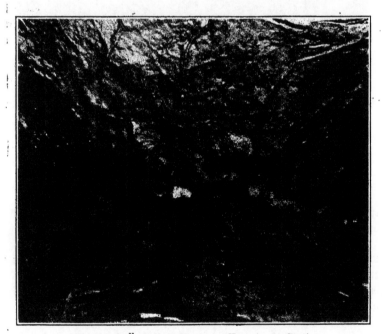

Fig. 13, Bulletin 207, Kentucky Experiment Station

the preparation of botulism antitoxin. In numerous experimental trials it was found that botulism antitoxin proved efficacious in protecting horses against an artificial infection of *B. botulinus* given per os and subcutaneously.

The protective quality of goat serum immune to *B. botulinus* against a fatal artificial infection of the homologous strain in

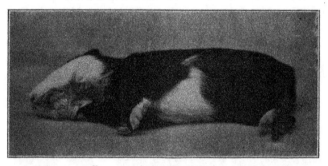

Fig. 14, Bulletin 207, Kentucky Experiment Station

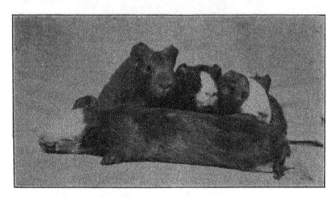

Fig. 15, Bulletin 207, Kentucky Experiment Station

guinea pigs is shown in Fig. 15. The three animals in the rear received varying doses of serum intraperitoneally on March 13th, followed on March 14th by 0.05 c.c. of toxin (unfiltered *B. botulinus* broth culture) per os. The same amount of toxin was also administered per os to an untreated pig. Death occurred in the control pig in approximately 24 hours, while the pigs receiving serum remained apparently healthy.

The protective quality of botulism antitoxin against the broth culture of the organism isolated from the cecum of horse No. 91 is shown in Fig. 16. Varying doses of serum were administered intraperitoneally on March 15th to the three pigs in the rear, followed on March 16th by 0.05 c.c. per os of the broth culture of the organism isolated from the cecum of horse No. 91. A control pig was simultaneously infected with the same amount of the broth culture. Fig. 16 was made on March 17th, on which day the control pig died. One of the serum treated pigs shown in this test died on March 24th. The other serum treated animals remained apparently healthy. Duplicate tests on guinea pigs with varying amounts of serum apparently provided protection against many times the lethal amount of the organism.

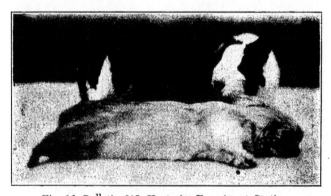

Fig. 16, Bulletin 207, Kentucky Experiment Station

Horses Nos. 98 and 99 received in wholesome feed 2 c.c. unfiltered broth culture of the anaerobic organism isolated from the cecum of horse No. 91 on March 6, 1917. These animals remained apparently healthy until the morning of March 8th at which time they were found in a decumbent and moribund condition. The preceding evening (March 7th) Nos. 98 and 99 consumed the grain but only a small portion of the hay allowed. Fig. 17 was made at 10 o'clock, March 8th. No. 98 died at 3 p. m. in the afternoon, while No. 99 survived until the following morning.

Horses Nos. 1002, 1003, and 1004 received two prophylactic injections of botulism antitoxin, followed by 4 c.c. (in doses of 1 and 3 c.c. at intervals of 9 days) of broth culture of the anaerobic organism isolated from the cecum of horse No. 91, in 1000 grams of

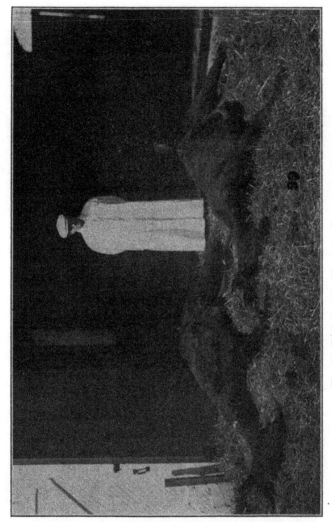

Fig. 17, Bulletin 207, Kentucky Experiment Station

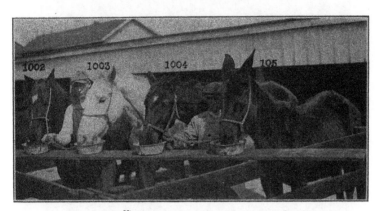

Fig. 18, Bulletin 207, Kentucky Experiment Station

wholesome oats. Mule No. 105 received the same amount of the organism, but no serum.

Fig. 19 shows the same animals with No. 105 in a decumbent position. Mule No. 105 displayed a marked resistance and continued to eat for approximately 9 days following ingestion of 1 c.c.

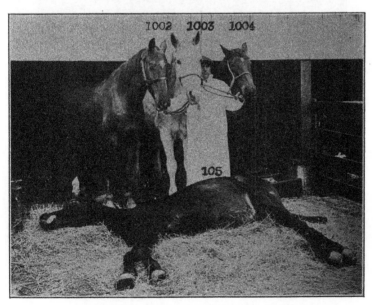

Fig. 19, Bulletin 207, Kentucky Experiment Station

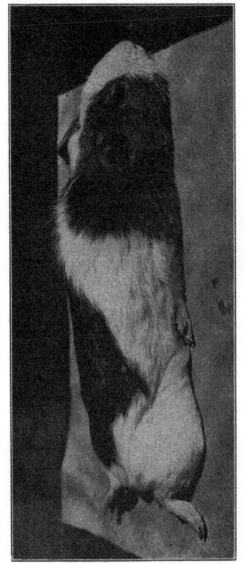

Fig. 21, Bulletin 207, Kentucky Experiment Station

broth culture but following the ingestion of 3 c.c. broth culture disguised in wholesome feed death occurred in 48 hours. The serum-treated horses, Nos. 1002, 1003 and 1004, remained apparently healthy and were released after 30 days' observation.

From the stomach of mule No. 105 an anaerobic organism resembling *B. botulinus* was regained which proved fatal when ingested by guinea pigs. In preliminary tests 0.5 c.c. of broth cul-

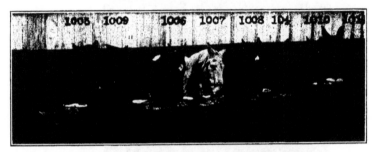

Fig. 22, Bulletin 207, Kentucky Experiment Station

ture was administered by the mouth to a guinea pig at 9:30 a. m. on March 30, 1917, resulting in death on March 31st at 3 p. m. Fig. 21 illustrates the prostrate condition of the animal 20 hours following the artificial infection per os.

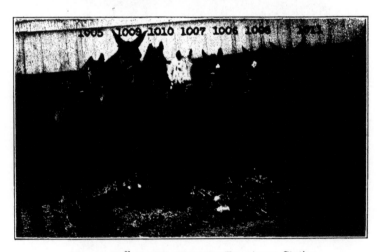

Fig. 24, Bulletin 207, Kentucky Experiment Station

To observe the effect of the sterile culture filtrate of the organism isolated from the cecum of horse No. 91 and its serological relation to *B. botulinus*, horses Nos. 1005, 1006, 1007, 1008, 1009, 1010 and 1011 were injected with botulism antitoxin and allowed to consume 2 c.c. of the filtered broth culture of the organism isolated from horse No. 91 in 1000 grams of wholesome oats 25 hours later.

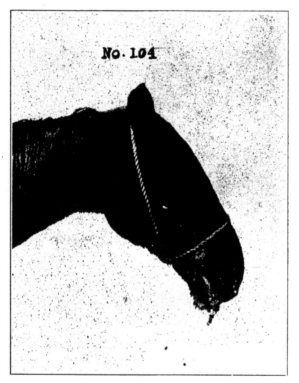

Fig. 23, Bulletin 207, Kentucky Experiment Station

Horse No. 104 received the same amount of the filtrate in feed simultaneously but was not injected with serum. Fig. 24 includes the same animals 7 days later, showing control in a moribund condition.

Control No. 104 4 days after ingesting 2 c.c. of the sterile broth filtrate, showed marked salivation and paralysis of the pharynx. (Fig. 23.) The symptoms in this animal were suddenly manifest, developing rapidly after the fourth day. Death occurred 7 days following the ingestion of the filtrate. The serum-treated horses remained healthy and were released in 30 days.

From water in which the oat hay was immersed a similar pathogenic organism resembling *B. botulinus* was isolated and to determine its relation, if any, to *B. botulinus,* tests were made upon guinea pigs. Three pigs received intraperitoneally varying amounts of sheep serum immune to *B. botulinus,* followed in 24 hours by 0.1 c.c. per os of the broth culture of the organism isolated directly

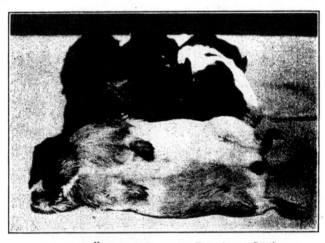

Fig. 26, Bulletin 207, Kentucky Experiment Station

from the oat hay water. The pigs receiving serum remained healthy, while the control pig succumbed in approximately 40 hours.

The protective quality of cow serum immune to *B. botulinus* was also observed by injecting three pigs intraperitoneally with varying amounts of serum, followed in 24 hours by an artificial infection per os of 0.1 c.c. of the organism isolated from the oat hay. (Fig. 26.) The serum-treated pigs remained healthy, while the control pig receiving the same amount of the broth culture by the mouth succumbed in approximately 18 hours.

Horse No. 1012 was given a prophylactic injection of serum immune to *B. botulinus* on March 20th. Horses Nos. 107, 112 and 1012 received 2 c.c. broth culture of the organism isolated from the oat hay March 21st. (Fig. 27.)

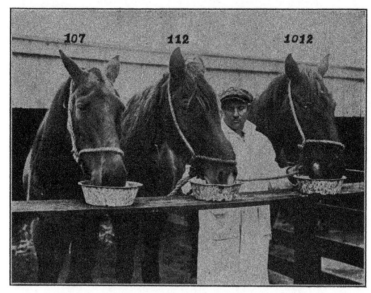

Fig. 27, Bulletin 207, Kentucky Experiment Station

On March 25th horse No. 107 was dull and stupid, with a noticeable impairment of the organs of deglutition. See Fig. 28. During the course of illness this animal salivated profusely. Mus-

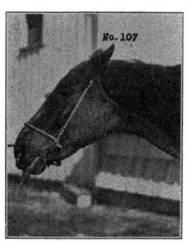

Fig. 28, Bulletin 207, Kentucky Experiment Station

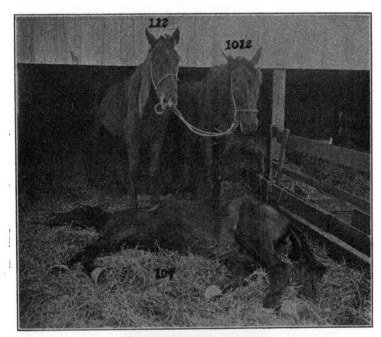

Fig. 30, Bulletin 207, Kentucky Experiment Station

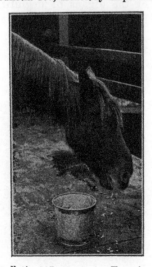

Fig. 31, Bulletin 207, Kentucky Experiment Station

cular weakness developed rapidly following the symptoms displayed on March 25th and the animal became permanently decumbent. Death occurred in No. 107 during the night of March
27th. Horses Nos. 112 and 1012 appeared normal. See Fig. 30.

Horse No. 112 showed no discomfort until March 30th, at
which time the feed was prehended slowly and with some difficulty,
though the appetite was apparently not impaired. Attempts to
drink were continuous but the water was returned through the nasal
passages. Corn was prehended, masticated and dropped upon the
ground. See Fig. 31. The symptoms continued and were possibly
augmented from this date, accompanied by marasmus.

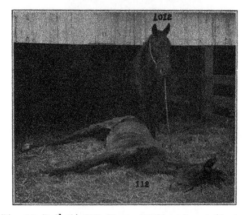

Fig. 32, Bulletin 207, Kentucky Experiment Station

On April 5th the animal (No. 112) became permanently decumbent and death occurred during the night. See Fig. 32. On
April 6th horse No. 1012 was to all appearances normal, though
on March 30th a transitory reaction was observed, at which time
antitoxic serum was administered. The manifestations soon subsided and the animal remained apparently normal and was released on April 30th.

Horses Nos. 1013, 1014, 1015 and 1016 received an injection of
botulism antitoxin on March 27th, and on March 28th, together
with untreated horses Nos. 109, 110 and 114 (See Fig. 33) were
each given 1000 grams of wholesome oats in which were mixed 2 c.c.
of the filtered broth culture of the organism isolated from the poisonous oats. Control horses Nos. 109, 110 and 114 all succumbed;

No. 109 died on March 31st, No. 110 on April 2nd, and No. 114 on April 7th.

The four serum-treated horses similarly infected and receiv-

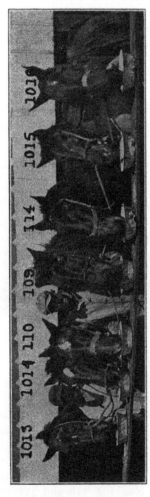

Fig. 33, Bulletin 207, Kentucky Experiment Station

ing portions of the same wholesome feed displayed no symptoms and were released after 30 days. See Fig. 34.

Following a sporadic outbreak of forage poisoning in mules in Carroll County, Kentucky, a corn ensilage was proved by feed-

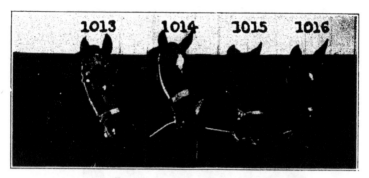

Fig. 34, Bulletin 207, Kentucky Experiment Station

ing tests to incorporate the causative factor of the disease. From the ensilage in question an anaerobic, Gram positive bacillus which in cultural and morphological characters seemed closely allied to *B. botulinus* (See Figs. 1 and 2) was isolated. In animal experiments it proved capable of engendering clinical forage poisoning in experimental horses and mules subsequent to ingestion of 2 c.c.

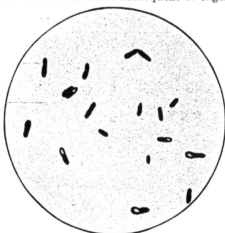

Fig. 1, Bulletin 208, Ky. Exp. Sta.

of the broth culture or the sterile filtrate of the broth culture, while .02 c.c. of the broth culture per os proved fatal to guinea pigs in 24 to 36 hours.

The apparent likeness of this organism to *B. botulinus* prompted the injection of animals with serum immune to *B. botu-*

linus, followed by artificial infection of the organism from the silage.

Three mature guinea pigs were given intraperitoneally on May 12, 1917, varying amounts of goat serum immune to *B. botu-*

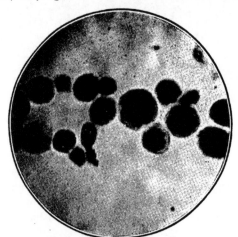

Fig. 2, Bulletin 208, Ky. Exp. Sta.

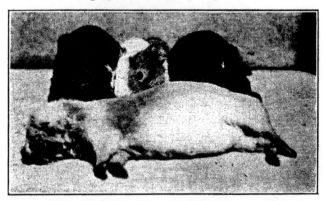

Fig. 3, Bulletin 208, Kentucky Experiment Station

*linus** and 24 hours later these animals received per os 0.1 c.c. broth culture of the organisms from the silage. A control **pig** receiving the same amount of broth culture but no serum died in 48 hours. (See Fig. 3.) The serum treated pigs remained healthy.

*N. B. S. Strain from Dr. Buckley, Washington, D. C.

The apparent serological relation of serum immune to *B. botulinus** to the filtered broth culture of the organism from the ensilage was observed in similar tests, wherein guinea pigs were apparently protected by intraperitoneal injection of the serum against

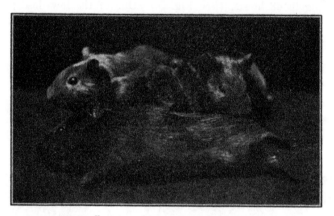

Fig. 4, Bulletin 208, Kentucky Experiment Station

an amount of the filtrate given by the mouth sufficient to cause death in a control pig in 3 days. Fig. 4 depicts the results of the filtered broth culture in an untreated pig while the serum pigs remained healthy.

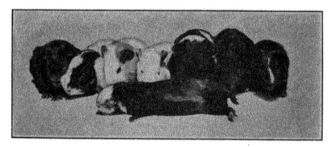

Fig. 5, Bulletin 208, Kentucky Experiment Station

The apparent protective quality in guinea pigs of serum immune to *B. botulinus** against the organism from the ensilage was followed by injecting serum immune to the organism from the ensilage into guinea pigs followed by a fatal amount of *B. botulinus.**

*N. B. S. Strain from Dr. Buckley, Washington, D. C.

Intraperitoneal injection of varying amounts of serum immune to the organism from the ensilage apparently protected guinea pigs against an amount of the unfiltered broth culture of *B. botulinus* given by the mouth which caused death in an unprotected pig in 48 hours. (See Fig. 5.) One of the low dose pigs, however, died in nine days after receiving the serum. The remaining serum-treated pigs remained apparently healthy.

The apparent protection afforded in guinea pigs against the organism from the silage by injecting serum immune to *B. botulinus* was followed by similar trials in horses.

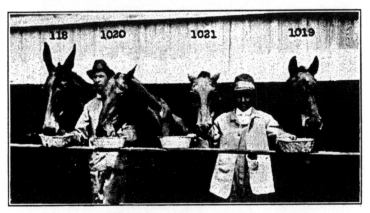

Fig. 6, Bulletin 208, Kentucky Experiment Station

Horses Nos. 1019, 1020, 1021, received an intravenous injection of botulism antitoxin on May 15, 1917. On May 16th these horses and an untreated mule, No. 118, were each fed 2 c.c. of the broth culture of the organism from the ensilage mixed with 1000 grams of wholesome oats. The animals were then allowed wholesome feed and water.

On the morning of May 17th No. 118 ate only a portion of the grain ration, while the three horses injected with serum appeared normal. At 10 a. m. No. 118 fell and could not regain a standing position.

At 3:45 p. m. the plate for Fig. 7 was made. No. 118 died at 3:30 p. m. The tongue was paralyzed and protruding from the mouth.

Post mortem examination showed gross lesions similar to those observed in animals naturally afflicted with forage poisoning.

From the preliminary studies, as extracted from bulletins 207-208 of the Kentucky Station, the writers are inclined to the belief that certain types of forage poisoning may result from the ingestion of feed contaminated with microorganisms resembling *B. botulinus*. The experimental results obtained by injecting animals with serum highly immune to *B. botulinus* as well as serum highly immune to organisms resembling *B. botulinus* isolated from poisonous forages followed by a fatal infection of *B. botulinus* or of the organisms closely resembling *B. botulinus* are suggestive of the possible value of serum in natural outbreaks of this disease.

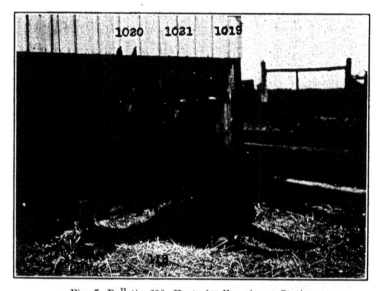

Fig. 7, Bulletin 208, Kentucky Experiment Station

It is not assumed that forage poisoning in all its phases result from infections of this type but the occurrence on forage of organisms resembling *B. botulinus* which, upon being artificially propagated in the laboratory have proven capable of engendering clinical forage poisoning in horses subsequent to ingestion, is regarded as contributive to our knowledge of the etiology of this disease. Supportive of this contention is the cultivation of *B. botulinus* and organisms resembling *B. botulinus* in forage extracts. The experimental evidence presented is supportive of the theory originally advanced by Dr. Leonard A. Pearson, while at the meeting of the

American Veterinary Medical Association in 1916 Drs. Buckley and Shippen pointed out the likeness of *B. botulinus* intoxication artificially induced in horses to sporadic forage poisoning.

———◆———

DISCUSSION

DR. EICHHORN: The so-called forage poisoning is a disease of considerable importance and the work of Dr. Graham plainly indicates that great steps have been made towards shedding light on the nature of the disease which up to date has baffled veterinarians. As Dr. Graham has pointed out, the work carried out by Drs. Buckley and Shippen has demonstrated that the *Bacillus botulinus* possesses pathogenic properties for horses and furthermore that the *Bacillus botulinus*, and especially its toxins, has repeatedly caused death of horses even when fed in small doses.

The symptoms manifested by animals artificially infected with the *Bacillus botulinus* or its toxins somewhat resemble those of forage poisoning. The inauguration of this work by Drs. Buckley and Shippen was undertaken under my direction and I followed it with the greatest interest since even initial investigations appeared to have established a relation between forage poisoning and botulinus intoxication. Not only cultures of these organisms but also the toxins alone when fed even in very small quantities to horses produced symptoms of forage poisoning. The remarkable feature in these experiments appeared to be that the feeding of only very minute doses of the toxins were required to produce symptoms to a condition which closely resembled forage poisoning.

Subsequent experiments have established that droppings collected from chickens after feeding them with cultures of the *Bacillus botulinus* have also repeatedly produced death in horses with symptoms of forage poisoning. These findings probably elucidated the experimental work which was previously reported by Dr. Graham on forage poisoning in which he found that chicken droppings contained in oats were responsible for losses in horses with forage poisoning. The work now reported by Dr. Graham has further advanced our knowledge on the etiology of the disease and has given us a definite knowledge on the causative agent of the disease. Besides, he even went further and demonstrated that a disease which in all particulars resembles forage poisoning may be successfully combated by protective immunization. As no doubt most of you know the *Bacillus botulinus* has been and is known as the organism causing sausage or meat poisoning and in the early work with this organism a serum.was developed for the treatment of this infection in human beings. No doubt, however, credit is due to Dr. Graham for furthering and developing it with regard to its application for animals. Besides such serum might possess great curative value for animals infected with forage poisoning.

There is only one more word. While these important factors have been established by him experimentally it will be of interest to undertake immediately further investigations along this line in order to establish whether actual outbreaks of forage poisoning occurring under natural conditions are caused by botulinus infection and whether the losses sustained from this disease are due to botulinus intoxication. It appears to me that this is the case but no doubt further work is required to establish it beyond a doubt.

DR. GOSS: The work of Dr. Graham is very interesting and shows quite conclusively that the forage poisoning with which he came in contact in Kentucky was due to the *Bacillus botulinus*. I have observed the different forms of diseases which have been called forage poisoning and have followed them carefully during the horse plague in Western Kansas and Nebraska. It has occurred in other places. There seem to have been more or less characteristic lesions in the brains of the horses. I did not get the symptoms as shown in this disease in Kentucky. There was usually a rise of temperature before the symptoms developed, more or less jerking, fall of temperature and increasing paralysis. On examining the brain, we found certain infiltrations which seemed to be quite characteristic of that particular disease. In some respects it was similar to Borna's disease, as described as existing in Europe, but there seems to be a different cause. We were unable to find intracellular or intramolecular bodies.

We have throughout the greater portion of the United States, or through the corn belt, the disease forage poisoning, which occurs where horses are allowed to eat quantities of moldy corn. In these cases we find large softened areas within the brain; the softened area nearly always occurs in the cerebrum; it may be on either side, or on both sides, and those cases are quite typical. The losses are very high indeed where we have had a bad visitation in a particular season.

There is a form of this disease where the fatality is quite high. The symptoms to all appearances are quite similar to those described by Dr. Graham. On examination of the brains of these animals no pathological changes are found, except indications of fatigue. In another instance, the animals did not show any increase in temperature, their temperatures were so normal that they were sleepy, and with paralysis, the tongue would hang out. The temperature would gradually go lower and lower until death resulted in the course of about 48 hours.

In another epidemic the animal showed symptoms more or less characteristic of influenza, and it had been diagnosed as influenza. The animals were eating fodder which was exceedingly moldy. The temperatures were high at first, and continued high, in this instance around 106 degrees; the heart beat was exceedingly rapid, and very weak, almost imperceptible, and nearly all the animals died within 48 hours. Unfortunately I did not get a post mortem on any of them. They were fed upon alfalfa, which looked quite good, but it had a peculiar odor, a sort of tobacco odor. That man lost about six horses. Out of eight or ten which were affected there were only three or four recoveries. We took some of the alfalfa to the laboratory and fed part of it to eight guinea pigs, and six out of the eight died. Further work was done in isolating the organism and we succeeded in isolating quite a number of organisms. This was done sometime ago before this work came out on *B. botulinus.* There is a possibility of an anaerobic, and I am wondering if it is a different form of anaerobic than the one found in Kentucky. In my observations there were only four forms of disease which were caused by feeding forage. The symptoms may be different but Dr. Graham's work will encourage, I think, further work along the line of isolating anaerobics, and it may be we do not do enough work in isolating organisms, as it is out of the ordinary technique of some laboratories.

DR. AMLING: There is no question in my mind that the condition is analogous to what we have in the East. I have had considerable experience and I find the same conditions from products eaten by animals and humans and in 99 out of 100 cases I say the conditions are due to fungi and poisons in the food.

I recall one case in particular—I know of several—that I had last summer. There was a poultry market where they bring in the poultry from the different markets, and keep and feed them for a few days. Across the street from a poultry market was a tumble down shack in which several people lived. The children would play about the gate and poultry plant. I found poultry showing conditions of paralysis. A little girl was stricken with disease and died a day or two afterward. I found a typical case of poliomyelitis in the poultry owner's horse which I was called to treat. I was associated, and am at the present time, with a gentleman named R. F. Hof, whom I consider one of the best bacteriologists and microscopists in the country, and he in each and every case has found these same bacilli, also micrococci and bacteria. These conditions passed along from one child to another. They all lead to the same termination—death in many cases. I do not suppose there was ever a time when we had the amount of fungi, molds, etc., that existed at that time all through the East. The cherries and berries could hardly be used; they were brought to the market on Friday or Saturday and by Monday, and in many cases in 2 hours, developed this mold. The merchants and producers all suffered severe losses because people would not buy. Berries would be bought in the afternoon or evening, placed in refrigeration, and probably served to a child the following morning with milk and sugar, which is a culture medium. The children were playing in the street, and there were changes in the atmospheric conditions, fogs, and variations of temperature many times of 40 degrees within ten hours. The children were perfectly healthy in the evening and the next morning after eating some of the berries they would appear to be afflicted with paralysis. There were intestinal troubles. There were gastric conditions and pains in head and cervical region (superior) and sudden death. There were many cases of inflation of the intestinal tract or stomach. In many of those cases a physician would be called, and a great many times he would diagnose it as a case of pneumonia. The distension of the abdomen and the pressure on the diaphragm minus temperature and the lower portion of the bronchial organs, caused a certain sound on account of the air retained there. The inhalation was probably free, and the exhalation probably arrested, causing pulmonary rales due to pressure on diaphragm due to gastric inflation, etc., which caused them to diagnose a condition of pneumonia, when pneumonia was not present. In many cases there was a lesion in the pulmonary tract (and pneumogastric). It was natural to find lesions there on account of the improper circulation of the air. These conditions I have found and have seen for many years. Most of these cases, to my mind, are brought about by various fungi, and a close and careful examination will usually find the cause.

Not many years ago I was called to several stock farms. There were quite a number of hogs, cattle, especially cows and their calves affected, and the first thing I did was to go over the ground. I found a lot of grain which I think was composed of kiln dried matter. It was supposed to be used in fattening cattle to kill, some to increase the milk supply, and the entire mass was impregnated with a dry fungus.

Another condition existed in a herd of very high grade Holsteins, some of the best in this country. A man lost several calves, and he sent the various parts of the organs down to us to examine. We found one and the same conditions in all of them, and the consequence was we investigated the feed and found the same fungi, also the bacteria, bacilli and micrococci always found present in the same condition. They had an enclosed space out in the country and were feeding, at that time, on fungus alfalfa, which I consider one of the most dangerous feeds for live stock. I do not know of any feed outside of corn that contains as many fungi as the alfalfa does, and takes as many of the elements out of the soil.

In another instance, we found on many farms a grade of bran which was supposed to be the very best grade that could be purchased. We found peanut shells ground up in it to increase the weight. Somebody was evidently making a large profit and in that peanut bran we found the same fungi.

Another instance, there was an infection among dogs some years ago. I found it in performing dogs which had eaten certain biscuits. The profession has not given sufficient attention to the question of feeds. The owner lost four or five dogs in probably 24 hours, and during the same time there were as many more paralyzed. When the owner got down through New England around Meriden three of them died in three hours. The veterinarians did all they could. The dogs were sent to Harvard, and no lesions whatever were found. The first thing I did was to look over the biscuit, and I found the same mold or fungus. I changed their diet and the condition was immediately removed. On two occasions there was a slight attack in the same group with the result that the owner had to purchase food at random when the supply gave out. In both instances the trouble was corrected by immediate correction of the diet and application of an intestinal antiseptic immediately administered. I kept them supplied for just such emergencies.

Dr. A. H. BAKER: I am particularly interested in this matter on account of the reference to the horses which died at Ottawa, Ill. Conditions surrounding that case were investigated by a scientist. It was at my suggestion that the scientist at the State University was called in. I recognized, when I was called there in consultation with a local practitioner, that we had cases of forage poisoning. Before I arrived five or six horses had died, and they all died with the symptoms that Dr. Graham described. The first symptom developed was pharyngeal paralysis, and the other conditions, including the recumbent position, in which the horse was unable to rise, and death in from 48 to 72 hours. We found on investigation that the owner had just started to feed from silos. The upper portion, a foot deep of that silo, was pretty moldy, he knew it was not fit for food and took it out, an l when it was dry he hated to throw it away, so he used it for bedding his horses, instead of bedding with straw, and to his surprise the horses ate this stuff. In the course of 24 to 48 hours they developed symptoms, showing a temperature and died in 2 or 3 days.

On investigation the scientists of the State University bought some old horses and fed this same stuff to them; the same symptoms developed and death ensued. They concluded that the moldy ensilage was the cause of the forage poisoning. In this connection we all know that some molds are harmless, while some molds are very fatal. I would like to suggest to Dr. Graham, now that he has started on this forage poison investigation, that he give us the result of a little further investigation, and enable us, if possible, to differentiate between poisonous and non-poisonous molds. It appeals to me particularly, because I believe forage poisoning is a very difficult problem for the practitioners to deal with.

Dr. Graham: The outbreak of forage poisoning at Ottawa, Illinois, referred to by Dr. Baker, was investigated by Professor H. P. Rusk and Dr. H. S. Grindley of the University of Illinois. If I an correctly advised, by a series of feeding experiments they were able to prove quite conclusively that the silage contained the etiologic factor in the outbreak which occurred on Mr. Alexander McLean's farm near Ottawa, Illinois. Feeding experiments that had been outlined and conducted during the summer months of last year were incomplete when it came time to refill the silo. The contaminated silage was covered with fresh silage. Separating the contaminated silage from the fresh silage was a layer of oil cloth. The new silage was fed by the owner with apparently satisfactory results. After removing the oil cloth covering, the contaminated silage was used in further feeding experiments conducted by Professor Rusk and Dr. Grindley during the past few months, at which time it was shown to possess its original toxic properties, and fatal results were consistently obtained in horses that were allowed liberal amounts of this feed.

Several horses in these tests were given anti-serum while three or four controls or untreated horses receiving similar rations succumbed after manifesting typical symptoms of forage poisoning. The results of their studies have not as yet been published, but from correspondence and first-hand observations during the course of the experiments it seems that the horses receiving serum were protected from the poisonous effect of the silage.

Replying to the question presented by Dr. Goss relative to the presence of gross lesions noted in the cerebrum of experimental horses, I might say that upon autopsy observations indicate the large areas of degeneration, or rather disintegration, to which Dr. Goss refers, are rarely present, at least not consistently so in our observations to date. The temperature of affected animals as a rule is not elevated. Numerous recorded temperatures of animals suffering from the disease, both naturally and artificially, indicate that some may show a high temperature while a larger number show a normal or sub-normal temperature.

. The relation of pathogenic molds to this disease have not been overlooked in our investigations but on the other hand numerous attempts have been made to determine the pathogenic properties of certain species of these organisms found upon animal feeds. The results obtained from time to time in this connection quite agree with the observations by different investigators relative to the role of the common molds in forage poisoning. It may be, however, that certain molds or other non-pathogenic organisms may be involved secondarily. In fact, laboratory experiments seem to confirm such a supposition, providing *B. botulinus* may be incriminated as the common etiologic factor in this disease. The occurrence of *B. botulinus* upon forage is apparently not indicated by the presence of molds yet it is possible that certain molds may favor the field for its growth and development. *B. botulinus*, in the presence of certain molds, will grow under aerobic conditions or even in distinctly acid medium, two cultural conditions which are not favorable to the development of *B. botulinus* independently. The modification brought about by secondary organisms in association suggests a symbiotic relation and there is little doubt that other saprophytic organisms as cited by Van Ermengem, Buckley, and Shippen, may create conditions favorable for the development of *B. botulinus* in nature, accompanied by the production of its specific toxin.

———◆———

SHEEP PESTS, PARASITIC AND PREDACIOUS*

B. M. UNDERHILL, V.M.D., University of Pennsylvania, Philadelphia, Pa.

It is said of sheep that they have ever been in the vanguard of civilization. As to this the history of the sheep industry in our own country affords an example. Moving constantly westward with the attraction to newer and cheaper lands, it came to occupy increasing areas of western range country until it seemed that wool and mutton production in any considerable scale belonged to the far-west. However true this may have been under past conditions, the decreasing extent of the ranges by their constantly increasing occupation has brought about a new era upon which must follow a more intensive system of animal husbandry. Under such a system sheep and wool production takes its place upon the higher priced land of the small farm where, with improved stock, better care, increased productiveness, and the attractive prices of an unsupplied demand, it should prove a profitable branch of farm industry. In certain localities this is already in evidence. The serious shortage in the supply of wool and mutton is not likely to be relieved, however, until familiarity with sheep and methods of caring for them becomes more general and certain elements of discouragement to the industry are eliminated or placed under more effectual control.

Reference to the 1915 report of the Pennsylvania Department of Agriculture will show the estimated number of sheep in Pennsylvania for that year to be 806,000, having an approximate total

*Presented at the annual meeting of the Pennsylvania State Veterinary Medical Association, Harrisburg, Pa., January, 1918.

value of $4,352,400.00. This estimate would indicate a decrease of
30% from the estimated number of sheep in the state ten years
earlier, there seeming to be a decline of about 3% per year.

The contribution of Pennsylvania to the present shortage of
American grown wool, as shown by the above figures, may be due
mainly to the lack of appreciation of sheep husbandry as a profitable branch of live stock industry. Two other factors, however,
weigh heavily as a contributing cause, if they do not in themselves
constitute the main one. These are the susceptibility of sheep to
parasites and the losses by death and injury from dogs. Both have
been besetting causes of discouragement to flock owners, dogs contributing to the pillage not only in a predatory sense but, in a less
degree, as carriers and disseminators of certain of the parasites
with which sheep are invaded.

The losses from the ravaging of flocks by dogs progressively
increases with increased density of human, and consequently of
canine, population. Pennsylvania, with its numerous towns and
industrial centers, has its concomitant quota of dogs, and this has
caused the dog problem as it relates to sheep to be peculiarly applicable to this state. Data compiled by the Bureau of Statistics
of the Pennsylvania Department of Agriculture relative to the
extent of this damage for the year 1914 set forth among other
summaries the following:

Total number of sheep killed................   5,187
Total number of sheep injured.............   3,813
Amount paid for sheep killed and injured....$ 46,640.70
Amount of dog tax collected................   147,815.88

These losses in killed and injured do not, however, represent
the entire damage. A flock once attacked becomes restless, excitable,
and for weeks afterward will rush about and become on the alert at
slight and harmless intrusions to which they would ordinarily give
no attention. The check in the normal gain of the flock from this
cause may be considerable and constitutes a loss for which the owner
is not reimbursed. A good sentinel against unwelcome intruders is
the sheep dog of America, the Scotch collie. This can be appreciated
by anyone who has seen a well-trained one at work; going about his
duties quietly, aggressively challenging any trespassing cur, and at
night warning the herdsman of lurking prowlers by his bark. A
poorly trained and bad-mannered collie, however, is worse than a
nuisance and should be classed with the common pack of sheep

damaging dogs. It is generally known that dogs that are well cared
for, both through their restraint and a certain lack of inclination,
are not likely to attack sheep. It is the unrestricted prowler, reverting in his night rovings to the predatory instincts of the wolf,
that is the offender, either alone or encouraged by a pack of similar
sneaking marauders. Such dogs should be hunted and destroyed as
are any other plundering wild beasts.

But let us hope that we are now at the dawn of a brighter day
for the sheep industry in Pennsylvania. On the fifteenth of this
January there went into effect an enactment of the last session of the
legislature which should pass the dog back into history as a serious
obstructor. In its main features this law provides that on or before
the fifteenth day of January of each year every owner of a dog
shall obtain a license with which there will be issued a metal tag to
be worn by the dog at all times. Between sunset and sunrise of each
day dogs are to be confined in such manner that they cannot stray
beyond the premises on which they are secured, unless under the
reasonable control of some person. A dog seen in the act of pursu-
ing, worrying or wounding any live stock, or attacking human beings, whether or not the dog bears the license tag, may be killed by
any person, and there shall be no liability on such person in damages
or otherwise for such killing. Under the duties of police officers in
the enforcement of this law it is stated that it shall be the duty of
every police officer to detain any dog or dogs which bear a proper
license tag and which are found running at large and unaccompanied by owner or keeper. For failure to perform his duty under
the provisions of this act, such police officer shall be liable to a pen-
alty of $2.00 for each offense. For the performance of this duty he
shall be paid the sum of $1.00 for detaining a licensed dog and the
sum of $1.00 for the killing of a dog. Any person violating or fail-
ing or refusing to comply with any of the provisions of this act shall
be guilty of a misdemeanor and, upon conviction, shall be sentenced
to pay a fine not exceeding $100.00 or to undergo an imprisonment
not exceeding three months, at the discretion of the court.

In these and in its further provisions we now seem to have a
dog law with teeth, let us trust that they will be equal to the canines
and carnassials of the carnivorous culprits. Be this as it may, its
effectiveness will depend upon the interest of citizens in seeing to
it that the law is enforced.

Clinical and laboratory experience has shown that sheep suffer more from parasitic diseases than from those caused by bacteria. With other herbivorous animals they share hostage to the larval stage of certain of the numerous intestinal parasites of carnivora to which infection their habit of grazing close to the ground perhaps has an exposing influence. Furthermore, their dense fleece and tender skin affords an attractive harbor for the sustenance and propagation of the mites and ticks with which they are externally beset.

Observed parasitism of sheep may exist in one or two individuals; more often it involves most or quite all of the flock, or the infestation may be of an enzootic or even an epizootic nature. From the viewpoint of the most prevalent form in which the problem presents itself, measures looking to the prevention of the spread of the parasitism from animal to animal in a flock and from flock to flock in a sheep-raising district are of prime importance. Treatment for the expulsion of the parasites from infested individuals is essential as preventing direct loss by death and by decrease in the productiveness of the animals. Furthermore, an animal which may have been thus completely rid of the specific parasite and its eggs will, of course, cease to be a menace to the flock from this source as long as the freedom lasts. Obviously, however, the danger of reinfection and spread are not removed by this treatment unless it is supplemented by measures applied to the parasite external to the sheep host, for the effectual carrying out of which a knowledge of the life history is essential. Unfortunately this life history is not completely known as to certain malignant roundworm species infesting sheep, though enough has already been determined upon which to base in most cases decidedly effectual procedures of control. It has somewhere been stated that it may be taken as an axiom in helminthology that each worm in the body develops from an egg or larva which has entered from without. Worms, unlike bacteria, do not go on multiplying indefinitely with the production of new adult generations in the same host. It follows, then, that preventive measures dealing with parasitism should be based upon the life history of the species to which such measures are applied. Where this is known wholly or in part and such knowledge intelligently taken advantage of, the problem of eradication or control becomes much easier of solution than it otherwise would be.

A case in point pertains to a parasite of sheep and other ruminating animals, the common liver fluke, *Fasciola hepatica*. It has been stated that previous to the working out of the life history of the fluke the loss in England from hepatic fascioliasis was for a time in the neighborhood of 3,000,000 head of sheep annually. The determination of the essential alternation of the fluke's parasitism between the sheep and snail host pointed the way for measures of control, consisting mainly in the elimination of snails by the elimination by drainage of places which harbored them, or in the limiting of the sheep to pastures free from standing water or overflow. Since the application of these simple preventive measures the loss from fascioliasis in England and other European countries has been greatly reduced. Apparently flukes have not been as prevalent among American sheep flocks as among those of Europe. To what extent this may be due to their being overlooked or to failure to report such cases cannot be determined, but it is probably true that whatever degree of actual immunity we enjoy from this pest may be largely accounted for in the fact that it has generally been the practice in this country to pasture sheep upon elevated and dry land rather than upon that which is low and marshy. There are, however, a sufficient number of cases of record to demonstrate the probability of fascioliasis becoming more prevalent with the growth of the sheep industry in the United States. There is, in fact, the possibility of its assuming in future years proportions of vastly greater economic importance than at present—even the dimensions of a ravaging plague—unless we are on the lookout for it and, where it appears, apply such measures as are indicated by the life history of the parasite.

The more serious symptoms in fascioliasis are usually among the lambs. Animals harboring but few flukes will give no evidence of functional disturbance, as has been demonstrated in slaughtering establishments where moderately infested livers have been repeatedly found in sheep in prime condition. In heavier infestations there is usually dullness, slow movement, and an inclination to lag behind the flock. Anemia is revealed in the paleness of the conjunctival mucosa, and there may be edematous swelling of the eyelids and perhaps of the brisket. Notwithstanding this the physical condition may remain good and, in fact there may be a tendency to fatten. Later, however, the symptoms become more aggravated, there is more edema in the dependent parts, the puffy conjunctiva forming a prominent ring around the cornea. With progressively diminished appetite there is loss of flesh, and, with the development of ascites, labored respiration, and diarrhea, the disease is at its maximum, usually reached about the third month after infestation.

Other flatworms infesting sheep belong with the family Taeniidae or tapeworms. In animals which do not eat flesh infestation with adult tapeworms is comparatively uncommon, and in no such case is the life history of the infesting species known. Of the domesticated herbivorous animals probably sheep most frequently harbor these worms, infestations being most prevalent in the flocks of our far western states. A species which seems to be peculiar to sheep among our domestic animals is *Thysanosoma actinioides* (*Taenia fimbriata*) which is readily distinguished by the long fringes on the posterior borders of the segments. Other species occurring in sheep and also in cattle are *Moniezia expansa, M. alba,* and *M. planissima.* These when fully developed vary in length from three to twenty feet or more according to species. In all the segments are much broader than long, and in all the cephalic armature of hooks is absent. As nothing is known as to their cystic forms, the manner in which animals become infested remains undetermined.

Unless the tapeworms are present in unusual numbers, taeniasis does not, so far as clinical experience goes, seem to cause serious disturbance in sheep. Lambs born in the winter and turned upon grass early, when pastures are wet with the spring rains, are most likely to suffer. Where losses occur in such cases they are generally due to malnutrition and digestive disturbances in highly susceptible or heavily infested lambs, the toxins elaborated by the worms contributing considerably in bringing about the morbid condition.

During the past summer two yearling lambs—one dead, one living—were brought to our laboratory from a flock near Philadelphia, among which some losses had occurred. The carcass, on autopsy, showed anemia, marked parenchymatous degeneration of the heart muscle, liver, and kidneys, spleen normal, pronounced catarrhal enteritis, and an acute lung edema. The small intestine contained a number of tapeworms of the species *Moniezia expansa* which were unmassed, the fragments when laid out having a total measurement of about one hundred feet. During the two days which the other animal lived it was very drowsy, refused feed and did not ruminate. The temperature and pulse were taken once, there, as recorded, being 104.4°F. and 150, respectively. Autopsy showed similar lesions to those of the first animal, the intestine containing tapeworms of the same species yielding a total length of about ninety feet.

Relative to toxins produced by intestinal worms, it is probably true that the effect upon the host does not necessarily depend upon the number of parasites present. The degree of virulence may vary with particular infestations, and, furthermore, there are undoubtedly cases of peculiar susceptibility, especially among young animals. It may be added in this connection that, as research workers in this field bring additions to our knowledge of the parasites and their pathogenic possibilities, evidences are being brought forth which point to the probability that certain verminous parasites, heretofore considered relatively harmless, are not so innocent as had been supposed and may be the primary offenders in certain conditions now assigned to other somewhat obscure causes.

Of the roundworms infesting sheep but two can be briefly reviewed within the present limits. Of these *Haemonchus contortus,* the species most commonly causing gastro-intestinal strongylosis, is probably responsible for driving more men out of the sheep business than any other adverse factor. The worm is thread-like, about three-quarters to one inch in length, and attaches to the mucosa of the fourth stomach and duodenum where it feeds upon the blood of its host. Infestations occur mostly among sheep which have access to low and marshy pasturage, young animals, as is the general rule in entoparasitism, being the greatest sufferers. Severe cases are accompanied by disorders of digestion and lead through loss of blood to pallor, dropsical conditions, and emaciation. Where a number of animals are involved any doubt as to the cause of these symptoms of a pernicious anemia may be cleared up by killing one and examining the fourth stomach. If there are heavy infestations this will reveal large numbers of the strongyles both free in the stomach's contents and deeply adhering to the mucosa, the latter showing the lesions of a subacute or chronic catarrh. It is significant as to the prevalence of the stomach worm that in sheep carcasses submitted to our laboratory for diagnosis it is the exception to find one entirely free from this parasite. It is often found in association with other parasitism, as strongylosis of the bronchi and lungs and nodular strongylosis of the large intestines, due probably to the fact that conditions which favor infestation with one are equally favorable to the other forms.

From what is already known of the life history of the stomach worm, it seems that infestation is direct, the larvae probably being taken up by the sheep with contaminated food and water. Becoming adult in the stomach, their eggs pass to the outside where they may hatch in a few hours or weeks according to more or less favorable conditions of temperature and moisture. Newly hatched larvae will not survive dryness or freezing, but if their vitality is sustained until they become surrounded by a chitinous sheath, they can then live under such conditions for a long period, and it is in this condition that they are infective. Becoming increasingly motile with a temperature rising above 40°F., and in the presence of moisture, as that from rain or dew, they make their way up the blades of grass to a position where they are readily taken up by the grazing ruminant. From the fact that the eggs and newly hatched embryos do not appear to be infective, and that dryness kills them before they reach their ensheathed or infective stage, it follows that the use of elevated pasturage with good natural drainage greatly reduces the chances of re-infestations. Systems of pasture rotation as a method of control are based upon the varying periods of time required for the newly hatched embryos to reach the infective stage under different mean degrees of temperature. At a constant temperature of about 95°F. this stage is reached in three to four days after the eggs have been passed. At 70° one or two weeks are required, while three to four weeks are necessary at about 50°. At temperatures below 40° the eggs will not hatch and larvae which may have reached ensheathment are inactive.

Under the usual climatic conditions of the northern part of the United States from November to March we are not apt to have a continuous temperature of over 40° for three weeks. There is, therefore, little chance of new infection from placing infected and noninfected animals together in clean lots or fields during this time. Based upon these findings, Ransom recommends a system of pasture rotation which is probably a very effective measure for the eradication of this parasite, although it involves considerable inconvenience. By this method animals which have been kept together from November through the winter, if removed in April to another clean field, may remain there for that month. In May the pasture is to be changed every two weeks. In June every ten days, and in July and August every week. In September the changes may be made as in June, every ten days, while in October a field may be occupied two weeks or more according to temperature. The following year the same pastures can be used in the same order of rotation, as any field which has not been visited by sheep, cattle, or goats for one year may be safely considered as free from infection.

In verminous bronchitis of sheep, due to the invasion of the bronchi by strongyles, *Dictyocaulus filaria,* a thread-like worm two to four inches in length, is in most cases the offender. Two smaller species—*Synthetocaulus rufescens* and *S. capillaris*—are responsible for deeper seated lung lesions and may co-exist in the same animal with the common invader of the larger air passages. Many cases of verminous bronchitis are complicated with gastric strongylosis. In post mortem examinations, therefore, the stomach should not be overlooked, as the stomach worms may be responsible for a proportion of the losses. The lung invasion may be light, in which case there may be no more manifestation of it than an occasional cough. In severe cases the cough is more frequent and becomes paroxysmal, a distressing dyspnea often accompanying the attack. The bronchial secretion expelled tends to be lumpy, and usually, though not always, contains the adult and embryo worms. Relative to the degree of infestation, these symptoms may pass to extreme difficulty in respiration, emaciation, pallor, edema of the larynx, muzzle and eyelids, and finally lead to the death of the animal in a state of complete prostration. The duration of such cases is influenced by the toleration of the affected animal. Very young lambs may succumb in a few days from the first observation of symptoms. Strong adults, on the other hand, are likely to gradually recover during a course of six to eight months. The majority of unfavorable cases, however, are among the lambs, and most of these will run a course of two to four months.

The lungworms deposit their eggs in the respiratory passages of their hosts, and most of the freed embryos are expelled with the bronchial secretion. Further than this little is known of their life history. It has been shown that under favorable conditions of warmth and moisture they molt at least twice, after which they retain their cuticular covering and in this condition may resist drying for a considerable period. It is probable that these larvae find their way to the sheep host with wet grass or with water from shallow collections upon the pastures. That infection cannot occur directly from animal to animal has been shown by Leuckart, Herms and Freeborn, and others, who were not successful in bringing it about by the introduction into the respiratory passages and stomach of bronchial mucus containing numerous embryos.

Prescribed limits will not permit even mention here of other internal and external parasites responsible for considerable losses among our flocks. But this whole subject of conditions adverse to the sheep industry has at the present time a side of broader importance than the purely economic one. It is stated that more than the entire wool production of the United States will be required for our armies. Relative to this the following figures are significant: in 1917 the wool crop of this country was 285,573,000 pounds, a decline of 4,619,000 pounds from that of 1914, and of 35,789,750 pounds from the crop of 1910. This in the face of the fact that from 1914 to 1916 there was a progressive increase of 187,323,399 pounds in our consumption of wool. As every ship will be needed for the transportation of our men and supplies to the countries at war, little can be imported to supply the tremendously augmented demand for an indefinite period to come. In view of these facts further comment as to the supply and consumption and sustained prices would seem unnecessary.

As this paper is addressed to an assemblage of veterinarians, it may be fittingly concluded with a word directing thought to the extent to which the welfare of the sheep industry must depend upon you. To you must logically fall the task of protecting our flocks from their worst enemy—the parasites. The efficient discharge of this responsibility calls for close study of more recent research in both the zoological and pathological fields of parasitology and a good working general knowledge of sheep as well. Superficiality has no place in the field of comparative medicine under present intensive systems of live stock husbandry. The appreciation of this by veterinary educators is indicated in the greater attention to the biological fundamentals and the bringing up of our courses to meet changing and more complex demands. Modern education in this branch of medicine requires that the student be fitted to intelligently co-operate with the advanced work of state and federal live stock sanitary organization, that he may so put his thought and training into action as to be an indispensable unit of service to his community in the eradication of such conditions as have caused the sheep industry to be almost completely abandoned in certain parts of the United States.

HORSE STRONGYLES IN CANADA

B. H. Ransom, Chief of the Zoological Division, Bureau of Animal Industry,
U. S. Department of Agriculture, and S. Hadwen, Pathologist, Health
of Animals Branch, Canadian Department of Agriculture

During the summer of 1917 a cooperative investigation of the disease of horses known as infectious anemia or swamp fever was undertaken by the Health of Animals Branch, Department of Agriculture, Dominion of Canada, and the Bureau of Animal Industry, U. S. Department of Agriculture. In this investigation a trip was made into the Province of Saskatchewan by one of the present writers (S. H.) and localities in other provinces were also visited. Besides data relating to swamp fever the trip yielded a quantity of interesting parasitic material from horses and it is the particular purpose of this paper to record some of the findings concerning nematodes parasitic in the large intestine. The material has been only partly worked up but sufficient has been done to give a fair idea of the species represented.

Until the appearance of the important monograph of Looss (1902) on the Sclerostomidae of horses and donkeys in Egypt knowledge of the various kinds of nematodes that occur in the intestines of horses was very imperfect. Looss showed that the strongyles parasitic in the large intestine of the horse comprise numerous forms, and described and figured nineteen distinct species representing four genera. Prior to Looss the text books recognized only two or at most three species and assigned them to a single genus, *Strongylus* or *Sclerostoma*. At the present time five genera are recognized and the number of species has been increased to twenty-six. That other species still remain to be described is quite evident to anyone who has examined in detail specimens of strongyles from the large intestine of the horse.

The genera to which the strongyles of the large intestine of the horse belong are as follows:

Strongylus Mueller, 1780 or 1784 (=*Sclerostoma* Rudolphi, 1809).

Oesophagodontus Railliet and Henry, 1902.

Triodontophorus Looss, 1902 (=*Triodontus* Looss, 1900 [not Westwood, 1845]).

Gyalocephalus Looss, 1900.

Cylicostomum Railliet and Henry, 1902 (=*Cylichnostomum* Looss, 1902'=*Cyathostomum* Molin, 1861 [not *Cyathostoma* Blanchard, 1849]).

[*Cylindropharynx* Leiper, 1911. This genus, two species of which have been described from the zebra in tropical Africa, is not yet known to be represented among the parasites of the horse.]

Very little has heretofore been published in America concerning the horse strongyles. Brief descriptions of the species found in Canada in 1917 (with the exception of the genus *Cylicostomum*) will be given in the present paper together with similar brief descriptions of the related species, not yet recorded in North America but likely to occur here. The genus *Cylicostomum* will be discussed only summarily as the Canadian material representing this genus has not been worked up in detail. In addition to a number of known species some new forms have been collected. Descriptions of these will be reserved for a future occasion.

Genus *Strongylus* Mueller, 1780 or 1784 (Type species, *S. equinus* Mueller).

Three species of this genus have thus far been recorded as parasitic in the horse and all three were collected in Canada during the summer of 1917. The adults of this genus can usually be easily distinguished because they are larger than most of the other forms that occur in the large intestine.

Species *Strongylus equinus* Mueller, 1780 or 1784.

The adults of this species measure, according to Looss, about 35 mm in length (male) and 45 to 47 mm (female). It is readily distinguished from the other two species of *Strongylus* occurring in the horse by the presence of three teeth in the base of the mouth capsule (two points on the dorsal tooth together with the two ventral teeth give the appearance of four teeth). *S. vulgaris* has one tooth and *S. edentatus* no teeth in the mouth capsule. According to Railliet (1915) immature forms of this species may be found in the pancreas and hepato-gastric ligament. Adults were collected at Lethbridge, Alberta, August 5.

Species *Strongylus edentatus* (Looss, 1900).

The adults (Looss's measurements) are 23 to 26 mm in length (male) and 33 to 36 mm (female). The absence of teeth in the base of the mouth capsule render this species easily recognizable.

Railliet (1915) states that immature stages occur in the subperito-
neal connective tissue of the right side of the body and in the testicles of cryptorchids. A male and female 25 mm and 30 mm in
length, respectively, were taken from the aorta of a horse examined
post mortem at Lethbridge, Alberta, July 5. Full grown adults
were collected at Lethbridge, August 5.

Species *Strongylus vulgaris* (Looss, 1900).

This is the smallest of the three species of *Strongylus* occurring
in the large intestine of the horse. The adult male measures 14 to
16 mm in length, the female 23 to 24 mm (Looss's measurements).
A single tooth is present in the base of the mouth capsule, but this
tooth is supplied with two prominent rounded projections so that
on casual examination there appear to be two teeth. According to

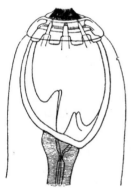

FIG. 1. *Strongylus equinus.*
From Looss (modified). X29

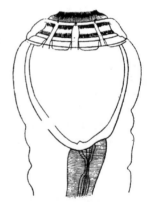

FIG. 2. *Strongylus edentatus.*
From Looss (modified). X29

Looss (1902) it is the immature stages of this species which are concerned in the production of verminous aneurisms of the mesenteric arteries and other branches of the coeliac axis. Railliet
(1915) states that the immature stages of *S. vulgaris* occur also in
sub-mucous nodules in the wall of the large intestine. Adults were
collected at Lethbridge, Alberta, August 5, and at Rosthern, Saskatchewan, August 31, in each case more numerous than individuals of the other two species of *Strongylus.*

Genus *Oesophagodontus* Railliet and Henry, 1902 (Type species,
    Oesophagodontus robustus [Giles, 1892] Gedoelst, 1903).

Only one species of this genus is known to occur in equines.

Species *Oesophagodontus robustus* (Giles, 1892) Gedoelst, 1903.

Length of male 15 to 16 mm, of female 19 to 22 mm. Mouth collar depressed, anterior margin tuberculated. Leaves of anterior leaf crown large, about 18 in number. Mouth capsule goblet-shaped, widest anteriorly; no dorsal gutter. Oesophageal funnel well-developed, the lining of its tri-radiate cavity modified to form 3 tooth-like structures, which do not protrude into the mouth capsule. Vulva 2.8 to 3.7 mm from the posterior end of the body. Dorsal lobe of male bursa lacking. Spicules end bluntly without

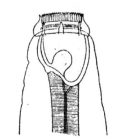

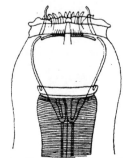

FIG. 3. *Strongylus vulgaris.* FIG. 4. *Oesophagodontus robustus.*
From Looss (modified). X29   From Boulenger (modified). X50

hook-like terminations. These few characters are taken from the more complete description given by Boulenger (1916). *O. robustus* has been recorded heretofore from India and England. It was collected at Lethbridge, Alberta, August 5, and Rosthern, Saskatchewan, August 31.

Genus *Triodontophorus* Looss, 1902 (Type species, *T. serratus* [Looss, 1900] Looss, 1902).

Looss originally described two species in this genus, *T. serratus* and *T. minor*. Sweet (1909) added a third species, *T. intermedius*, found in a horse in Victoria, Australia. This species was later collected in England by Boulenger (1916) who enlarged upon the description given by Sweet. Boulenger also described two other species collected from horses in England, namely, *T. tenuicollis* and *T. brevicauda*. In 1902 Railliet and Henry referred to the presence of *Triodontophorus* in France but did not mention the species. Linstow (1904) recorded *T. serratus* as present in India and Leiper (1910) recorded it as occurring in England. In Canada

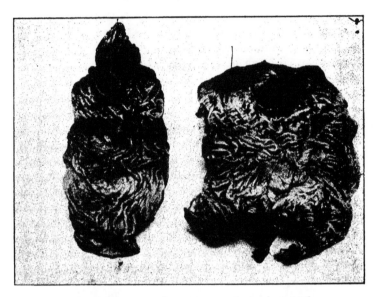

FIG. 5. Ulcers in colon of horse. From photograph.

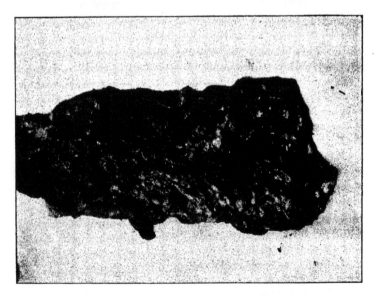

FIG. 6. Ulcer in colon of horse, showing worms (*Triodontophorus tenuicollis*).
From photograph.

during 1917 neither of Looss's species was collected, but forms were found corresponding to each of the other three species.

From the standpoint of the pathologist an interesting fact concerning this genus, apparently not heretofore noted, is its relation to ulcerations of the mucosa of the colon, one of the species

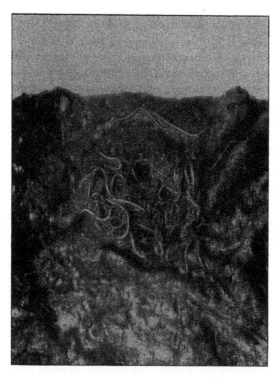

FIG. 7. Same as Fig. 6, magnified. From photograph.

at least (*T. tenuicollis*) being associated with and probably responsible for ulcers found in the mucosa of the colon of a horse examined post mortem at Lethbridge, Alberta, August 5. (Figs. 6, 7.) The same species was also associated with ulcers found in the colon of a horse at Regina, Saskatchewan, July 20 (Fig. 5). Except for the presence of the worms the ulcers are very similar in appearance to those observed in hog cholera. From the ulcer shown in Figs. 6, 7, twenty-five individuals of the species *T. tenui-*

collis were removed. The armature of the mouth capsule of the forms belonging in the genus *Triodontophorus* is rather formidable because of the presence of three well-developed blade-like teeth, and it seems quite likely that these teeth play an important part in the production of the ulcers with which the worms have been found associated.

Species *Triodontophorus serratus* (Looss, 1900) Looss, 1902.

Average length of male 18 mm, of female 25 mm. The mouth collar is slightly depressed at the margin. The margins of the capsule teeth are denticulated. The vulva is more than 2 mm from the posterior end of the body. The dorsal lobe of the male bursa is short. These few characters are taken from the more complete description given by Looss (1902). The species was not found among the horses examined in Canada in 1917. It has been recorded from Egypt, India, and England.

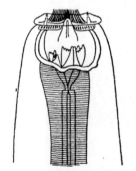
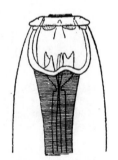

FIG. 8.   *Triodontophorus serratus.*   FIG. 9. *Triodontophorus minor.*
From Looss (modified).   X104   From Looss (modified).   X104

Species *Triodontophorus minor* (Looss, 1900) Looss, 1902.

Average length of male 13 mm, of female 14 mm. The mouth collar is depressed at the margin. The margins of the capsule teeth are only insignificantly denticulated. The vulva is about 0.7 mm from the tip of the tail. The dorsal lobe of the male bursa is long. These few characters are taken from the more complete description given by Looss (1902). The species was not found among the horses examined in Canada in 1917. It appears to have been recorded only from Egypt, having been found in one of 30 horses examined by Looss. Looss notes that it is remarkable for its habitat in the last, thickened portion of the large loop of the colon, all the other species of horse strongyles observed by him having been found in the cecum and first third of the large loop of the colon.

Species *Triodontophorus intermedius* Sweet, 1909.

Length of male 14.5 to 15.5 mm, of female 16.5 to 18.7 mm. The mouth collar is circular in profile. The margins of the capsule teeth are denticulated. The vulva is 1.45 to 1.7 mm from the posterior end of the body. The dorsal lobe of the male bursa is short. These few characters are taken from the more complete description given by Boulenger (1916). *T. intermedius* has been recorded heretofore from Australia and England. It was collected at Saskatoon, Saskatchewan, July 14, Lethbridge, Alberta, August 5, and Rosthern, Saskatchewan, August 31.

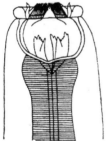
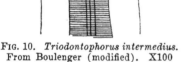
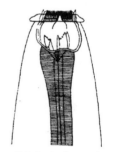

Fig. 10. *Triodontophorus intermedius.* From Boulenger (modified). X100

Fig. 11. *Triodontophorus tenuicollis.* From Boulenger (modified). X100

Species *Triodontophorus tenuicollis* Boulenger, 1916.

Length of male 13.5 to 19 mm, of female 16 to 19.5 mm. The mouth collar is depressed at the margin. The margins of the capsule teeth are denticulated. The vulva is 0.46 to 0.56 mm from the posterior end of the body. The dorsal lobe of the male bursa is short, sharply marked off from the lateral lobes. These few characters are taken from the more complete description given by Boulenger (1916). *T. tenuicollis* has been recorded heretofore from England. It was collected at Regina, Saskatchewan, July 20, and Lethbridge, Alberta, August 5, and is the species concerned in the production of the ulcers shown in figs. 6, 7.

Species *Triodontophorus brevicauda* Boulenger, 1916.

Length of male 13.5 to 14 mm, of female 16 to 17 mm. The mouth collar is high and erect, attaining its greatest breadth anteriorly. The margins of the capsule teeth are not denticulated.

The vulva is about 0.3 mm from the posterior end of the body. The dorsal lobe of the male bursa is long. These few characters are taken from the more complete description given by Boulenger (1916). *T. brevicauda* has been recorded heretofore from England. It was collected at Saskatoon, Saskatchewan, July 14, Lethbridge, Alberta, August 5, and Rosthern, Saskatchewan, August 31.

Genus *Gyalocephalus* Looss, 1900 (Type species, *G. capitatus* Looss, 1900).

Only one species of this genus is known.

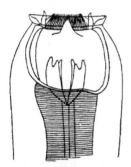   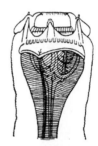

FIG. 12. *Triodontophorus brevicauda.*   FIG. 13.   *Gyalocephalus capitatus.*
From Boulenger (modified). X100   From Looss (modified). X104

Species *Gyalocephalus capitatus* Looss, 1900.

Length of male 7.5 mm, of female 9.5 mm. Leaves of anterior leaf crown very numerous, slender, pointed. Mouth capsule very short and relatively broad. No trace of a dorsal gutter. Anterior portion of esophagus very wide, middle portion slender. Oesophageal funnel almost hemispherical in shape, supported internally by apparently six strongly arched longitudinal ribs starting from the mouth capsule and converging posteriorly toward the commencement of the tri-radiate lumen of the esophagus. Vulva about 0.7 mm from the posterior end of the body. Prebursal papillae very long, form supporting rays of the male bursa. These few characters are taken from the more complete description given by Looss (1902). *G. capitatus* has been recorded heretofore from Egypt by Looss who collected a single pair of specimens from the colon of a mule, from France by Railliet and Henry (1902), and from England by Leiper (1910). It was collected at Lethbridge, Alberta, August 5, and Rosthern, Saskatchewan, August 31.

Genus *Cylicostomum* Railliet and Henry, 1902 (Type species *C. tetracanthum* [Mehlis, 1831]).

This genus, as constituted at present, contains a larger number of species than any other genus of horse strongyles, and the worms that belong to it are much smaller in size on the average than the worms of any of the other genera in question. These facts render specific determination as a rule more difficult than in the case of the other genera, especially since a considerable number of species is likely to be present in the same individual host. A study of each specimen under a high power microscope is usually necessary for a determination of its species. Following are the named species of *Cylicostomum* occurring in the horse and other equines:

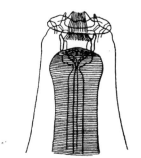 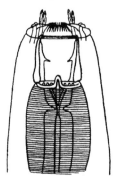

FIG. 14. *Cylicostomum labratum.*   FIG. 15. *Cylicostomum poculatum.*
From Looss (modified). X190   From Looss (modified). X190

Cylicostomum tetracanthum (Mehlis, 1831), *C. labratum* (Looss, 1900), *C. labiatum* (Looss, 1902), *C. coronatum* (Looss, 1900), *C. bicoronatum* (Looss, 1900), *C. poculatum* (Looss, 1900), *C. calicatum* (Looss, 1900), *C. alveatum* (Looss, 1900), *C. catinatum* (Looss, 1900), *C. nassatum* (Looss, 1900), *C. radiatum* (Looss, 1900), *C. elongatum* (Looss, 1900), *C. auriculatum* (Looss, 1900), *C. mettami* (Leiper, 1913), *C. euproctus* (Boulenger, 1917), *C. insigne* (Boulenger, 1917), and *C. goldi* (Boulenger, 1917).

Altogether, so far as appears from the literature available, seventeen named species of *Cylicostomum* occur in the large intestine of the horse and other equines (mule and ass). As already noted some new species belonging to this genus were collected in Canada during 1917, but descriptions of these will be left for a future paper.

Most of the species of *Cylicostomum* thus far recorded as parasites of the horse measure in the adult stage less than 15 mm in length, several less or scarcely more than half this size. A prominent circular mouth collar is present surrounding the mouth opening, more or less distinctly set off from the rest of the body. The mouth collar is regularly rounded, slightly flattened or depressed, or (in one species) with its outer edge projecting forward. Inner surface of mouth collar occupied by the anterior or external leaf crown, consisting of narrow flattened leaf-like processes with pointed or rounded tips, ranging in different species from 8 to 42 in number. Mouth capsule sub-cylindrical in shape usually broader than long but may be longer than broad. Posterior or internal leaf crown comes off from inner surface of mouth capsule near its

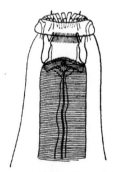

Fig. 16. *Cylicostomum coronatum.* From Looss (modified). X190

anterior border, and is composed of elements varying from small inconspicuous tubercles to long flattened leaf-like processes. Dorsal lobe of male bursa set off from the lateral lobes by a distinct notch. Dorsal rays of bursa large, split down or almost down to the roots of the externo-dorsal rays, each with two lateral branches of about the same size as the posterior portions of the rays themselves. Externo-dorsal rays closely approached to the postero-lateral rays, with their terminal portions turning off backwards more or less suddenly from their main course at an obtuse angle. Genital cone well developed, usually bluntly conical, but sometimes long and almost cylindrical. Spicules long and slender, equal in size, terminating posteriorly in a double hook, one branch of which bends sharply backwards. Vulva of female closely approached to the anus. The adult cylicostomes, according to

Looss, do not adhere to the mucous membrane, are not bloodsuckers, and feed upon the matter found in the contents of the intestine of the host, such as vegetable debris, the ciliates usually found in large numbers in the cecum and colon, nematode ova, etc. According to Railliet (1915) the immature stages of the cylicostomes occur encysted in the mucosa of the intestine.

From the material collected in Canada during the summer of 1917, besides some new species, twelve species of *Cylicostomum* have thus far been sorted out, namely, *C. labiatum*, *C. labratum*, *C. poculatum*, *C. catinatum*, *C. coronatum*, *C. bicoronatum*, *C. calicatum*, *C. radiatum*, *C. nassatum*, *C. elongatum*, *C. insigne*, and *C. goldi*. All of these were collected from the large intestine of horses examined post mortem at Lethbridge, Alberta, August 5, and Rosthern, Saskatchewan, August 31. *C. insigne* was found only in the Lethbridge horse; *C. elongatum* and *C. coronatum* only in the Rosthern horse; the others were present in both cases.

The writers are indebted to Mr. L. N. Garlough of the Zoological Division, Bureau of Animal Industry, for assistance in sorting out the specimens of the various species of *Cylicostomum* represented in the Canadian material, and to Dr. A. E. Cameron of the Entomological Branch, Ottawa, for assistance in field work.

BOULENGER, CHARLES L. 1916. Sclerostome parasites of the horse in England. 1. The genera *Triodontophorus* and *Oesophagodontus*. *Parasitology*, Cambridge (Eng.), v. 8 (4), June 30, pp. 420-439, figs. 1-7, pl. 22, figs. 1-7.
———— 1917. Sclerostome parasites of the horse in England. 2. New species of the genus *Cylichnostomum*. *Parasitology*, Lond., v. 9 (2), Feb., pp. 203-212, figs. 1-5.

GEDOELST, L. 1903. Résumé du cours de parasitologie. ix+107 pp. 8°. Bruxelles.

GILES, GEORGE M. J. 1892. On a new sclerostome from the large intestine of mules. *Scient. Mem. Med. Off.*, India, Calcutta, pt. 7, pp. 25-30, 1 pl., figs. 1-14.

LEIPER, R. T. 1910. [Exhibition of specimens of entozoa.] *Proc. Zool. Soc.*, Lond. (1), June, p. 147.
———— 1911. Some new parasitic nematodes from tropical Africa. *Proc. Zool. Soc.*, Lond. (2), June, pp. 549-555, figs. 140-144.
———— 1913. A new cylicostome worm from the horse in London. *Vet. J.*, Lond. (460), v. 69, Oct., pp. 460-462, figs. a-c.

VON LINSTOW, O. F. B. 1904. Nematoda in the collection of the Colombo Museum. *Spolia Zeylanica*, Colombo, v. 1 (4), Feb., pp. 91-104, pls. 1-2, figs. 1-27.

LOOSS, ARTHUR. 1900. Die Sclerostomen der Pferde und Esel in Egypten. (Notizen zur Helminthologie Egyptens. 3). *Centralbl. f. Bakteriol., Parasitenk* [etc.], Jena, 1. Abt., v. 27 (4), 5. Feb., pp. 150-160; (5), 12. Feb., pp. 184-192.
———— 1902. The Sclerostomidae of horses and donkeys in Egypt. *Rec. Egypt. Govt. School Med.*, Cairo, pp. 25-139, pls. 1-13, figs. 1-172.

MEHLIS, E. 1831. Novae observationes de entozois. Auctore Dr. Fr. Chr. H. Creplin. *Isis* (Oken), Leipz. (1), pp. 68-99, pl. 2, figs. 1-18; (2), pp. 166-199.

MOLIN, RAFFAELE. 1861. Il sottordine degli acrofalli ordinato scientificamente secondo i risultamenti delle indagini anatomiche ed embriogeniche. *Mem. r. Ist. Veneto di sc., lett. ed arti*, Venzia (1860), v. 9, pp. 427-633, pls. 25-33.

MUELLER, O. F. 1784. Zoologica Danica seu animalium Daniae et Norvegiae rariorum ac minus notorum descriptiones et historia. v. 2, 1 l., 124 pp. 8°. Lipsiae.

RAILLIET, A. 1915. L'emploi des médicaments dans le traitement des maladies causées par des nématodes. *Rep. 10. Internat. Vet. Cong.*, Lond. (Aug., 1914), v. 3, pp. 733-749.

RAILLIET, ALCIDE, and HENRY, A. 1902. Sur les sclérostomiens des équidés. *Compt. rend. Soc. de biol.*, Par., v. 54 (4), 7 fév., pp. 110-112.

RUDOLPHI, C. A. 1809. Entozoorum sive vermium intestinalium historia naturalis. v. 2 (1), 457 pp., pls. 7-12. 8°. Amstelaedami.

SWEET, GEORGINA. 1909. The endoparasites of Australian stock and native fauna. Part 2. New and unrecorded species. *Proc. Roy. Soc.*, Victoria, Melbourne, n. s., v. 21, pt. 2, Mar., pp. 503-527, pl. 29, figs. 1-9.

BLACKLEG AND ITS PREVENTION*

G. A. JOHNSON, Sioux City, Iowa

Blackleg is an acute infectious disease of cattle, known under a large number of different names. While other ruminants are not immune to the disease, it is not common among any of them.

Some authors state that swine sometimes suffer from blackleg, but we are inclined to believe this a mistake in diagnosis and that the supposed cases of blackleg in swine are some other form of emphysematosa, as there are several other conditions that are caused by other gas forming bacilli that more or less closely resemble true blackleg.

This opinion is based largely upon the fact that it is quite a common practice among farmers of many localities of this country to feed the carcasses of animals that have died of blackleg to their swine without producing a single case of blackleg in the swine, so far as we have been able to learn.

Blackleg and anthrax were considered one and the same disease until Bollinger, in 1875, and Feser, in 1876, demonstrated that they were two separate and distinct diseases, blackleg being due to the *Bacillus Chauveaui* and anthrax due to *Bacterium anthracis*.

---

*Presented at the 30th Annual Meeting of the Iowa Veterinary Association, Ames, Iowa, January, 1918.

Blackleg, to a certain extent, is a localized septicemia, somewhat similar in biologic principles to tetanus. It is usually characterized by local emphysematosa of the subcutaneous and muscular tissue, accompanied by septicemia. The period of incubation in natural infection is usually from 3 to 5 days and the disease usually runs a fatal course in from a few hours to three days.

SYMPTOMS. In well defined cases there is loss of appetite, and cessation of rumination. The temperature does not give much information because it may be as high as 105, 106 or even 107 degrees F., while in other cases it does not go over 104 degrees F. Stiffness is an early symptom and in the majority of cases the animals manifest uneasiness by lying down and getting up, which is done with more and more difficulty as the disease progresses. In the majority of cases tumefaction in some part is present; especially in the later stages of the disease, the swelling is not very painful and usually presents the well known crackling sound upon manipulation, but in a typical case this may be absent. The history of the herd is of value in gaining a diagnosis, i. e., has there already been a loss indicating blackleg? Are the premises known to be infected with blackleg, etc.?

POST MORTEM LESIONS. As is well known this disease is characterized by a local emphysematosa of the striated musculature of some part of the body, as the shoulder or hip, with the formation of more or less gas. Upon excision there is usually found an exudation of dark or black bloody serum. Just underneath the skin the striated muscles present a more or less darkened or black color. There are usually small cavities filled with gas, giving the muscle a spongy feeling and appearance, and as a rule these parts do not contain an excess of moisture. However, there are cases where there is less gas and more exudation. But the diseased parts always present a very pronounced characteristic odor, described by some as sour-like, or like rancid butter, while others describe it as a sweetish, rancid smell, but not like rancid butter.

In typical cases there is little change in the visceral organs except the liver which is frequently affected by the formation of small ochre yellow centers ranging from 1/16 to ½ inch in diameter, and of dry-like consistency. But in a typical case we may find the musculature of any part affected, as the throat, one masseter muscle, etc., while in extreme cases the characteristic muscle changes appear to be absent. In such cases there are likely to be more or less reddish patches on the serous membranes, frequently diphtheritic-like growths, especially on the pleura and pericardium. In these cases the visceral organs are likely to be engorged and more or less congested. It would appear that such cases might be termed generalized, while the ordinary case is usually localized and circumscribed. But owing to the fact that in some instances it assumes a rather generalized form, a post mortem of these atypical cases is not complete until all voluntary musculature of the body has been examined. The blood is always dark and firmly clotted, especially in the heart. This fact is of great assistance in differentiating blackleg from anthrax. Again there is little tendency in anthrax to the formation of emphysematous swelling, and also the lack of blackleg odor.

The distinguishing differences between blackleg and malignant edema are, the odor which is fetid in malignant edema and the very moist musculature. It should as a rule be easy to differentiate between blackleg and hemorrhagic septicemia, but an atypical or generalized case of blackleg might be mistaken for a case of cutaneous hemorrhagic septicemia and vice versa. But if we remember that in blackleg the emphysematosa is usually in the heavier muscles, while in hemorrhagic septicemia it is more in the dependent parts as the brisket, belly, etc., and that the fluid in hemorrhagic septicemia is more of a serous nature, usually containing less hemorrhage, we may be able to differentiate these conditions without the aid of a microscope. On the other hand it should be borne in mind that it is possible to have both these diseases in the same herd if not in the same animal, in which case it would be advisable to immunize against both diseases.

Shortly after the discovery of the causative agent, *Bacillus Chauveaui*, it was closely studied and an attenuated virus vaccine was produced, that was capable of producing more or less immunity in susceptible animals, and under variously modified processes large quantities of these vaccines have been produced and used from that time until now.

That these vaccines were of more or less merit and filled an important field is attested by the millions of doses that have been used. In fact they were the best and only remedy of merit on the market until recently. But as is always the case with attenuated viruses, the results have not always been what were desired.

The field experiences have demonstrated that in some instances these vaccines kill a certain percentage of the calves vaccinated, while in others they do not protect for any length of time. In some instances herds were vaccinated four or five times in a year and still losses continued; especially has this been true of late years, when the available ranges and pastures have been over-crowded with stock, which has a tendency to increase exposure and consequently the prevalence of the disease.

NEWER VACCINES. Recently a new line of vaccines has been developed and placed upon the market so that it is not necessary now to rely upon the old time attenuated viruses. These newer vaccines are germ free and consist of aggressins, true and artificial, and blackleg anti-serum.

GERM FREE BLACKLEG VACCINE. The germ free blackleg vaccine is an aggressin. Briefly, it is prepared as follows: supposedly susceptible calves are inoculated with a virulent strain of pure blackleg virus and the disease allowed to run its natural course. The carcasses of such animals that die within forty-eight hours after inoculation are taken into the laboratory, properly prepared and inspected, and if found free from harmful invaders, the diseased tissues are removed, and the serum and juices from these diseased parts are collected and purified by filtrating processes, etc., so as to render the finished product absolutely sterile. The fact that the animal dies of blackleg within forty-eight hours after inoculation indicates that large quantities of toxins and antigens are produced.

In order to assure sterility of the product each serial lot is thoroughly tested by three separate and distinct processes, the fermentation tube test, the culture media test, and the guinea pig test. These tests are carried out according to the regulations prescribed by the Bureau of Animal Industry.

The product must stand each of these tests perfectly before it is offered for sale. It should also be tested on guinea pigs or calves for potency. Thus we have in the germ free vaccine an absolutely sterile product that contains all the products of virulent blackleg bacilli generated in the natural way. It is harmless, even in quantities twenty or more times the size of the regular dose. It requires handling the animal but once. It may be used on any sized or aged animal and under varied conditions, such as at time of branding, dehorning, castrating, etc. It will produce a lasting, if not a permanent immunity. However, it requires from five to ten days to produce its full immunizing effect, during which time the animal may contract the disease.

More recently an artificial aggressin has been put upon the market under the name of blackleg filtrate. It is prepared by growing the blackleg bacilli on artificial media in the laboratory, and purifying by filtration, etc., but as this product is still in the experimental stage and some inoculation tests and field reports do not fully bear out the claims put forward for it, we prefer to reserve judgment pending more definite information.

BLACKLEG ANTI-SERUM. This is produced by hyper-immunizing horses by repeated injections of increasing doses of virulent blackleg virus. After hyper-immunization is complete, the blood is drawn, clarified, filtered, etc., and after being tested for purity and potency, is ready for use.

This serum has more or less curative value when used in the early stages of the disease, but the very nature of blackleg precludes successful medication in most cases, hence it is not advisable to build false hopes about a cure. Better play "Safety First" and vaccinate with the germ free vaccine before the herd becomes infected.

This serum is also used in conjunction with blackleg virus to produce immunity, but this does not appear advisable for three reasons:

1st. It does not produce as lasting immunity as does the germ free vaccine.

2nd. It is much more expensive and requires handling the animal twice.

3rd. Virus should never be used unless necessary, because of the danger of not only producing an occasional death, but also of contaminating the premises and thereby increasing infection and perhaps creating new centers of infection.

On the other hand, blackleg anti-serum has a place in a limited field and that is where a virulent type of blackleg has broken out in a herd of valuable cattle. Then it is advisable to give a large protective dose (30 to 60 c.c.) of serum. This should check further development of the disease within the herd, or render such animals as might develop the disease, within 24 hours to 48 hours after treatment, more amenable to curative serum treatment. Then to follow this protective dose of serum in about fifteen days by giving a regular dose (5 c.c.) of germ free blackleg vaccine. The reasons for making the injection of the germ free vaccine approximately fifteen days after administering the serum may be briefly stated as follows: the serum and germ free vaccine are antagonistic, the one counteracting the other, hence if the vaccine is given before the serum has been largely eliminated (which apparently takes about 15 days) the one will counteract the other. On the other hand, if we wait too long after the effect of the serum has passed away, the disease may develop again. By this method the spread of the disease within the herd should be checked and a lasting immunity produced with a minimum loss of animals, with absolutely no danger of spreading or producing disease. A still better method, where conditions are favorable, is to take the temperature of all animals at time of treatment and such as show a temperature of 104 degrees F. or better, should be given a much larger dose (100 to 300 c.c.), according to indications. This method has been followed in several instances with very gratifying results. But it can be seen that it is rather expensive to be used in ordinary herds and can be followed only where conditions are reasonably favorable for handling the animals.

Another method of handling a herd already affected with blackleg is to administer the germ free vaccine in regular sized dosage, and keep very close watch of the herd for about ten days and should any of the animals present any symptoms of blackleg, immediately administer a curative dose (300 to 500 c.c.) of serum. This is not so certain, but may be cheaper than the first mentioned method.

In attempting to produce immunity by means of an attenuated virus, a materially different biological principle is involved than that involved where a germ free vaccine is used. Where an attenauted virus is used (it makes no difference whether it be blackleg, anthrax, smallpox or whatever disease) it is supposed to produce a mild or modified form of the disease, which stimulates the production of antibodies in the animal. This involves a number of vital points, the two most important of which are the proper attenuation of the virus, and the proper condition of the individual to be treated.

Regarding the virus, if it is attenuated too much, it will not produce any reaction (disease), whereas if it is not attenuated sufficiently it may produce so violent reaction as to prove fatal.

Regarding the condition of the individual, if its resistance to the disease should be very low, it would suffer a strong reaction which might prove fatal, or if its resistance should be very high, the individual would suffer little or no reaction and hence acquire little or no immunity. But should the attenuation be just right and the individual in the proper condition, then the proper reaction or degree of disease will take place and more or less immunity be acquired. But being hedged in by so many uncontrollable factors, the strangest part is that there are not more failures. Another fact that should never be lost sight of is that every time any virus vaccine is used, the virus of the disease in question is being introduced on the premises, and until we know much more about biology we have no assurance that it may not result in harm. In other words, it should be considered dangerous. In using these virus vaccines in herds affected with blackleg, it is about the same as using virus alone in a cholera infected drove of swine. But when a germ free or sterile vaccine is properly administered, there is absolutely no danger of conveying any disease. The theory upon which germ free blackleg vaccine produces immunity, briefly stated, is that the antigens contained therein stimulate the production of antibodies in the individual, or in other words, it is the product of the germs that stimulate the production of the antibodies which render the animal immune.

ADMINISTRATION. The most essential point to be observed in administering germ free blackleg vaccine is cleanliness. Have clean, sterile syringes and needles, draw the vaccine direct from the container into the syringe, as there is always danger of contamination where it is turned from the original into any kind of container, and then drawn into the syringe. Disinfect the seat of injection with some good agent as tincture of iodine.

Intramuscular injections of germ free blackleg vaccine insure a little quicker absorption, but are more painful and upon the whole have little or no advantages over subcutaneous injection.

Blackleg serum should be injected intramuscularly, especially in case there is any localized swelling, when it should be injected in and about the swelling, not to exceed 30 c.c. in one place. Some have advocated intravenous injection, but as the serum is from a different species of animal, it may be slightly dangerous.

The following data procured from the owners of the cattle indicate the results that are being obtained with germ free blackleg vaccine:

No. Herds	No. Head	Year Vaccinated	No. died of Blackleg since Vaccination	
			1st day	After 10 days
12	1887	1915	0	0
8	3320	1916	0	0
	25000	1917	5	0

Thus it will be seen that as far as we have any data the animals retain their immunity.

The most remarkable fact is that out of the several hundred thousand doses of the germ free blackleg vaccine that have been used this year there has not been a single animal reported lost from blackleg later than 8 days after vaccination, and but a very small fraction of 1% during the first eight days after vaccination, and all such loss was in herds where there had been losses from blackleg previous to the herd being vaccinated with the germ free blackleg vaccine, or in other words, in infected herds.

———•———

CONSERVATION SLAUGHTER*

W. W. DIMOCK, Ames, Iowa

By conservation slaughter is understood the slaughter of all animals that are in danger of death or deterioration from injuries and disease, or for various reasons are unprofitable, that their flesh may be utilized for food. Further, conservation slaughter should be carried out on all animals even though the flesh is unfit for human food; provided, (1) that they are suffering from any condition that is incurable, (2) that the time and expense make treatment unprofitable, (3) that during the time of sickness they expel from the body highly infectious material that contaminates the quarters and thus exposes other animals. All such animals are to be utilized as explained below.

The plan for conservation slaughter is to be carried out in connection with the general movement and necessity to conserve the food supply of the nation and to stimulate increased production. A few unprofitable animals in each herd and flock of the state make a total, the consideration of which is worthy of our most serious attention. Data at hand show that in the

*Presented at the 30th Annual Meeting of the Iowa Veterinary Association, Ames, Iowa, January, 1918.

herds and flocks of Iowa there are many hundreds, even thousands of animals that are being kept at a very serious loss in these times of high feed costs. A few such animals in the past have had no appreciable effect upon the economic question of live stock production in Iowa, and largely so because of the great quantities of food stuffs that were available at a comparatively low price. At the present time, however, when we stop to consider the high cost of all food stuffs consumed by animals and the rapid increase in the retail price of all meat food products, it is forcibly brought to our attention that there is a great and unnecessary economic loss sustained from keeping among the flocks and herds of the state, animals sick in a way that makes them a source of danger to their fellows or that will finally result in their deterioration or death, or that are not up to a reasonable minimum production, or that are from any cause decidedly unprofitable. All are fully aware of the desirability of making provision for the most satisfactory disposal of such animals. Many of the animals coming under the class mentioned above may be disposed of for food purposes through the regular channels of sale. However, if any individual shows evidence of ill health, or is suffering from an injury or local disease, the sale price is very materially less than the actual value of the animals for food purposes, and again, the condition of the animal may be such as to make it impossible to ship any distance. In order that all animals still fit for human food may be utilized for such purposes, and the owner receive at least the approximate value for food purposes and thus in every way possible help to prevent loss and at the same time conserve the meat food supply, I believe that we should make every effort possible to handle them under what we may term "conservation slaughter".

Before attempting to handle animals that would naturally come within this field, it will be necessary to inform the owners and live stock dealers of the state concerning the purpose and necessity of starting a movement of this kind, and to give more or less specific directions to the owners and veterinarians of the state regarding the inspection of animals desirable to ship or to be handled locally under conservation slaughter.

In carrying out conservation slaughter at the present time I would propose that it be accomplished or undertaken, in general, in one of the three following ways:

First, that when possible all animals that are to be disposed of for purpose of conservation shall be shipped to a point having an abattoir that maintains federal inspection.

Second, that slaughter be carried out in connection with a local or municipal slaughter house, or on the farm, and the carcass inspected by a competent local veterinarian.

In cases where animals are slaughtered under the general plan suggested in connection with conservation slaughter, the inspection of the carcass should in all cases be performed according to the rules governing inspection as carried out by the meat inspection service of the Bureau of Animal Industry, United States Department of Agriculture. In case the meat from animals killed under the plan of conservation slaughter in local abattoirs or on the farm is to be offered for sale, the veterinarian making the inspection should be approved by the executive officer of the Animal Health Commission of the State of Iowa.

The classes of conditions for which the majority of animals so affected may with safety be used for food purposes under conservation slaughter are:

First. Accidental injury of healthy animals. For example, broken legs, wire cuts, hook wounds, or deep wounds from any cause, the location or nature of which makes recovery uncertain or unprofitable.

Second. Local diseased conditions or diseases that remain local throughout their course or that have little or no tendency, especially in the early stages, to become general in character and that have from experience been shown to be of no danger to the human when the flesh is used for food following removal and condemnation of the affected part or parts. For example, actinomycosis of cattle, caseous lymphadenitis of sheep, scirrhous cord of pigs, granular vaginitis of cattle, polyarthritis of pigs and many organic diseases.

Third. That class of diseases that are local and chronic in nature but tend to cause loss of condition in the animal, thus materially reducing its production and often finally terminating in death, either because of marked changes in the part affected or because of the frequency of secondary infection. For example, parasitic diseases where the parasites tend to localize in some particular organ or part, as nodular disease of sheep, echinococcus in the liver of the pig, pulmonary strongylosis, scabies, chronic organic diseases, paralysis of pigs, chronic local inflammations, tumors, etc.

Fourth. Systemic and constitutional diseases that do not in the early stages necessitate condemnation of the carcass, but that do upon becoming generalized render the carcass unfit for human food and necessitate total condemnation. For example, rachitis, sniffles or infectious rhinitis in pigs, tuberculosis, leukemia, anemia, and diseases of the nervous system.

Fifth. Those acute and chronic non-infectious diseases that not infrequently result in the death of the animal, such as a choke, urinary calculi, rupture, arthritis, acute indigestion, intestinal intussusception, etc.

Sixth. Those acute infectious conditions for which there is no cure and for which prevention is uncertain or inadvisable, the disease spreading more or less rapidly and often causing death of a large number in the herd or flock. For example, hog cholera, swine plague, hemorrhagic septicemia, stomatitis, foot and mouth disease, etc. The slaughter of animals to prevent their becoming infected in the case of an outbreak of an acute specific infectious disease in the herd or flock must be carried out with great care, and this applies particularly to those herds that are in a fattened condition and ready for market.

Seventh. Those animals that are economically unproductive, including non-breeders and unprofitable producers. For example, sheep, cattle and swine that fail to breed because of some malformation, or because of some diseased condition of the ovaries, uterus, or udder, or animals that have become non-breeders from any of the various complications associated with infectious abortion. Many such animals can be recognized upon a thorough physical examination. Examples of unprofitable producers other than for breeding purposes are to be found in cows that are being kept for dairy purposes, and animals for fattening purposes that fail to make proper gains because of type or constitutional condition.

The great importance of the object to be obtained from the carrying out of conservation slaughter is further supplemented by the saving of stable room, time spent in care, and feed stuffs that sick and unprofitable animals consume without making any gain in flesh, or producing in a way that makes them profitable. Many of the sick animals will finally die, resulting in almost a total loss of both the animal and the food that had been consumed.

In the Service and Regulatory Announcements published by the Bureau of Animal Industry, United States Department of Agriculture, are found in the last few numbers many items dealing with the conservation of meat products as being carried on by the Federal Meat Inspection Service. In the issue of October 20, 1917, is found as follows:

"For the purpose of promoting the conservation of meats and products the bureau's conservation committee visited a number of representative plants, conferred with the proprietors and operators of official establishments, and studied operations and procedures to see how such conservation might be promoted consistent with approved meat inspection methods."

As a result of the above, they report on the following phases of conservation:

LEAN MEAT. All careless and inefficient trimming of pork cuts, and the unnecessary loss of particles of lean meat left on the fat trimmings are to be avoided as much as possible. This lean meat has little value as fat but a maximum value as meat for food.

FATS. The committee recommends that where possible, all fats should be so handled as to conserve them for food purposes, that is, that no edible fats shall be permitted to become inedible through failure to properly handle them.

CANNING OPERATIONS. That all canned products shall be inspected immediately after filling. All leaky cans to be soldered and resterilized within the time prescribed by the regulations (6 hours) so as to prevent their spoiling and thus conserve the contents for food purposes.

CURED MEATS. It is suggested that every establishment do everything possible so that losses from curing may be reduced or entirely prevented.

Other suggestions made were that great care should be taken in connection with the proper handling of meats so as to prevent their becoming soiled, and spoiling from lack of proper refrigeration, especially in connection with transportation; also to avoid packing of meats in unsuitable containers for shipping.

There is also a note on the rough handling of live stock suggesting that the managers of slaughter houses and stock yards prevent, so far as possible, the rough handling of live stock, thus reducing the number of bruises, this entailing a loss since bruised meat has a value for tankage only.

In the Service and Regulatory Announcements for October 11, 1917, there is a statement on the use, preparation and handling of meat passed for sterilization. In the past, our inspection service has in the main recognized only two classes, and as a rule the establishments have been prepared to handle only the two classes, these being "U. S. Inspected and Passed", or passed unconditionally, and "U. S. Inspected and Condemned" as unfit for food. At the present time the Bureau (Meat Inspection Service) is recommending that certain meats be passed for sterilization (U. S. Inspected and Passed for Sterilization) providing the establishment has facilities for properly sterilizing the meat, the rule being, that it shall be heated to a temperature not lower than 170° F. for a period of not less than 30 minutes and that the product shall be prepared and marketed according to the requirements of the Bureau.

In the Service and Regulatory Announcements for July 3, 1917, under the heading, "Conservation of Meat Food Supply", is given a full statement regarding the purpose, object, and necessity for the conservation of meat. It is believed that conservation of a material nature can be accomplished without surrendering the purpose for which inspection is maintained.

Since the government, through its Federal Meat Inspection Service, in cooperation with the abattoirs of the country, is doing all in its power to conserve the meat products of the country, it would seem that the state, county, town, municipality, and the farmer should take an active part in attempting to bring about conservation, and that the state and its representatives that are in a position to do so should furnish the farmer, live stock owners, and the veterinarian with the information necessary to accomplish this without in any way endangering the live stock interests as a whole or the health of the consuming public.

SUPPLEMENTARY—CONSERVATION OF HIDES, FATS, AND BY-PRODUCTS. Considering the great importance and almost vital necessity of fats as used in connection with the war, provision should be made for the utilization of all animals that die or are killed because of sickness from a condition that renders their flesh unfit for human consumption, through arrangements to save the hide, render the carcass to obtain the fat, and prepare the refuse for tankage or fertilizer. During the last few years, in many of the large and small towns and cities of the state, rendering establishments have sprung up and are doing a profitable business. However, there is room for the introduction of many other such establishments. These establishments, in my opinion, should be licensed and every stockman in the country should be informed regarding the advantage of having the men connected with these rendering plants call for all dead or dying animals, that the carcass may be salvaged. I further believe that the state, through its Animal Health Commission, should supervise the type of conveyance by which dead animals or diseased animal tissue may be transported from the farm to the rendering establishment, and also supervise the general sanitary condition of the establishment itself. Personally, I can see no reason why, for the present at least, pigs dying of cholera or animals of hemorrhagic septicemia, and from most of the other infectious diseases could not with safety, if carried in a properly constructed tank, be transported from the farm to the rendering establishment and utilized for grease and tankage. Pigs dying from hog cholera are utilized for such purposes where the carcass can be used without being transported from one point to another.

DISCUSSION

DR. K. W. STOUDER: This subject of "Conservation Slaughter" is indeed a timely and very practical one for discussion. We are told that fats are very essential to the conduct of war, and yet it is easy to compute that in hog losses alone, Iowa in one year, when disease was not particularly prevalent among our swine, saw more than 1200 tons of fat absolutely wasted, and this is estimating that each hog carcass would have yielded only 10 lbs. of fat. If these fats were worth 10 cents per pound, which is easily below the present market for inedible grease, we have lost about a quarter of a million dollars in hog fats, to say nothing of the proteins which would be by-products of the rendering and exceedingly valuable hog feeds, and worth at least another $100,000 or more, at present prices.

Our Extension and Veterinary Investigation Departments have had reports from practically all parts of Iowa showing heavy losses at times among other classes of live stock, particularly hem. orrhagic septicemia among cattle. In some of these cases because of fear on the part of the owner not even the hides are saved, much less the carcass fats and by-products, yet a well organized render. ing service could have saved labor, fats and glycerine, and lessened the spread of infection. Modern invention has improved methods and increased savings materially in all branches of business, and we must soon expect to see the truck with tank constructed box going out over areas of country collecting the carcasses of animals for rendering, for they are proving practical where used already. It occurs to many of us that adoption of such a system should be speeded up, and the plan extended and perfected so that not only the dead carcasses may be salvaged, but that the unprofitable animal, the accidentally injured, and the chronically sick but still partially valuable animals may be easily and cheaply disposed of under a system which utilizes their complete value, and yet most certainly protects the consuming public as well as the surrounding live stock from disease exposure.

These possible economies are well known to every veterinarian. Few others are informed regarding their extent and it is your duty to your country to see that these savings of fats are made in your community just as far as possible. The furtherance of such plans by assisting capable and experienced rendering concerns to find suitable locations, the education of the stock owner to utilize such plants and service, and the posting of ourselves upon the subject of meat inspection until we can give good advice as to the salvage in a carcass fit for human food, can be one of our contributions to the welfare of our country at this time.

DR. CHAS. MURRAY: There are two forms of conservation discussed by Dr. Dimock which impress me as deserving of emphasis, viz.: emergency slaughter of animals on the farm and utilization of fats from animals dead through accident or disease. In the work of our department, we are frequently called upon by correspondence to render a decision as to the advisability of making some use of animals destroyed or dead of disease. These requests come mainly from the laity and the increase in numbers of such inquiries leads me to conclude that they are ready to do their part in conservation of such material. Samples of meat are frequently received with a request that they be examined to determine their suitability for food. These samples come from fat animals that have choked, frozen parts of their bodies, or met with accidents that render them unable to get around, etc. We are in poor position to render a decision except from the history given, for the parts sent are invariably muscle from a part of the body entirely removed from that affected by the injurious agent. Here, it seems to me, is the opportunity for the local veterinarian. He is in a position to inspect the carcass and to make an intelligent decision in the matter. He is in position to encourage his clients to make use of such material as is fit for food, and the client can well afford to pay him liberally for his time and services.

There is an increasing sentiment among stock men to utilize the carcasses of animals for food for hogs or for the fat. I believe every farmer can well afford, in case he does not have the advantage of a collection system for dead animals, to construct a crude, low priced rendering plant where he can render out the fats to be sold at a remunerative price, and cook the fleshy part of the carcass for food for his remaining animals. The price realized from the sale of the fat will pay well for the time and labor necessary for cooking the carcass, and the fact that when the process is completed the carcass has been satisfactorily and safely disposed of ought to be of additional value in that sanitation is thus properly preserved.

DR. J. I. GIBSON: I have been interested in this paper because I have been giving the subject serious consideration. I believe conditions and circumstances as they now exist make it the duty of all owners of breeding animals to keep only such animals as are proven breeders, of course, including young animals which are most certain to prove breeders. I believe it is the duty of all owners at this time to sacrifice such animals as have proven barren and to keep in their places sure breeders or young animals to be tried out as breeders. The cattle men (breeders of pure-bred cattle) have always carried in their herds animals favored on account of their blood lines that will not breed and are, therefore, a bill of expense and are not proper animals to sell to any purchaser other than the packer or butcher. With the increased demand for meat all such barren animals should be sent to slaughter, thereby increasing the meat supply and conserving the feed heretofore consumed by the barren animals that are entirely worthless from the breeder's standpoint. I believe every farmer in Iowa should increase his breeding herds of cattle, sheep and swine, and that no more worthless, barren animals should be carried from year to year in our breeding herds.

I am also interested in the supplementary part of Dr. Dimock's paper on the conservation of hides, fats and by-products of our dead animals. I figure the hides, fats and by-products of the dead animals in Iowa properly conserved will bring to our people about $10,000,000 a year. From what information I can gather only about 10 per cent of these valuable products is conserved by the rendering plants now in operation in the state. About half of the value of these carcasses is represented in the fats, the balance in the hides, tankage, fertilizer, and by-products. These commercial fats now bring about $15.00 per hundred.

The fats contain a percentage of glycerine which varies from 4 to 12 per cent and would average 6 per cent glycerine. Glycerine is worth from 75 cents to $1.00 per pound and is liable to continue to rise in price, especially during the existence of the war. Glycerine is the real cause of the present high price of all fats. Glycerine is used in the manufacture of explosives, therefore, no argument should be necessary to convince the people of the state and nation that all fats carrying a percentage of glycerine should be conserved and the glycerine extracted, lest there come a time in this great world struggle between autocracy and democracy when there might not be sufficient glycerine available to the United States and our allies for the manufacture of sufficient explosives to destroy the Hun or drive him back across the Rhine. Any laws existing upon our statute books that require the burning or burial of the valuable animal carcasses should be disregarded by the War Department, and an order should be issued commanding the people of this and all other states to conserve all fats from animal carcasses, in order that the glycerine might be extracted therefrom and an ample supply of this valuable product conserved for the purpose of administering a sound threshing to the Teuton armies. The scarcer the supply of glycerine the higher the price will be of all these fats. I estimate an annual waste of 20,000 tons of non-edible fats and grease in the State of Iowa, which I believe should be conserved and could be saved without interfering with the sanitary work of the state in the control and prevention of the spread of diseases of live stock. The rendering process will sterilize the products and thereby render them harmless. I therefore hope to see some action taken by the War Department calling for the conservation of all animal fats.

PROBLEMS OF TICK ERADICATION
Personal Influence of the Inspector

Dr. W. H. Dalrymple
Department of Veterinary Science, Louisiana State University
Baton Rouge, La.

(The following is an abstract of a highly instructive address delivered by Dr. Dalrymple at the conference of Bureau inspectors engaged in tick eradication work held at New Orleans, Louisiana, January 15-18, 1918.)

THE MAN IN AUTHORITY. One of the most desirable and valuable qualifications in the man with authority is first of all an accurate knowledge of the work over which he presides and the gift of being able to handle other men satisfactorily. Although a man may be a master in the details of his work, yet if he is lacking in the personality and tact necessary to success his manner is more liable to repel than attract people to him, with the resultant lack of cooperation afforded him and consequent hindrance to the accomplishment of the ends desired.

It is generally conceded that the greatest obstacle to the most successful prosecution of veterinary sanitary work, in which may be included tick eradication, is the gross ignorance of the people as to the procedure and the ultimate result sought. Antagonism is displayed despite the fact that the work is carried on for their individual benefit and that of the community and state in which they live. And yet, without some effort being consistently and continuously exerted to dispel such ignorance, final success must of necessity be considerably delayed. Hence in this particular phase of the work success depends largely upon the men in authority being endowed with personal magnetism and tactfulness.

(Dr. Dalrymple at this point related several entertaining instances in his early work as a veterinary inspector in Ireland in connection with contagious pleuro-pneumonia. These reminiscences illustrated very forcibly the value and importance of tolerance and tactfulness in inspiring confidence in the people, and securing their good-will and cooperation.)

OBSTACLES TO TICK ERADICATION. Anyone who has been in touch with tick eradication since the beginning of the campaign knows the trials and tribulations through which he has had to pass and the many obstacles which have incessantly confronted him. While many of these have been overcome there still exist, and will to the end, those of a similar character which must be tackled.

In mentioning a few of these obstacles I think we may give ignorance, which might be extended to gross all-around ignorance on the part of the laity, the very first place. Ignorance concerning the true object to be attained; ignorance regarding the fever tick and its life habits; ignorance concerning the methods of procedure for the destruction of the parasite and the fever with it; and ignorance as to the value of the work to the individual cattle owner, etc.

It appears to me, that with an average amount of tact, and a little more condescension, if you will, a great deal of this ignorance might be dispelled by a little man-to-man and heart-to-heart talk concerning the various phases of the problem. In other words letting in the true light to the darkened understandings, for the normal individual, even with the densest sort of comprehension, may be made to see and understand if only the problem is clearly explained to him and more particularly if it is done in a tactful way and in a manner which appeals to the man, arouses his interest, and gains his confidence, friendship, and good-will.

True, suspicion is a dominant factor with many of these people. This, too, is born of ignorance, through erroneous information proffered by similarly ignorant or suspicious individuals. Once ignorance is dispelled, suspicion also will gradually vanish.

The lack of cooperation is a tremendous obstacle in the prosecution of this important work; and where are we to place the cause for this want of sympathy, if not in the ignorance of so many of our people? Cooperation suggests correct understanding and enthusiasm; and once the people get understanding through enlightenment, cooperation is bound to follow. It cannot be otherwise; a man may be ignorant, but that is no indication of his being a fool, to his own detriment, if once he sees the light.

SELFISH OBJECTORS. There is another class of people who, although they may not be wholly ignorant of conditions, yet for selfish personal reasons frequently obstruct the progress of tick eradication. I refer to the man with cattle but with insufficient or no pasture of his own and depending for the sustenance of his cattle upon free range or the generosity of his neighbor. This man fears a stock law which he considers would interfere with his business, and for purely personal reasons he has no sympathy with the work and blatantly calls out for "personal liberty", which he seems to interpret as the right to selfishly benefit himself at the expense of his neighbor and everybody around him. Then we have the unpatriotic citizen who seems to object to contribute his due share to taxation through legitimate assessment of his cattle, which he believes the work of tick eradication would force him to do. We are all familiar with these obstructionists, and time will, of course, eventually straighten them out through the general enactment and enforcement of suitable legislation. This desirable result, however, may be very materially assisted by accurate information judiciously and tactfully imparted to the people themselves.

There is another class of obstructionist who bobs up periodically and who, unfortunately, is rather effective in his methods. I refer to the little politician with some petty political office in view. This man carefully feels the pulse of his community regarding the tick eradication question, and if he finds that ignorance prevails and consequently an aversion to the work, he loses no opportunity to add to this ignorance and to strengthen the people in their spirit of aversion. He simply plays upon the credulity of the uninformed, so that he may successfully ride into office through their votes.

This class of citizen usually knows better, but his campaign is conducted in an absolutely selfish manner, without any regard whatever for the real good of his neighbors or for the successful development of his community or of his state. He is a dangerous man, however, because through his sophomoric campaign talks and speeches he is frequently able to sway the minds of the people, and in some instances the minds of the local authorities in the county, whose assistance and cooperation are so much needed to successfully carry on the work, by posing as the "friend of the poor farmer" against imaginary governmental aggression.

Even in a case of this kind there is a remedy. The "toxin" of ignorance must be carefully combated by the judicious use of the "antitoxin" of knowledge. In other words our poorly informed people must be educated, so that they may be able to think intelligently for themselves and base their conclusions upon proved facts.

SUMMARY. As this whole matter appears to me, it would seem to resolve itself into two main issues, viz.:

1. The fact that great ignorance still prevails concerning the work of tick eradication, and which must of necessity be dispelled before we may hope to reach the goal of tick-freedom in the shortest possible time; and

2. That the only feasible method to accomplish this, as I see it, is through the education of the people; which I believe will largely devolve upon the county inspector, who is presumed to come into daily contact with the cattle owners in his immediate locality.

This would suggest, therefore, that the inspector must not only be familiar with every phase of the work, but he should be an educator—shall I say of the kindergarden type? because it should be remembered that his "pupils" are but babies in knowledge of the problem he is trying to solve. He should be patient, tolerant, and sympathetic, but withal he should be firm, and he should be a student of human nature, so that he may draw the people to him through being able to adapt himself to their various idiosyncracies, their peculiarities of temperament, etc.

Education, therefore, is the surest weapon we possess with which to bring the tick fight to a "peaceful issue" in the shortest time possible, because it will bring with it all other measures necessary to accomplish the final result.

I fully realize, of course, the magnificent work that has already been done in the face of all the obstacles mentioned, and no doubt others which I have failed to allude to. There is a great deal yet to be accomplished, and there is still an immense amount of gross ignorance, and what I have said is more in the nature of an appeal to those who expect to be in the fight during the remainder of the campaign.

Finally, we must always bear in mind that this country is at grips with the most powerful (military) and relentless foe which possibly the world has ever known, in the greatest conflict of which there is any record in history, and on the outcome of which depend momentous consequences. Therefore, everything that it is possible to do to conserve and increase the food supply in meat and meat-food products at this time of stress, and for some time in the future, should be done, not alone from the standpoint of patriotism but as an absolute necessity, in fact a war measure. I am of the opinion that the successful early completion of the work of tick eradication in the South will be one of the most potent factors in aiding our country and our associates in the war to decide the conflict favorably.

MAKE YOUR MONEY FIGHT.

—Under Federal supervision there were dipped in Louisiana during the month of March about two hundred thousand cattle. There were constructed during the month 813 dipping vats although the state-wide law, governing the work of tick eradication, did not become operative until April 1. There are now 3478 vats in operation in the state.

—Announcement is made of the marriage of Miss Mabel E. Williams to Dr. Edward F. Sanford, New York City, February 14.

—A Cornell Veterinarians' Club was recently organized at New York City with a membership of nineteen. Dr. Cassius Way was elected president, C. V. Noback, vice president; L. Price, secretary-treasurer.

—The following-named veterinarians have been added to the force engaged in hog cholera work in the State of Illinois with headquarters at Springfield, Illinois: Drs. Howard L. Deuell, Theodore M. Bayler, Albert M. Meade and Grant B. Munger.

—LIBERTY LOANS STRENGTHEN THE LIBERTY LINE.

CLINICAL AND CASE REPORTS

DIAPHRAGMATIC INTERCOSTAL RUMENOCELE IN A CALF

Walter J. Crocker, Philadelphia, Pa.

From the time of birth until destroyed the calf in the illustration manifested a swelling which occupied almost the entire side of the body. It varied in size from a lump as big as a man's fist to a small tub. At times it entirely disappeared. On palpation it sometimes presented the consistency of mush, at other times it felt like a balloon.

The animal was destroyed and autopsied immediately. The diaphragm was displaced forward and adhered to the thoracic wall

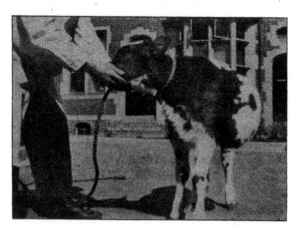

on the left side for a distance of six inches. A slit-like opening, 15 cm. long, appeared in the diaphragm and last intercostal space and showed white fibrous margins. A large portion of the rumen passed through this opening in the diaphragm and intercostal muscle into the subcutaneous tissue forcing it together with the skin outward to the formation of a large sac. The rumen in the sac contained gas and soft food material. The rumen was not adhered to the subcutis but was easily forced back into the abdomen. No evidences of strangulation were present. In this case the hernial ring was constituted of a congenital opening in the diaphragm and last left intercostal space. The hernial sac was formed by the subcutis

and skin. The hernial contents consisted of a portion of the rumen.
Thus the pathologic anatomical designation diaphragmatic intercostal rumenocele.

Other organs and tissues presented no alteration.

OBSERVATION ON TREMBLES (MILK SICK) IN COWS, TRANSMITTED TO MAN BY MILK AND MILK PRODUCTS

H. R. SCHWARZE
Bacteriologist, Department of Agriculture, Springfield, Ill.

On May 29th, 1917, a report was received by the State Veterinarian in Department of Agriculture, Division of Animal Industry
and Veterinary Science, from Mr. O. S. H., Atwood, Ill., stating that he had a sick cow on his farm, located two and one-half
miles northwest from town.

The local veterinarian had been called to treat the case. On
making an examination they were unable to make a positive diagnosis, but thought it might be some form of indigestion and treated
the animal accordingly.

Mr. O. S. H. further stated that his son became ill about the
same time the cow first showed sickness. The son was taken to
St. Mary's Hospital at Decatur for treatment and died after several days' illness. The physician attending the son thought he was
suffering from some plant poisoning.

That being the case, Mr. O. S. H. thought the boy might have
contracted the disease from the cow and would like to have the
Department make an investigation.

On the 30th day of May I proceeded to Atwood to investigate
the trouble existing on the farm owned by Mr. O. S. H. On my
arrival at Atwood, I called on the local veterinarian who was in
attendance on the case, and the two of us went out to the farm to
see the sick cow. We arrived at the farm about one o'clock. When
we went to the barn we found the cow had died a short time before
our arrival.

The history of the case, according to the owner, was that this
Jersey cow, aged 4 years, giving a good flow of milk, had been kept
in a clean, warm barn all winter and spring up to May 1st, during
which time she had received nothing but dry food. On May 1st,

he turned her out to pasture. On the 20th day of May, the cow began to show stiffness and her flow of milk dropped from three gallons normal to one and one-half pint.

The local veterinarian was called the same evening to see the cow. The symptoms described by the veterinarian in charge were, drooping of head and ears, stiffness, irregular gait, dullness, irregular pulse, respiration slow, temperature about normal, drank water freely, slight appetite, cessation of rumination, eyes glazed, membranes congested, bad-smelling breath and constipation. The diagnosis made by him was some digestive trouble, and the patient was treated accordingly with laxatives and stimulants.

However, the animal did not improve, but seemed to be on the decline with all the former symptoms more marked. On the third day she preferred the recumbent position to standing up. When made to rise she would get up with difficulty, trembling of entire muscular system would take place. Walk was very irregular, general stiffness. When leaving her alone she would again take the recumbent position and the trembling would stop.

Whenever the animal was disturbed and excited the former symptoms would present themselves. As time went on the symptoms became more aggravated until she was unable to rise, with absence of normal reflex, gradually going into coma, followed by death on the ninth day.

On post mortem examination we found the body still warm with rigor mortis complete. The skin appeared quite smooth, the eyes appeared glassy and mucous membranes showed congestion; membranes of mouth and tongue normal. When opening the body a peculiar acidulous odor was detected, the blood was tarry black in color, did not coagulate but rather jellied, lungs and heart normal. The gastro-intestinal mucosa seemed to be slightly congested with the exception of the abomasum. The mucosa of this organ was greatly congested. The contents of the stomach and bowels seemed to be drier and harder than normal with the exception of the abomasum. The contents of the stomach were more liquid than normal (no doubt due to the various drenches the cow had received.) The liver was slightly enlarged, showing fatty degeneration; spleen and kidneys normal; bladder contained an abnormally large amount of urine. The urine had a very strong acidulous odor, yellow in color, specific gravity 1025, acid reaction.

In connection with the sickness of this cow, the son of Mr. O.

S. H. became ill on the seventh day of May, 1917. Their local physician was called the 20th to treat the boy. However, the trouble did not respond to the treatment, but his condition was growing more serious. Consequently they took him to St. Mary's Hospital at Decatur for treatment. On investigation it was found that the boy consumed a great deal of milk, which was taken from the cow before any symptoms were noticed. In fact, the father stated that milk was the boy's principal diet.

The boy's symptoms, as described by his father, were similar to the ones manifested in the cow. Glassy appearance of the eyes, congestion of mucous membranes, dullness, nausea, vomiting, stiffness and constipation.

On the 26th day of May, 1917, Mr. H. P. H., who lives across the road from his brother, O. S. H., became ill. The same physicians were called to treat him. He was treated at home and not taken to a hospital like the former patient. We went over to see Mr. H. P. H., but were not allowed to go in the room with him. We talked to Mrs. H. P. H. about the case, and the symptoms she described were that he was very weak, listless, complained of stiffness, nausea and vomiting spells, breath had a bad odor, and a peculiar appearance of the eyes.

When asked whether Mr. H. P. H. consumed much milk before he became ill, she said that he did not consume any, but that he was fond of cream, home-made cheese and butter of which he had consumed considerable.

The milk products that were consumed by Mr. H. P. H. were made of milk taken from two cows that did not show any symptoms of trembles. However, they were kept in a pasture adjoining the one where Mr. O. S. H. pastured his cow.

These two cows were taken from their pasture as soon as the trouble was suspected.

The symptoms described by the physicians in charge of the boy were, the patient complained of stiffness of the back, a foul-smelling breath, constant vomiting, no rise in temperature, obstinate constipation, pupils dilated, conjunctiva congested, knee jerks were present but gradually became absent. The Babinski sign was always marked, a lumbar puncture was made, the Nonne Apelt test applied with negative reaction. Urine gave a marked acetone reaction. He refused all food, gradually became weaker, went into coma and died the tenth day.

The symptoms manifested by Mr. H. P. H. were the same as the former. However, no lumbar puncture was made and Nonne Apelt test applied. Mr. H. P. H. recovered after a long siege of illness.

It was further found that there had been a previous case of trembles on this farm. In the year 1915 there was a sick cow on this farm, which showed the same symptoms recognized in Mr. O. S. H.'s cow. This cow died. She was owned by Mr. O. S. H., who also became affected and died. Also his child became affected but recovered after a long illness.

The milk and carcass of the cow were fed to hogs. These also developed the disease and died.

The pastures where these animals were kept was a twenty-acre timber tract, divided in two ten-acre lots by a wire fence. One lot was used by Mr. O. S. H. for his cow, the other by Mr. H. P. H. for his two cows. The lay of the land was flat with a swail in the north center which was divided by the fence so that each pasture had about the same amount of low land. There was no domestic grass of any kind present. However, there was a large crop of weeds, such as low larkspur, mandrake, buch brush, burdock, iron weed, poke berry, Indian turnip, poison ivy, horse weed and a number of other plants I was unable to identify.

The interesting feature of these cases, to the writer, is that the same symptoms were manifested by all of the patients.

FALSE PREGNANCY; PULMONARY DRENCH; TUMOR ON OVIDUCT*

T. H. AGNEW, Pasadena, California

False pregnancy in four goats of a herd of thirty. These goats were bred and were with kid to all appearances. At the termination of pregnancy, labor pains developed, the water bag burst, but no kids were present. They regained their normal condition in seven to nine days, and are again bred and now believed to be from two to four months pregnant.

Called to a cow about 2:30 P. M. She did not appear well that morning. The owner, an experienced cow man, gave her a dose

---

*Presented to the Los Angeles Veterinary Medical Association at its February meeting.

of salts, without any apparent discomfort to her at the time. Upon examining her, found pulse 80, temperature 94, tongue protruding, and breathing very short. She died in four hours, and the post mortem revealed the fact that the dose of salts had passed into the lungs.

Cocker bitch, four years old, has had five or six attacks within a year of what seemed like colic. When examined, by palpation of the abdomen, found what seemed to be an enlarged ovary. Decided to operate. On opening abdomen, found attached to Fallopian tube a three-sided tumor, about two and one-half inches long, resembling a Brazil nut in shape, quite hard and enclosed in a cyst. This was removed and the bitch has had no further attacks of pain, several months having elapsed since the operation.

"A PECULIAR CASE OF LAMENESS"

ERNEST F. JARDINE
Basseterre, St. Kitts, B. W. I.

Sometime in the month of September I was called to see a lame mare. The animal was supposed to be about 5 months with foal. Had been lame about 4 days and thought it was due to the shoeing so animal was taken to the shoeing smith. Nothing was found in the hoof to reveal the cause. Shoes were replaced. Then had the animal led out of the stable, which had a decline, to the ground.

Mare walked perfectly well out of the stable, also along the ground when led, backed all right. I searched the hoof and found nothing. In fact, I told the owner the animal was not lame. He then said, she is all right like that, but trot her and she goes rather funny. I then had the mare trotted, and the animal, instead of placing the left hind leg on the ground at all, held it up in the air the same way as a dog does when he has anything wrong with his leg.

It wasn't a fracture, it wasn't a nail or anything in the hoof; manipulating the limb from the external angle of the ilium, along the sacral region, etc., to the hoof, the animal showed not the slightest sign of any pain. Naturally the owner wanted to know, not so much, he said, as to what was the matter with her, as he was to know whether she would get right or not. I was at a loss as to what to say, but told him I thought the trouble was in the crural muscles, and about a month's rest would help her. I advised warm fomentations to the crural region morning and night for one-half hour at a time, and prescribed a stimulating liniment of ammonia, turpentine, tincture of arnica and soft soap and water, to be rubbed in after fomenting.

I saw the owner about six weeks later and he told me the mare was all right again. Whether the treatment, or nature, effected the cure, or whether the trouble was really in the crural muscles or not, I will not venture to say.

SUCCESSFUL TREATMENT OF TETANUS

MAJOR FRED FOSTER
Post Veterinary Hospital, Fort Sam Houston, Texas

For the treatment of tetanus, attention is invited to a recipe given herewith that has proved successful in an experiment by Capt. W. W. Richards, V.C., N.A., and First Lieut. Asa R. Andrews, V.C., N.A., in a test made at the Post Veterinary Hospital, Fort Sam Houston, Texas.

One mule, weight 1000 lbs., admitted to the hospital February 19th, 1918, with a well developed case of tetanus; rigid condition of the ears; elevated condition of the tail, the whole musculature involved; marked condition of the membrana nictitans on the least excitement; was able to open mouth sufficiently to prehend and masticate food. The following treatment was used:

Placed in a comfortable box stall, loose, put on a bran mash diet, drinking water *ad libitum*.

February 19th, intravenous injection of 4 ozs. 3% solution sulph. magnesium.

February 20th, 6 ozs. 3% sol. sulph. magnesium.

February 21st, 8 ozs. 3% sol. sulph. magnesium.

February 22nd, 8 ozs. 3% sol. sulph. magnesium.

February 23rd, no medication.

February 24th, 8 ozs. 3% sol. sulph. magnesium.

February 25th, no medication.

February 26th, 8 ozs. 3% sol. sulph. magnesium.

February 27th, no medication; able to eat off the floor.

February 28th, such a marked improvement discontinued medication.

March 4th, placed in corral where he could take voluntary exercise.

March 14th, returned to duty.

(No other medication used outside of the magnesium sulphate.)

That the experiment may be given further tests so as to prove its worthiness, it is desired to bring it to the attention of other veterinarians.

THE CARE OF THE FEET

Capt. John H. Gould
Division Veterinarian, 88th Division, Veterinary Corps

Where horses and mules are allowed to run in corrals that are poorly drained, muddy, not properly cleaned, and polluted with stable refuse, thrush, hoof rot, and even canker of the foot are apt to develop. Animals under these conditions should have their feet cleaned by use of a blunt pointed hoof hook, or other blunt instrument, at least twice each week. If there is discovered any signs of decay in the frog or other part of the foot, the whole plantar surface should be treated with an application of pine tar. The tar should be tucked into the bottoms of all crevices, and, if such crevices are deep in the middle or lateral commissures of the frog, a small pledget of oakum should be tamped in over it as an additional protection and to assist in retaining the tar.

Frayed portions of horny frog and loose scales of sole should be removed, as they harbor filth and dirt. If the foot is unduly large, by reason of lack of care in trimming, the excess horn should be removed and the foot should be properly leveled.

In cases where the cracks and crevices in the frog are deep and cause lameness, equal parts of pine tar, oil of tar and turpentine may be used to advantage.

Great care should be exercised in keeping corrals and stables free from stable refuse and mud holes, but barring the possibility of such a perfect condition of corrals and stables, the feet of all horses and mules should be regularly cleaned out in order that any deviation from the normal may be determined before it reaches the stage whereby it becomes serious enough to incapacitate the animal for duty.

From past experience with large numbers of animals, I should predict that unless unusual care is taken to guard against the condition mentioned, that there will be a great number of animals in our cantonments and remount stations affected with thrush in varying degrees of intensity. And this more particularly as the frequent freezing and thawing attendant to the variable weather of the spring months approaches, preventing to a great extent the thorough cleaning of the corrals, open sheds and stables.

ABSTRACTS FROM RECENT LITERATURE

POLL EVIL. Capt. J. A. Mathison. *Veterinary Journal.*— The concise record of a number of cases of poll evil that came under his observation and which proved interesting by the different conditions of the parts met with in the disease.

Three cases were due to parts of the occipital bone being loose and driven in the tissues of the poll. Removal of these pieces and efficient drainage was followed with recovery in 24-$_{35}$ and 59 days.

In another case a piece of shrapnel was found lodged in the occipital region.

In two cases resection of the ligamentum nuchae was resorted to and demanded 12 and 23 days for recovery.

In seven cases, where the ligament had remained healthy but where the pus had burrowed underneath, recovery varied between 12 and 102 days in the hospital.

In two cases the abscesses were superficial to the ligament and recovered in 10 and 32 days.

In nine cases resection of the ligament was performed and diseased portion removed. These remained under treatment between 46 and 65 days.

Of the whole number treated, 17 were geldings, and the balance mares.   A. L.

TUBERCULAR ARTHRITIS OF THE CERVICAL VERTEBRAE. Lieut. W. G. Burndred, A.V.C.—A very old Australian mare was suffering with stiffness and was unable to pick up food from the ground. No history of her case could be obtained. One day it was noticed that she was unable to lower her head to drink water from a stream. When examined she was found with impairment of motion in the neck, in the region of the 6th and 7th cervical vertebrae. She manifested pain on pressure of the region or when forced motion was executed. The mare was placed under observation. Tuberculined she showed manifest reaction. Mallein test was negative. Destroyed, after the diagnosis of tuberculosis was made, she only showed the articular surfaces of the 2d, 3d, 4th, 5th and 6th cervical vertebrae with their articular surfaces studded with small gelatinous nodules of the size of pin's head. Those between the 6th and 7th vertebrae were covered one-half with similar nodules, larger in size, the other part being adherent and covered with granulations. No tubercles were found in any of the organs of the body. The lesions of the articular surfaces were primary lesions of tuberculous condition of the articular surfaces.   A. L.

GOITER IN A DOG. Horace Roberts, F.R.C.V.S. *Veterinary Journal.*—A fox terrier had two large swellings on the upper part of the neck. They interfered with his breathing. The dog was of a very nervous nature. An operation was not likely to be accepted on account of a previous fatal result obtained on this dog's mother. Internal administration of thyroid gland was suggested. One tabloid of one grain which contains not less than 0.05 per cent of iodine was given every evening for three hundred consecutive evenings. After this long treatment the goiter was found quite normal, the respiration was natural, there was no more cardiac impulse and on stethoscopic examination of the heart, there was found a regular function.   A. L.

NECROTIC VAGINITIS IN CATTLE. G. Mayall, M.R.C.V.S. *Veterinary Journal.*—Three cases are recorded by the author. One lived five days and died. A second lived a week and died. The third lived ten days and recovered. The treatment consisted in the removal of the cleansing, injections and swabbings of the vagina with a solution of mercury iodide and mercuric chloride bougies were inserted. Internal antiseptics were given in linseed tea. The author remarks that there seems to be an intimate connection between this complaint and the retention of the afterbirth, and he believes that the disease is a necrotic one as seems to be considered by some authors.   A. L.

NOTES ON THE TREATMENT OF MANGE. Vétérinaire Aide-Major Chatelain, 1st Class. *Recueil Médecine Vétérinaire*, January 15th, 1918. (Translated by Major L. A. Merillat, Veterinary Hospital, A. P. O. 731.)—Of all the ailments that hinder the effectiveness of a campaign, mange is the most tenacious and widespread, presenting difficulties both as regards the cure of the affected animals and the administration of remedial measures.

Nearly all of the remedies recognized or employed by veterinarians bring good results. Some are rapid and some are slow but all of them cure well enough.

The rapidity of the cure varies according to the pains taken in administering the treatment and the best results, as in all medication, all things being equal, occur when the practitioner applies the treatment himself.

These things being agreed the points to be considered in the treatment of mange in an army in the field are: 1st, the rapidity of application; 2nd, the curative effects of the remedy; and 3rd, the cost.

FIRST—THE RAPIDITY OF APPLICATION. Not only the time required in treating the diseased skin must be considered but also the preparatory treatment such as clipping, because all the remedies that have a fatty base require clipping before being applied. Clipping in a campaign presents great difficulties. There is usually only one clipper in a unit and since the clipping of a horse is a long tiresome job, especially when affected with mange, the affected subjects and suspects cannot be treated as rapidly as they should be. Then again the fatty substances are difficult to spread in winter when hardened by cold, and the time required for the men to wash their hands and that consumed in washing the cured animals must also be computed. Furthermore the price of soap and pomades still further show the disadvantages of such treatment. Price and time are important factors in a campaign, where it is always essential to work fast to check the spread of the disease.

For these reasons those remedies which do not contain fatty bases should be preferred because (except in horses with heavy coats) the therapeutic treatment can be administered without clipping, so that the treatment of a large number of horses can be done in a short time. Rapidity of treatment is therefore also an important factor.

SECOND—THERAPEUTIC EFFECT OF THE REMEDY. In a general way it might be said that the effects of medicaments are analogous. Some are perhaps more active than others, but always the enthusiasm with which they are administered manifestly influences the results. Most all veterinarians have had good results with remedies which, when handed to others to administer, have been less effectual. It is therefore futile, in the interest of the sick, to recommend a new remedy if it will not be enthusiastically administered. The author has kept in mind the need of improvising practical formulae. Because of the difficulty of getting supplies one formula must often be substituted for another.

THIRD. As stated above pomades are effectual but they have three disadvantages: (a) the necessity of clipping; (b) very careful application and subsequent care; and (c) the expense.

It is therefore preferable to substitute products and compositions other than those which have appeared in the professional journals. A rational and effectual remedy that has given excellent results both economically and therapeutically is the sulphur bath given by means of the dipping vat, but to make this treatment satisfactory in war it would be necessary to build veterinary hospitals with dipping vats within 20 kilometers of the front in order that all animals affected could be treated.

In lieu of the dipping vat, and when it becomes necessary to meet the emergency of treating an animal in the field showing suspicious depilations I conceived a succedaneum that has given happy results, consisting of cresyl, soap, polysulphure, carbonate of potash and carbonate of sodium. When these are mixed promiscuously they generally cause an insoluble and inert precipitate. The following plan of dispensing removes this obstacle. These formulae, in addition to giving rapid and excellent results, yield a homogeneous emulsion. When allowed to stand it separates into two layers: a green, moss colored one below that is opaque and an orange colored one above that is transparent. It has a powerful therapeutic effect and can be used as well by the practitioner as in war. It is indispensable to always shake the mixture well before using.

PREPARATION. Solution C. Cresyl, 250 gm; hot water, 1000 gm.

Solution D. Polysulphate, 100 gm; hot water, 1000 gm.

Solution A. Potassium carbonate, 40 gm; sodium carbonate, 10 gm; hot water, 1000 gm.

Solution B. White soap, 40 gm; hot water, 1000 gm.

Take one part of Solution A and add one part of Solution B and shake violently; add one part of Solution C and shake again, then add one part of Solution D and shake violently for several moments.

METHOD OF APPLICATION. Wash the horse all over with a wisp of hay and water, and when wet incorporate in the wisp 15 grams of black soap and rub it in briskly all over the body to make the soap lather penetrate to the skin. Let the lather dry a quarter of an hour and then wash off the soap. Now without drying the horse rub the solution into the coat with gentle friction and let it remain for two days and then wash well with white soap.

(Dose: 100 grams for a horse affected all over the body.)

RESULTS. In benign cases one application and in bad cases two to three applications suffice to cure animals affected all over the body, providing they have not been treated with remedies of an irritating nature which have burned the skin and caused the formation of crusts. Immediately after the first application a pronounced amelioration is noticed.

Of the 54 horses treated in this manner all but two were cured promptly.

This treatment is effectual and exceedingly practical where better methods, such as dipping and sulphuration, are not possible to carry out. The word polysulphate is a word used to designate a product entering into nearly all mange remedies that is chemically a pentsulphate of potassium. L. A. M.

A NOTE REGARDING MYIASIS, ESPECIALLY THAT DUE TO SYRPHID LARVAE. Maurice C. Hall. *Arch. Int. Med.*, v. 21 (3), March, pp. 309-312.—This paper records an additional case of myiasis due to rat-tailed larvae in man and summarizes the cases to date. There appear to be at least 17 records claiming the presence of syrphid larvae in the digestive tract of man, one record claiming their presence in the nostrils of man, and two records claiming their presence in the diseased vagina of cattle. The case of rat-tailed larvae in the vagina of a cow, published by Bruce in the *Journal of the A. V. M. A.* for October, 1917, is the second case of the sort, the first case having been published by Hall and Muir in the *Archives of Internal Medicine* in February, 1913. There is a note regarding the occurrence of live rat-tailed larvae in February in Colorado at an altitude of 9,000 feet. M. C. HALL.

EXPERIMENTS ON THE TREATMENT OF RINDERPEST WITH VARIOUS DRUGS. William Hutchins Boynton. *The Philippine Agricultural Review*, Vol. X, No. 3, 1917.—So called cures for rinderpest have been found lacking in curative power. Highly susceptible animals were used in all the experiments. A highly virulent strain of virus was used to inject the animals upon which the drugs were tried. In the localities where cures for rinderpest had been reported the recoveries of animals without such medication were very high.

Twenty different drugs were used. An 0.85 per cent solution of sodium chloride, warmed to about 41°C. was used to dilute the drugs for intravenous and intraperitoneal injection whenever the dilution was necessary.

Strychnine, nitroglycerin, and echinacoid stimulate animals passing through immunization by the simultaneous method. These drugs are practically useless against rinderpest contracted in the usual way. Only two animals out of a total of over fifty recovered from the disease when treated with the various drugs. The drugs had no curative power for the animals suffering from rinderpest.

HAYDEN.

ACUTE ARTICULAR RHEUMATISM IN THE HORSE—RHEUMATIC FEVER. V. S. *Veterinary Journal.*—A seven-year-old big Shire gelding was taken lame suddenly and grew worse rapidly with considerable swelling from the hock down to the fetlock. His temperature went up to 106°, his pulse was 60, the conjunctiva was injected and the urine slightly colored. Diagnosis was made of acute rheumatic fever with endocarditis. Submitted to alkalines, salicylate and digitalis. The horse was put in slings but his condition grew worse and though its temperature went down a state of collapse set in and he was destroyed. At the post mortem there was found acute synovitis of the fetlock with furrows on the articular cartilage, erosion on that and on the os suffraginis and the sesamoids. The heart had a boiled and streaky look with commencing vegetations of the endocardium of the left auricle just above the insertion of the mitral valve.   A. L.

TWO CASES OF TETANUS. Ernest Morgan, M.R.C.V.S. *Veterinary News.*—A brief record of a well bred mare, cast from the army, which had run away a fortnight before and sustained some cuts about the legs. The symptoms were well marked although she could take enough food to keep her alive. Chloral in four dram doses given daily twice a day brought her to an uninterrupted recovery, although she had been kept in a loose box with open windows in a slaughter house where daily killing was carried on.

The other case was not so fortunate. An eight-year-old bay mare had no perceptible wound and yet showed marked tetanic symptoms. On the 3rd day she had swellings between the fore legs and under the chest. On the 6th day had a strong jugular pulse. She could lay down frequently and rise without difficulty. She ate slowly and practically she seemed to improve but finally she got down and was killed. At the post mortem a decolorized clot extending into the arteries was found with also an extensive valvular disease of the heart. A. L.

ARMY VETERINARY SERVICE

THE ARMY VETERINARY SERVICE

MAJOR RAINEY, British Army Veterinary Service

The present work and organization of the Army Veterinary Service afford a striking instance of what can be achieved in a short while when science is adequately assisted by finance and in other ways given facilities fairly completely to develop its latent possibilities. The existing war is the first recorded in military history in which the veterinary service of the Army has been permitted and assisted to carry out a definite scheme of its own generation, and it is this fact which gives most interest to a critical examination of results as they stand today.

The British nation has been blamed by other nations and by its own citizens for its disregard, in the past, of science, but the Royal Army Medical Corps and the Army Veterinary Corps of the present constitute a powerful argument for those defenders of British sanity who maintain its capacity to adapt to practical needs ideas which other, possibly more imaginative, nations have visualized more fully, but have not always in the last resort so completely developed. The old English proverb, ''Sharp's a good dog but Holdfast's a better'', may perhaps be taken to express this national characteristic.

Primarily, an Army Veterinary Corps must justify its cost on economic grounds. The humanitarian factor, although it plays an important part in the practical work of the corps, cannot for purposes of war on a modern scale be held alone to justify the cost of so extensive an undertaking as the Army Veterinary Corps of the British Army of today.

It is not possible at this stage to draw up a balance sheet that would accurately or even approximately show what dividend the Nation derives from its capital outlay in this respect, but the following figures present, it is thought, a fair *prima facie* case in favor of an Army Veterinary Service as an economic factor in war:

(a) The total wastage* among horses and mules of the British forces at home and expeditionary forces abroad, including losses from enemy gunfire and all other causes whatsoever, during the year ending December 31st, 1916, amounted to 1C% of the total animal strength.

(b) The total wastage among horses and mules of the British forces during the year 1912 (i. e., during peace) amounted approximately to 14.80% of the total animal strength.

These figures mean that in spite of continuous losses from enemy gunfire, and from the inevitable chances and vicissitudes of war, the annual wastage among probably the largest number of horses and mules ever collected together has, during the last complete year of war, actually been less than the rate of wastage in time of peace. This, notwithstanding the fact, bemoaned by humanitarians, that the bulk of the animals have been standing night and day in the open exposed to all weathers, whereas in time of peace all Army animals are stabled under the best hygienic conditions.

The average annual mortality among Army animals participating in the South African War, 1899-1902, exceeded 55% per annum for the whole war.

There was no Army Veterinary Corps in those days. The Army Veterinary Department, as it was then, consisted of only a few officers and Auxiliary Civil Veterinary Surgeons whose duties for all practical purposes were limited to professional attendance upon such sick and wounded animals as chanced to come within their narrow official scope.

Proposals for a better organization, indeed for any adequate organization, were coldly received. The military chiefs of those days, in common more or less with the rest of the community, had little confidence in their veterinary advisers and relied largely

---

*The expression "wastage" includes deaths, destructions, missing and castings for destruction or sale. The mortality alone in 1916 was 9.47%.

upon the time honored fallacy that all such subsidiary technical matters were of slight, if any, military importance.

Considerations of more legitimate military importance may have led, in 1899-1900, to a Cavalry campaign for which no hay was thought necessary, resulting, for example, in that memorable occasion on which a Brigade of Cavalry marched out from Bloemfontein under 100 strong, the remainder *hors de combat* for the most part from bulk starvation and consequent debility of their horses.

Major W. E. Watson, D.S.O., 6th Dragoon Guards, who marched out with the "Brigade" on that occasion, places the strength of effective mounted men as low as fifty.

It is not, however, claimed that the South African War of 1899-1902 and the present European War are exactly parallel cases in a veterinary point of view. It is not necessary to make such a claim since there is a wide enough margin between an annual equine mortality of 9.47% and 55% to permit of considerable departure from the parallel, without affecting the validity of a statement that on the whole the better results of the present war in equine matters are chiefly attributable to the work of the Army Veterinary Service.

If the South African War was one of marching and countermarching, then this war has been one of hauling and straining to drag vehicles and guns of all descriptions through tenacious mud, under conditions of the greatest hardship and discomfort. Moreover, although there has been little of cavalry work in France, Egypt has afforded opportunity for some extensive operations in this respect, and, in the fighting against Bulgaria during 1916 very heavy work was required of the pack-transport animals. Statistical returns for the German South West African Campaign and Rebellion, August, 1914, to July, 1915, and for the subsequent period, July, 1915, to March 1st, 1916, show an annual mortality at the rate of 9.09% among animals (horses and mules) of the Union forces.

The conditions of this campaign were similar in most respects to those of the South African War, 1899-1902, with this considerable difference that the Union Government were careful to include in their forces an Army Veterinary Corps, identical as far as possible in its organization and proportionate strength with the Army Veterinary Corps of the Imperial Army.

There are thus three distinct figures from which deductions can be made:

1. Those of South African War, 1899-1902, with an annual mortality of 55%.

2. Those of German South West Africa, 1914-1915, annual mortality of 9.09%.

3. Those of the European War, 1914-15-16, inclusive of campaigns in France, Egypt and Salonika—annual mortality under 10%.

If it may be permitted to indulge in a little loose algebraic discussion, then:

Let 'A' be taken to mean an Army at war.
Let 'B' be taken to mean an efficient Army Veterinary Corps.
Let 'C' be taken to mean the peculiar conditions of a South African War.
$A+B-C$ = an annual equine mortality of 9.47%.
$A+B+C$ = an annual equine mortality of 9.09%.
$A-B+C$ = an annual equine mortality of 55%.

The above very simple equations certainly appear to indicate that plus B, otherwise an efficient Army Veterinary Corps, bears an important relation to mortality among Army animals in war.

It is true of course that there is an economic limit to the dimensions and utility of an Army Veterinary Service or of any other administrative service, but that point does not seem yet to have been worked out by calculations. It would appear to be important actuarially to establish precisely what proportion expenditure on each administrative service should bear to the cost of an Army or other National undertaking as a whole, so as to be productive in the long run of the best economic results.

This is a field of scientific inquiry, so far as military operations are concerned, in which little or nothing has been accomplished. At the beginning of the war there were published in the daily newspapers letters from ill-informed and distressed humanitarians in which statements were made to the effect that an Army horse lasted only for a few days after arrival at the front. How unnecessarily these good people distressed themselves and a sympathetic public may be deduced from the above announced annual death-rate which, it is believed, gives the war horse five years' expectation of life after being posted to the British expeditionary force.

The officers of the Army Veterinary Corps are graduates of British and Colonial veterinary colleges, with the exception of

Quartermasters appointed for duty as such to Veterinary Hospitals, Horse Convalescent Depots, Base Depots of Veterinary Stores and Schools of Farriery.

As there exists a good deal of misconception among the general public concerning the degree of professional education required for purposes of graduation as a duly qualified Veterinary Surgeon, it may here be stated that the curriculum of a modern veterinary college extends over four years, that is one year less than the period required for graduation as a practitioner of human medicine and surgery. The curriculum embraces the same subjects as those of the medical student modified or extended where necessary to meet the different requirements of the domesticated animals. It is estimated that about 40% of the entire veterinary profession of this country are now employed as officers in various capacities with the Army Veterinary Corps. The numbers of officers and other ranks, A.V.C., available for duty on mobilization in August, 1914, were: Officers, 109; other ranks, 322, including reservists. Today there are over 1200 officers and considerably more than 20,000 N.C. Os. and men, exclusive of native Indian and Egyptian subordinate personnel. The personnel of the Army Veterinary Corps is, therefore, like that of other branches of the service, chiefly composed of officers and men who have joined the colors since the outbreak of war. No man passed fit for service with front line combatant units has been accepted for enlistment in the Army Veterinary Corps (Regulars) since September, 1915, and of those enlisted prior to that time nearly 3,000 have been transferred to R.N. and B.F.A. and replaced by Class B recruits. As far as possible men accustomed to horses were enlisted, but this source of supply proved to be limited in view of the prior claims of combatant arms, so that it has been necessary to train *ab initio* what appeared most unlikely material. Fortunately the material proved better than official fears. What was lacking in experience was found fruitful in intelligence, and the impression has been gained that for instruction in scientific principles it is as well to have intelligent virgin soil as painfully to have to modify the little knowledge that in veterinary matters especially "is a dangerous thing".

The present personnel as a whole is keen, enthusiastic, and imbued with those ideas of humanitarianism and helpfulness which are essential to useful work among dumb and comparatively stupid animals.

The work of the Army Veterinary Service comprises:

1. The examination for soundness of all animals prior to their purchase for the Army.

2. Care of remounts on board ship.

3. Prevention and control of contagious and other diseases among all Army animals.

4. Treatment of minor cases of sickness and injury under regimental arrangement with the unit to which the animals belong.

5. Evacuation to veterinary hospitals of all cases of sickness or injury that cannot be treated properly with the unit, or that, for military reasons, it is not desirable to retain with the unit.

6. Maintenance of an efficient standard of horse-shoeing throughout the Army.

7. Supply of veterinary medicines and equipment.

8. The training in schools of farriery of shoeing-smiths and cold-shoers required for the Army.

9. Careful observance of and advice upon all matters directly or indirectly affecting the welfare of the Army horse, e. g., stable-management, forage and feeding, watering, etc.

The policy of the Army Veterinary Service is well expressed in the adage, "prevention is better than cure". The importance of prevention in military matters is paramount, and herein veterinary medicine diverges widely from human medical practice. This becomes apparent when one remembers that the horse cannot help himself but is entirely dependent upon the observation and foresight of those whose work it is to fend for him.

Veterinary and medical practice run side by side so far as hygiene, sanitation and antisepsis are concerned, but the point of divergence is where the man can report himself "sick" and the horse cannot. This means that if the horse is to be adequately protected he must be inspected at least once daily by someone who is competent to detect incipient symptoms of disease.

It does not require much imagination to realize the enormous amount of work and organization involved in arranging for this service alone in connection with a military horse strength of many hundreds of thousands.

The difficulty in detecting the first symptoms of disease in a horse is considerable and no small degree of experience is necessary before this difficulty can be overcome. This fact is particularly brought home to those concerned in dealing with outbreaks of equine influenza and pneumonia. In this class of disease, the greatest scourge of the equine race under conditions of domestication, frequently there is in the early stages little or no abnormal symptom apparent to the unskilled observer. A horse to such may appear in good health although at the time a clinical thermometer will register a rise of 5° F. if the temperature of the animal be taken. It is hardly necessary to add that if taken out and worked in this condition, as only too often happens, the animals will subsequently either die or become so seriously ill as to necessitate several weeks of careful treatment.

Remounts, that is, unseasoned horses, are peculiarly liable to this class of disease, so much so that practically every horse undergoes an attack subsequent to purchase and prior to commencing his military training. The Army Veterinary Service took early steps to combat this potential cause of wastage by enforcing the rule that in no case was any remount to be embarked on a ship or transferred from a Remount Depot unless his temperature had been taken and found to be normal not later than the day immediately preceding his journey. This simple measure alone has probably saved the lives of thousands of horses. In addition to the above rule instructions are that when an outbreak of pneumonia or influenza occurs in any unit no horse of the unit is to be worked on any day during the existence of the outbreak unless his temperature has been taken and found normal.

The foregoing technical information is given as an instance of the complexity and far reaching possibilitiies of equine preventive medicine.

Horses on Board Ship. There is no branch of administration in which the Army Veterinary Service has better justified its existence on economic grounds than in connection with the care of and arrangements for horses and mules on board ship.

At the outbreak of war it became evident that a large number of horses and mules would have to be purchased in other countries and brought to England by sea, and the Veterinary Directorate at the War Office undertook to provide veterinary surgeons to take charge of the animals during the voyage to this country. Veterinary surgeons were also sent out with the Purchasing Commission to examine the animals before purchase and to make such arrangements subsequently as would ensure that only healthy animals were placed on board ship for conveyance to this country or

elsewhere as might be required. One veterinary surgeon and a
carefully selected lay assistant were allotted to each ship carrying
horses or mules.

The appointment of an assistant, in addition to a veterinary
surgeon to each ship proved a fortunate arrangement as it was
found possible after a year's experience to place many of the assistants in sole charge of the animals, and to withdraw a corresponding number of veterinary surgeons for duty with Divisions
of the new armies at a time when the problem of finding sufficient
veterinary officers for the latter was acute.

For purposes of convenience both veterinary surgeons and lay
assistants, when acting in sole charge of horses on board ship, are
described as "conducting officers". These conducting officers have
done invaluable work. Many of them have been continuously employed on horse-ships since October, 1914, and have become trained
experts of the highest order.

During the first few months of the war the losses on board ship
were somewhat heavy, averaging about 3% for a short period. It
is now rare to lose 1%. Ship after ship arrives in port after the
voyage across the Atlantic with at most one or two animals lost on
the voyage and often none. Even on the long sea route from
Canada to Mediterranean theatres of war the loss has seldom
amounted to 1%. Including the above mentioned heavy losses
during the first few months of the war the total average loss on
all horses and mules shipped from the beginning of operations to
the present date barely exceeds 1%. These excellent results are
attributable in part to the pains taken to ensure the animals being
in good health when shipped, in part to the expert care bestowed
on the animals on board ship, and in part to the improvements on
horse-ships that have been carried out during the war as the result
of suggestions and recommendations received from conducting
officers. A notable improvement in this connection has been the
adoption of a system whereby animals are carried free in pens,
each pen containing about five horses or mules. Formerly all Army
remounts were carried in narrow stalls, each animal having a stall
to itself of a maximum width of 2 feet 6 inches.

The pen gives more freedom of movement, better facility for
sanitation and ventilation, and even permits an animal, desiring
to do so, to lie down for a while.

Incidentally an important economy has been effected in that
far less timber is required for constructing pens than stalls.

The foregoing is only one instance of the many problems that have been tackled successfully as. the outcome of keen and zealous observation and research on the part of conducting officers.

Conducting duty during this war has naturally not been devoid of stirring and perilous incident. In July, 1915, the S. S. "Anglo-Californian", carrying 925 horses from Canada to England, was attacked off the coast of Ireland by a German submarine. After three hours' shelling and the death of the captain the ship put into Queenstown in a leaky and battered condition. Of the 925 horses on board 26 were killed by shell fire. The remaining 899 were ultimately landed at an English port in good condition owing to the gallant behavior of the civil veterinary surgeon, Mr. F. Neal, who, although he had every opportunity to leave in the ship's boats at the same time as the subordinate staff, remained at his post and tended the horses almost single-handed until the ship was conveyed into port. He also attended the wounded on board during the engagement. In recognition of these services brought to notice by the Admiralty, Mr. Neal was presented, with the approval of the Treasury, with a gold watch suitably inscribed to commemorate the occasion.

The foregoing is but a single instance of numerous acts of heroism and devotion to duty on the part of conducting officers.

The following extract from the diary of a veterinary surgeon who has acted with distinction as conducting officer since October, 1914, will give some idea of the nature and importance of this work:

S. S. MECHANICIAN, 9TH VOYAGE EX MONTREAL, 958 HORSES, AUGUST 10TH, 1915—DAILY REPORT

A. E. BOYER, M.R.C.V.S., Veterinary Surgeon in Charge

On voyage out all decks were thoroughly cleaned and disinfected. The whole of parting boards, floors, ceilings, stanchions, breast boards, etc., after being scrubbed and disinfected were sprayed with 10 per cent solution of creolin previously to being whitewashed. All mangers were scrubbed with caustic soda and disinfected.

Tuesday, August. 10th, 1915

Commenced loading at 8:30 a. m. and finished at 1 p. m. 978 horses were sent, and I, in conjunction with Mr. McEcheran, the veterinary surgeon employed by the Remount Commission, rejected 20, consequently we are sailing 20 horses short. The causes of rejection were as follows:

1 injury to foot, old abscess under wall.

1 suspicious of the contagious dermatitis.

2 cases of strangles well developing.

16 cases of temperatures over 102 degrees.

I took on board over 30 with high temperatures, varying from 100 to 102 degrees.

2 p. m.—Tour of whole ship. Several horses very dull. Saw men allotted to sections, and went over same.

8 p. m.—Tour of whole ship. Saw every horse; found several cases, for which I sent salines. Temperatures very bad; there is no wind. Several horses slightly blowing and sweating. Outside temperature, 69 degrees.

1 Tween, 84 degrees	4 Tween, 76 degrees	Horses do not look very promising tonight, but it is due to the heat. Have every port open, all wind scoops out, and all wind sails up. Can do no more, only hope for some wind.
1 Orlop, 80 degrees	5 Tween, 84 degrees	
2 Tween, 80 degrees	6 Tween, 80 degrees	
2 Orlop, 82 degrees	6 Orlop, 80 degrees	
2 Hold, 76 degrees	6 Hold, 80 degrees	
3 Tween, 80 degrees	7 Tween, 82 degrees	
3 Orlop, 82 degrees	7 Orlop, 80 degrees	

Wednesday, August 11th, 1915

3 a. m.—An awful night. Called out by night watchman. Several horses blowing with heat, one a bad case of congestion; had 9 moved to more airy positions.

7 a. m.—Tour of top deck. With one exception all cases doing well. Not a breath of wind. Horses looking very dull.

10 a. m.—Tour of whole ship. Temperatures very high. More horses moved. Saw every horse, very worried with heat; had all parting boards out and started mucking out.

2 p. m.—Another tour of whole ship. Temperatures still high; no wind. Horses all look jaded and weary, and are without exception the most sick and sorry horses I have ever had.

8 p. m.—Tour of whole ship. Saw every horse; moved 5 tonight. Temperatures a trifle better, but still high. If this heat continues shall be sure to have some losses. Am praying for a breeze. Outside 64 degrees.

		These are a little better than they have been all day; had 84° in one part today. This has been without exception the most worrying day I have ever had. The horses are a poor lot and seem to crack up and start blowing at 80°. Had I not moved them to the top I am sure I should have had 2 or 3 deaths from congestion to record tonight.
1 Tween, 76 degrees	4 Tween, 68 degrees	
1 Orlop, 74 degrees	5 Tween, 78 degrees	
2 Tween, 72 degrees	6 Tween, 74 degrees	
2 Orlop, 74 degrees	6 Orlop, 76 degrees	
2 Hold, 70 degrees	6 Hold, 76 degrees	
3 Tween, 72 degrees	7 Tween, 76 degrees	
3 Orlop, 76 degrees	7 Orlop, 72 degrees	
(B 14578)	A 2	

Thursday, August 12th, 1915—Nice breeze blowing

7 a. m.—Tour of top deck. All cases moved from below doing well and feeding.

10 a. m.—Tour of whole ship. Temperatures little better; saw every horse; discovered Case 11, pneumonia, also Case 10, strangles, abscess on shoulder, opened same; ship being thoroughly mucked out. Other cases doing well.

2 p. m.—Another tour. Saw every horse; all mucking out finished; ship very sweet; temperatures good, horses looking better; have hopes now, but there are a lot showing signs of a febrile condition. Case 11, pneumonia, got temperature down from 106.4 to 105 degrees, panting, slightly easier. Ship in good form.

8 p. m.—Another tour. Saw every horse; ship cool and sweet: discovered Case 13, showing slight pain in feet; had him moved to place where he could lie down; temperature not up, pulse only slightly. All temperatures good tonight. Pneumonia case slightly better, temperature down to 104. Outside, 58 degrees.

1 Tween, 70 degrees	4 Tween, 62 degrees	Found two Ventilators were not trimmed; altered same, and in 15 minutes a drop of 2 degrees.
1 Orlop, 68 degrees	5 Tween, 70 degrees	
2 Tween, 66 degrees	6 Tween, 68 degrees	
2 Orlop, 70 degrees	6 Orlop, 64 degrees	
2 Lower	6 Hold, 74 degrees	
Hold, 68 degrees	7 Tween, 70 degrees	
3 Tween, 66 degrees	7 Orlop, 70 degrees	
3 Orlop, 70 degrees		

Friday, August 13th, 1915—Fine day, nice breeze

7 a. m.—Tour of top deck. All feeding and doing well; had Case 5, a poor, miserable black gelding with strangles, boxed off, so that he could feed without being worried by others and receive special diet.

10 a. m.—Tour of whole ship. All cases doing well; ship being mucked out; saw every horse; called to Case 15, colic, gave draught.

2 p. m.—Tour of whole ship. All cases doing well; mucking out all finished; ship sweet and cool; colic case better.

8 p. m.—Tour of whole ship. All cases doing well except laminitis, which is still in pain, all four feet being affected; temperature not bad, and although high, the ship is very sweet. Have great hopes, but shall not relinquish my vigilance. I miss my assistant, who was sent to take a ship from Newport News. Outside, 55 degrees.

1 Tween, 68 degrees	3 Tween, 62 degrees	6 Orlop, 66 degrees
1 Orlop, 67 degrees	3 Orlop, 68 degrees	6 Hold, 70 degrees
2 Tween, 64 degrees	4 Tween, 60 degrees	7 Tween, 68 degrees
2 Orlop, 70 degrees	5 Tween, 70 degrees	7 Orlop, 68 degrees
2 Hold, 66 degrees	6 Tween, 70 degrees	

Saturday, August 14, 1915—Fine day, nice breeze

5 a. m.—Called to Case 16, colic, gave draught.

7 a. m.—Tour of top deck. All doing well; opened strangles abscess, Case 5, very large and putrid, disinfected stall; colic case still in pain, had him moved to top deck.

10 a. m.—Tour of whole ship. All cases except colic doing well; fear it is a case of severe impaction. Saw every horse, opened strangles abscess; Case 6, had stall disinfected; temperatures good, horses looking very well; mucking out done, and ship thoroughly clean; lines disinfected at 11 a. m. Pneumonia case little better, laminitis the same.

2 p. m.—Tour of whole ship. Saw every horse; colic case still in pain, passed catheter and gave enema; all others doing well.

8·p. m.—Tour of whole ship. Colic case little better, had good passage; all horses except pneumonia and laminitis look very well, and I have great hopes; temperatures excellent tonight. Outside, 54 degrees.

1 Tween, 65 degrees	4 Tween, 56 degrees	Arranged with Chief
1 Orlop, 62 degrees	5 Tween, 63 degrees	Officer and fixed a wooden
2 Tween, 62 degrees	6 Tween, 62 degrees	air-shoot with a wind
2 Orlop, 64 degrees	6 Orlop, 60 degrees	sail attached, to run into
2 Hold, 60 degrees	6 Hold, 66 degrees	dead end of No. 6 Hold;
3 Tween, 59 degrees	7 Tween, 60 degrees	it at once brought the
3 Orlop, 62 degrees	7 Orlop, 62 degrees	temperature down 4 degrees.

10 p. m.—Colic case better, horse out of pain and nibbling a little food.

Sunday, August 15, 1915—Fine day, nice breeze

12:15 a. m.—Called to Case 18, colic, gave draught and left instructions.

7 a. m.—Colic case better. Tour of top deck; all doing well.

10 a. m.—Tour of whole ship. All cases doing well; mucking out finished at 10:30; ship very sweet.

2 p. m.—Tour of whole ship. Saw every horse; all decks cool and sweet, all horses looking well; cases doing as well as can be expected.

8 p. m.—Tour of whole ship. Discovered Case 17, influenza, temperature 106.4; gave draught and moved to a better position. Saw every horse; all cases doing well; temperatures very good tonight. Outside, 57 degrees.

1 Tween, 66 degrees	4 Tween, 60 degrees	Considering the outside, these are excellent.
1 Orlop, 65 degrees	5 Tween, 64 degrees	Undoubtedly this is the
2 Tween, 66 degrees	6 Tween, 64 degrees	best ship on the trans-
2 Orlop, 68 degrees	6 Orlop, 68 degrees	port for keeping venti-
2 Hold, 66 degrees	6 Hold, 70 degrees	lated when you have a
3 Tween, 68 degrees	7 Tween, 65 degrees	little breeze.
3 Orlop, 64 degrees	7 Orlop, 66 degrees	

Monday, August 16th, 1915—Wet, but good wind blowing

7 a. m.—Tour of top deck.

10 a. m.—Tour of whole ship. Saw every horse; mucking out done; had several poor weedy horses moved to better positions. Pneumonia case progressing favorably. Laminitis case no worse. Influenza patient's temperature down to 104 degrees. Ship very sweet, and unless something unforeseen occurs, I hope to land every horse.

2 p. m.—Tour of ship. All patients about the same. Wind rather strong, but it is keeping the ship cool, and we have plenty of fresh air in all parts.

8 p. m.—Tour of ship. Saw every horse; all patients progressing. Pneumonia case, temperature lower. Influenza case, temperature 104.6 but is feeding a little. Ship cool and sweet. Temperature good. Called to colic case; gave draught. Outside, 58 degrees.

1 Tween, 64 degrees	4 Tween, 60 degrees	Owing to rough sea on weather side we have had to have the Orlop deck ports closed, but so arranged the wind sails that we kept them cool.
1 Orlop, 64 degrees	5 Tween, 65 degrees	
2 Tween, 63 degrees	6 Tween, 66 degrees	
2 Orlop, 66 degrees	6 Orlop, 69 degrees	
2 Hold, 65 degrees	6 Hold, 70 degrees	
3 Tween, 66 degrees	7 Tween, 66 degrees	
3 Orlop, 66 degrees	7 Orlop, 68 degrees	

Tuesday, August 17th, 1915—Fine day, light breeze

7 a. m.—Tour of top deck. All patients doing well. Regret to say Case 5, strangles, has an abscess forming on the shoulder, otherwise he was doing well.

10 a. m.—Tour of ship. Saw every horse. Discovered two more cases of strangles and one influenza. Patients progressing, although one influenza case causes a little worry. Mucking out finished 10:30. Ship sweet, but wind is dropping.

2 p. m.—Tour of ship. Saw every horse. Wind almost dropped; some holds rather warm, but sweet. Only three cases causing anxiety; others all doing well.

8 p. m.—Another tour. Saw every horse. Ship rather warm, and several horses slightly blowing; had 10 moved to top deck and more airy positions. Gave night foreman list to watch horses, and orders to move them upon the slightest sign of blowing. My cases do not seem quite so well tonight. Am hoping for a wind to spring up. Feel rather anxious tonight. Outside temperature, 62 degrees.

1 Tween, 74 degrees	6 Orlop, 71 degrees	4 Tween, 64 degrees
2 Tween, 72 degrees	7 Tween, 72 degrees	6 Tween, 70 degrees
2 Hold, 70 degrees	1 Orlop, 71 degrees	6 Hold, 73 degrees
3 Orlop, 74 degrees	2 Orlop, 73 degrees	7 Orlop, 72 degrees
5 Tween, 70 degrees	3 Tween, 68 degrees	

Wednesday, August 18th, 1915—Fine day, nice breeze

7 a. m.—Tour of top deck. All horses moved better. All patients, except bad influenza case, doing well.

10 a. m.—Tour of whole ship. Wind getting up; all mucking out done at 10:30. Saw every horse, discovered another bad influenza case, and two more cases of strangles; all looking and doing well, except Case 17, which is causing some anxiety; ship very sweet.

2 p. m.—Tour of ship. Saw every horse; ship nice and cool and sweet; all cases progressing, except 17.

8 p. m.—Tour of whole ship. Saw every horse; all patients seem a little better tonight; temperatures are down, except pneumonia case, which has gone up to 103°, but pulse is good at 60. Nice breeze blowing, and ship very cool and sweet, although I have four patients very bad; with ordinary luck and care I hope to land every horse. We are 745 miles from Avonmouth at noon today. Temperatures good tonight. Oustide, 61 degrees.

1 Tween,	70 degrees	3 Tween,	67 degrees	6 Orlop,	68 degrees
1 Orlop,	68 degrees	3 Orlop,	70 degrees	6 Hold,	70 degrees
2 Tween,	66 degrees	4 Tween,	62 degrees	7 Tween,	68 degrees
2 Orlop,	66 degrees	5 Tween,	65 degrees	7 Orlop,	70 degrees
2 Hold,	66 degrees	6 Tween,	63 degrees		

11 p. m.—Called to Case 28, colic; gave draught and left instructions, only mild case.

Thursday, August 19th, 1915—Fairly strong wind

7 a. m.—Tour of top deck. Last night's colic case better; all horses doing well, except Case 27, causing a little worry.

10 a. m.—Tour of whole ship. Saw every horse; opened three strangles abscess in cases; all patients doing well; Case 17 a little better. All mucking out done by 10:30, and ship cool and sweet.

2 p. m.—Tour of whole ship. Saw every horse; all patients progressing.

8 p. m.—Tour of whole ship. Saw every horse, and although there are one or two cases which cause a little anxiety, I have great hopes of landing every horse. We expect to reach Avonmouth early Saturday morning. Ship very cool and sweet tonight; and not a single horse blowing. Outside, 62 degrees.

1 Tween,	69 degrees	3 Tween,	66 degrees	6 Orlop,	66 degrees
1 Orlop,	65 degrees	3 Orlop,	68 degrees	6 Hold,	70 degrees
2 Tween,	66 degrees	4 Tween,	63 degrees	7 Tween,	68 degrees
2 Orlop,	67 degrees	5 Tween,	64 degrees	7 Orlop,	70 degrees
2 Hold,	66 degrees	6 Tween,	64 degrees		

Friday, August 20th, 1915—Fine day, nice breeze

7 a. m.—Tour of top deck. All patients doing well. Called to Case 30, colic; gave draught; also to Case 34, ditto. Case 27 still worrying.

10 a. m.—Tour of whole ship. Saw every horse. All doing
well. Discovered Case 35, an injury to off coronet which is forming a quittor. Mare in much pain; gave draught. Mucking out
all finished 10:30, and horses being well groomed. Have great
hopes of landing all.

2 p. m.—Tour of whole ship. Wind dropping a little; hope
it will spring up again. All doing well.

8 p. m.—Tour of whole ship. Saw every horse. Being in the
submarine zone, all orlop ports are closed, and the wind having
dropped, these decks are rather warm, but the ship is sweet. Two
cases only worrying, 27 and 35. Hope to unload tomorrow. Outside, 62 degrees.

1 Tween, 72 degrees	4 Tween, 66 degrees	These are, I am afraid, going to rise as the wind is still dropping. I have put on extra watchmen with lamps (as we are sailing all lights out to-night), with instructions to move to upper deck any horse showing the least sign of blowing. My cases number 35 all told, tonight.
1 Orlop, 71 degrees	5 Tween, 71 degrees	
2 Tween, 70 degrees	6 Tween, 69 degrees	
2 Orlop, 72 degrees	6 Orlop, 74 degrees	
2 Hold, 69 degrees	6 Hold, 74 degrees	
3 Tween, 70 degrees	7 Tween, 73 degrees	
3 Orlop, 70 degrees	7 Orlop, 74 degrees	

*Saturday, August 21st, 1915—Anchored in Walton Bay at 6:30
A. M. to await tide*

7 a. m.—Tour of top deck. All patients progressing, and others
looking well.

10 a. m.—Tour of whole ship. All patients doing well. Saw
every horse. Mucking out done by 10:30; all sails and alleyways
disinfected, and mats laid down for unloading. Although I have
about five for hospital, I anticipate not losing one. Ship rather
warm; breeze very light.

2 p. m.—Have just heard that we are not to unload until tomorrow morning. This disheartens me after working hard with
the horses all the voyage and, having the utensils put away and
ship thoroughly cleaned, must make arrangements to feed again
tonight and tomorrow morning. Ship very warm; no wind.

8 p. m.—Tour of whole ship. Regret to find temperatures are
rising; several horses blowing, and in getting one out to take on
top deck have been severely kicked on the knee and disabled *pro
tem.*; my head foreman has completed my round. As far as I can
see no ship has come from the dock, and the authorities could have
unloaded us this afternoon had they made an effort. I have five
serious cases which may take the wrong turn owing to the heat,
and a record spoiled. Have put on extra watchmen with the foreman with instructions to take every horse to the weather deck upon
the slightest sign of blowing. Have persuaded the horsemen to

get up at 2:30 a. m. to again muck out and disinfect the ship before going into dock. My knee is very painful, and I hope nothing
happens in the night. Am very sick at not being unloaded today.
The temperatures are getting bad, there is no wind, and the ship
being anchored, makes it worse. Outside, 63 degrees.

1 Tween, 74 degrees	4 Tween, 68 degrees	
1 Orlop, 76 degrees	5 Tween, 80 degrees	
2 Tween, 76 degrees	6 Tween, 77 degrees	
2 Orlop, 76 degrees	6 Orlop, 76 degrees	These I am afraid,
2 Hold, 73 degrees	6 Hold, 77 degrees	will get higher.
3 Tween, 76 degrees	7 Tween, 74 degrees	
3 Orlop, 74 degrees	7 Orlop, 73 degrees	

On the whole, the horses have improved on the voyage, and
are far and away in better condition than when I received them,
but there are quite a lot weary and showing signs of temperatures,
which tonight will not improve. I sincerely hope I shall be able
to land them all, not having lost one up to now.

August 22nd, 1915—Ship docked 4:30 A. M.

7 a. m.—Tour of top deck. All doing well. My knee being
still painful, my head foreman went all over the ship, and all is in
order. The mucking out was finished at 4 a. m.

9 a. m.—Commenced to unload. Landed every horse, obtaining certificate that their condition was very good. Finished at
11:30 a. m.

I attribute the success of this voyage to the fact that the ship
was mucked out every day and that special care and attention was
paid to the ventilation. I cannot speak too highly of the chief
officer, Mr. Dingle, who entered into the ventilation problem with
great zeal, and devised many little schemes to get fresh air into
bad corners. I am sure without his assistance and cooperation I
should never have got through without losing one or two.

This ship is undoubtedly one of the best in this transport
business, both as regards facilities for working, appointment and
ventilation. The holds and decks are lofty and the alleyways wide.

A. E. BOYER, M.R.C.V.S.

Work of A.V.C. at the Front. The work with Divisions in the
front line and field units and elsewhere is largely of a preventive
and first-aid nature. In each Division in addition to the Mobile
Veterinary Section of which, later, there is a definite number of
officers and non-commissioned officers, Army Veterinary Corps,
distributed as evenly as possible throughout the fighting units,
just as are Medical officers and N.C. Os. of the R.A.M.C. These
veterinary officers and N.C. Os. are responsible for carrying out
simple first-aid treatment and for deciding what cases are slight
enough for "duty and dressing", and what should be handed over to

the Mobile Veterinary Section of the division for evacuation to veterinary hospitals on the lines of communication. They carry out the constant inspections of animals mentioned in the earlier portion of this article as being indispensable to prevention of diseases, both contagious and non-contagious among animals. Relatively the number of bullet and shell casualties among horses and mules is small as compared with similar casualties among officers and men, because the animals are as far as possible kept behind the firing-line.

In a big Cavalry action naturally matters would be different, but this form of warfare on a big scale still is awaited so far as the British forces in this war are concerned. Horses fare better than men in so far as their thicker skin and bulkier tissues offer greater resistance to projectiles and splinters, but worse than men in that economic considerations and mechanical difficulties often render it necessary to destroy horses for wound conditions which at most would maim a man. Open wound dressing is necessarily for the most part practiced in the field. Bandaging is only practicable to a relatively small extent. Under the best conditions it has not on the whole been found a suitable form of dressing for the unclean type of wound met with on active service, and in the case of equines it is most difficult to apply a bandage to any situation other than the lower extremities of the limbs that will not speedily become displaced and thus a positive evil instead of a hypothetical good. Certainly bandaging appeals strongly to the popular imagination. There is an effective cleanly appearance about a freshly bandaged wound which catches the eye of the journalistic artist and, through his efforts, that of the general public.

In point of actual results, however, it has been found better to disregard superficial appearances and to enlist the bactericidal aid of the oxygen of the atmosphere.

What is probably the best form of field dressing for horses discovered up to the present is as follows: Foreign bodies are removed from the wound as far as possible without probing. Shreds of damaged tissues certain to die and decay if left *in situ* are similarly removed with the dressing scissors. The wound is then gently cleansed with antiseptic wool, facilities for downward drainage of discharge are established and the dressing is completed by painting all exposed tissues with tincture of iodine.

It would not be permitted in an article of this kind to state fully how the personnel of the Army Veterinary Corps is disposed throughout a Division; suffice it to say that every animal is able to receive at all times the expert attention of this personnel. No horse is permitted unnecessarily to suffer. If it is evident that he cannot be restored to usefulness within a reasonable period then he is painlessly destroyed on the spot. If his injury or disease is amenable to treatment he is evacuated without delay to a base hospital containing facilities for the most up-to-date and scientific methods of treatment.

The Mobile Veterinary Section is a complete Veterinary Unit, allotted to a Division, corresponding in many ways with a Field Ambulance of the Royal Army Medical Corps. The duty of this unit is principally to collect from fighting formations in its Divisional area all injured, sick and debilitated animals requiring to be sent back to the large veterinary hospitals on the lines of communication. It also acts as a dressing station and undertakes the collection from the base of veterinary medicines and equipment. These stores are then distributed by the section as required to divisional combatant units, a system which has proved far more convenient and expeditious than that in vogue in the earlier stages of the war when each unit in the field received its supplies independently from Base Depots of Veterinary Stores. Approximately half of the personnel of the Mobile Veterinary Section is utilized in the duty of collection of sick and first aid treatment, including injection when necessary of tetanus antitoxin; the other half forms what is known as the Railway Conducting Party. This party is responsible for safe conveyance of the patients from the nearest available railhead to the Veterinary Hospital at the Base and first-aid attendance *en route*. On its return from the base the conducting party brings with it the medicine and equipment required for distribution to Divisional Units, as mentioned above. Not all the patients collected by the Mobile Veterinary Section are sent to the base; when the division is stationary milder cases are retained and treated by the section and ultimately returned cured to units.

Veterinary Hospitals and Convalescent Horse Depots. These are situated on the line of communication and at the various bases of the Expeditionary Forces, in addition to many established in Home Commands.

An overseas veterinary hospital is established to deal at one time with 1250 cases or a greater number, its organization being such as to permit of ready expansion. The personnel allowed for each hospital is sufficient but not extravagant, having in view the important principle that an administrative service should be an economic dividend-paying proposition.

It is interesting to reflect that on mobilization the then diminutive Army Veterinary Corps was sufficiently hard put to it to find skilled subordinate personnel for one veterinary hospital as at present constituted, whereas there are now about thirty such, apart from Camel Hospitals and Convalescent Horse Depots, all staffed with competent highly trained personnel.

Each hospital is subdivided into wards and each ward as far as possible is appropriated to the treatment of a separate class of injury or disease. To the most skilled surgeons is given the care of wound cases; officers who have specialized in microscopic work have charge of the cases of parasitic skin disease and microbic affections. Similarly each non-commissioned officer has definite duties allotted to him according to the capacity he displays for a certain kind of work.

The treatment of parasitic skin disease alone presents an enormous problem. From earliest history parasitic skin disease has ever been the distressing accompaniment of war. Horses, like men, suffer from the depredations of lice but a far worse scourge of the former is in the disease known as mange.

This disease, caused by a microscopical insect parasite which attacks skin and in one species burrows under the surface of the skin gives enormous trouble. The intense irritation that occurs causes the affected horse to lose flesh rapidly unless promptly and efficiently treated. One veterinary hospital with the British Expeditionary Force is practically confined to the treatment of this disease alone. In the earlier stages of the war each case had to be separately treated by hand, involving an enormous amount of labor, but now there are established in many veterinary hospitals specially constructed dipping baths capable of dealing rapidly and easily with any number of patients. The bath is a long trench-like affair, dug into the ground and lined with concreted material, impervious to water. The bath is filled up to a certain height with a solution or mixture of the medicaments found most efficacious in destruction of the mange parasite and kept by means of steam of precisely that temperature ascertained to be necessary for the best results in the treatment. Matters are so arranged that the horse on plunging into the bath is completely immersed in the solution whence he emerges, having traversed the length of the bath, by upward incline to the dripping pens.

The principal trouble in regard to mange is to find a solution or mixture of medicaments that will destroy the parasite and its eggs without injuring the skin of the patient. Unless care is taken to observe both these conditions injury to the skin to a serious extent may supervene, so that the remedy proves "worse than the disease".

To eradicate mange entirely from an Army in the field has so far proved impossible, but in this war it is kept well under control and has never got the upper hand, as it did in the South African War, 1899-1902, when it caused heavy mortality and inefficiency.

The great progress in methods of treatment of mange made by the Army Veterinary Service in the present war is scientifically gratifying and economically important. It has in fact, as a disease, ceased to be a terror and now only remains a nuisance. In the British Expeditionary Force 80% of all cases of disease, including wounds, admitted to veterinary hospitals are returned to duty in due course. Of the remaining 20% a considerable proportion are painlessly destroyed, and sold at a good price to the local inhabitants for human consumption. In this country the percentage returned to duty from veterinary hospitals is naturally higher in proportion as the conditions obtaining at home are more favorable than those nearer the firing line. The absolute wastage both overseas and at home is thus kept down to a low monetary figure.

Each veterinary hospital is an entirely self-contained unit responsible not only for the treatment of 1250 horses and mules, but for the discipline, training, payment, and general welfare of over 400 non-commissioned officers and men. Apart from medical and surgical treatment the horse and mule patients have to be fed, watered, groomed, shod, exercised and generally cared for in such a way that they will be fit for duty at the front or elsewhere when discharged from hospital. All animals thus discharged for duty are sent straight to remount depots where they are classified and posted again for service to various branches of the Army as may be most suitable.

The selection of adequate sites for veterinary hospitals has been a difficult business. Apart from the large area required, questions of accessibility to railway stations, good water supply, facilities for disposal of manure and carcasses, called for serious consideration. A horse normally needs for drinking purposes alone about 8 gallons of water a day in addition to the requirements for surgical and other purposes. In the opening months of the war the veterinary hospital was necessarily for the most part an open air institution. Not at once could there spring into existence the present admirably constructed stables, operating sheds, shoeing forges, exercising tracks, store houses and other carefully devised arrangements for the convenience and comfort of animals and men.

Although it is true that horses tied up in the open will, if well fed and rugged, and provided with moderately mud-free standings, keep in good health and flesh, it is nevertheless impossible in the climatic conditions of Northern Europe to obtain the best results in these circumstances so far as veterinary hospitals are concerned. Among reasons that contribute to the desirability of some sort of overhead cover for sick horses, there stands out prominently the fact that it is not reasonable, humanly speaking, to expect men to give to patients standing in the open in wet weather the individual care and attention which are essential to successful veterinary work. Moreover, during the winter months, at least, covered accommodation is absolutely necessary for the adequate treatment of mange which, as already stated, forms a constant and considerable proportion of equine patients in time of war. To deal efficiently with this disease it is necessary to clip the animal all over, to wash or "dress" them frequently, and to leave them unrugged during the course of the treatment, as rugs harbor infection and facilitate spread of the malady. It is evident that grave loss of flesh and condition must occur if unclipped and recently "dressed" animals are exposed day and night to wintry weather while tethered and without protection or shelter of any kind. Condition is easily lost but hard and tedious to restore. A really emaciated animal takes many weeks and even months to recover sufficient muscular bulk to fit him for the heavy exertion of military duty at the front. The financial expenditure represented by covered accommodation for veterinary hospitals is therefore repaid in preservation of condition and consequently accelerated convalescence. In veterinary as in most other matters "time is money", as practically every horse delayed in hospital has to be replaced in the unit whence he comes by a fit horse from a remount depot. Shelter and a moderate amount of warmth are great aids in the restoration of condition as well as in preventing the loss of it. Food has not only to build up the tissues but to maintain the body temperature, and the more is diverted to the latter service the less is available for the former. On a standard minimum food ration, therefore, it is important for body building purposes to keep the patient warm.

Especially during the winter in France and Belgium, when the universal mud throws heavy strain upon gun teams and transport animals by reason of the great difficulty in dragging vehicles over the shell torn swamp-like ground, a constant stream of debilitated and war-worn horses and mules pours into the veterinary hospitals from divisions at the front. These animals for the most part are not diseased but merely weakened through loss of muscular and other tissue. For such horses the comfortable surroundings and shelter of the hospital act like magic. Except in the case of old animals, in a comparatively short period the hollow sides fill out, the coat resumes its normal bloom and the returning strength and spirits give evidence of restored vitality. These results could not be attained in double the time were covered accommodations in winter not available.

Old animals, if debility is at all advanced, recuperate slowly even under the best conditions, so slowly indeed that it is often economically necessary to destroy them rather than to keep them until again fit for work. This lack of resiliency in the old animal renders it most undesirable to purchase for war purposes any horse that has passed the prime of equine life. The period of a horse's life during which he is at his best for military purposes is very brief. If under six years of age he is highly susceptible to all forms of equine contagious disease and stands the hardship of a campaign badly. If over twelve years, although resistant to contagious disease, he has generally lost the elasticity and recuperative powers necessary to enable him to "pick up" quickly after a severe bout of work. Therefore it is that military veterinary hospitals receive an undue proportion of the old horses of an Army especially in the winter months. It would be ungracious to proceed to any description of the buildings of the veterinary hospitals without referring to the assistance afforded in this respect by the Royal Society for the Prevention of Cruelty to Animals. This admirably organized society has labored throughout the war to assist the Army Veterinary Service in its efforts to promote the welfare of the Army horses and as a logical consequence the efficiency of the armies in the field. Naturally the objective of the society is humanitarianism but the active practice of a genuine, if in a technical point of view irrelevant, good inevitably leads to increased efficiency at some point or other. Benevolent societies like the R. S. P. C. A. and Y. M. C. A., whose objectives at first sight may appear widely removed, are in effect working towards the same end—efficiency. Science, religion, secular benevolence and philosophy, in so far as they are all striving for a positive good are aiming for the same goal, and their progress is only limited by the degree of truth on which their policy and excursions are based.

A crank, that is, an individual who conducts a more or less violent crusade on behalf of a doctrine or belief based on erroneous premises, is more dangerous in his friendship than in his enmity to any of these spheres of useful activity. This reflection brings us back to the wisdom of Solomon and Socrates, who exhorted their generations above all things to "seek wisdom—get understanding".

That country or state which devotes most attention and gives most support to science better described as exact knowledge must, other things being equal, be the most successful in its undertakings whether in peace or war. It is futile in this connection to claim that the demoralization of modern Germany is attributable to overmuch cult of science. The scientists of Germany, like other classes of the Hun community, are harnessed to the Juggernaut of militarism. Those who dictate the high policy of the German Empire are not scientists, but relatively ignorant despots who have employed for evil purposes a force painfully elaborated by the research of scientific men primarily working for the benefit of humanity.

In November, 1914, the Army Council accepted an offer from the society to start a fund for the purpose of hospital requisites for sick and wounded horses, under the title of "The R. S. P. C. A. fund for sick and wounded horses". The Duke of Portland consented to act as chairman of the committee formed, in accordance with the sanction of the War Office, to work in close cooperation with the Army Veterinary Department and supplement the recognized supplies for Army Veterinary Services.

This fund has up to the present collected over 100,000 pounds which has been spent on building veterinary hospitals as required, supplying special horse tents, horse drawn ambulances (for all the veterinary hospitals and for the mobile veterinary sections attached to each division of the British Army) besides presenting motor horse ambulances for the armies themselves. The fund has also provided Bentail corn crushers and chaff-cutters with petrol engines for all the hospitals in France, and has supplied a large number of clipping machines, hand-clippers, dandy brushes, curry combs, Vermorel sprayers, etc., as required.

The first hospital built in 1914 was for 1,000 horses and was constructed of wood and galvanized iron, with wooden mangers and wooden water-troughs. It consists of a series of buildings, each with accommodation for 50 horses and a double expense forage store. It was found that wooden structures required a great deal of repair, and it was also thought that in case of advance or retirement the steel constructed shelters would be more advantageous, as they could be unbolted and removed to some other situation. Therefore, the other three hospitals, built very much on the same plan, but increased to 1250, have been made of steel or cast iron throughout, with roof and centre divisions of corrugated iron. The mangers of the latter are of pressed steel and run down the central divisions, and the stables are fitted with bales. The flooring consists, in the majority of cases, of ashes and railway sleepers, though where it has been possible to make them they have been constructed of cement. Each building has been supplied with a guttering round the eaves and has two drinking troughs, in the majority of cases made of galvanized steel, but latterly these have been replaced by troughs made of reinforced concrete. Each horse has a space of 5½', length of building 144', width all over 28', minimum height 8', height of ridges 11'. The fund has also provided the hospitals with dining huts, officers' mess, and kitchens with stoves and boilers; also ablution rooms, men's mess rooms with larder, scullery and kitchen, Quartermaster's stores, bath rooms for the men, with douches. Administrative offices, consisting of C. Os.' office, clerk's room, guard room and cells; Quartermaster's office, saddlers' shops, carpenters' shops, pharmacy and stores, drying sheds, dressing sheds and stores (four to each hospital). Sergeants' mess, Sergeants' bathroom, operating sheds and forage and chaff cutting sheds with corn crushers and chaff cutters complete. The fittings for the hospitals have been complete in every detail, including, where it was considered necessary: laboratories for microscopic work, cameras for research work, sterilizers for operating purposes, dressing boxes to contain liniments, bandages, etc., for each ward.

In all cases the fund has provided the complete material and the labor has been found from the Army Veterinary Corps men themselves. This has worked admirably, because after the stables had been erected a certain number of the personnel of each hospital could, for the time being, be employed on constructing buildings under the guidance of Mr. A. H. Fass, who has done splendid honorary work in superintending the erection of the various hospitals given by the fund.

The fund also provided the necessary buildings for 500 horses at No. 1 Convalescent Horse Depot; these buildings are very similar to the ones provided for the hospitals, and they have recently been added to increase the accommodation to 750 horses. In all, hospital accommodation—including stabling for 500 horses at the isolation hospital, Woolwich—for nine thousand five hundred horses have been presented through this fund.

It should be pointed out that the advantage of accepting such voluntary aid is that the work can be carried out under the guidance of the Works Department, but without adding to or hampering that department at a time when it is already overwhelmed with work; therefore, the important question of accommodation for sick and wounded horses can be dealt with immediately, and does not have to wait its turn with all the other work which has to be seen to.

Another supply from the fund which has been of great use to the corps, is that of "Vermorel" sprayers, seventy-eight of which have been issued to all the hospitals and mobile veterinary sections. These are not only of great utility for dressing and cleansing wounds, but also for disinfecting railway trucks in which the horses have been brought railhead, thus preventing the possibility of spreading contagious diseases.

The fund has also presented motor-lorries for conveying fodder and other supplies to certain of the hospitals, and it is by these various aids that the utility of the fund has been established. To the Chief Secretary of the R. S. P. C. A., Hon. Captain E. G. Fairholme, the Army Veterinary Service is greatly indebted for the

enthusiastic and efficient way in which he has organized and coordinated the work of the fund so as to adapt its resources with a
minimum of waste or friction to the immediate needs of the service.

What has been described in detail concerning veterinary hospitals and the assistance of the R. S. P. C. A. applies chiefly to the
hospitals of the British Expeditionary Forces, but the guiding
principles of the military veterinary hospitals are the same in
commands at home and in the expeditionary forces.

The detail is modified to meet local requirements. In Egypt,
for example, it is neither necessary nor desirable to provide cov-.
ered accommodation to the same extent as in northern Europe.
The hospitals in Egypt, moreover, are manned largely by native
Egyptian personnel, thus effecting an important economy and
saving in man-power. In addition to the standard veterinary hospitals for horses and mules there are established in Egypt, hospitals for camels, organized on lines similar to the former, and also
principally manned by native Egyptian subordinate personnel.
There are three of these camel hospitals, each established to deal
with 1250 camels. The veterinary service in Egypt includes in its
organization a mobile veterinary section (apart from the usual
divisional mobile veterinary section), having a roving commission.
It was found necessary to provide this special unit on account of
the widely extended disposition of the forces of Egypt and the
long journeys occurring in the transit of animals to and from veterinary hospitals.

The veterinary services working with the British forces in
German East Africa have had, in addition to normal professional
work, to cope with various problems of the most difficult nature.
It was considered advisable, in view of the many specific diseases
affecting cattle and equines in East Africa, to hand over the conduct of the Army Veterinary Services in that country to the permanent veterinary staff of the British East African Administration. The chief veterinary officer of the staff was appointed to the
Army Veterinary Corps, with temporary rank appropriate to the
proper discharge of his responsibilities, and with power to nominate for temporary commissions in the Army Veterinary Corps,
such veterinary surgeons on his staff as he considered most competent to assist him. The arrangement proved to be a fortunate one,
as these officers brought to their military duties a knowledge of the
local diseases obtained by years of residence and research work

among live stock in that country. The well equipped veterinary laboratory at Nairobi was placed at the disposal of the Army Veterinary Service, and many problems were worked out therein with results that have been helpful in the difficulties attending the operation of cavalry and transport in regions beset with fly-borne diseases of the most fatal character.

Among other duties the Army Veterinary Corps has to undertake the collection and care of cattle for fresh meat and transport requirements of the forces. These cattle have been kept comparatively free from rinderpest and other local diseases by inoculation with sera prepared in the Nairobi laboratory and by various measures scientifically ascertained to have protective powers. It is not, perhaps, too much to say that a considerable portion of the success attending the operations in German East Africa is fairly attributable to the highly skilled services of the Civil Veterinary Staff, working under the auspices of, and in coördination with the Army Veterinary Service as a whole. The diseases encountered include South African horse-sickness, rinderpest, tsetse-fly diseases, surra, epizootic lymphangitis and anthrax, a sufficiently formidable list to deal with in addition to the normal scourges of war.

Glanders and Mallein. To describe fully the work done during the war by the Army Veterinary Service in connection with the control of glanders alone would require greatly more scope than that of this entire article.

As is now fairly generally known, glanders is a particularly deadly equine disease of insidious nature and is highly infective. Records of this disease date back to Hippocrates and Aristotle, and from earliest history it has caused important losses among horses in times of war. The reasons for its predominance in time of war are partly the same as those which cause most infectious diseases to multiply at such times, but notably a tendency to assume a virulent form when by reason of hardship or food shortage the constitutional bodily resistance of the animal is reduced. An outbreak of glanders occurring in peace among well-fed, highly conditioned otherwise healthy animals spreads slowly and with difficulty, on account of the physiological resistance it encounters; in war, on the other hand, an outbreak occurring among war-worn or debilitated animals will speedily assume most serious proportions unless adequate means are adopted to check it. Fortunately an adequate means now exists in mallein, a substance composed of

killed cultures of the glanders bacillus to which has been added
glycerin and carbolic acid.

When mallein is injected by means of a hypodermic syringe
under or into the skin of a horse affected with glanders a reaction
takes place in which a swelling forms at the site of inoculation
and a marked rise of temperature occurs within twenty-four hours.
If the horse is not affected with glanders no reaction occurs. As
glanders may be dormant in an apparently healthy horse for
months, ready to break out in an acute rapidly fatal form at any
moment, the value of a means whereby the latent disease can be
readily detected becomes easily apparent.

Mallein has been freely used in the present war with the result that the mortality from glanders has been less than 1% of the
total mortality from equine disease in general. Every remount is
tested with mallein as soon as purchased. Animals arriving from
Canada or elsewhere after purchase are again tested. In brief,
the test is applied at every period in the animal's career found
from past experience to be associated with an outbreak of glanders.
Last but not least animals cast and destined to be sold are tested
with mallein before sale so as to avoid the possible chance of transferring to the civilian community an infected horse that may develop acute glanders subsequently to sale and thus spread disease
to the detriment of national welfare. Naturally all this mallein
testing means a great deal of anxious work and drudgery. There
are few duties of which the Army veterinary surgeon becomes so
heartily sick as this incessant testing of horses with mallein. Nevertheless it has to be done and results show that for the most part
it is done skilfully and thoroughly. The operation itself is practically painless, most horses take no notice of it, and there is in a
healthy animal no painful sequel such as may occur after vaccination or inoculation for enteric in man.

Formerly all mallein for the purpose of the British Army was
obtained from the Royal Veterinary College laboratories in London, but at an early stage of the war it was decided that the Army
Veterinary Corps should undertake the preparation of the mallein
required and that the laboratory of the Army Veterinary School
at Aldershot should be used for this purpose. Accordingly an
officer of the Special Reserve of the Army Veterinary Corps, a
trained bacteriologist, was appointed to carry out the work and
matters proceeded satisfactorily till at the height of its activity

the laboratory was turning out 80,000 doses of mallein a month. This could have been maintained, but an interesting development in the history of mallein lessened the need for the variety of mallein hitherto in use. This development occurred as the result of research by French veterinary surgeons who discovered that a very much smaller quantity of a differently prepared mallein injected into the skin of the eyelid sufficed to give a more delicate and, in the opinion of many operators, a more certain test for glanders. The dose of the original mallein injected under the skin of the neck was from 15 to 20 drops, whereas for the eyelid test with the French mallein about two drops are sufficient. A much finer needle is used for the latter so that the greater sensitiveness to pain of the eyelid is automatically compensated. If an animal is glandered a swelling of the eyelid speedily occurs, after injection, accompanied by a more or less profuse discharge from the eye; no reaction is seen if the animal is healthy. For some time the new mallein was all obtained from French sources, but recently the laboratory of the Army Veterinary School has commenced to prepare it and no difficulty is anticipated in turning out an equally reliable preparation of identical nature.

During the last two years only two cases have occurred in which a cast Army horse or mule has been found to be affected with glanders after transfer by sale to the civillian community, notwithstanding the large numbers of Army animals that have been so disposed of during this period. Perhaps this fact constitutes the best evidence that could be offered of the efficiency of the mallein test and the way in which glanders among Army animals has been controlled by this and other means.

Horse Ambulances. The application of horse ambulances to military purposes has been an interesting and useful feature of the present war. During peace, horse ambulances have for some time past been used by the Army Veterinary Corps in connection with station veterinary hospitals but it is believed that the present war is the first in which they have been taken into the field.

Two chief kinds of horse ambulances are used at present, motor horse ambulances and horse-drawn vehicles. The motor horse ambulance was first used overseas at a busy port where the veterinary hospital was necessarily located on a height some distance from the quay. When dealing with animals sick or injured by some accident on the voyage, it was found that some rapid and powerful means of transport was desirable to convey the patients with the least possible delay from the ship's side to the veterinary hospital. Help was forthcoming in an officer from the committee of the Home of Rest for horses at Cricklewood acting in conjunction with the R. S. P. C. A. to supply a motor horse ambulance if the Director of Transport at the War Office would agree to allow the motor firm selected to release from combatant requirements a suitable chassis. In due course this permission was obtained, a body constructed to carry at one time two patients was fitted to the chassis, and the ambulance was despatched overseas. Needless to say, it proved a great success.

Since then other motor ambulances have been supplied by the R. S. P. C. A. as required. It has been necessary for military reasons to keep the number within low and definite limits so as not unduly to encroach upon the prior claims of combatant branches of the service and of the R. A. M. C. for chassis and petrol. No such considerations, however, have hindered the adequate supply of horse-drawn vehicles for ambulance purposes, and these are now included in the equipment of all veterinary hospitals and many mobile veterinary sections. Apart from the humanitarian aspect these motor ambulances play an important economic part in facilitating the removal to veterinary hospitals of numbers of horses and mules that would otherwise have to be destroyed. Injuries to the foot bulk largely in the list of troubles to which the war horse is particularly subject. Of this class of injury the principal cause is the extraordinary liability of iron nails lying on the ground to attach themselves to and penetrate the sole and frog of the horse's foot. Most of the material conveyed to the troops overseas is packed in light wooden cases and in the process of opening and ultimately burning these, nails become distributed broadcast. Every possible effort has been made to prevent this distribution, but military exigencies are such that this phenomenon is to a large extent inevitable. The extent of injury to the horse caused by picked-up nail naturally varies according to the degrees of penetration and the amount and nature of infective dirt carried into the wound at the time of, or subsequent to, the accident. Very often the accident causes no obvious lameness at the time and, especially in the presence of mud, the condition may escape observation until, perhaps, one morning the affected animal is found so lame as to be unable to bear any weight on the foot. This occurs by reason of the rapid formation of pus, resulting from infection of the wound, within the rigid horny capsule of the foot, causing pressure on the sensitive structures within. First-aid is at once administered by paring away the horn over the wound, liberating the pent-up discharge and applying an antiseptic dressing, but the horse remains very lame and unable to walk without much pain and distress. The question of his removal to a railway station for dispatch to hospital is solved by the horse ambulance. In this he travels in comparative ease the distance to the station, and having completed the railway journey, is again conveyed in comfort in an ambulance to the veterinary hospital, where his foot receives more particular attention and he is soon on the high road to a speedy recovery.

The cases of picked-up nail, that is, the cases of injury to the foot of Army horses from this cause, in France alone, number several hundred a week. Attempts are being made to devise a movable metal protection to the sole of the foot that will prevent penetration by nails without being too heavy or difficult to adjust, and it is hoped that in due course a satisfactory outcome of the experience will result. In the meantime the horse ambulance probably justifies its provision and maintenance on account of this item alone.

Army Schools of Farriery. Army horses working on modern macadamized roads have to be shod well and frequently if they are to remain effective and therefore at duty. A set of shoes will often barely suffice a horse in a gun-team for 100 miles of modern road work, i. e., about five days constant but not severe marching.

If an army fights on its belly, it is certain that a horse does all its work on its feet, and for military purposes in western Europe an unshod horse is useless. While the New Armies formed during the first year of war were still "on paper" it was foreseen that unless extraordinary steps were taken there would be a very serious shortage in the Army of men able to shoe horses. Accordingly every possible means was utilized to obtain shoeing-smiths. This was before the days of conscription and in order to get as many as possible of the experienced blacksmiths scattered throughout the country to join the Army, high rates of pay and attractive prospects of promotion were offered. This measure sufficed to relieve immediate needs but it was clear that for future purposes much more comprehensive arrangements would have to be made. The supply of ready-made blacksmiths suitable for the Army was com-

paratively small. The motor-car, by replacing horses for many
purposes both in town and country, had hit the art of farriery
very hard and the village smithy had for some time fallen off in
attractiveness to young men seeking a trade to follow. Obviously,
therefore, the thing to do was for the Army to train its own shoeing-smiths, or at any rate to get soldiers trained as shoeing-smiths
in some way or other. The question of training was taken up
eagerly. Wherever opportunity offered young soldiers volunteer-
ing for the work were placed under training in military and civilian forges. Classes of instruction were started in veterinary hospitals, remount depots, etc. The Borough Polytechnic Institute,
Bermondsey, gave considerable assistance by organizing large
classes of instruction in cold-shoeing at Herold's Institute, Bermondsey. The great demand was for shoeing-smiths for Royal
Field Artillery and Infantry Transport. The cavalry were fairly
well off, as they were able to train, with the assistance of older
farriers called up from the reserve, under regimental conditions,
sufficient recruits for their purposes. The Army Service Corps
were also well off, as the great majority of blacksmiths coming into
the Army from civil life in the early months of the war were enlisted by special arrangement in the A. S. C. Also the A. S. C.
were in a position to undertake the training of considerable numbers of cold-shoers and shoeing-smiths in their regimental forges,
which were already established at most pre-war military stations
in this country. Presently, as might have been expected, it was
discovered that a grave lack of uniformity existed in the degree
of proficiency displayed by the newly trained men. Some of the
new "cold-shoers", as they were officially described, were fairly
useful, others proved after trial to have only a superficial and
theoretical knowledge of the work. Meanwhile the rapid growth
of the New Armies and the necessity for quick replacement of casualties occurring overseas called for an ever increasing number of
adequately trained cold-shoers and shoeing-smiths.

　. Briefly, the difference between a cold-shoer and a shoeing-
smith is one of degree, in which the latter has the advantage. The
cold-shoer knows enough about shoeing to take off and nail on
shoes and carry out what may be described as "minor repairs".
The shoeing-smith is a complete artificer able to make a shoe as
well as to adapt it to its destined purpose.

　In the early summer of 1915 the Army Veterinary Department

of the War Office offered to establish and organize Schools of Farriery, each school to be capable of turning out about 1,000 cold-shoers every three months. This offer was accepted and steps were taken forthwith to form three Army Schools of Farriery in this country. At the same time a small School of Farriery came into being on the lines of communication, British Expeditionary Force, under the auspices of the Veterinary Directorate overseas.

The schools have all been working at high pressure since the winter 1915-16 and have given the utmost satisfaction. The system of instruction and standard of examination are uniform and each pupil must give definite proof of competency before he is "passed out" of the school and becomes entitled to the extra-duty pay earned by qualified artificers. A modern Army School of Farriery is a busy affair. With nearly eighty forges going, each fire serving for the instruction of about half a dozen pupils, a daily shoeing of some hundreds of horses, the school is on a par with other gargantuan institutions arising out of the war. Great ingenuity has been displayed by the instructors in devising means of a dummy or artificial nature to assist in the early stages of tuition. A simple but highly effective apparatus varying in form but similar in principle has been introduced to which the foot from a dead horse can be firmly attached. The apparatus with foot attached can then be manipulated and moved through varying angles in exactly the same way as a blacksmith manipulates a horse's foot and leg in the course of shoeing. The learner thus begins on a dummy of infinite patience and insensitiveness to pain should the former be clumsy in his early efforts to nail on a shoe.

The schools are located in the vicinity of remount depots and large garrisons so that there may be an ample supply of Army horses for purposes of instruction and demonstration. The assistant instructors are largely drawn from retired and re-enlisted Army Farriers. In addition to tuition in the art of shoeing, the pupils go through a short course in first-aid surgery of the horse's foot, so that they may know what to do in case of need arising out of their own inexperience or some fortuitous circumstance beyond their control. Questions on this subject form part of the qualifying examination. About two months' concentrated training at a farriery school enables a man of fair average intelligence and manual dexterity to qualify as a "cold-shoer". Not less than three additional months of training are needed before a pupil is qualified to pass out as a "shoeing-smith".

It is correct to speak of the ''Art'' of shoeing. A competent farrier must be at least somewhat of an artist to be able after a brief scrutiny of a foot so to shape the glowing iron by a few blows of the hammer as to bring its curves into true accordance with those of a hoof that may and often does present abnormality of outline. A skilled farrier scorns over-precise mensuration. At most he will register the greatest breadth or length of a foot by breaking off to the required length a piece of straw to correspond with such dimension. Subsequently with only this piece of straw, and the image reflected in his trained memory, to guide him he will make a shoe that on being fitted will often be found to require no alteration whatever. The Schools of Farriery cannot produce this degree of excellence after five months of training, but they can and do turn out a very useful artificer whose transition to artist is only a question of native capacity and time. In the achievement of this end the problem of how to supply a hastily collected Army of modern dimensions with a sufficiency of forge-artificers has been satisfactorily solved.

In the course of description of any form of honest endeavor the narrative is apt to take on a highly laudatory tone and thus to convey the impression that, wherever else there is shortcoming, at any rate the subject under review is perfect. If such an impression has been conveyed by the foregoing notes it is fortunately not too late to correct it. The Army Veterinary Service, in common with all other organizations dependent for their success upon the individual efforts of human beings, contains a normal proportion of seekers for the line of least resistance, faint-hearted fighters in the struggle against disease and inefficiency. An Army, like a Nation, gets pretty nearly what it deserves in the way of scientific assistance. The vast possibilities of sanitation and preventive medicine are as yet dimly realized even by veterinary surgeons themselves, much less by those who have not at all considered the matter. The many hundreds of debilitated horses pouring every week into veterinary hospitals could be reduced by one-half, were the personnel of the Army Veterinary Corps and that of other Arms concerned with horse-management universally alive to the prior necessity of prevention as distinct from cure of disease. In the professional tendency, inherent in most practitioners, to devote the mind principally to the ''healing art'' rather than to the practice and propagation of the principles of horse management, hygiene and sanitation, lies no small share of the causes that come between perfection and the Army Veterinary Service of today.

It has not been possible in the scope of this article to go closely into detail; the attempt has been made rather to give a general idea of the objective and routine of the Army Veterinary Service. In connection with the views expressed and the demonstration offered of what can be achieved by assisting and encouraging scientific work it is pathetic to reflect that the chief and original source of veterinary service in this country, the Royal Veterinary College of London, is struggling barely to maintain its existence. The arrival of the modern motor vehicle naturally has caused a great falling off in students whence formerly the college derived the bulk of its income. Unassisted at the present time in any way by the state, its funds, such as they are, depreciated by the war, its benches depleted of students, the college has indeed fallen on evil days.

The Royal Veterinary College of Ireland derives liberal financial assistance from the Department of Agriculture and Technical Instruction, and the Edinburgh Veterinary College is substantially helped by the Scottish Education Department, but the English parent college is left to its own resources.

In comparison with the assistance that is given to medical education and all sorts of technical education it may, in view of the above facts, be fairly stated that the Royal Veterinary College has been sadly neglected. Veterinary surgeons are not wealthy men, they pursue an idealistic rather than a profitable profession and are not, therefore, in a position to enrich by endowments the source of their professional education, as so frequently occurs in the case of the Arts and other learned professions.

The enormous amount of valuable national service performed by veterinary surgeons is for the most part overlooked or hidden away in the corner of some Departmental Blue-Book. Even if Armies pass away and there is no more war, the flocks and the herds of the Empire will always require the assistance of the veterinary profession. A Board of Agriculture or Colonial Administration would be handicapped indeed without its veterinary advisers and executive. Assistance cannot, therefore, be denied to the Royal Veterinary College on the grounds that the motor car has banished forever the national need for expert veterinary surgeons. To meet the argument that the present is no time for incurring further public expenditure it may be stated that the college could be kept above water by appropriating to its needs the annual emoluments paid from the coffers of the State to any one of many dispensable people holding appointments of doubtful utility but indisputable dignity.

———◆———

—Captain Ernest W. Hogg, entering the Veterinary Reserve Corps June, 1917, has attained a captaincy and has been assigned as Division Veterinarian at Camp Meade, Md.

—First Lieut. Charles M. Stull has been transferred from Fort Bliss, Texas, to the 1st Cavalry, Douglas, Arizona.

—Dr. Curtice C. Bourland has been transferred from Fort Oglethorpe, Ga., to the 80th Field Artillery, Camp MacArthur, Waco, Texas.

—Lieut. Ivan G. Howe, Camp Greene, Charlotte, N. C., has received a commission as First Lieutenant.

—First Lieut. J. L. Ruble, formerly at Fort D. A. Russell, Wyo., is now at 2d Brig. Headquarters, 15th Cavalry Div., Fort Bliss, Texas.

—Dr. Nelson N. Lefler, formerly of Batavia, N. Y., has received a commission as Lieutenant in the Veterinary Reserve Corps and has been ordered to report at Camp Greenleaf, Fort Oglethorpe, Georgia.

—Second Lieut. J. J. Martin, formerly at Fort Riley, has been transferred to Camp Funston, Kans.

—First. Lieut. A. A. Leibold is with the American Expeditionary Forces, France.

—First Lieut. Julius Stotchik, formerly at Leon Springs, Texas, is now with the 21st Field Artillery, Camp MacArthur, Waco, Texas.

—Majors L. A. Klein and A. L. Mason, who went to France on a special mission last November, have completed their work and returned to Washington.

—Lieut. Charles C. Dobson, formerly of Muncie, Ind., is now at Headquarters 76th Infantry Brigade, Camp Shelby, Miss.

—Lieut. Joseph F. Crosby has been transferred from Camp Sevier, S. C., to Fort Sill, Okla., 1st Field Artillery.

—Lieut. Henry H. Haigh, formerly of Philadelphia, Pa., is now with the American Expeditionary Forces in France.

—Lieut. C. W. Likely, formerly with the 341st Field Artillery, has been recently appointed First Lieutenant and transferred to the Command of the Mobile Veterinary Section, No. 314, at Camp Funston, Kans.

—Dr. M. W. Scott has been transferred from East St. Louis, Ill., to Front Royal, Va., on Influenza Control, with temporary headquarters at Louisville, Ky.

—Captain Ross A. Greenwood, formerly at Camp Meade, is with the American Expeditionary Forces.

—Dr. Ralph B. Stewart has been recently promoted from Second Lieutenant to First Lieutenant and has been transferred from Camp Dodge, Ia., to the 310th Cavalry at Fort Ethan Allen, Vt.

—Lieut. Raymond Lamb, of the British Machine Corps, after three years' service, has won the Military Cross for gallantry at Beersheba, Palestine. Lieut. Lamb is the son of Dr. Percy Lamb, formerly of Colorado.

—Lieut. R. O. Stott has been transferred from Douglas, Arizona, to the Auxiliary Remount Depot, Fort Bliss, Texas.

—Lieut. Harve Frank has been transferred from Chicago, Ill., to El Paso, Texas.

—Lieut. H. E. Torgersen has been transferred from Fort Douglas, Utah, to the Remount Depot at Deming, Texas.

—Major D. H. Udall has been transferred from Fort Oglethorpe, Ga., to Camp Grant, Rockford, Ill., as Division Veterinarian.

—Major E. B. Ackerman and Lieutenants Muldoon and Claris have been transferred from Fort Oglethorpe, Ga., to Camp Lee, Va.

—LIBERTY LOANS STRENGTHEN THE LIBERTY LINE.

—Dr. L. H. Wright, assistant professor of physiology and pharmacology in the School of Veterinary Medicine at College Station, Texas, has resigned to accept a position as research worker in the University of Nevada and State Experiment Station at Reno, Nevada.

—Dr. F. Edward Isaacson, formerly Animal Pathologist at the Maryland Agricultural Experiment Station, has accepted a position with the Lederle Antitoxin Laboratories at Pearl River, N. Y.

—MAKE YOUR MONEY FIGHT.

AMERICAN VETERINARY MEDICAL ASSOCIATION

DR. HILTON ELECTED TO EXECUTIVE BOARD

On Wednesday evening, April 10th, 1918, the post-card ballot which was recently made to select a member of the Executive Board for the First District was counted. The result of the count of the ballots shows that Dr. George Hilton of Ottawa, Ont., Canada, was elected to this position. Those acting as tellers were Drs. J. T. Hernsheim, S. E. Bennett and H. B. Raffensperger, Resident State Secretary for Illinois.

L. ENOS DAY, Acting Secretary.

THE PHILADELPHIA MEETING

Active preparations for the 55th annual convention of the American Veterinary Medical Association are being made by the local committee of arrangements.

The meeting will cover four days, August 19th to 22nd, and will be held in Philadelphia with headquarters and meetings at the Bellevue-Stratford Hotel.

T. E. Munce, General Chairman of the A. V. M. A. Committees, has appointed sub-committees with the following chairmen :

Finance—H. B. Cox......................Philadelphia
Hotel and Reservation—D. E. Hickman....Philadelphia
Program—C. M. Hoskins.................Philadelphia
Entertainment—Fred Stehle, Jr..........Philadelphia
Ladies' Auxiliary—Mrs. H. B. Cox........Philadelphia
Transportation—F. H. Schneider..........Philadelphia
Registration—Thomas Kelly..............Philadelphia
Clinic—Wm. J. Lentz....................Philadelphia
Press and Publicity—W. S. Gimper.........Harrisburg
General Chairman—T. E. Munce...........Harrisburg

Meetings of the several committees have been held at which definite plans were formulated indicating that a comprehensive program including new features, in addition to the customary general and joint sessions and section work, will be presented.

Matters pertaining to the activities of the Army Veterinary Corps will be an especially interesting portion of the program. It is expected that the Army Veterinarians will be represented by leading members of the profession from the armies of the Entente Allies in addition to those from our own forces.

The veterinary phase of sanitary police work in the cantonments at home and on the battle fields abroad has suddenly assumed an importance never before accorded it; and it will be interesting to all members of the A. V. M. A. to learn from those directing this work, of the successful efforts made to meet the emergency of rapidly expanding armies.

Every effort will be made to overcome any inconveniences of travel and entertainment that may arise from the war situation and a record breaking attendance at the 55th convention is expected.   W. S. GIMPER.

REDUCED FARES FROM PACIFIC COAST TERRITORY

The question of authorizing special excursion fares from Pacific Coast territory to the East during the coming season was given consideration by the Trans-Continental Lines at a conference held in March and it was decided to refrain from authorizing such fares because the facilities of the railroads are being taxed to the utmost in moving troops, munitions, fuel, food and other essentials. The indications are that demands in that relation will increase rather than decrease.

The action stated does not, however, deprive delegates from the Pacific Coast of reduced fares since they may take advantage of regular nine months excursion fares which are in effect daily from Pacific Coast Common Points—California and North Pacific Coast—to eastern terminals of Trans-Continental Lines. These tickets are sold at a substantial reduction from double the one way fares and are on sale daily. They are limited for return within nine months from date of sale. These excursion fares approximate two cents per mile in each direction and are about one fare and one-third. These excursion tickets are sold only from the States of California, Nevada, Oregon, Washington and British Columbia.

EXPANDING OUR JOURNAL

For some time it has been quite apparent to the writer, at least, that our editor is handling a situation practically unsupported and unaided that is beyond what should be required or expected of any one individual, particularly in face of the fact that he has important duties to perform aside from the publication of the JOURNAL.

It has, speaking in all frankness, been somewhat of a mystery just how our editor has managed under existing conditions to make such a good showing.

In this connection it is suggested that the time is at hand or is fast approaching when our JOURNAL will have to be enlarged and contain a greater variety of matter to meet the requirements and fancies of men following the different specialties presented by veterinary science.

If this be true, it is manifestly obvious that if our editor is at present performing a large task, his burden should not be increased but rather should be lightened.

We have two suggestions to remedy the existing conditions and to prepare for the future: first, that all A. V. M. A. Resident State Secretaries be required to assume among other things the duties of associate editors and that the president, when selecting state secretaries, choose men who have an aptitude, and who are in a position to assist our editor in collecting news and literature that will enable us to make our JOURNAL more attractive and valuable; second, that a business manager be secured whose duty it would be to look after the advertising, printing, subscriptions and other commercial details incidental to the successful publication of a JOURNAL such as ours.   R. A. ARCHIBALD.

ASSOCIATION MEETINGS

CONFERENCE ON TICK ERADICATION

The greatest gathering ever held in conference for the advancement of the work of eradicating the cattle fever tick was held in New Orleans, January 15 to 18, at the St. Charles Hotel in their spacious convention hall, the session lasting four days with an attendance of approximately 300 workers and veterinarians from all southern states where the work is still in progress.

The convention hall was profusely decorated with the National emblem. The meeting, being called to order, was opened with singing of the Star Spangled Banner by the assemblage, followed by an address of welcome by the Mayor of New Orleans, the Honorable Martin Behrmann.

Dr. R. A. Ramsey, chief of the B. A. I. tick eradication forces, addressed the conference on "Organization of the Bureau and the

Need of Cooperation Between Its Employees'' in a manner which indelibly impressed its import on the minds of all fortunate enough to be present and obtain the benefits of the doctor's wide range of experience.

, The work of eradication of the cattle fever tick from the South has taken a wonderful impetus in its progress in the last few years; Kentucky, California, Missouri, Tennessee and Mississippi have made entering wedges clean through to the Gulf Coast, splitting the solid South from the federal and state quarantine bondage and a greater part of other states have been cleaned, leaving only 48 per cent of the square mileage originally quarantined that yet remains to be worked.

All eyes are on Louisiana this year and Dr. E. I. Smith, Inspector in charge of the Louisiana forces, in a well worded and comforting address, gave the conference "impromptu" his field experiences as applied to administrative duties as Inspector in Charge, and the assurance that Louisiana would make a drive this year that would put it Over the Top in eradication of the tick.

The reception accorded Dr. W. H. Dalrymple of Louisiana was synonymous with his national reputation as a veterinarian and an address teeming with originality of thought and masterly in delivery was heard by the assemblage with enthusiastic applause.

All of the southern states were represented by their respective state veterinarians. Dr. C. A. Cary of Alabama was attentively listened to, as the doctor always has something good to divulge. Dr. Peter F. Bahnsen of Georgia, "the man with the punch", in true characteristic style brought repeated applause.

Compelling dipping when public sentiment will not mold to voluntary action was the theme of Dr. R. E. Jackson, Inspector in Charge of Alabama, and the doctor knows how to handle this matter to perfection. There being no state-wide tick-eradication law in Alabama, the doctor has shown that he is a past master in the art of injunction, for by his regulation device, cattle can only be moved with his permission out of the counties in his state that are not eradicating the tick. Like Dewey at Manila he has them bottled up until they agree to eradicate.

A missing personality was conspicuous by its absence in that of Dr. J. A. Kiernan, now chief of tuberculosis eradication, who, on former gatherings of the tick eradication forces, wielded the gavel with a vim and vigor that carried the business along on schedule time. The anonymous question box idea, although introduced with the best of intentions to bring out knotted problems to be untangled by the conference, had a reacting anaesthetizing effect on the assembly; restoratives were applied in the assignment of two old generals in tick eradication work to do picket duty and see that no one lapsed into coma. Doctors Charles Becker of Alabama (sweet under all circumstances) and J. B. Reidy, Inspector in Charge, of Texas, enlivened the dull siege through which we were passing with characteristic stimulations.

The singing of the last stanza of the song "AMERICA", led by Dr. C. Becker, closed the conference *"sine die"*. A general handshake and "adieus" were given all around, the meeting declared a huge impetus to the workers in tick eradication to renewed effort and greater confidence; all then left for their various fields of assignment in the new and greater South.

EDWARD HORSTMAN, Veterinary Inspector.

NORTHEASTERN PENNSYLVANIA VETERINARY CLUB

Dr. T. E. Munce, Acting State Veterinarian for Pennsylvania, and Dr. A. E. Wight, U. S. Department of Agriculture, Bureau of Animal Industry, addressed a joint meeting of the Northeastern Pennsylvania Veterinary Club, the Cattle Breeders and County Agents, with reference to the Accredited Herd Movement, at Hotel Sterling, Wilkes-Barre, Pa., on Thursday, March 21st.

Dr. Howard C. Reynolds, of the International Correspondence Schools, Scranton, Pa., acted as chairman. Chas. F. Johnson, Superintendent of the Luzerne County Industrial Home at Kis Lyn, Pa., gave the opening address, setting forth in a brief way the necessity of the breeders, county agents and veterinarians becoming more united in their efforts to fight a common enemy (tuberculosis). Dr. Munce gave a paper on the "Eradication of Bovine Tuberculosis and Accredited Herds", referring to the work that is being done by the State Live Stock Sanitary Board of Pennsylvania in regard to controlling the disease. Dr. Wight outlined the work that the Federal Department is doing with reference to the Accredited Herd Movement. He stated that twenty-seven of the states had already taken up the Accredited Herd Movement and were working in conjunction with the federal authorities in an effort to eradicate the disease in thoroughbred herds. Dr. Henry

W. Turner of Pittsburgh opened the discussion of Dr. Munce's and Dr. Wight's paper, and also referred to his experiments in seven-day retesting. Dr. Weaver of State College, Dr. Brunner of Harrisburg, Dr. Ridge of Somerton, Dr. Church of Wilkes-Barre, Drs. Paget and Helmar of Scranton, and Mr. A. J. Anderson, Editor of the *Pennsylvania Farmer* of Philadelphia, also took an active part in the discussion.

Many of the most representative breeders of registered cattle were present and expressed their willingness to cooperate with the state and federal authorities in carrying out the Accredited Herd Movement. Mr. George Carpenter, one of the most prominent breeders of Guernsey and Holstein cattle in Northeastern Pennsylvania, a man who has had wide experience in the dairy and cattle business, was present and gave a fine talk, bringing out that tuberculosis was one of the most vital things with which the dairymen and breeders had to contend, and also showed his willingness to go along with the state and federal authorities in their effort to control the disease. Mr. Conygham, of the Conyghams Farms at Dallas, Pa., and Mr. Benj. Covey of the Elmview Farms, Elmhurst, Pa., gave very enthusiastic talks and showed a keen interest in the movement. Mr. Engle, County Agent of Susquehanna County, and Mr. Sloan, County Agent of Bradford County, both gave interesting talks. Mr. Sloan extended an urgent invitation, requesting Dr. Munce and Dr. Wight to attend the Bradford County Breeders Association meeting to be held sometime in August.

Those in charge of the meeting were very much pleased with the enthusiasm with which the Accredited Herd Movement was received and feel that the work will progress rapidly as soon as the state and federal authorities have their working forces thoroughly organized. H. C. REYNOLDS.

—LIBERTY LOANS STRENGTHEN THE LIBERTY LINE.

—Educational and demonstrational work in connection with hog cholera has been inaugurated in the State of Mississippi; Dr. Hugh L. Fry in charge at Jackson, Miss.

—The Tifton Packing Company of Tifton, Ga., has been granted inspection of its products with Dr. James I. Martin in charge.

COMMUNICATION

EMPYEMA OF THE CHEST

Editor Journal of the American Veterinary Medical Association:
Ithaca, N. Y.

In the April number of the JOURNAL there appeared a very interesting and instructive case report by Dr. D. D. LeFevre of Newark, N. Y., entitled "Empyema of the chest and gangrenous necrosis of lungs", which was "read at the 10th Annual Conference for Veterinarians, Ithaca, N. Y., January, 1918".

Dr. LeFevre is to be congratulated upon his methods in handling this case. It is evident that through the employment of heroic measures—measures from which many practitioners would have shrunk—he secured really remarkable results. As intimated in his report, there is a paucity of literature on thoracic surgery in our veterinary text books, and the little that is described is not calculated to cause the practitioner to approach the subject with enthusiasm.

Dr. LeFevre states that "both sides of the chest seemed to be about two-thirds full of some kind of fluid * * * not wishing to run any chance of getting the other side of the chest infected, the canula was immediately withdrawn * * * by percussion it was found that the liquid extended to nearly the same height on both sides of the chest, but it was at a much lower level than formerly. Either the partition between the two halves of the lungs had become ruptured or the liquid from the left side had seeped through the partition into the right side".

Although Dr. LeFevre does not make it quite clear, he no doubt meant, when he said that the fluid "had seeped through the partition", that it passed through the natural openings in the posterior mediastinum about to be mentioned in quoting from Chauveau, Sisson, and Strangeways. Therefore it would not have been necessary for the "partition between the two halves of the lungs" to have "become ruptured" to have brought about the bilateral affection described.

Chauveau: "The posterior mediastinum * * * its inferior part, always deviated to the left, is extremely thin, and perforated by small openings, which give it the appearance of fine lace work."

Sisson, after noting that these apertures are "sometimes absent", makes the following statement: "the character of the pleura here probably explains the clinical observation that in the horse, fluid exudate resulting from unilateral pleurisy is usually present in both pleural sacs in like amount."

Strangeways: "The posterior mediastinum is cribrated inferiorly, several openings leading from one pleural sac to the other. This arrangement is *peculiar to solipeds,* and explains the fact that in these animals there cannot be pleural effusion confined to one side of the chest."

My old "Courtenay", published years ago—which in reality is a compilation of notes on theory and practice delivered to his students for many years by the late Professor Andrew Smith—in discussing hydrothorax in the horse, states that "In cases where copious effusion has taken place, the fluid freely passes from one side of the cavity to the other, there being free communication between the sides, except when closed by bands of lymph".

My only excuse for this communication is that it seems worth while to draw particular attention to the peculiar anatomy of the posterior mediastinum of the horse, and the importance of keeping in mind this peculiarity from a clinical standpoint.

J. P. FOSTER,
Mayo Clinic, Rochester, Minn.

Editor Journal of the American Veterinary Medical Association:
Ithaca, N. Y.

I have been reading the JOURNAL of recent dates relative to the eating of horses and I have formulated for your JOURNAL the enclosed article which I trust you will feel disposed to print in your next issue, and I think you will unless you have to get Dr. Hoskins' O.K.

With kindest regards, I am

Sincerely yours,
MARK WHITE.

EATING OF HORSES NON-AMERICAN

I have noted the recent advocates of the eating of horses' flesh in the JOURNAL of recent issues, but I, as a veterinarian, native born American, am not in sympathy with this movement and I believe that I voice the sentiment of the majority of veterinarians and Americans.

The eating of horses and dogs is a foreign custom and it will be hard for us Americans to get the consent of our minds to eat our horses, we are too humane and love the horse next to man.

The veterinarian usually is a humanitarian at heart and the best friend of the humane societies, if not he has missed his calling and should not have studied veterinary medicine and is doomed for to fail at his vocation.

We, as veterinarians, should be the last to advocate the killing of our horses for food and the publicity of such in our journals reflects seriously upon us as a profession and will certainly hurt us.

Dr. W. H. Hoskins evidently has an appetite for the steak cut from his old grey mare, but you and I will gladly let him feast alone. We are all aware of the excessive development of Dr. Hoskins' political faculty, but now his stand for Americans eating horses would appear as if he was either boarding at a "Foreign Boardinghouse" or else was seeking publicity at the expense of the veterinary profession.

As evidence of Dr. Hoskins' humanitarian faculty being somewhat atrophied, may be shown by the fact that while I was a student at the University of Pennsylvania, I had occasion to visit Dr.
Hoskins' hospital and was shocked to see him advocate and open
abscesses with the hot iron and he insisted that this was the most
scientific method. This inhuman treatment would explain why he
would enjoy horse steak for supper, but I for one will let him eat
alone.

In the countries where they eat horses and dogs they are very
cruel to these animals.

REVIEW

VETERINARY POST MORTEM TECHNIC

WALTER J. CROCKER, B.S., V.M.D.
Professor of Veterinary Pathology, School of Veterinary Medicine,
University of Pennsylvania
8° Cloth, xiv+233 pp., 142 illustrations. J. B. Lippincott Co., Philadelphia
and London. $4.00 net.

This attractive volume is a welcome addition to American
veterinary literature. It was written as a manual for the use of
college students. If I am not mistaken it will prove to be of even
greater value to those, no longer in college, who need to refresh
their memory or to learn an orderly procedure for making an autopsy.

The titles of the chapters give an idea of the scope of the
work. Chapter I, General Considerations; Chapter II, Autopsy
Room; Chapter III, Post Mortem Instruments; Chapter IV, External Examination; Chapter V, Internal Examination of the
Horse; Chapter VI, Internal Examination of Ruminants; Chapter VII, Internal Examination of Swine; Chapter VIII, Internal
Examination of the Dog and Cat; Chapter IX, Internal Examination of the Mouse, Guinea Pig, Rabbit, Fowl and Elephant; Chapter X, Technic and Description of Organs; Chapter XI, Post Mortem Protocol and Report.

In the third chapter nearly sixty different instruments are illustrated and their use described briefly. Everyone will not agree
with the author's statement that in autopsy work the tendency to
use a butcher knife is to be avoided "since systematic post mortem
work is not butchery". The instruments used by those whose
business is commercial post mortem work are well adapted for the

purpose for which each is used and they are economical. The price of special post mortem instruments is excessive. In the chapter on the internal examination of the horse directions are given for performing the autopsy with the horse lying on the right side. Other authors give also the method of procedure when the cadaver is lying on its back and when lying on the left side. The statement is made that in cases of digestive disorders the autopsy should be performed with the horse lying on its back so that a possible twist of the intestines might be discovered. I must confess that I have never seen a case where having the horse lying on its back made the slightest difference. By the time an autopsy on a horse is made the intestines are under sufficient pressure to change their position when the abdominal cavity is opened. There might possibly be an occasion when it would be embarrassing not to be able to make an autopsy of a horse lying on the left side. The important thing is to be able to make a systematic autopsy. It is certainly better to know one method than to have a vague impression of two or more.

Clear, detailed directions are given for each step in making an autopsy. The method to be followed in different stages of the autopsy and in opening the several organs after they have been removed from the cadaver is illustrated from photographs of fresh specimens. The book is well illustrated. The paper and print are excellent.

This book is the only one on this subject available to those using the English language. It seems something bordering on the obvious to say it is the best book of its kind procurable. It is much needed and deserves a hearty welcome. S. H. B.

—Make Your Money Fight.

—Dr. R. N. Shaw has removed from Boston to North Amherst, Mass.

—Veterinary Inspector J. S. Oldham has been transferred from Ashland, Ala., to Falfurrias, Texas, for work in tick eradication under Dr. J. B. Reidy, Inspector in Charge.

—Dr. W. A. Curtis, who has been at Iloilo, Philippine Islands, has returned to this country. His address is Chanute, Kans.

—Liberty Loans Strengthen the Liberty Line.

NECROLOGY

ALEXANDRE FRANCOIS LIAUTARD, M.D., V.M.

Alexandre Francois Liautard died at his home, Bois Jerome, France, April 20th, 1918, in his eighty-fourth year.

Born in Paris, February 15th, 1835, Dr. Liautard in his early youth entered the famous veterinary school at Alfort, France, from which institution he graduated in 1856, and after serving three years in the French Army, came to America to practice his profession, and reorganized the New York College of Veterinary Surgeons in New York City, which had been chartered in 1857. At the same time he studied medicine at the University Medical College, in New York City, and received his degree of Doctor of Medicine in 1865.

He was one of the organizers of the United States Veterinary Medical Association, and recorded the first official report of that organization, having been selected to act as secretary at the sessions of that first meeting on June 9th and 10th, 1863, where seven states were represented. It was at this meeting, when this noblest of men and skilled veterinarian, a graduate from a seven-year course veterinary school and at the time a student in medicine, surrounded by the forty men who with him were organizers of our national association, all earnest of purpose, mostly self-made men, and while veterinary practitioners, but few regular graduates, that Dr. Liautard, with the generosity and breadth of character that were his attributes, suggested as the motto of the association, *Non Nobis Solum*—not for us alone—which he afterward adopted as the motto of the American Veterinary College, and which is still the motto of the consolidated schools in New York City today. Another example of his nobility of character and self-sacrifice, was when, in 1913, the American Veterinary Medical Association made him Honorary President on the occasion of its fiftieth anniversary in New York—he being the only living charter member— he denied himself the pleasure of being present to remain at the side of his invalided wife in France.

Dr. Liautard served as president of the United States Veterinary Medical Association from 1875 to '77 and again from 1886 to '87. When the United States Veterinary Medical Association decided it needed an official organ, Dr. Liautard was selected as its editor; and after some years, when he had made of it an interesting and important organ of the veterinary profession, the association decided to pass it over to him as his own periodical. This step in no way detracted from the value of the *American Veterinary Review* (which he named it) to the association, but on the contrary added to it, and at the same time increased its value to the American veterinary profession in general, which, under Dr. Liautard's editorship, it guided and molded both in and out of the association; and when the *Review* was again taken over by the American Veterinary Medical Association some forty years later, it still found Dr. Liautard the senior editor, and he never ceased to contribute richly to it up to the time of his death.

Dr. Liautard's entire life was devoted to veterinary education. In 1875 he severed his connection with the New York College of Veterinary Surgeons, where he had been Dean, Professor of Anatomy, Operative Surgery, Clinical Director, etc., since 1860, and organized the American Veterinary College, where he filled the same role until the amalgamation of the two schools as a department of New York University in 1899 under the name of the New York-American Veterinary College, when the late Professor William J. Coates became his successor.

In addition to his college work, Dr. Liautard was constantly working in the preparation of text books for the veterinary profession and was the author of a long list of standard works.

As an anatomist and teacher of anatomy he never had an equal. Holding various colored crayons in his left hand, he would stand before a black board and lecture by the hour; at the same time, accurately drawing in colors the subject of his lecture, placing in each part while describing it; and at the completion of his lecture a beautiful colored plate surrounded by the names in white chalk would remain behind him on the board for the students to study. Many of them who had had training in drawing, copied them in their note books. And up to the time of his death, although in his eighty-fourth year, in addition to his activity and keen interest in veterinary education and veterinary matters generally, he followed with close interest the work of the school of which he was the founder.

In 1884 Dr. Liautard was decorated by the French government as *Chevalier du Merite Agricole.*

As founder of the first veterinary school in America and as one of the founders and first secretary of the United States Veterinary Medical Association, he justly merited the title of Father of Veterinary Medicine in America, accorded him by the American veterinary profession.

The principles that he unconsciously instilled into all who came in contact with him, the memories of his nobility of character, the school which he founded, his museum of rare pathological specimens and his library of more than three thousand volumes which have formed the foundation of a library that bears his name in the city of his activities, form a part of the priceless legacy that he has left to the American veterinary profession. Although at an age when his death might have been looked for at any time, the announcement of it comes as a shock from which it is difficult to recover. It is indeed difficult to realize that Alexandre Liautard is dead. His name has been associated with the American veterinary profession and the national organization from the very beginning and during their entire growth and development, and his loss to them will be as sad as it is inestimable; yet, at his age we must not wish to deny him his retirement from the turmoil of the world to the peaceful rest he so well deserves. *Requiescat in pace.*

Dr. Liautard is survived by a loving and devoted daughter, Mrs. Louise M. Boyer.

ROBERT W. ELLIS.

To the editor the death of Dr. Liautard is a great personal loss. From the beginning of our acquaintance after a personal visit eleven years ago, there has been an irregular correspondence which became more intimate when the *American Veterinary Review* was taken over as the official JOURNAL OF THE AMERICAN VETERINARY MEDICAL ASSOCIATION. His interest in the JOURNAL and its success was unlimited. His long life was devoted to unselfish service for the profession he loved. Modest and unassuming, he gave of his best without thought of reward. It is doubtful if the younger generation of our profession realizes in full its profound obligation for the great work he initiated here and the interest he has always maintained in our advancement.

- The nobility of his character is evidenced by his active interest in the Franco-Belgian Relief Fund,of which he was one of the originators, which, with our own Allied Relief Fund, stands as a memorial to his great heart. The sufferings of others and the victims of injustice and oppression aroused in him a responsive thrill of sympathy which translated itself into active relief.

He was one of the great world forces in the veterinary profession. True and loyal to the best ideals with unselfish service, it may well be said of his career in unlimited measure: "Well done, thou good and faithful servant." P. A. F.

JOHN KING

John King, V.S., Carlyle, Saskatchewan, a member of the American Veterinary Medical Association.

ERNEST C. DINGLEY

Dr. Ernest C. Dingley, Philadelphia, Pa., a member of the American Veterinary Medical Association, died November 26, 1917.

BLAIR W. TRUAX

Dr. Blair W. Truax, Burr Oak, Kans., a member of the American Veterinary Medical Association, was killed in an automobile accident.

MISCELLANEOUS

—Veterinary Inspector Robert Thumann has been transferred from Orangeburg, S. C., to Kansas City, Mo.

—The graduating exercises of the Kansas City Veterinary College took place April 23.

—Dr. M. H. Leininger has left Vernon, Ala., and will supervise tick eradication work in three counties with headquarters at Andalusia, Ala.

—Dr. C. A. Klein has removed from Cincinnati, Ohio, to Omaha, Neb., S. S.

—Dr. A. M. Eichelberger will be located at Kipp, Alberta, until next November, where he is interested in a large wheat and live stock ranch. His practice at Shreveport will be conducted by Dr. G. A. Cunningham of New Orleans during his absence. Dr. Frank Collins of Monroe will fill Dr. Eichelberger's place as Secretary of the Louisiana State Board of Veterinary Medical Examiners.

—Dr. T. M. Bayler has removed from Waterloo, Ia., to Bloomington, Ill.

—The next meeting of the Hudson Valley Veterinary Medical Society will be held at Hudson, N. Y., May 1, 1918.

—Dr. John T. Myers has removed to Aurora, Ill., in charge of the government supervision of the plant of the Aurora Serum Company, vice Dr. P. C. Hurley, resigned.

—The work for the control and eradication of hog cholera in the State of Ohio has been placed under the supervision of Dr. Charles H. York, in cooperation with the State Veterinarian. The educational and demonstrational work in Ohio still remains under the supervision of Dr. L. P. Beechy.

—Dr. Joe H. Bux is in charge of educational and demonstrational hog cholera work at Little Rock, Ark., vice Dr. V. W. Knowles, resigned.

—Dr. Harry W. McMaster takes the place of E. B. Jansman, resigned, at the abattoir of the Fesenmeier Packing Company, Huntington, W. Va.

—Dr. Ralph Graham has changed his headquarters from Sedalia, Mo., to Jefferson City, Mo.

—Dr. Lyman B. Dunlop is inspector in charge of federal meat inspection at Salt Lake City, Utah, in place of Dr. Frederick H. Thompson, assigned to tuberculosis eradication with headquarters at St. Paul, Minn.

—Dr. John W. Logan succeeds Dr. B. J. Cady as inspector in charge of educational and demonstrational hog cholera work in the State of California with headquarters at Berkeley, Calif.

—Dr. E. D. Harris, formerly of Casseton, N. D., is now associated with the Florida Live Stock Sanitary Board at Tallahassee, Florida.

—Dr. George R. Teeple has removed from Fort Morgan to Denver, Colo.

—Dr. A. H. Davis has been transferred from Chicago, Ill., to Cheyenne, Wyo., for work upon scabies and dourine.

—Dr. R. W. Gannett of Brooklyn, N. Y., has been appointed to the State Board of Veterinary Examiners, to fill the unexpired term of Dr. W. Reid Blair.

—Dr. F. M. Kearns has sold his practice at Lebanon, Ky., to Dr. R. E. Taylor of Chilton, Ky. Dr. Kearns has removed to Hillsdale, Ind., to engage in farming and stock raising.

—MAKE YOUR MONEY FIGHT.

JOURNAL
OF THE
American Veterinary Medical Association
Formerly American Veterinary Review
(Original Official Organ U. S. Vet. Med. Ass'n)

PIERRE A. FISH, Editor   ITHACA, N. Y.

Executive Board

GEORGE HILTON, 1st District; W. HORACE HOSKINS, 2d District; J. R. MOHLER, 3d District; C. H. STANGE, 4th District; R. A. ARCHIBALD, 5th District; A. T. KINSLEY, Member at large.

Sub-Committee on Journal

J. R. MOHLER   R. A. ARCHIBALD

The American Veterinary Medical Association is not responsible for views or statements published in the JOURNAL, outside of its own authorized actions.

Reprints should be ordered in advance. A circular of prices will be sent upon application.

VOL. LIII., N. S. VOL. VI.   JUNE, 1918.   No. 3.

Communications relating to membership and matters pertaining to the American Veterinary Medical Association should be addressed to Acting Secretary L. Enos Day, 1827 S. Wabash Ave., Chicago, Ill. Matters pertaining to the Journal should be sent to Ithaca, N. Y.

COMMUNITY OF INTEREST

The origin of clubs, societies and associations may doubtless be traced to those who felt they possessed aims, ideals and interests in common exclusive of, or in addition to, individual interests. Efforts at reform, advancement of a cause, recognition and promulgation of ideas are promoted and attained when backed by the strength of massed effort rather than by weak individual effort. In professional lines there is also the element of unselfishness, in which there is willingness to give, from one's experience, aid that will assist in the uplift of other members of the profession. In this day and age there is little or no argument over the advantages derived from organization. Educational benefit, solidarity and strength develop and the cause is advanced.

Granting the desirability of such organizations in times of peace, it is equally evident that their benefits are quite as advantageous in time of war, although from the nature of conditions there may be more irregularity and variation in carrying through the procedure near the battle front. The organization of the Somme Veterinary Medical Association in the region of active warfare in France by the allied veterinarians indicates a realization not only of ordinary advantages but of special advantages which may accrue by meeting and discussing diseases and conditions which are more or less peculiar to the war and the area involved.

The VETERINARY JOURNAL has published in its April number a partial account of the proceedings of the first conference, held January 12: At this conference a number of British and French veterinary officers were in attendance and devoted their time to presenting and discussing papers on glanders, epizootic lymphangitis, ulcerative cellulitis, periodic ophthalmia and the control and treatment of mange and other contagious skin diseases. A spirit of friendship and comradeship already existent has been intensified; generous cooperation strengthened and true community of interest realized. War-time friendships are strong and lasting and compensate to some extent for the horrors and realities of war.

Ever alert to the interests of American veterinarians, the late Dr. Liautard, upon hearing of the organization of the Somme Association, took steps to inquire if American participation would be acceptable. In his Chronicles in our May issue he promised to inform us later of the result. Death has written *Finis* to his Chronicles, but the VETERINARY JOURNAL assures American veterinarians of a hearty British welcome and it is to be hoped that some of our veterinarians may be stationed in localities where they may avail themselves of the benefits of the organization. A number of our veterinarians are already in France and doubtless many more will be there before the war is over. Conditions will be new to them and opportunities to benefit from the experience of their colleagues, who have been so much longer in the field, should be of material advantage in mastering the problems they will encounter. A free interchange of ideas is of inestimable value and affords mutual encouragement. The experience gained will serve for future use, for there will be a never-ending warfare against disease.

It is a matter of grateful recognition that one of the last acts of Dr. Liautard's useful life was an effort to cement more firmly the bonds of friendship between the veterinarians of our country and those of his native land and of Great Britain and to put our profession upon a truly cosmopolitan basis.

P. A. F.

EUROPEAN CHRONICLES

Bois Jerome.

A DIFFERENTIAL DIAGNOSIS.—Major Veterinarian Doctor J. Rogers has written a communication to the Societe Centrale upon the differential diagnosis of calculus and coprostasis in horses; this differentiation is not only a simple clinical success but has great importance, as it permits the possessor of a calculus to be sent to the slaughter house and thus reduces the loss to the owner. The differentiation between the ailments can be made almost immediately or within a few hours.

The article deals successively with the symptomatology of calculus obstruction and the elements of differentiation between this and stercoral obstructions.

The evolution of the calculus has three stages. The last of which is its stoppage when inclosed in the intestine. In this stage three forms may be manifested: the *convulsive,* the *soporose* and the *flatulent.*

In the *convulsive,* essentially characterized by a crisis of convulsions, the animal, in the intervals, presents nothing to indicate the severity of his condition. When the crisis comes, there are spasms, contractions, tetanus, etc., more or less explicit in nature and affecting only one muscle or several and assuming the aspect of a regular epileptiform crisis. These last a few seconds, a few minutes or even a quarter of an hour. Sometimes it is only a spasm of the levator muscle of the upper lip or cloni of the inferior, trembling at the eyes, shaking of the muscles of the neck, of the trunk or perhaps of the limbs; pleurothotonos, opisthotonos, spasms of the great oblique muscle of the head, nystagmus, etc. All are manifestations characteristic of this convulsive form. The tympany takes place later.

In the *soporose* form, the principal clinical manifestation is a semi-comatose condition. There is generally observed hypertension of the facial artery and myosis. The horse lays down carefully and the decubitus is accompanied with moans. It occurs most frequently and for a long time, on the side of the lesion. There are also some slight convulsive motions. Tympany is late.

In the third form, the *flatulent,* tympanitis appears after a

---

*Doctor Liautard's last contribution was sent under date of April 3 and was received April 26, eight days after his death.

few hours and the manifestations are those of intestinal indigestion.

To establish the differential diagnosis, the doctor first describes that of the intestinal obstruction.

If the horse has not passed any fecal matter for a few hours, 6, 12, or 18, the obstruction is of course suspected and if rectal exploration is made, when the arm is withdrawn, it is found covered with a coat of coagulated mucus. This is what he calls the *"arm sign"*. It is a very important one. The presence of the mucus on the thermometer (*thermometer sign*) is also convincing. The arm sign is the proof of the presence at that part of the intestine of a cream-like intestinal secretion, which is also observed in intestinal obstruction. It is positive a few hours after the beginning of the stage of complete obstruction.

Rectal exploration gives also other indications. Some are positive, the *palpation* of the *calculus* or of an egagropile situated in the floating colon; or again of aggregates of egagropiles, which are also decisive in the diagnosis. *Stercoral masses* may also be detected. These are more frequent with calculus than with coprostasis.

The finding of a collection of stercoral matter is not sufficient to eliminate the presence of a calculus as it may have taken place back of that obstacle and give rise to a *pseudo coprostasis*. It may also be borne in mind that a *pseudo-relaxation* may occur of the matter accumulated back of the calculus. All evacuations occurring after a few days of retention must be followed by lasting improvement to prove coprostasis.

A summary of the elements of the differential diagnosis may be considered as follows:

In *calculus*, the horse lies down, either exclusively or by preference and for a long time, upon his side, even on the side where the calculus is situated. On the side he prefers, the animal seems to have less pain while when lying upon the other he seems to suffer greatly.

In *coprostasis* the horse lies *indifferently and alternately on either side*. At the beginning of the evolution of the calculus there is generally a marked period of great agitation which does not occur in coprostasis.

The signs offered by *auscultation* differ also. If a calculus is situated in the zone that can be auscultated, one detects a great hyperactivity in the intestines. There are murmurs, borborygmus and various sounds in one part of the zone and not existing in the other, an obstacle existing between them and forming a barrage. Besides these signs the practitioner may also perceive strong and energetic contractions of the intestines which push forcibly the liquids collected in front of the obstacle.

In *coprostasis* on the contrary the intestines are quiet, contract softly and with less energy than in calculus, except in cases where there is a condition of enteroplegia or enteroparesis.

A very marked difference is sometimes observed in the intestinal activity on one side or the other of the abdomen. It is thus that under the influence of a calculus, the left side more often presents a spasm or paresis, while on the right there is hyperactivity. The *intestinal hemiparesis* in cases of obstruction is more marked in calculus.

In *calculus* there is at times mydriasis, at others myosis, but a state of contraction or dilatation is very marked.

In *coprostasis* the pupil is paranormal for a long period which precedes the stercoremia, which is accompanied with mydriasis.

In *calculus* the conjunctiva is generally redder than yellow. It is the contrary in coprostasis.

One of the best elements of differentiation is that furnished by the relation between the pulse and temperature.

In *calculus* there is dissociation between them.

In *coprostasis* they are both in perfect accord.

Finally as Dr. Rogers says: do not neglect the influence of the work to which the animal has been submitted, his age, his hygienic condition and living. Calculus may be recognized without exclusion of the possibility of egagropile.

ON GLANDERS.—The value of the oculo-reaction in the diagnosis of glanders has been the subject of many writings, its advantages and its objections have been extensively discussed and yet it is interesting to add an opinion of any authoritative value. The record made in the *Revue Generale* of Panisset of the various contributions gathered from continental journals may be of some interest.

Among the contributions there is one from Veterinary Major Schneider, who, having studied the different methods of clinical and experimental diagnosis, states as follows the preference he has for the *conjunctivo-reaction*, a new name which is presented in place of the one accepted before, the *oculo-reaction*.

"The conjunctival test is an exceptional method, simple, quick, sure and without danger. Any practitioner can resort to it without special material or instrument. A glass rod, a brush or a syringe is sufficient. It demands little time and is very economical. With it occult or latent glanders can be detected as surely as with any other method.

It can be applied as well in isolated cases as in collective examinations, when horses are imported, as well as in civil or military gatherings, etc.

The presence of fever or any other diseases is no contraindication, an important fact in importation. It can be invalidated only in cases of purulent catarrh of the conjunctiva.

It will reveal prematurely a recent infection of glanders.

In cases of doubtful reaction, the examination of the blood can be immediately resorted to, without being obliged to wait perhaps three months as with the subcutaneous injection method.

The reaction is clearly specific when compared with other methods of malleination and as to the hematologic examination; its record for error is the smallest of all.

The conjunctivo-reaction has been used for several years and is said to be considered in Central Europe as the best method of malleination and also the surest and simplest of the auxiliary means of diagnosis of glanders.

There are, of course, errors referred to this method as well as others, even if at a minimum. A Doctor Schnurer gives the subject his consideration and states how and when the errors may be attributed in the two peculiar conditions of (1) a positive reaction with healthy horses and (2) a negative one in diseased cases.

In the former, the following may be considered:

(1) *Premature appreciation.* Immediately after the deposit of mallein upon the conjunctiva, there takes place a specific inflammation of the mucosa, followed quite often, after 6 to 8 hours, with a secretion which simulates the positive reaction.

(2) *Traumatic conjunctivitis* caused by the presence of sand, dust, lime or rubbing against the walls of the stable due to the itching following the application of the mallein.

(3) *Inflammatory condition* already existing as in periodic ophthalmia, strangles, etc.

(4) *Insufficient careful post mortem* which fails in bringing to evidence lesions often very small and difficult to discover.

For the latter, that of the negative reaction in glandered animals, there are:

(1) *Insufficient* contact of the mallein. The mucous membrane of the conjunctival sac of the lower eye lid must have been touched by the mallein and the application must be strong.

(2) *Erroneous appreciation* of the nature of the lesions discovered, principally in the skin and walls of the nasal cavities.

(3) *Removal* of the purulent conjunctival secretion by the horse's rubbing or external agency.

(4) *Test applied* during the period of incubation; the reaction not being generally obtained until two or three weeks after the infection.

(5) *Presence of very advanced lesions.* If all the above conditions are eliminated the proportion of errors becomes insignificant.

CONTAGIOUS VESICULAR STOMATITIS.—Director Vallée of Alfort has lately presented at the Societe Centrale a statement from Veterinary Major Jolly upon a small epizootic which he has observed in the army.

In his remarks the Director stated that this was a new contribution to the study of an affection which appeared to be unknown in France before the war, but has been described as observed in Germany and Italy and has received an excellent description in the work of Hutyra and Marek.

The origin of the cases, observed in France, was without doubt from North America brought by the importation of horses. According to the information published by the Bureau of Animal Industry of Washington, it was shown that the disease existed extensively in 1915 in the stations where the French and English governments had gathered thousands of animals for exportation.

The contagiousness of the disease is not to be discussed and the observations from American sources have proved the easy transmissibility of the infection to bovines. In these, the manifestations are such that they might be considered as of foot and mouth disease. A marked differential fact is the non existence of digital and mammary localization, so regularly noticed in aphthous fever, and again the resisting power of swine and sheep to the infection.

The communication of Major Jolly was then ordered for publication. It gave a long description of the history of the outbreak, of various manifestations that were observed, of the progress and duration of the disease and of the treatment, which was followed by rapid recovery and consisted in repeated washing of the mouth with boric and bicarbonate solutions and with glycerinated collutories of chlorate of potassium and honey.

Experiments made by Jolly on inoculation and contagiousness gave him only doubtful results.

The report ends with the consideration of three principal and exceptional points noticed in this outbreak:

(1) The pyretic value of the toxins as well as their toxicity was practically nil. The elevation in the temperature was very slight, the severe cases were very few and there was no mortality.

(2) It was noticed that the appetite remained good, although in half and often two-thirds of the cases the mucous membrane of the tongue had disappeared.

(3) The very great rapidity of the reparative process on the tongue was also very important. In some cases it took place with truly astonishing rapidity. There were, however, exceptions and in some horses five or six weeks were necessary to complete the cicatrization. In other cases the proliferation of the cicatrical cells, instead of proceeding regularly from the periphery to the center of the wound, took place by spots of epithelial neoformations at the center of the wound.

———◆———

FILARIASIS OF THE WITHERS IN HORSES.—Professor Law in his excellent work on Veterinary Medicine gives brief mention of the *Filaria reticulata* of the ligamentum nuchae and Professor Wallis Hoare in his work speaks of *Filaria cervicalis* and consequently Captain John Robson, M.R.C.V.S. of the A.V.C. in France states that he cannot claim any originality in the discovery of the parasite. He has nevertheless published in the *Veterinary Record* of Feb. 23rd a very interesting and complete article, probably the first thorough record of the definitive pathological conditions produced by the filaria which he has frequently discovered in the numerous cases he has had occasion to treat in his practice in Western Australia.

The article of Mr. Robson begins with a few preliminary remarks relating to the history of the cases he had observed, then he enters into the etiology of the disease and comes to his discovery, how he observed the parasite and gives the description of it. The symptomatology is then given in full.

"Horses may contract filariasis of the withers at any age, old animals appear to be just as susceptible as the young. Generally the first noticeable sign of its presence is a slight swelling of one or both sides of the scapula and about three inches beneath the mane. The swelling is not painful on palpation, although the animal is somewhat stiff and guarded in his head movements and avoids lowering the neck too much. This swelling may remain stationary but as a rule increases to a moderate extent during the following few weeks, gradually involving the region in front of and over the withers in a more or less uniform enlargement, which persists for months sometimes.

In favorable cases this gradually begins to subside and a natural depression results. Atrophy and wastage of the tissues involved is a marked feature of this stage; its extent depending on the severity of the infestation. Very commonly a quite noticeable depression on the median line, and capable of holding two or three tablespoonfuls of water, is left between the antero superior angles of the scapula.

After a time the most severe cases show a more or less pronounced pointing at some part, usually about the front or top of the withers and a sinus results which may remain discharging a small amount at intervals, often for some months, and then eventually heals up.

A few of the worst cases develop rapidly from the beginning, burst, discharge and become practically fistulous.

Quite a number of horses infested with the filarial parasite recover naturally. It undergoes calcareous encystation. But in some subjects the condition may become aggravated and a real fistula remains."

The treatment is the conclusion of the article of Mr. Robson. It can be summarized in free incisions, long ones in the median line or close along the sides of the mane, on one or both sides. All diseased tissue, fibrous, osseous or ligamentous must be removed. Calcareous deposits must be scraped off. Full drainage must also be resorted to. Hemorrhage is abundant and is controlled by packing, which is removed 24 hours after the surgical interference. It was proved by experiments that it was better not to protect the wound by outside dressing, but once the granulations were started to resort only to free exposure to the air with the use of astringents.

BIBLIOGRAPHY—MALADIES DU PORC (DISEASES OF SWINE)—by Doctor G. Moussu, Professor at the Veterinary School of Alfort, published by Asselin and Houzeau of Paris.

In my last chronicle I announced this work; it is now my pleasure to present it to our readers, as a very interesting and well prepared book likely to be of essential use to breeders and veterinarians.

In this important treatise we are first introduced to the buildings for pigs, kennels with drawings and a presentation of the arrangements necessary to the comfort of the animals. All the dispositions necessary for the feeding of the occupants are also well considered.

A special chapter follows this introduction on the choice and care of sows used for reproduction. The various conditions and care pertaining to gestation, accouchement, feeding in the early life of young, and the weaning, all of which will prove most interesting reading to breeders.

Surgery forms the basis of the next chapter. Castration of the adults and younger subjects, and cryptorchidism are treated and accompanied with several plates. The accidents pertaining to castration are also fully considered.

The balance of the work is of great importance, viz: the pathology, divided as it is in chapters most instructive and valuable and bringing before the readers all that pertains to the subject.

First comes the diseases of the digestive apparatus which are manifested clinically by symptoms quite easily recognized. Constipation and diarrhea are followed by the ailments of the mouth, namely, the various forms of stomatitis, scorbutus. Then the diseases of the stomach, intestines and liver, with indigestion, jaundice, gastro-enteritis, infectious hepatitis, various forms of intoxication, as carbonate of sodium, chloride of sodium, germinated potatoes, and phosphorus.

The diseases due to parasites form the next important chapter: echinococcosis, distomatosis, intestinal helminthiasis. Then anal imperforation, prolapsus recti, ascites and mesenteric pneumatosis demand the attention of the reader.

The diseases of the respiratory apparatus are considered:

acute contagious coryza, various forms of throat troubles, the anginas, pulmonary congestions, bronchitis, pneumonia and its varieties of enzootic and specific forms.

In the consideration of the diseases of the apparatus of locomotion, osseous cachexia and osteomalacia form a beautifully illustrated chapter with photographs and colored plates which are typical and deserve attention.

In the parasitic affections of the muscles, cysticercus and trichinae occupy most of the chapter.

The diseases of the nervous system are treated briefly: abscess of the encephalon, chorea and epilepsy.

The various forms of herniae, the many varieties of skin diseases, a description of the urinary and genital apparatus brings the work to its end with a consideration of infectious diseases.

The work of Doctor Moussu embraces almost the entire field of porcine pathology, at least in its practical application. The book represents a great progress and is a valuable addition to veterinary literature.

The publishers have kept the volume small in size. It is well gotten up with good illustrations, especially the colored ones, and if the contents have been gathered in the limited space of about 250 pages, it can be said that the quality has not been sacrificed for quantity and the motto *Multum in Parvo* is fully and widely realized.

Veterinarians and swine breeders will surely read the work of Professor Moussu.   A. L.

—Dr. S. E. Springer has removed from New Orleans, La., to Durango, Colo.

—Dr. T. S. Rich has been transferred from Detroit to Lansing, Mich.

—Dr. Peter A. Franzmann has removed from Chicago, Ill., and is in charge of federal meat inspection at Davenport, Iowa.

—Dr. Frank G. Miller is in charge of the meat inspection station at Lewiston, Idaho.

—Drs. Herbert K. Moore, Carlton R. Osborn and Carl H. Fauks have been added to the veterinarians employed in Oklahoma for the control of hog cholera.

ANIMAL PARASITES AFFECTING EQUINES*

C. P. FITCH

The subject of parasitology is receiving more and more attention in the curricula of the various veterinary colleges and by
practitioners. The profession is gradually coming to realize the
importance of animal parasites in the sanitary as well as the economic aspect of all our domestic animals. Infectious diseases
cause a tremendous total loss in the country, a great deal of which
could be prevented provided the proper preventive measures were
applied. The same statement applies in a large measure to parasitic
diseases which are usually less well understood by the profession
at large than are the common infectious diseases of bacterial origin.
At the present time considerable agitation is being made to dis-
seminate knowledge on this very important subject and this symposium is a very decided step in the right direction.

There is one phase of parasitology which should receive more
attention by writers of text books for veterinarians. This is the
nomenclature. Zoological terminology is constantly changing. The
law which governs these changes is that of priority. The first
name given to a parasite is the one to be finally adopted. Another
feature which changes the names is the fact that further study of a
group of parasites sometimes shows that instead of there being one
species there are a number of different ones and this of course
breaks the group up into several species each of which has its own
particular name. This can no better be illustrated than by the
Sclerostomes. When Müller in 1784 described this group of worms
he gave to them the name of *Strongylus equinum.* de Blainville
in 1828 renamed the group *Sclerostomum equinum.* It was not,
however, until the masterly study of Looss in 1900 that it was
shown that there were a very large number of different species included in this group and from this time on several scientists have
studied this group and verified his conclusions. Notable among
these are Albrecht and more recently Boulenger.

It is unfortunate that this condition in the terminology exists but it is a natural sequence and must be met in the best possible way. It is, however, very confusing to the student and to the

*Presented at the 54th Annual Meeting of the American Veterinary Medi-
cal Association, August 20-24, 1917, Kansas City, Mo.

practitioner as well to find several names relating to the same parasite. Teachers of parasitology and likewise of veterinary medicine should take great care to use the best accepted terminology and to point out the synonyms which may be used to designate the same species.

Furthermore, some of our best text books of veterinary medicine are translations from foreign languages and the parasites which are found in Europe may and often do vary considerably from those which are common here. This fact must be taken into consideration when using these books for beginners in the subject of medicine.

The parasites affecting the horse can be divided into two main groups, those affecting primarily the skin, the (1) external parasites and (2) internal parasites, those found within, as in the abdominal or thoracic cavity, affecting the various internal organs, etc.

EXTERNAL PARASITES. The flies, gnats, ticks, lice and mites are the more common parasites affecting the skin of the horse. In certain localities, especially in swampy places, mosquitoes become a pest to the equine family.

The flies can be conveniently divided into three main groups (1) biting flies, (2) bot flies, (3) those causing cutaneous myiasis. In the first group those belonging to the genus *Tabanus* are the largest and most voracious. The large black horse fly (*T. atratus*), which is often an inch in length, causes the animal severe irritation and if it attacks in large numbers the loss of blood due to the bites of these insects is considerable. The green headed horse fly, *T. lineola,* (often called the lined horse fly) is a somewhat smaller species but nevertheless very predacious and seems to be widely disseminated throughout the country. Of the other species of Tabanidae which are less widely scattered, *T. costalis, T. stygius, T. punctifer* and *T. striatus* which seems to be the common one found in the Philippines, should be mentioned. These insects cause not only great irritation due to their sucking the blood of the animal attacked but also they may transmit mechanically the causes of infectious diseases such as anthrax and also protozoa, for example, *Trypanosoma evansi,* the cause of surra. In this connection also should be mentioned *Glossina morsitans* or the tsetse fly which transmits *Trypanosoma brucei* or the cause of nagana. There are a number of species which are less common than the foregoing, the most frequent of which are *Haematopota pluvialis,* the rain breeze fly and *Chrysops calcutrens,* the blinding breeze fly.

The stable fly or *Stomoxys calcitrans* is probably the most widely scattered of the biting flies. This insect is slightly smaller than the common house fly and can be seen nearly always during the warm weather sucking blood from the horse preferably from the legs. This insect as well as the Tabanidae may transmit mechanically the causes of infectious diseases.

A fly somewhat closely related to the foregoing and often found on the horse is *Hematobia serrata* or the so-called horn fly. This insect is still smaller than the stomoxys and is found most commonly on cattle.

The bot flies are widely distributed in this country. It is commonly supposed that *Gastrophilus equi* is the most common species but in New York State it would seem from the examination of the larvae that *Gastrophilus nasalis* is quite as frequent. *Gastrophilus hemorrhoidalis,* the so-called "red tailed" bot fly, is not frequent here although it has been observed. The larvae of this insect attach themselves to the right as well as to the left sac of the stomach, to the mucosa of the duodenum and sometimes to that of the rectum. Here it causes a very injurious pruritus. *Gastrophilus pecorum* is said by Herms to be rare or absent in the United States.

It is usual to find the larvae of these insects on post mortem examination and they are generally considered not to cause any particular harm to the host. One cannot, however, observe the injuries caused by these parasites to the mucosa of the stomach and intestines, especially when they occur in rather large numbers without considering what significance such extensive loss of the secretive and absorbtive mucosa must play in the digestive process. It is quite likely that certain of the colics that are obscure in origin can be traced to the destruction of the mucosa by these parasites. Death also may result from their presence. Two cases among others may be cited in this connection. In one the horse died from rupture of the stomach due to the occlusion of the pylorus by the larvae of the Gastrophilus. The other animal died of toxemia due to icterus. The larva of one of these parasites had attached itself at the opening of the hepatic duct into the duodenum and prevented the outflow of bile. The Seyderhelms also claim that the larvae of these parasites are the cause of swamp fever or infectious anemia. This, however, due to the researches in this country and abroad, does not seem probable.

In the treatment of this group of parasites many agents have been used. Among the most efficient seem to be turpentine in rather large doses followed by an aloes ball and carbon bisulphide administered in capsules.

Equines are not attacked so extensively by the "flesh flies" as are some other species of domestic animals notably sheep and cattle. Horses and mules are occasionally infested by the larva of these insects which get into wounds causing the most severe irritation. Among the insects which should be mentioned in this connection are *Chrysomyia macellaria* or the screw worm fly particularly common in the south and central west, *Calliphora vomitoria*, the blow fly, *Lucilia caesar*, the blue bottle fly, *Sarcophaga carnaria*, the flesh fly, and sometimes the ordinary house fly or *Musca domestica*. The larva of any of the above may be occasionally found in wounds. Careful cleansing of the wound with a disinfectant will not always remove these larvae and picking them out with forceps has often been resorted to.

The gnats are especially troublesome in certain parts of the United States and by attacking the animal in swarms often lead to death. Their bites are especially painful, especially when the relatively small size (1-4 mm.) of the insect is taken into consideration. The economic losses are great as given by Washburn, the State of Tennessee lost $500,000 worth of stock in a single year. The more important species of this insect are *Simulium pecuarium* or the buffalo gnat, and *Simulium venustum* or the common black fly. Williston states that there are seventy-five described species of this group of parasites. Fly repellants such as oil of citronella, smudges, etc., serve to keep these insects away to some extent.

There are but few ticks which are of any particular importance among the parasites which attack equines. None of these as yet have been proven to transmit an infectious disease to the host as does the Texas fever tick to cattle. In the northeastern United States ticks are relatively uncommon on equines and are practically ignored. In the southern and western parts, however, these parasites are quite common. The species which should be noted are: *Ornithodorus megnini*, the spinose ear tick often found in the ears of horses and mules; *Dermacentor electus*, the so-called "dog tick", although commonly found on the dog occasionally gets on equines and causes considerable irritation; *Ixodes ricinus,* the castor bean tick, also occasionally is found on horses. There are a number of other species of ticks which in certain localities are found on equines but these parasites are not widely disseminated.

Phthiriasis or "lousiness" is a relatively common affection, especially among those animals which are not kept under the proper sanitary conditions. There are two kinds or classes of lice which attack the horse. The sucking louse, which is the larger, has a long pointed head and belongs to the genus Hematopinus. This parasite, by means of its rostrum, pierces the skin of its host and sucks the blood. The other class belongs to the genus called the Trichodectes. They are the biting lice usually smaller than the above and live on scales and debris of the skin. These lice have a round, broad head and can readily be told from the sucking lice.

There is but a single species of sucking lice which attacks equines, *Hematopinus macrocephalus (asini).* There are two species of the biting lice, *Trichodectes pilosus* and *Trichodectes equi (parumpilosus).* The name of this latter species is *equi* and not *parumpilosus* as given by Hall, according to the very extensive researches of Harrisen.

Under ordinary conditions there is very little difficulty in diagnosing a case of lousiness in the horse. The animal usually shows itching and on parting the hair the parasites are readily found.

The treatment advised varies widely according to the individual veterinarian. Clipping the animal should be the first procedure. The insecticides, either in the form of dusting powder or dips or even ointments may be applied. Among the common dusting powders, those containing pyrethrum, sulphur, naphthalin and a variety of other products are the ones usually employed. Of the dips used those prepared from the coal tar products are in the most common use. Recently Hall has tried experiments showing that sodium fluoride is a very efficient dusting powder to destroy the biting lice but is of no value in destroying the sucking lice.

The more important diseases of parasitic origin in equines are due to infestation by one or another form of mite producing what is commonly called *mange.* This disease is widely disseminated in this country and probably exists more or less in all localities. The present world war has called particular attention to mange because it spreads so rapidly among a group of horses and on account of the difficulty of affecting a cure. During the past year many articles have appeared in the English and French veterinary journals on this disease.

The common form of mange in horses is the Sarcoptic. The mite causing the disease is technically known as *Sarcoptes scabiei* var. *equi*. It is quite small, about 225 μ long by 170 μ broad, and lives in burrows in the skin. There are two forms of mange. The sarcoptic and psoroptic (the common form in sheep), it is much more difficult to effect a cure in the former because the mite dwells so far beneath the outer layers of the skin. The different parasiticides do not penetrate to the place where the parasite is found. The symptoms produced by this mite are an intense itching followed by the loss of hair and scales in the infested areas. The part to be first attacked seems to be the withers. From here it may spread over the whole body. The hairs on the affected part at first stand erect and bristly. Due to constant rubbing and biting, open sores and vesicles may be found.

It is not always easy to distinguish symptomatically between sarcoptic mange and different forms of eczema. The only positive method is to make scrapings from the affected areas and examine them microscopically for the presence of the mange mite or the ova. Several precautions should be taken when making an examination for mange. First select a locality that has shown recent infestation from which to get the material. Second *scrape deep*. The mites live far below the surface in burrows. Third, if possible, make the examination before treatment is begun. The scrapings should be placed in a test tube or other convenient glass container and 10% caustic potash added. This dissolves the scales and debris. Several drops of this material are placed on a glass slide and a cover glass placed over them. The specimen is then examined under the low power (16 mm.) objective of the microscope and care should be taken not to ignore the eggs which are often found in abundance. A quick method is to boil the scrapings and caustic for a minute, then centrifuge and examine the sediment. We have used this method at the college for many years with good results. It has recently been described by Sheather.

All kinds of treatment have been suggested and used for mange. Recently, during the concentration of equines on account of war and the resulting frequency of mange, many new and novel

methods have been suggested. Among these should be mentioned
the "air cure" of Berton, a French veterinarian in the army.
This treatment simply consists of turning affected animals out to
pasture and leaving them there day and night, at the same time
providing plenty of good water, grain and hay. These are absolutely
necessary to get the animal in good condition when the doctor
says the mange disappears. This takes from two to three months
and has proved effectual in a large number of cases. Tutt, an
English veterinarian, recommends the following: Clip **when**
necessary, including the *tail*. Singe also if possible. Wash the
animal with a solution of liq. cresol, comp. 1-40 in water. Wash
out all soap and dry thoroughly. The following day apply the
following:

> Sulphuris .... ℥ iv
> Ol. picis .... ℥ i
> Ol. cetacei......................... O i

This should be well brushed in but too much friction must be
avoided. If well applied the dressing need not be disturbed until
the sixth day when it should be washed off. One dressing often
effects a cure and the most severe cases are cured by three applications. Champetier recommends the following to be applied to
an animal affected with mange:

> Pentasulphide of potassium......   40 gms.
> Nicotine ....   1 gm.
> Sodium arsenate ....   2 gms.
> Water ....1000 gms.

The ingredients must be thoroughly powdered before attempting to
dissolve them.

Other agents commonly used are common sulphur ointment,
sulphur dip, formalin 10%, creosote and Vienna tar liniment—

> ℞   Picis liquidae
> Sulphuris sublimate..............aa ℥ iii
> Sapo mollis
> Alcoholis ....aa ℥ vi
> **M**

In order to prevent the occurrence of this disease Tutt recommends
the following, applying particularly to the army:

"(1) Attend to the grooming; (2) frequent inspection of *all*
animals; (3) isolation of newly joined remounts for 21 days; (4)
all cases of 'skin irritation' to be isolated until cured. This may

be due to: (a) neglected grooming; (b) lice; (c) mites from other sources, e. g., bedding, forage, buildings occupied by fowls. (5) Disinfection of all standings *before* putting animals into them. This is to be carried out as often as possible.''

The principle to be observed in the treatment of mange is first to soften the scabs and scales by washing and then apply a parasiticide in such a manner that it will penetrate to the mites.

The other forms of mange sometimes found on equines are the so-called Symbiotic or leg mange and the Psoroptic mange. The parasites causing these affections are known technically as *Chorioptes bovis* var. *equi* (Symbiotes) and *Psoroptes communis* var. *equi*. They are much less common than the sarcoptic variety. The chorioptic mite attacks the region of the pastern, the hollow of the heel and the fetlock. The psoroptic mite usually is found on the rump, poll, back or where there is the thickest hair. Law states that this is by far the most common form of mange. In our experience in this locality it is much less common than the sarcoptic.

The treatment of these forms of mange does not differ materially from that given for the sarcoptic. It is much easier usually to effect a cure as neither of these latter mites bore into the skin but live on the scales.

INTERNAL PARASITES. The important parasites which are found within the body of the horse belong to the phyla of *Nemathelminthes* or the round worms. There are a few flat worms which are occasionally found in equines and these, of course, belong to the *Platyhelminthes*.

A worm which may be found in the epithelium of the oesophagus of the horse is known as *Gongylonema scutatum*. It can be noted as a zigzag yellowish line from 1-2 inches in length, especially in the thoracic portion of this organ. Ransom and Hall showed that the intermediate hosts of this parasite were dung beetles of various species. They worked, however, with the varieties of this parasite found in cattle and sheep.

The two true stomach worms of the horse are *Habronema* (*Spiroptera*) *microstoma* and *Habronema* (*Spiroptera*) *megastoma*. The *microstoma* is the largest of the two, a cylindrical whitish worm from $\frac{1}{2}$ to $1\frac{1}{2}$ inches in length, is usually found free in the stomach but also may be attached to the mucosa. The *megastoma* is a smaller, grayish white worm from $\frac{1}{4}$ to $\frac{1}{2}$ inch in length. This parasite burrows beneath the mucosa of the stomach and forms small bunches or, as they are commonly called, "tumors". These vary in size from ¼ to 2 inches in diameter. In the center of these growths galleries are noted which contain a cheesy, necrotic material and the worms are usually one to five in number. The galleries communicate with the inside of the stomach by means of very small openings through which the worms can . sometimes be squeezed. The growths caused by these parasites may, if situated near the pylorus, hinder the outward passage of food. If they are very numerous they also undoubtedly interfere with the digestive process. They are generally considered, however, of little pathogenic importance.

Ascaris megalocephala, the large round worm affecting equines, is often referred to as the "common stomach worm". The normal habitat of this parasite is the intestine but by migration it is often found in the stomach. This is by far the largest parasite found in the digestive tract of equines. It is cylindrical in form, tapers at both ends and ranges in size from 3 to 4 inches in length up to 18 to 20 inches. The head of this worm is furnished with three lips which in the larger forms can be made out with the unaided eye. The ova are spherical, measuring from 90-100 μ. They pass out with the feces and develop in water or moist earth. They are extremely resistant to heat or cold and will live for a year or even longer in the ground. This parasite does not seem to have an intermediate host but infestation takes place directly through the digestive tract by consuming food contaminated by the ova. An examination of the feces should show the ova if the animal is infested. Young animals which are unthrifty when kept under fair conditions are very apt to be infested by this parasite and a simple feces examination will make the diagnosis clear.

The symptoms shown by an animal harboring these worms are varied. In most cases of a mild infestation no symptoms are noted. If large numbers of the worms are located in the intestinal tract the animal will show various symptoms of digestive disturbance as colic and diarrhea. The animal is unthrifty in appearance, anemic, pot bellied, rough coat, etc. Thum specifies the colics caused by this parasite as follows:

"(1) Illeus verminosus; (2) enterospasmus; (3) invagination; (4) enteritis verminosa; (5) perforation of the intestine.

"Thum records his observation on two fatal cases of illeus verminosus (obturation colic) due to ascarides. Anterior to the obturation there was an enormous dilation of the bowel, with constriction posterior, and gangrene at the point of obstruction. Young animals are more subject to this disturbance.

"Enterospasmus was observed in a two-year-old foal attacked with severe colic characterized by marked tympany and constipation, wihout visible cause. Death from peritonitis followed in five days. ·On autopsy a long constricted portion contained numerous ascarides. It is reasonable to assume that a normal peristalsis would have carried the worms beyond the constricted part, and that the spasms hindered peristalsis. Diagnosis here, as in human medicine, can be made positive during life only through laparotomy.

"Intestinal invagination occurs when a piece of intestine is in a state of spastic contraction and is telescoped by the part immediately behind.

"Verminous enteritis originates from the areas to which the worms are attached. Defects in the mucosa are surrounded by an inflammatory zone that may lead to the formation of ulcers and finally necrosis with perforation. They may also perforate a bowel that is ulcerated from some other cause."

In all cases which show these symptoms we wish to impress the importance of making a feces examination to determine whether intestinal parasites are the cause of the disturbance. Oftentimes animals which are infested pass these worms and they are so large they are easily noted.

Treatment for this parasite is much more efficient than for some others, to be described later. Many vermifuges are used. Among the more common are tartar emetic, sometimes employed as follows:

    ℞   Antimonii et potassii tartratis........iv ℨ
        Sig. Dissolve in a pail of water.

Give 1/3 at 6:00 a. m., at 7:00 a. m. and at 8:00 a. m. before feeding. Turpentine in linseed oil is a common and efficient drug to expel these worms. Areca nut, iron sulphate and arsenious acid are also often employed. Care must be taken to avoid reinfection. Clean water and clean food must be provided. The stalls and mangers should be cleaned and disinfected, and the animal, provided it has the habit, should be prevented from eating its bedding.

Pin worms are among the most common parasites found in the intestinal tract of equines. These parasites are known techni-

cally as *Oxyurus curvula* and *Oxyurus mastigodes*. The former
is the smaller of the two, the latter being commonly called the
"long tailed" oxyurus. It is quite probable that further study
will show these worms belong to the same species. They vary in
length from ¾ to 2 inches. The female is thick at the anterior end
and gradually comes to a fine point posteriorly. The worms are
grayish white in color. The posterior part is made up almost entirely of ova. The ova are oval, asymmetrical, having at one end a cup-
like projection known as an operculum. They are present in large
numbers in the feces of animals infested by these parasites.

The normal habitat of these worms is the cecum, colon and rectum. An animal, if infested, usually passes large numbers of the
worms and they can be recognized during the act of defecation.
Sometimes they fail to pass out of the anus and are crushed in the
sphincter ani. The whitish material thereby liberated from the
worm collect in crusts about the anus and is often observed particularly in old horses. If one makes a microscopical examination of these crusts they are found to be composed almost entirely
of ova.

The symptomatology produced by this parasite does not differ
markedly from that described under the ascaris. Certain features
are rather distinctive, however. The pruritus ani is usually more
intense, the presence of the grayish crusts around the anus and the
presence of the worm in the feces, especially during the act of defecation, are usually distinctive. These points are as a rule sufficient upon which to base a diagnosis. In case of doubt a feces
examination will usually give positive results.

In the treatment of this parasite the same agents are used
as for the ascaris. It should be remembered, however, that vermicides given per orem have to pass through nearly the entire intestinal tract before coming in contact with the parasite. In this way
they become much diluted and are thereby less efficacious. High
enemata of weak disinfectants, such as 1% creolin combined with
the oral administration of vermifuges, is the most efficient treatment. This must be continued over a considerable period if all of
the parasites are to be removed. A mild infestation with these
worms seems to cause no particular harm and in our experience
it is exceedingly difficult to completely rid an animal of the parasite. Whether this is due to the lack of efficiency of the vermicides
or to reinfestation is usually difficult to state. We have found.

however, that an agent which will keep down the numbers of these worms and yet probably will not completely rid the animal of them and also an agent that can be administered continually is better in the end than some of the more vigorous drugs. An old remedy which we have found very efficient is to keep before the animal continually a mixture of equal parts of common salt and wood ashes. We do not claim that this will destroy all the parasites but after a thorough cleaning out by the use of the drugs given above, then keeping the above mixture before the animal, seems to prevent a heavy infestation returning.

The most important group of intestinal parasites affecting equines both from the standpoint of economic importance as well as frequency are those belonging to the so-called Sclerostomes. The disease caused by these parasites has been known in this country for the past century. It is widely distributed not only here but in Europe and other foreign countries.

The species of this parasite was first described by Müller and named by him *Strongylus equinus*. This was in the latter part of the 18th century. Goeze, a few years later, describes what he considers the same parasite and calls it the "palisade worm". Rudolphi in 1803 gave a more detailed description of the parasite and called it *Strongylus armatus*. In 1828 de Blainville studied this group and called it the *Sclerostomum equinum*. Up to this time no divisions had been made, all the worms being included in one species. Mehlis in 1831 recognized that the small forms were not the same as the larger ones and he established a new species which he called *Strongylus tetracanthus*. Poeppel in 1897 called the larger form *Strongylus neglectus*. It, however, remained for Looss in 1900-01, working in Egypt, to carefully study this group and place it upon a clear scientific basis. Following his work we find that of Albrecht and more recently Boulenger.

The terminology and classification of this group of parasites to be here given follows the work of Looss. We wish to point out, however, that little if any careful systematic work has been done in this country on this exceedingly important group of worms. At least if such work has been done we have as yet been unable to find a published account of the same. It is quite possible that when this group of parasites is carefully studied here we shall find that the species present differ in certain respects from those found abroad. There seems to be no more fertile field open to investigators of parasitology than this group of worms.

Sclerostomum equinum, Müller, is the largest member of this genus. It ranges in length from ¾ to 2¼ inches. The color is usually reddish brown and the body is straight and rigid. Mouth is obicular, widely open and has two concentric rings, the outer of which has six papillae and the inner chitinous denticles. From the inside of the mouth capsule there arise four, or more correctly three, teeth. One of these, arising from the walls of the dorsal gutter is divided into distinct points. The other two arise from the oesophagus. The ova are 90 μ by 50 μ, oval in shape and when seen often contain an embryo or at least are segmented. The normal habitat of the mature parasite is the cecum and large colon of equines. It is often found attached to the mucous membrane of these organs. The immature forms (larvae) of this parasite have been found in the walls of the blood vessels, frequently in the pancreas, liver and lungs.

Sclerostomum edentatum, Looss, is smaller than the foregoing. It varies in length from ¾ to 1½ inches. Head is globular and divided off from the rest of the body. The mouth capsule is cup-shaped and is devoid of teeth. It is usually a dark gray or brownish in color. The habitat of the adult form is the colon and cecum. The immature forms are found in various places, in the peritoneum, pleura, free in the peritoneal cavity, in the ligaments of the liver and in the muscles of the fore arm (Railliet and Henry). They have not been found in the blood vessels.

Sclerostomum vulgare, Looss, is the smallest of the three. It is found from ½ to 1 inch in length. Head is not set off from the remainder of the body. Buccal capsule provided with two teeth. The adult forms occur in the cecum and colon and may be attached to the mucous membrane. According to Looss, Railliet and Henry, and others, this is the most common species found abroad. The immature forms cause the verminous aneurisms which are so commonly met with in branches of the mesenteric artery. They are also found in the mesenteric lymph glands, in the submucosa of the cecum and other places.

We desire here to point out the important fact that nodules due to the larvae of this group of parasites may be and often are mistaken for those due to glanders.

Cylichnostomum tetracanthum, Looss, is much smaller than the three preceding forms. It is from ¼ to ½ inch in length, whitish to gray in color. Mouth capsule is shallow and outwardly is provided with leaf crowns. It is found usually in the ceeum and never attached to the mucous membrane. In distinction to the three foregoing species this worm is not a blood sucker. The food of these parasites consists of a mealy substance probably debris, according to Looss, from the mucosa of the intestine due to the action of a secretion poured out by these worms. The worms are almost always found in rather close juxtaposition to the inside wall of the intestine and by pouring out a chemical substance which acts on the mucous membrane destroys the secretive and absorbtive action of this organ. The pathological action of this parasite seems to be entirely chemical.

Looss describes a number of other species of parasites under this same genus (Cylichnostomum). He also describes several other worms under the genera Tridontophorus and Gyalocephalus. These parasites were found in equines. There is very little doubt that when a careful study of this group is made in this country that it will be found that these species and also probably new ones are present here. We have identified in animals post mortemed at the college parasites belonging to the three genera of Sclerostomes here described and *Cyl. tetracanthum.* It is impossible in a paper of this kind to devote the space to these parasites which is merited by their importance. The description of these worms just given and of the disease caused by them which is to follow we realize is incomplete in many particulars. The following account of the manner of infestation, the development of the larvae, and the disease produced is largely taken from the account of Albrecht.

Albrecht found sclerostomes as intestinal parasites in nearly every horse examined and believes this represents the usual condition. Eggs were found in the feces of 42 army horses out of 44 examined: 18 of the 42 also carried eggs of *Ascaris megalocephala.* Post mortem examination of the digestive system usually revealed numerous specimens of *Scl. vulgare* and *Cyl. tetracanthum*, less frequently *edentatum* and *equinum*. These were most numerous at the junction of the cecum and colon.

Material for investigation consisted of eggs and larvae taken from mature females, and from the feces. Eggs of *Cyl. tetracanthum* are larger and narrower than those of the other three species, which cannot be differentiated. In feces they are always found singly, are elongated, have a thick wall, and are colored yellow by the bile pigment of the intestines.

: : Development of the egg depends on the amount of oxygen and
heat. At ordinary room temperature 2 to 3 days is required for
the development of the embryo and separation from its covering.
In a few days eggs are no longer found in the feces, one only
finds embryos, which are best termed larvae. The larvae are
curved, have a long thread-like tail and a conical anterior end.
The cuticle of the youngest larvae is very delicate, but soon increases in thickness. After a time the outer cuticle gradually
loosens until the larva is free in the old cuticle within which it
moves freely. This form may be termed the ripe larva. While
the larva in its earlier stages is non-resistant, especially to drying,
it now becomes highly resistant and survives in fecal balls that are
completely dry on the surface. In a 0.5 per cent formalin solution
they remain active after twenty-four hours.

Distinct variations in the different larvae are not present until after 2 to 3 weeks' growth, but in a warm temperature they may
develop in a few days. The larvae of the *tetracanthum* have a long
tail, the anterior end of the body is more pointed, and there is a
sharp demarcation between the body and the tail. The intestinal
canal is shorter than in *vulgare*. Larvae of *vulgare* are somewhat
thicker than *tetracanthum*, the anterior end less pointed, the posterior end gradually passes into the thread-shaped tail which is
shorter in proportion to the body. In *S. tetracanthum* the intestinal canal is enclosed in 8 to 9 cells, *Scl. vulgare* in 32 cells, mo-
saic in form and arranged in double rows.

After moulting the body retains its length, but the tail is
lost; it is now known as the rhabditis form (rod-shaped) and has
a short posterior end.

In Albrecht's investigations the larvae remained in their
sheaths for 8 to 9 months when kept in feces or water. When they
are placed in a moist oven at 35°C. for several days many are
separated from the sheath. According to Railliet this process of
moulting occurs in 15 to 20 days, but the observations of Albrecht
indicate that this first moulting process does not usually occur in
the outer world, but after entering the host. After moulting the
dried larvae possess great vitality and were observed to retain
life for five months in ordinary water without special nourishment.

Sclerostomes in fresh feces were confined to eggs in a state of
division; they were never found just before or immediately following the first moult. In the intestinal contents of slaughtered horses

larvae were found in only one case, but many sexually mature individuals were found, especially at the junction of the cecum and colon. The larvae may be found in fecal matter three days old, and in contaminated straw. When one places a fecal ball that is at least three days old in a glass dish, pours over it a physiological salt solution or pure filtered water so that the bottom is covered with a few mm. of liquid, the larvae soon wander to the water and with good light may be seen with the unaided eye. They have the appearance of small worms, move actively, and through the entanglement of their tails may form distinct balls.

It is probable that the larvae are taken through the digestive tract. Segmented or embryonic eggs ingested with food or water are not capable of further development. The process of wandering from fecal balls to water occurs in pastures, where under proper moisture conditions the larvae become attached to grass. Animals at pasture are more subject to infestation than when hitched in stables, though the habit of nibbling dirty straw in stables is a common method of ingestion.

As in all parasitic diseases the gravity and nature of the disease and the intensity of the symptoms are in direct proportion to the number of invaders. A few sclerostomes seem to cause no symptoms. *Scl. vulgare* and *Cyl. tetracanthum* are largely infestations of young horses. Larvae that cause aneurisms in the anterior mesenteric artery cause lesions that remain during life. In addition to causing embolisms, larvae that wander as individuals into the terminal vessels of the intestines give the first impetus to intestinal diseases (colic). Under ordinary development the ingested larvae, without intermediate carriers, develop directly through several moultings into sexually mature individuals in the intestines. In other cases larvae leave the intestines via the blood stream and are carried to the greatest variety of body organs where they should be regarded as strayed individuals. It is highly improbable that the development of the sexually mature *Scl. vulgare* depends on the passage of the larvae through the mesenteric arteries.

It is very important to find means to prevent the ingestion of larvae with the food and thus prevent the migration of the parasites to the intestinal arteries of the horse. Diagnosis is highly important in providing for prophylaxis, and it is very easy to determine the presence of sexually mature parasites in the intestinal canal through finding eggs in the feces. With a pincette remove from a fresh ball a piece about the size of a pea. Place it on a slide and separate it with a few drops of clean water. After bringing to a thin film examine with a 100 to 150 magnification. Short forms of eggs indicate the three large species, while long oval eggs characterize *Cyl. tetracanthum*. The following method of diagnosis may also be used: Place a ball of the suspected feces in a clean vessel and protect against drying, let it remain 8 to 14 days, pour over it clean water until it is completely saturated and a small amount of water remains in the bottom of the dish. After a few hours pour off the water and examine it for larvae. In warm weather the larvae are usually present in 5 to 8 days, or the process may be hastened by keeping the fecal ball in a warm moist place.

After larvae reach the arteries and tissues they are not accessible, so that their suppression in the intestines assumes great importance. All infested animals should be kept from pastures until free from parasites. Carefully remove all feces from the stables, and prevent fecal contamination of food and water, though water is not the most frequent carrier of the larvae. In all intestinal diseases of the horse more attention should be paid to an examination for parasites and eggs. As a vermifuge Albrecht considers turpentine with linseed oil more effective than tartar emetic, which has little or no effect on intestinal sclerostomes. Horses given maximum doses of tartar emetic may still carry eggs of sclerostomes in their feces. The administration of 80 c.c. of oil of turpentine in 500 c.c. linseed oil has been followed by the expulsion of numberless ascaridae and many sclerostomes. Since the color of the sclerostomes so closely resembles that of feces one must examine the latter very carefully for expelled individuals. Sclerostomes are best destroyed by burning since thousands of larvae may develop within a dead female.

Of the other parasites affecting equines probably *Filaria papillosa* (*equina*) is most often found. This is a long slender, round worm from 2 to 5 inches in length and white in color. It is found most commonly free in the abdominal cavity. It may also be found in the eye, in the scrotum and in any of the serous cavities. As a rule this parasite causes no trouble. In the eye and scrotum, however, it may lead to local inflammation. No effective treatment has ever been devised.

Verminous bronchitis in the horse is a rare disease in this country. It is caused by *Dictyocaulus arnfieldi*.

Bull has recently described a disease of horses in Australia characterized by granulomatous swellings around the urethral orifice of the glans penis or sheath. He finds the cause of this condition to be a larval nematode of the genus Habronema. A somewhat similar disease in this country commonly known as "Bursatti" has been described as being caused by a fungus.

Ransom describes a worm which is closely related to *Habronema microstoma*, which likewise occurs in the stomach of the horse. This parasite has its larval stage in the ordinary house fly. Ransom calls this parasite *Habronema muscae*.

Of the flat worms or Platyhelminthes which infest the horse three species of tape worms have been described. They are known as *Anoplocephala plicata*, *Anoplocephala perfoliata* and *Anoplocephala mamillina*. They are all unarmed parasites, having a large head and found usually in the small intestine. It is not known what animal contains their intermediate stage. The tape worms are very infrequent among equines and are of little pathologic significance.

Among the protozoa *Trypanosoma equiperdum*, the cause of dourine, is the most important in this country. It seems to be one of the trypanosomes which is transmitted by direct contact. It cannot be denied, however, the possibility of its also being transmitted by some insect. The Sarcosporidia which occur in the musculature, especially that of the heart, are not uncommon on post mortem examination of equines. Among the fungi those that cause ring worm or *Trichophyton tonsurans* and the Actinomyces are probably the most frequently found.

A few references not including the standard Text Books of Parasitology:

ALBRECHT, A. Zur Kenntniss der Sklerostomen beim Pferde. Zugleich ein Beitrag zur diagnose. Vorbenge und Bekämpfung. *Zeit. f. Veterinärkunde* (909), H. 4, s. 161.

BANKS, N. The Acarina or mites. *Report No. 108. U. S. Dept. of Agriculture.*

BERTON, M. La Gale et la cure d'air. *Rev. Gen. de Med. Vet.*, T. XXV (1916), p. 531.

BOULENGER, C. L. Sclerostome parasites of the horse in England. I. The genera *Triodentophorus* and *Oesophagoclontus*. *Parasitology* (1916), VIII. Sclerostome parasites of the horse in England. II. New species of the genus *Cylichnostomum*. *Parasitology* (1917), Vol. IX, p. 203.

BULL, L. B. A granulomatous affection of the horse. Habronemic granulomata (cutaneous Habronemiasis of Railliet). *Jour. Comp. Path. and Ther.*, Vol. XXIX (1916), p. 187.

CHAMPETIER. Le traitement de la gale. *Bul. de la Soc. Cent. de Med. Vet.* (1917), p. 68.

FAYET, M. Du Diagnostic de la Gale Sarcoptique Equine sur le Font. *Rev. Gen. de Med. Vet.*, T. XXV (1916), p. 539.

HALL, M. C. Notes in regard to horse lice, *Trichodectes* and *Haematopinus*. *Jour. Am. Vet. Med. Ass.*, Vol. IV (1917), p. 494.

HARRISEN, LAUNCELOT. The genera and species of mallophaga. *Parasitology*, Vol. IX (1916), p. 11.

LEVENVUE, M. G. Equides Strongylidosis. *Rev. Gen. de Med. Vet.*, T. XXIV (1915), p. 593.

LOOSS, A. The sclerostomidae of horses and donkeys in Egypt. *Rec. Egyptian Gov. School of Med.*, Cairo, Vol. I (1901), p. 27.

RAILLIET, A. ET HENRY, A. Sur les Sclerostomiens des Equides. *Compt. r. de la Soc. de Biologie*, (1902), p. 110.

RANSOM, B. H. The life history of Habronema muscae (Carter), a parasite of the horse transmitted by the house fly. *Bull. No. 163, B. A. I., U. S. Dept. of Agriculture.*

RANSOM, B. H. AND HALL, M. C. The life history of *Gongylonema scutatum* *Jour. of Parasitology*, Vol. II (1916), p. 80.

SHEATHER, A. L. An improved method for the detection of mange acari. *Jour. Comp. Path. and Ther.*, Vol. XXVIII (1915), p. 64.

THUM, H. Askaridiasis beim Pferde und Schweine. *Zeit. f. Tiermedizin.* Bd. XVIII (1914-15), s. 503.

TUTT, J. F. D. Some notes on skin disease of the horse. *Veterinary Record*, Vol. XXIX (1917), p. 461.

PARASITES OF SWINE*

W. L. HOLLISTER, Avon, Ill.

Parasitism of swine is with the average country practitioner one phase of swine disease that is shamefully neglected. Cholera is successfully combated with serum and virus, mixed infection of pulmonary and other types are gradually being eradicated through bacterial vaccine treatment, but wormy pigs are in most localities considered a matter of course, and the feeling that a hog is not a hog without worms is taken for granted.

With kerosene and gasoline gradually, maybe I had better say rapidly, taking the place of horses in the country as well as the cities, the hog becomes a more important factor as a means of furthering the veterinarian's income, and adding to his real worth in his community.

In presenting a paper on this subject it is the intention of the writer to confine himself to what he considers a practical discourse on the harmful parasites that come within the average practice of the country veterinarian.

---

*Presented at the 54th Annual Meeting of the American Veterinary Medical Association, August 20-24, 1917, Kansas City, Mo.

Many parasites infesting swine are rarely if ever found in America and for this reason will not be mentioned in this paper. To facilitate description we will divide them into three classes, as follows:

CLASS No. 1. Those parasites infesting the external or cutaneous surface of body..

CLASS No. 2. Those parasites infesting intestinal tract.

CLASS No. 3. Those parasites infesting the body tissues.

Phthiriasis, or lousiness, is the most common parasitic condition of swine. The hog louse, *Hematopinus suis*, is the largest of all lice infesting domestic animals, is a blood sucker and produces direct irritation and if in great numbers causes an unthriftiness due to extraction of blood from the animal and constant distress from its persistent attacks. In some localities swine are infested with fleas, "Siphonoptera", and are a constant menace to the well being of swine.

Lousiness is easily remedied, but only temporary unless constant vigilance is maintained as is also the case with fleas. Nearly all of the recognized dips on the market are effective, also crude oil as it is now possible to apply it by means of the patented rubbing posts by which a constant supply of oil is kept on hand for the hogs' use.

Personally, I have found a Naphthalene powder, dusted in the nests at cleaning time, the cheapest and most satisfactory method, as it kills those already on the hogs and as it is kept permanently in the nests and hog houses, it destroys the young lice as fast as hatched.

Mange exists in two forms, Demodectic and Sarcoptic. Demodectic mange is caused by the *Demodex folliculorum "suis"*, a microscopic parasite infesting the hair follicle. This type of mange usually spreads very slowly, and only a few animals in the herd are affected. The lesion produced is that of denuded areas, especially on the thin skin of the abdomen and legs with pustules in which the parasite exists, many of them in each pustule. Owing to the nature of this mange, treatment is difficult and very unsatisfactory. The most practical method to pursue is to sell infested animals and clean and disinfect the premises.

Sarcoptic mange, caused by Sarcoptic Scabei "Suis", a microscopic parasite which burrows into the skin usually around the ears and eyes or on the inner side of the forelegs and thighs. It forms a heavy scab which, when rubbed off, leaves denuded and thickened skin from the intense irritation. Unless affected animals are segregated from the others nearly all will become affected.

Sarcoptic mange may be quite successfully treated with the lime and sulphur dip, or nicotine treatment.

Under class No. 2. Those parasites infesting the intestinal tract are five in number, namely:

(1) *Ascaris suis.* (2) *Esophagostoma dentatum.* (3) *Trichocephalus crenatus.* (4) *Echinorhynchus.* (5) *Trichina spiralis.*

Ascaris suis is the parasite that gives us the feeling that a hog is not a hog unless wormy, for he is present in practically every hog. A long white or pinkish parasite pointed at either end, and is usually found in the small intestine, but in badly infested herds is found in the stomach and large intestines. It is not uncommon to find the lumen of the small intestine entirely obstructed by these parasites, also the hepatic duct. They cause an unthriftiness in the hog due to direct absorption of the nutrition.

The *Esophagostoma dentatum,* a small white or grayish white parasite infesting the submucosa of the large intestine, if in large enough numbers, cause diarrhea and emaciation.

The *Trichocephalus crenatus* is a whip-like blood sucking worm, found firmly attached to the mucous membrane of the intestine. They are not at all common in this country, but when present in large enough numbers cause diarrhea, indigestion, and general unthriftiness.

The *Echinorhynchus gigas* has been sometimes called the tape worm of the hog, owing to the transverse markings, giving it a segmented appearance. The ova pass to the ground in the feces and are ingested by the larvae of the May beetle. Hogs ingest the May beetle larvae, which, upon entering the digestive tract of the hog, passes to the mature stage and attach themselves to the intestinal wall by means of hooklets. Small nodules occur at the point of anchorage which, viewed from serous surface of the bowel, appear as a nodule resembling a tubercle and may be mistaken for tuberculosis.

The *Trichina spiralis* can only be partially discussed under the heading of Parasites Infesting the Intestinal Tract, and again considered under the heading of those parasites infesting the body tissues.

When the encysted larvae of the Trichina is eaten the larva is liberated and becomes a mature parasite in the intestinal tract of the hogs. The mature female deposits her ova and the same are hatched in the intestinal tract of the hog from whence these larvae migrate through the intestinal wall to the various tissues of the body where they become encysted larvae and remain as such.

The intestinal irritation by the mature parasite causes diarrhea and the migrating larvae may cause pruritis, stiffness of gait, painful respiration, but is rarely fatal in the hog. Treatment of these various intestinal parasitic conditions should always include preventive treatment which is sanitation. Good, clean and well disinfected premises are rarely if ever infested but such conditions do not always exist.

Probably more money has been spent by hog raisers for so-called worm eradicators and condition powders without any beneficial returns than upon any other diseased condition of his live stock. There are various drugs used in ridding pigs of worms, such as santonin, creosote, turpentine, areca nut, worm seed, and others.

A very good way to treat pigs under 100 lbs. is to diet pigs for 24 hours in a dry lot and then dose each pig separately with 2½ grs. each of santonin and calomel put up in capsule form using a canine balling gun to administer. Have attendant hold pig as if to vaccinate in axillary space; if badly infested repeat in 7 to 10 days. After the herd has been freed of worms have the lots well cleaned and refuse burned or buried and then as a preventive treatment, feed coal slack 4 parts and sodium chloride 2 parts in self feeders or boxes so that it will be kept constantly before them.

Class No. 3. Those parasites infesting the body tissues. Under this class we have the *Strongylus paradoxus, Trichina spiralis* —"larval form"—*Cysticercus cellulosae,* larval form of the *Tenia solium,* the *Distoma hepaticum, americanum* and *lanceatum, Sarcocystis miescheri,* all of which from certain view points are of interest; but as we are considering them, the *Strongylus paradoxus* and *Sarcocystis miescheri* are, with the exception of the larval form of Trichina, which has already been mentioned, may cause muscular soreness, the only ones of real interest.

The *Strongylus paradoxus* is a white or brownish white thread-like worm, one to one-half inches in length, and occasionally claimed to be of numbers sufficient to cause bronchial pneumonia.

Treatment is of very little avail, further than isolation of diseased hogs and disinfection of sleeping quarters.

The *Sarcocystis miescheri*, sometimes called the kidney worm, is very common in southern hogs, and while it is not considered a dangerous parasitic condition, it is claimed by some that it may cause a weakness of the back by destroying the muscle fibre. Treatment is of little avail.

Owing to the fact that the general practitioner has so little time for careful study of the life history of the various parasites infesting domestic animals, I feel that many here are much more capable of carrying the discussion of this paper to a profitable end, and I expect little of my paper other than a means of promoting discussion.

PARASITES OF SHEEP[*]

A. D. KNOWLES, Missoula, Montana

In order that the veterinary practioner may successfully treat and control parasitic infections of sheep he must have an intimate knowledge of the different parasites together with their life history and the modes of attacking their host, the sheep.

In order that he may have a satisfied client he must certainly differentiate in his diagnosis between the various parasitic infections in order that the most economical measures may be pursued and a prognosis may be given which will assist the owner to make calculations for the successful handling of his diseased flock.

The time allotted for this article is too brief to admit of giving the description and life history of every parasite to which the sheep is subject, therefore it will be my purpose to give the description and characteristics of the more important parasites together with the treatment and sanitary regulations in common use and a few case reports taken from my own practice.

The blood-sucking parasites, both external and internal, produce the greatest injury to their hosts, the greatest economical loss to the sheep owner and are as a rule the more difficult to control both by therapeutic treatment and sanitary regulations; it is not sufficient, therefore, that the attending veterinarian find ticks or

*Presented at the 54th Annual Meeting of the American Veterinary Medical Association, August 20-24, 1917, Kansas City, Mo.

lice on the sheep but he must exhaust every means of diagnosis to determine whether or not the animals are also affected with scab parasites.

It is not sufficient, when examining an unthrifty flock, to be satisfied with finding external parasites, but symptoms of internal parasites should be looked for and if the veterinarian cannot determine their absence positively by clinical symptoms he should demand an autopsy.

In the post mortem the veterinarian should not be satisfied with finding the tape worm in the intestines, the fluke in the liver or the bot in the frontal sinuses, but he should exhaust every means of diagnosis for the isolation of the more dangerous blood-sucking parasites of the stomach and intestines, and the lungs.

I have known veterinarians to have made mistakes in diagnosis in these very things which resulted in dissatisfaction between practitioners and their clients.

Ectozoa. The *Oestrus ovis* is not a true parasite yet it must be taken into account in considering the parasitic affections. The adult, slightly larger than the house fly, is very active during the summer months and causes excitement and restlessness of the sheep in its endeavors to propagate its species by depositing its larvae in the anterior nares. This annoyance to the sheep causes the flock to run and refuse to feed with a resultant loss of condition.

The larvae, having migrated to the frontal sinuses, appear to cause no symptoms of disease until several months after their attachment and only when they have reached such dimensions that their size causes irritation of the mucous membrane and is evinced by a mucous discharge from the nostrils, sneezing and coughing, and in extreme cases with loss of appetite, separation from the flock and remaining in the recumbent position. Treatment of this affection is only practicable in valuable sheep and in small flocks, and is not followed with satisfactory results as a rule. For protection against the adult fly the smearing of the sheep's face and nose daily with some substance objectionable to the fly, such as fish oil, oil of tar, or a preparation composed of sulphuric acid, drachms six—turpentine, ounces two—and cottonseed oil, pints two, is the best treatment that can be pursued.

For treatment of the larval disturbance, inhalations of sulphur fumes, steam inhalations of turpentine, or the coal tar disinfectants, or resorting to the operation of trephining the sinuses and extraction of the larvae with forceps, constitute the known methods.

The other varieties of ectozoa include the skin parasites and in them the symptoms of restlessness of the animals caused by skin irritation is similar but varies as to the degree of irritation and general injury to the animals.

The *Melophagus ovinus*, sheep tick, is not a true tick but may spend its life on the original host; it is a blood-sucker and also consumes the wool fat. This is the commonest ecto-parasite of the sheep; it causes more or less irritation to the skin and is believed by many veterinarians and sheep owners to be a greater menace to sheep raising than all other ectozoa. The young of this parasite is brought forth in the form of pupae in a flexible case which is cemented to the wool of the sheep and allows the young to escape after a month.

These parasites are easily destroyed by dipping the sheep in any of the commonly used dips and, therefore, the cheaper dips, such as those made from coal tar, are sufficient and it is not necessary to heat the water in order to destroy the ticks.

Sheds and corrals where infected sheep have been kept must be thoroughly disinfected and all litter burned.

It is advisable to dip sheep infected with this parasite immediately after shearing, especially where they are to be removed to summer pastures apart from the infected premises.

PHTHIRIASIS. Of the lice-infesting sheep there are two varieties—blood-sucking and biting, or wool-eating, lice.

While the wool-eating lice cause the host more or less uneasiness, their greatest damage is to the wool which becomes matted and frequently falls off leaving bare patches of skin.

The blood-sucking lice cause great uneasiness of the affected sheep which is indicated by scratching with the hind feet, rubbing against other animals and objects and by biting themselves and pulling out tufts of wool.

The diagnosis of phthiriasis in sheep is easy, but the practitioner should not be satisfied with finding ticks and lice on sheep but should exhaust every means of diagnosis to determine the absence of scab parasites.

Ticks and lice on sheep yield readily to the ordinary commercial sheep dips, but it is my opinion that where it is desired to eradicate these parasites completely from a flock they should be dipped a second time after the lapse of ten days. Some flockmasters in Montana are accustomed to dipping their sheep at shearing time and again the following October in order to avoid ''feeding the ticks''.

SARCOPTIDAE. Of the three varieties of scab parasites of the sheep the Psoroptes is the most common and most contagious; of the other two the Sarcoptes, which is confined principally to the head, and the Symbiotes, whose natural habitat is the feet and legs, are rarely met with in ovines and will not be given special consideration in this article.

The veterinary inspector, or practitioner, is frequently confronted with an owner and employees who will not only give no assistance in diagnosing scabies among a flock of sheep, but who have culled out every animal which gave any indication of infection and destroyed or secluded such animals from the inspection of the veterinarian.

It is, therefore, up to the official inspector to find the ''bug'' and demonstrate it to the anxious but unwilling flockmaster.

If the flock is confined in a corral or shed a little patience upon the part of the inspector and close observation of the flock will usually reveal some suspicious action—soiled spots on the wool from saliva where the animal has bitten itself may be the first symptom seen, or a sheep will be seen to bite at its side or some part of the body, or to rub against another animal or some stationary object with considerable energy. If watched for a time this animal will be seen to repeat the symptoms and when his attention, and that of the flock, has ceased to be engaged by the presence of strange persons or things, more attention will be given to the scab parasite and the real typical symptoms of scabies may be seen.

It may require much patient examination upon the part of the inspector to locate the parasite. It may crawl right out of the first scraping of skin and wool or it may require a hand lens to demonstrate it. But I have usually found that the owner was much impressed when the parasite was demonstrated on a glass slide under the microscope after soaking the scrapings in caustic potash solution.

When magnified by the use of the microscope the legs look so large and the head with its rostrum so prominent that the layman is usually surprised at the facilities which this parasite has for punishing its host, and becomes an advocate of treating the animals, and a willing assistant.

The only way to destroy all of the scab parasites on a sheep is to immerse the animal in a solution which contains some chemical that will destroy the life of the parasite. There are a number of such chemicals but it is important to use such solutions as will give the very best therapeutic results with the least damage to the sheep and its wool.

There are two formulae which seem to meet all of the requirements and are used extensively in America for treating sheep scab. They are lime and sulphur and tobacco and sulphur. The dip must be kept at a temperature of from 100 to 105 degrees F., and the sheep must remain in the solution for at least three minutes. The treatment must be repeated within from ten to fourteen days in order to destroy the parasites which hatch after the first dipping.

After the second dipping if the sheep can be driven immediately to fresh range and not allowed to come in contact with infected sheds, corrals or range, there is little danger of a recurrence of the scab among them but the flock should be kept under observation for not less than three months and not allowed to mingle with other sheep during that period.

The sheds, cars and corrals, where infected sheep have been, should be disinfected and any of the chemical disinfectants may be used in sufficient strength to kill the parasites; it must be used in solution and all woodwork and floors saturated with the disinfectant. All litter must be burned and infected range should not be used for several months. The time which may be required for the parasites to die without animal nourishment is indefinite and, so far as I know, has never been determined.

ENTOZOA. The endo-parasites of the sheep are the greatest economic menace to the sheep industry. The fact that their modes of attacking this animal are insidious is the principal reason why the diseases caused by these internal parasites gain such degrees of intensity before their discovery in a flock.

The predisposing conditions which favor parasitic affections are youth, old age, innutritious and damaged food, unsanitary sheds and corrals, too close confinement, low marshy pastures, contaminated drinking water and exposure to cars or yards where infected sheep have been kept.

Of the several internal parasites of the sheep each has its peculiar organ or tissue to live in and will not survive if confined to any other part of the body. Some are oviparous and their eggs must pass out of the body to favorable conditions of soil and moisture. Some are ovoviviparous and are enabled to propagate their species within the organ of their choice and the young mature without leaving it, while others must leave the body in one form or another, be taken into the body of another animal where they must spend a part of life before returning to the original host for further development.

With the exception of the *Oestrus ovis,* already referred to, the *Coenurus cerebralis* and the *Distomum hepaticum,* the internal parasites of sheep belong to either the round or flat worms.

As I understand it the liver fluke is not of much importance in America and will not be considered in this article.

The *Coenurus cerebralis,* the "gid" parasite of the sheep, has its natural habitat in the nerve centers, especially the brain. This parasite has caused considerable loss among the flocks of the northwest, especially in Montana, where the sheep are ranged in large bands and controlled by means of dogs, which harbor the *Taenia coenurus,* which is the parent of the *Coenurus cerebralis.*

The propagation of this parasite is carried out by the passing of the ripe segments of the tape worm of the dog, with the feces, to the ground where great numbers of ova in each mature segment are taken in with the food by the young sheep. The eggs are readily dissolved by the digestive juices liberating the embryos which attach themselves by means of hooklets to the walls of the alimentary tract, then pass into the blood vessels and are carried by the circulation to the nerve tissues which afford a favorable medium for the growth of the *Coenurus cerebralis.*

The injury to the host is caused by the growth of the embryo in a cyst and it is the pressure on the brain, caused by the increasing size of the cyst that causes the interference of sensation or locomotion of the sheep; and if several parasites happen to be affecting the animal at the same time death is certain to follow.

The symptoms exhibited by the sheep are those of aberration of the brain, such as turning in a circle, holding the head abnormally high or low, interference with locomotion or complete paralysis.

Diagnosis consists in finding the *Coenurus cerebralis* in the

·brain. Treatment is unsatisfactory and is confined to the operation of trephining the cranium and extracting the larvae from the
cranial cavity. Prophylaxis consists in the total destruction of
the heads of all dead sheep in order that the brains containing the
Coenurus cerebralis may not be eaten by dogs and also by treating the suspected dogs for tapeworms.

TAENIASIS. There are twelve varieties of tape worms known
to infect the intestines of sheep and the life history of them is not
known—it is known, however, that sheep grazing on certain swampy
pastures become infested with these worms.

The *Taenia fimbriata* is the most common type found in
America and in its relation to the sheep is not unlike the other
varieties.

Tape worms derive their nourishment from the absorption of
the food in the intestinal canal of the sheep; the worm attaches
itself to the mucous membrane of the small intestine and grows by
segments shedding the ripe segments impregnated with ova to
pass out with the feces. Some of these worms grow to a length of
fifteen feet and where a large number infest the same animal their
volume interferes with the passing of the food in the intestines, in
addition to the nourishment which their host is deprived of by
their presence.

The symptoms of tape worms in sheep are anemia, enlarged
abdomen, "pot belly", intermittent appetite, great thirst, trailing
behind the flock, diarrhea, great prostration and death.

The diagnosis is made by recovering the segments of the tape
worm in the feces or by autopsy and recovering the worm from the
intestinal canal.

NEMATODA. The order Nematoda includes the families Filar-
iadae and Strongylidae which are the most injurious parasites of
the sheep and probably cause greater economic losses than all the
other parasites of the sheep combined. These thread worms are
blood-suckers, multiply rapidly, have wonderful vitality outside
the body of the sheep, are insidious in their attacks and persistently undermine the health of the ovine. The sheep is subject to
infestation with two varieties of lung worms, the *Strongylus filaria*
and *S. rufescens;* the former a white thread-like worm from two
or three inches long, infests the bronchi of the sheep, is oviparous
and the eggs must pass out of the body and fall in favorable surroundings to hatch and bring forth the larvae. Damp earth is

favorable to the growth of this parasite but after the young is hatched if it happens to be in water containing decomposing vegetation it soon perishes. If, however, the water in which it falls is uncontaminated the worm thrives and moults within two weeks. Should it then dry up it may remain for several months a live germ which, when taken into the body of a sheep, will grow and propagate its kind.

The *Strongylus rufescens*, a thread-like worm somewhat smaller than the former, inhabits the bronchi and bronchioles of the sheep. It is oviparous and the eggs hatch in the bronchi; the young worms develop to maturity where they are hatched, frequently causing irritation of the lung tissue resulting in hepatization and abscess of the lung.

Symptoms—anemia, coughing in spasms, especially upon rising or exercising, muco-sanguinous discharge, asphyxiation.

Diagnosis: The Strongyli or their ova may be recovered in the nasal discharge and examined under the microscope or the worms may be located in the bronchi by post mortem.

Lesions produced: The trachea and bronchi contain more or less mucous which is frequently tinged with blood; the bronchioles are usually filled with mucous and often pus is found in some of them; there is usually hepatization of areas of lung tissue and abscesses of varying dimensions containing specimens of the worms.

Of the Strongyli infesting the alimentary tract of the sheep there are two varieties, *S. contortus* and *S. ostertagi*. They are both oviparous and their eggs pass out to the ground where they hatch in two or three days, under favorable conditions; the embryo moults twice and is then prepared to withstand several weeks of vicissitudes of the weather; it is found attached to blades of grass which favors its chances for being taken into the stomach of its host.

The *S. contortus* is about an inch long, thread-like in appearance, the male somewhat smaller than the female. It is found attached by hooklets to the mucous membrane of the abomasum and small intestines. In addition to injuring the sheep by sucking its blood, it produces a certain amount of inflammation of the mucous membranes which interferes, in certain measure, with digestion and assimilation of food.

The *S. ostertagi* is slightly smaller than the former, and are found in small nodules in the mucous membrane of the abomasum and small intestines.

. Symptoms: In an affected flock there will be seen some individual sheep lagging behind the bunch, the flock as a whole will
look unthrifty, sick ones will be seen to scour and constipate alternately, the wool is dry, the skin and visible mucous membranes
pale, the animal is thin and weak, exhausts easily, has a varied
appetite and drinks frequently.

In an infected flock the percentage of deaths is large although
the losses do not usually occur in bunches, but one or more daily
succumb to the disease.

TREATMENT. The treatment of the internal parasites of
sheep need not differ for the different varieties of tape and round
worms nor for those affecting the lungs from the intestinal varieties. It has been my experience that sheep badly affected with one
variety of internal parasites also harbor two or more; and frequently lung, intestinal, flat, and round worms all abound in the
same animal.

The modes of entrance of all the internal parasites of the
sheep are similar and the sanitary and prophylactic measures to be
adopted will answer for all varieties.

It is almost impossible to completely disinfect pastures or
corrals contaminated with the internal parasites of sheep and it is
desirable, in addition to disinfecting them as thoroughly as conditions will permit, to move the sheep to fresh ground or range at
least every two weeks. This is practicable in the range states of
the West and especially where sheep range in the National forests,
as they are never camped in the same place more than one week at
a time and are, therefore, on fresh pastures all of the time.

Where it is impossible to move sheep frequently to uncontaminated pastures, whatever treatment is to be pursued must be
continued as long as the sheep are confined on the infected ground.

In taking into consideration treatment of the internal parasites of sheep the veterinarian must not lose sight of the anemic
condition of the animals, their depraved appetite and their opportunities for reinfection.

To be successful in treating internal parasites of sheep whatever medication is used must be administered to each animal.
Where the treatment is given in the food or drinking water there
will always be some animals which will refuse such treatment or
will take so little that they will continue to harbor the parasites
and remain a source of danger to other members of the same flock.

In addition to treating sheep with the object of destroying the parasites such medicines and food must be used as will best build up its normal resistance to the parasites. Some of the chemicals which are known to be destructive to internal parasites are impractical for use. For example, where administered in the feed in which only part of the animals get the treatment or where skilled services are required like administering the treatment intratracheally.

Volatile substances such as turpentine, gasoline, benzine and chloroform, and treatment with fumigations or steam inhalation which may be used for treating lung worms, in my practice, have no advantages over volatile vermicides administered by the mouth which are partly eliminated by the lungs and destroy the lung worms in that way.

For a number of years I have depended upon the use of turpentine for the treatment of internal parasites and have met with entire satisfaction in the treatment where the flocks would be frequently moved to fresh ground.

The treatment which I have followed is composed of the following formula: Three pounds of common salt is dissolved in three gallons of water and a half pound each of nitrate of potash and powdered ginger are added and the mixture steeped at a temperature of 160 degrees F. for several hours, stirring occasionally. When the emulsion has cooled to 100 degrees F. twenty-four ounces of turpentine are added and the mixture stirred until thoroughly mixed.

The dose of this mixture is four ounces for an adult sheep. Upon beginning the treatment on a flock of diseased sheep I direct that the treatment be administered, by drench, after fasting twelve hours and repeated twice, three days apart, and that the treatment be given once a week as long as the sheep continue to remain exposed to infection.

If the flock can be moved every week or two the treatment should be continued until there are no remaining symptoms.

I have used this treatment on a great many different flocks of sheep during the past number of years. Have frequently found lambs in the feed-lot in the fall of the year affected with lung worms and have directed their treatment with this turpentine emulsion and have invariably received good reports, the sheep taking on a thrifty appearance and gaining flesh rapidly.

In the year 1908 I had occasion to treat a flock of 1300 grade Oxford sheep. They were running in two bands 100 miles apart and had been separated only a few weeks when I was called to see the flock of young sheep consisting of yearlings and two-year-olds. Some hundred sheep had died out of 500 and there were a great many sick ones, a few dying each day. Autopsies revealed the presence of round worms, both in the lungs and alimentary tract, also the tape worm in the intestines. In addition to bronchitis the autopsies revealed pneumonias with multiple abscesses in the lungs. The older members of the same flock were not so badly affected, although the sucking lambs of some two or three months old showed the disease. These sheep were given the turpentine emulsion as described above and the treatment was repeated weekly for about two months. All of the increase from this flock of sheep was used for breeding purposes and scattered among the flocks throughout the country and the same band of sheep was kept together for a number of years to my knowledge, their increase being kept continuously for breeding purposes with no reports of losses or recurrence of the parasites. I will say that these sheep were changed every two weeks to fresh ground during the first summer and were never returned to the farms which they were on when they were affected with the worms.

I have never treated a bunch of sheep infected with internal parasites with this formula which did not show improvement, but in some flocks which were not changed from their original inclosure sickness among them increased upon suspension of the treatment, and it is my opinion that where animals cannot be changed several times to fresh ground and watering places, they will have to be treated continuously.

BIBLIOGRAPHY

KAUPP, B. F. Animal Parasites and Parasitic Diseases.
LAW, JAMES. Veterinary Medicine.
NEUMANN-McQUEEN. Parasites and Parasitic Diseases of Domestic Animals.

DISCUSSION

MR. C. C. KNOBLOCH: Dr. Fitch laid great emphasis on the terminology of our parasites. So far, this country has done so little work in parasitology that we have accepted without question all work done in Germany. Dr. Fitch, in his illustrated lecture this morning, referred to the sclerostomes, properly called *Strongylus*, according to the Bureau. I might say here in all earnestness that if terminologists, especially teachers of parasitology, will go to the Bureau they will have little trouble in getting sraightened out. I have found and described nineteen species of *Strongylus*. Ransom gives twenty-seven, but he quotes the work of Looss in 1900 in Egypt. That work describes the parasites of horses in parts of the body which they do not inhabit in the United States. You can question my statement if you wish, but if you accept that you will see the need of original research along these lines.

Dr. Fitch, this morning, showed especially one he called *Strongylus edentatus*. That is manifestly a mistake, because edentatus means without teeth. We do not find that form of species in this country at all. There is no record of toothless sclerostomes in the United States.

I am not a veterinarian, but I was sent up here by authority from the State to talk just a little on this, and put before the profession the idea that the research work on these worms is to be started in the hotbed of parasites in Oklahoma.

I have taken my Master's and partial Ph.D. in studying these worms, and if I can work in harmony with the veterinary profession, which I am certainly going to try to do, I know it will be appreciated by the Bureau and I am sure it will be appreciated by the State Board of Agriculture.

Dr. Fitch: In my talk this morning I think I emphasized the necessity for men in our veterinary schools to make a special study of parasites. Very little work has been published in this country on this phase, particularly with reference to the *Strongyli* of horses.

There is one error I wish to correct and that is in regard to *Strong. edentatum*. I have found this parasite and identified it. This fact has never been published, however, and the gentleman was correct in saying that, as far as he knew, the parasite had not been found in this country. I have identified three Strongyli, i. e., *Strongylus equinum*, *S. vulgare* and *S. edentatum*.

Mr. Knobloch: I own that the parasites in the northern states of the country show greater variations than those in the South. Most of my work has been done in the South and I stand corrected. You should have sent in your work to some central bureau so that all of us would have had the benefit of it.

Dr. Hall: I feel very much disposed to criticize the entire association for the present condition of our knowledge of parasites in the United States. There is no topic in veterinary medicine that I know of that is handled by veterinarians in practice and at their scientific meetings with so little regard for the actual state of the world's knowledge upon the subject, as this subject of parasites. If you had a practitioner or laboratory man come before you and refer to bacilli as micrococci, you would hoot him, I think. I do not believe you would be any more tolerant. Yet, in actual practice you call every sort of large worm *Ascaris* without regard to the fact that there are hundreds of species that you are lumping together without any regard to their life histories or their effect upon the host.

I am certain that this symposium on parasites, owing to the emergencies of one sort and another that have arisen, has come before you at a time when most of you are somnolent or verging on coma. I do not think we are in a position to take up the topic at this late stage with other things coming on for our consideration and do it justice. I simply wish to say that you do not know how ignorant the veterinary profession of America is in regard to the entire subject of parasites. The question of nomenclature has been raised here, and as I say, you would never tolerate in your naming of bacteria what you accept in the subject of parasites.

The subject of parasites is more important than you think; it is more important to you in your practice than you think. Acute febrile diseases come on quickly and you are called in. You notice fever symptoms and you make your diagnosis on the clinical picture and treat it according to the more or less prevalent methods. But you have any number of cases in your practice where there are afebrile conditions, with no clear clinical picture—merely an unthrifty animal. In the case of the young animal it falls off in health rapidly and dies because of the fact that the young animal cannot tolerate the insult and injuries due to the presence of worms in the digestive and respiratory tracts, whereas the older animal can stand such treatment. But you do not recognize that afebrile condition as parasitic. You make any number of other diagnoses, but you do not adopt the modern method of diagnosis.

The idea of making an examination of the feces and finding parasite eggs is simple compared with a bacteriological examination, yet you men who take a swab and secure culture from a case and have a bacteriologist report to you the strain of bacilli you are dealing with are stumped utterly by parasitic cases. The idea of taking a scraping from a case of mange, macerating it for ten minutes in caustic potash, and examining it for mites, does not occur to you—you guess it is mange. And when you get into the field of cutaneous diseases you are in a good place to guess. The parasitic diseases are the most easily diagnosed of diseases, but you do not take the trouble to diagnose them. You could with little trouble eliminate the parasitic diseases and then guess at the rest of them, but you do not take the trouble because you are used to doing it the other way. You take your terms in parasitology from your clients, who talk about "wolf in the tail" and "hollow horn", when the nomenclature on worms is as superior to that as your diagnosis in the terms of pathology is superior to that of the farmer who has not made a study of it. When the zoologist comes to you and says, "That is not *Sclerostomum* but *Strongylus*," you say, "What is the use, why do you want to bother with all those silly names?" There is a reason. The genus *Ascaris* probably has a thousand species, and there would be just as much sense in keeping those thousand species under one head as there would be in filing the correspondence of all your clients under the name Smith and then sorting them out every time you wanted to look up a letter from a certain client.

The one idea I feel like contributing to this meeting is that you are ignorant on the subject of parasitology and you are not even ashamed of it. The zoologist deals with animals; he has his code and he tries to live up to it. There is a reason why we take the oldest name. It is the only one we can pick on a fixed objective basis. The question is often asked, why we do not keep the common name? What is the common one? The common one in France or Belgium is not the common one here. It is just the same as taking the most common terms of diagnosis, the farmer's terms, and using them yourself. When the zoologist comes into the field of veterinary medicine make him live up to your code in terminology and the ethics of the profession. When you are in a field like parasitology, a medico-zoological field, you must conform to the code of the medical man and the zoologist.

The subject of life histories of parasites is of great importance; unless you know the life history as you should know it, prophylaxis is a difficult matter; when the life history is known, you can find a weak spot somewhere. When we learned that the causative agent of Texas fever lived in the tick, we studied the tick and found that this tick could be found on the cow with great certainty, and that it did not wander off to rodents and miscellaneous other animals, and that made it possible for us to confine our attention to the ticky cow. It simplified the whole thing; when you dipped your cow you got rid of Texas fever. In South Africa they have ticks that do not stay on the cow, but are found on the rodents and other animals, and they wander high, wide and far; we are fortunate that we do not have them.

Another thing I have tried to emphasize in a paper recently is the importance of manure disposal as a factor in controlling parasitic diseases. The parasites of the gastro-intestinal tract produce eggs which pass out in the manure. The parasites of the respiratory tract produce eggs that are coughed up and, in the main, as the saliva is swallowed, pass out in the manure. You should look on all manure of our domestic animals as bearing parasites, because most of our animals have parasites and their eggs pass out in the manure.

We owe a great deal in this country to the work of the Bureau of Animal Industry on life history. The very beautiful and classical work of Smith and Kilborn on Texas fever is an illustration. We owe a great deal to the work of Dr. Charles Wardell Stiles, although his work led him into the field of human medicine, where his work has been adequately recognized by the medical profession. And we owe a great deal to his successor, Dr. B. H. Ransom, who has done some beautiful work. He is a most admirable, careful, conscientious, painstaking worker and his work on stomach worm in sheep, trichinosis, cysticercosis and other things will become classics. If the A. V. M. A. appreciated what he has done in this field, as it should, it would elect Dr. Ransom an honorary member of this association, and feel honored in doing so. You pay so little attention to parasitology that you do not know what good work has been done in this country.

I believe we should know more about the distribution of parasites in this country, but you cannot know anything about the distribution of parasites unless your identification is practically correct. A gentleman has recently said that some of our sclerostomes have not been properly reported; if they were reported by the average veterinary practitioner I would not put much confidence in it, but would assume it was a sclerostome and not go any further. But you are going to do better after awhile, you are going to get out of this slip-shod way you have been practicing, because you cannot go on doing it that way. We are outgrowing it. Incidentally, the gentleman stated that *Strongylus edentatum* does not occur in the United States. I have collected this parasite a number of times and there are many specimens in the Bureau collection at Washington.

I made an investigation for the United States Bureau of Animal Industry in 1913, looking up the distribution of some diseases, and it appeared at that time that a nodular worm, which had been confined previously to the eastern and southern parts of our country, was spreading west and had reached as far as Kansas; it may have spread further by this time. This is an important disease. You all know that the intestines of sheep are used as sausage casings. The western sheep furnish a good grade, free from worm nodules, and the southern and eastern sheep furnish a bad grade because of this nodular worm; if this disease continues to spread, it will cause considerable loss in this one matter of sausage casings. But unless you know something about parasitology, you cannot recognize or check the disease.

It also appears that our fringed tape worm from the liver of sheep is losing ground in this country and is now vanishing, and I think it will disappear without any particular steps being taken to eradicate it. That I take to be due to the breaking up of the free range. While the life history of this worm is not known, I think the breaking up of the free range has interfered with the life cycle; that the sheep no longer keep in touch with the intermediate host essential to the life history of the worm.

Just a word about treatment, we know so little about that.

The entire subject of anthelmintics needs overhauling and revision. I worked on this subject in the Bureau of Animal Industry for over a year and have continued that work at Detroit, and it is surprising to find how ineffective the average much-used anthelmintic is when you put it to the acid test of killing the host animal after treatment and finding what worms are left. You give a dose of the anthelmintic and you get some worms, and you think that is all the animal had, but when you kill the animal you find out differently. The milder doses will have to be continued day after day to get effective results. There seems to be a disposition among veterinarians and medical men to believe that one anthelmintic is good against anything. Oil of chenopodium, American worm seed, is a specific for the ascarid group, but it won't remove tape worms. It will once in a while, but that is not what you want; you want dependable efficiency.

Just another thing; there is a very common belief that mineral mixtures, containing wood ashes, lime, salt, and so forth, are efficacious in preventing and curing worms, and that this is especially true of worms in hogs. When I was in the Bureau, W. D. Foster and I carried on experiments to test this. The Bureau was not entirely satisfied with our conclusions to the effect that these mixtures were no good from an anthelmintic standpoint, so they repeated the experiments, and they may have continued to repeat them after I left the Bureau. But I will tell you what I think about these mixtures personally, and that is that they are not worth a continental. If you want to feed a mineral mixture to your pigs because they need it in their business, to build up their bone, or increase their appetite, or keep them happy, why do it. If you want an anthelmintic, get one. I have given anthelmintic medication in slops in flock or herd treatment, but I do not think it is any good; anthelmintics are seldom effective when given by cafeteria methods. It would be nice if such methods were effective. No one wants to get out and run down an "ornery" 200-pound sow and hold the brute while it is given an anthelmintic, but I do not know of any way to give one except to fast the animal, clear the digestive tract of food material as much as possible, and then give a well selected anthelmintic in sufficient dose under the best possible conditions, if you want results.

I think that is probably sufficient for one afternoon. Understand, that I am not cross or angry. I am good natured, but I wish I could stir you people up to a realization of the fact that you are "kidding" yourselves when you think you are taking the subject of parasitology seriously, because you are not. If anyone came to address you on the same basis in bacteriology that you use in parasitology, you would not stand it.

DR. MERILLAT: I am glad to have one so eminently prominent in the parasitic world as Doctor Hall, endorse the position the officers of the American Veterinary Medical Association took last summer when we decided to take up the study of parasitology seriously. It is to be hoped that the future officers of the association will take their cue from this splendid address and that we will all prolong our studies until we come to a realization of its importance.

Dr. KNOWLES: I wish to come to the defense of the practitioner in this matter. If every practitioner were to study parasitology as Doctor Hall indicates, most of us would not have time to take care of the regular practice; however, the thought is right and parasites should have more attention from the veterinary practitioner.

It seems to me the thing we need is some thorough investigators who will put in their time studying parasites and give the profession the results of their work. Our government will need to do some of this work that has been carried on by European countries in the past. If some system of studying this very necessary subject of parasitology can be carried out so that the practitioners may have the advantage of it, it will be of value, but practitioners cannot conduct investigations in private practice.

I will state that I have used copper sulphate, iron sulphate, and arsenic in the feed in the treatment of intestinal parasites in sheep, but the treatment did not prove satisfactory for the reason, perhaps, that the animals did not eat it regularly and also that they were kept on the same infected ground. As was stated in my paper, whatever treatment is used for destroying parasites in sheep, should be administered at regular intervals to each animal separately.

I once had a herd of 300 Angora goats under treatment for intestinal parasites and after giving the emulsion, referred to in my paper, I advised removing the flock to uncontaminated ground, but that was not done at the time so the copper sulphate compound was given in the feed but after a month the sheep were again showing the effect of the worms and the turpentine emulsion treatment was resumed with satisfactory results, and continued for several weeks when the flock was removed, in the spring of the year, to another farm where no further trouble was reported.

Dr. HOSKINS: I wish to express my great appreciation of the remarks of the gentleman from Oklahoma and Dr. Hall; and I wish to add to it this fact, that those who are in the practice of veterinary medicine in the large cities, who have practiced for a quarter of a century, and have enjoyed a large equine practice, are now confronted with a new situation.

I was fortunate enough during the last six or seven years to have associated with me my younger son, and while in a period of ten years more than 80 per cent of the practice I had enjoyed passed away through the advent of the automobile, the association of my son and the gain because of the study and knowledge of parasitology and infectious and contagious diseases of dogs and cats enabled us, during that period, to keep up as large an income during that six or seven years as I had enjoyed during a period of twenty-five years. I wish to confess it was not because of knowledge I possessed.

I fully recognize, as pointed out by Dr. Hall, that the time has come when my clients ask me to pass on diseases of dogs and cats that bear evidence of parasitism where my knowledge and opinion might last for a little while, but would not last against that of my son who would stick to the microscope and would not make a diagnosis until he had made a proper examination.

This field is an immense one; it is a tremendous field in the large cities. So there is not only the opportunity but there is the reward that is going to come which we are all seeking in our work. I indeed feel that I have greatly profited by hearing Doctor Hall and the gentleman from Oklahoma, and I hope we will all take the lesson home to ourselves.

Dr. J. F. Mitchell: I met, in connection with my business in Anaconda, an entomologist, William Moore, from St. Paul. This gentleman told me that he was working on the parasitic diseases of the soldiers in the European trenches. We all know about the typhus fever killing a great many Serbian soldiers and that the lice have spread to the British and French soldiers on the western front.

Among other things he told me that the British soldiers were now wearing around their necks, bags of asafetida, naptha and iodoform, and this combination made fumes which worked down into their clothes and killed the lice. It seems that the American soldiers do not wear their leggings as tight as the European soldiers, so that it is impossible to hold enough fumes in their clothing to kill lice. A student got a dose of crabs and he was given this compound and he wore it around his neck. It drove the crabs down and the next morning he found that his legs were all raw around his garters. The crabs had become numbed, fallen down to his garters where the fumes having dispersed they came to life; the student then became disgusted and used blue ointment.

There are very many available substitutes that will kill lice on sheep. I know a man who worked on about fifty sheep in a small tight building, and at an expense of about $1.50 he killed the ticks on those sheep; their wool was four inches thick.

The dipping of sheep in Montana and other northwestern states in winter has brought serious consequences. It really kills a number of the sheep in Montana. The United States Government advises the dipping of sheep every so often when they are infected with sheep scab.

If we can get the same results by fumigation, it will remove the danger of immersing the sheep in dips when the weather is very cold.

Prof. William Moore has published six papers on this subject, though his results have not been so far as I know largely checked up by field work, they are certainly very important to sheep owners who handle pure bred animals.

DR. CHASE: I wish to add my approval to the very able remarks that have been given expression to today by Doctor Hall and the gentleman from Oklahoma. I wish to add my most hearty approval to the action of the association which this gentleman from Oklahoma represents, and say that the veterinary profession, I am sure, will stand behind him and help him. He can depend upon us to do our part in making his research a success. The importance of this subject has only of late years been made manifest; it is a question that has been more or less obscure; the importance of it has not been made felt until recently. This, I believe, is the first time in the history of the association that it has ever taken up a whole session in the discussion of parasites, and it shows the trend of the times.

The Bureau of Animal Industry, in its last bulletins, has laid down that the veterinary colleges throughout the United States must provide in the curricula a certain prescribed number of hours for the consideration of parasites in order that they may turn out proficient and qualified meat inspectors.

The important part that parasites play has been shown to be great. They often obscure a correct diagnosis if you are not cognizant of their importance in the production of disease.

The importance of parasites in the transmission of disease has been shown in many instances, and the researches of the times show that they play a much more important role as we learn more of the diseases. Malaria we know is produced by the mosquito. Yellow fever was absolutely eliminated in our Canal Zone by the knowledge that Col. Goethals possessed of yellow fever being carried and disseminated by the mosquito. By protecting his men from the mosquito he saved the lives of the workers in that zone, which had theretofore been impossible of habitation by white men.

We know also that the tape worm, the most fatal internal parasite perhaps, is carried and disseminated by a number of other insects. The fly is a carrier of the tape worm larvae which, when taken into the body of the animal in its food, develops into the mature worm. The dog louse also carries the larvae of the tape worm, and in its course it will produce the mature worm in a like manner.

I wish to say that much good can be done by giving time and attention to the thought that is necessary to be given to this subject. The fact of our giving this subject the consideration we have at this meeting shows that we are waking up to the importance of it. The Bureau is giving it more consideration and it is a subject that the coming young veterinarian will be required to know and he will be called to account for a lack of knowledge of the subject such as has been shown this afternoon by a large portion of this body.

DR. QUITMAN: I wish to say, first of all, that no one present has appreciated the remarks of Mr. Knobloch and Dr. Hall more than I, and I heartily concur particularly in Dr. Hall's condemnation. However, I also concur most heartily in the defense of the practitioner. The specialists expect the practitioner to see the veterinary profession through their eyes. I make the mental calculation that to become proficient in the different branches as they would have us, we would have to extend our college courses to seventeen years. I wish to say to Doctor Hall that I think he is in error when he says that in order to eradicate intestinal parasites the animal must be freshly pastured and a well-chosen anthelmintic administered, and that is the only way you are going to get rid of the parasites. I take issue with him on that after twenty-five years of close observation. I do not know a single anthelmintic that would eradicate the parasite that would not destroy the mucous lining. That takes essential treatment, but it will have to be administered over and over again to remove the long tape worms.

I do not advocate the administering of anthelmintic drugs or vermifuges or vermicides in the slop of pigs, because you cannot regulate the dose. If these pigs could be fed some drugs—sulphate of copper is splendid, sulphate of iron is useful, but my choice is arsenic given for a long period of time—you would get rid of worms more quickly; say extended over a period of two months.

DR. HALL: I would like to set myself straight on this matter and say that I entirely sympathize with the viewpoint of the average practitioner. His proposition is that he has to do the practical thing, satisfy his client, cure the patient if possible, get his fees and make a living. That is a straight, clean-cut proposition; and I am not at all of the notion that it is up to you gentlemen as practitioners to sit down and study parasitology now, not for a moment. What I tried to say this afternoon was simply this—that Dr. Knowles and Dr. Hollister and Dr. Fitch had to tell you just about what is in the text books, but reduced to the simplest terms they could put it in, in order that you could understand it. The fact that they had to do so is in itself a criticism of the present state of your knowledge on the subject. I do not think it is up to you practitioners now to start in and reform the situation; but I think it is up to the veterinary colleges to teach parasitology as it should be taught, with some regard for accuracy, and that the men who go out in the future should go out with a better equipment than you have. You practical men who are in the business making a living can go downstairs and take an intelligent part in a discussion of serum therapy that would lose me. You are more skilled in diagnosis of lameness and other common ailments. You could do as well in practical parasitology. It is out of the question that you practitioners should study parasitology now, or that I should have the capacity for clinical diagnosis that others have. But it is possible for colleges in the future to turn out students who will have these qualifications.

In regard to Dr. Quitman's statement, there are some worms you can get rid of, certain species, with a proper anthelmintic where you can do practically a 100 per cent job. I have killed in the course of my investigations, probably, between two and three hundred dogs. The way we do is to give the dog a treatment; the feces of that dog are collected the next morning and broken up and carefully screened and washed, and the worms picked out and counted and identified carefully. We repeat the collecting on the second, third, and fourth days; and sometimes it is repeated for three months to see what happens in the three months. On the fourth day we usually kill the dog and the test of the anthelmintic efficiency consists in seeing how many worms are left. It is astonishing how little efficacy there is in some drugs.

That treatment Dr. Quitman has advocated may be very excellent and in some aspects I know it is. For instance, in dealing with whipworms in the cecum of dogs, at times the treatment will get them, other times it will not. But if you give a grain of santonin day in and day out for a week and repeat this after a week you ultimately get the worms out of the cecum. Of course, you have to figure what the treatment will do to the dog. When you use arsenic on a horse you get systemic results that you have to consider. You can push arsenic to the point where it ceases to be a remedy.

—Dr. E. V. Hoover has removed from Defiance to Lima, Ohio.

—Dr. Robert O. Rothermel is in charge of federal meat inspection at Reading, Pa.

—Dr. Edwin Laitinen has removed from Texarkana, Ark., to North Colebrook, Conn.

—Dr. Hugh L. Fry, formerly at Kendalville, Ind., is for the present at Jackson, Miss.

—Dr. R. Banister has removed from Letts to Alert, Ind.

—Dr. H. Greeder has removed from Luxemburg, Wis., to Enid, Okla.

—Dr. H. Cardona has removed from Milbank, S. D., to New Orleans, La.

A BOTHRIOCEPHALID TAPEWORM FROM THE DOG IN NORTH AMERICA, WITH NOTES ON CESTODE PARASITES OF DOGS

Maurice C. Hall, Ph.D., D.V.M., and Meyer Wigdor, M.A.
Research Laboratory, Parke, Davis and Company, Detroit, Michigan

Although at least four species of bothriocephalid tapeworms have been reported from the dog in various parts of the world, there were no records of the sort from the United States until recently. The first record of which we are aware is one by Van Es and Schalk (1917), who report what they call *Dibothriocephalus latus* from a dog at Agricultural College, N. D. Their specific determination is apparently casual, being only incidental to work on anaphylaxis, and is presumably based on the fact that the worm was a bothriocephalid tapeworm and that *D. latus* is one of the commonest and best-known of these worms from the dog. We wish to report another case of the occurrence of a bothriocephalid tapeworm in the dog in this country.

Four specimens of a species of bothriocephalid worm were collected by us from the small intestine of an experiment dog, No. 140, at Detroit on July 27, 1917. These specimens are all small, measuring respectively 7.5, 14.5, 16 and 36 mm. in length and very narrow, the largest specimen being less than 2 mm. wide. The head of the largest specimen is 1.64 mm. long; that of the next largest is 1.5 mm. long; that of the next largest is 1.37 mm. long; that of the smallest is 1.66 mm. long. The width of the head is about 0.4 mm. in the narrow transverse diameter across the bothridial aperture and about 0.7 mm. in the dorsoventral diameter from the external margin of one bothridium to the external margin of the other. There is no neck, the head arising directly from the anterior margin of the first segment. In stained toto mounts, the primordia of the genitalia appear 3 to 3.33 mm. posterior of the head (Fig. 1). They first appear as diffusely spherical objects, later becoming dumbbell-shaped, the dumbbell subsequently elongating. There are no eggs present in any of the strobilae and the genitalia appear to be immature; it is possible that they are abortive and sterile. Malformations and displacements of the genitalia are common. The last normal segment of the largest worm, about 7 mm. from the posterior end, is 558 μ long

and 1.34 mm. wide. In the next largest worm, the largest segment, not far from the posterior end, is 668 μ long and 833 μ wide.

The bothriocephalid cestodes of the dog were at one time re-

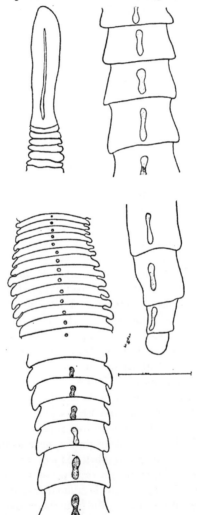

FIGURE 1. *Diphyllobothrium americanum*
Camera lucida sketch of portions of strobila

ferred to the genus *Bothriocephalus* Rudolphi, 1808, of which the
type is *B. punctatus* (Rudolphi, 1802) Rudolphi, 1810, from vari-

ous fish. They were later referred to the genus *Dibothriocephalus* Luehe, 1899, of which the type is *D. latus* (Linnaeus, 1758) Luehe, 1899, but in 1910 Luehe regards his genus *Dibothriocephalus* as a synonym of *Diphyllobothrium* Cobbold, 1858, of which the type is *D. stemmacephalum* from *Delphinus phocaena*, and the bothriocephalid worms from the dog are now generally referred to *Diphyllobothrium*. These worms are briefly described as follows:

D. latum attains a length of 2 to 9 meters. It has a head 2 to 3 mm. long according to Braun (1906) and Fiebiger (1912) and 2 to 5 mm. long by 0.7 to 1 mm. wide according to Neveau-Lemaire (1912). These writers agree that the neck is thin, its length depending on the state of contraction. It would appear from the fact that our strobilae are only a few centimeters long, instead of several meters, and that the heads are only 1.37 to 1.66 mm. long and 0.4 to 0.7 mm. wide, and from the fact that they have no neck, that we have a form other than *D. latum*, and we believe that such is evidently the case.

In this connection it is interesting to note that Nickerson (1906) notes a case of *D. latum* in a child born in Minnesota and who had never been out of that state, the first record of an infection with this worm where the infection is known to have been acquired in this country. Nickerson says the head of the worm was 1.75 mm. long and 0.9 mm. wide. These figures are intermediate between those given for *D. latum* and those for our specimens. Nickerson states, regarding *D. latum*: "There are no reports of its being found in American dogs, cats or foxes—the other animals which are known to serve as definitive hosts for the parasite." He also states: "Larvae of *Dibothriocephalus* do occur in American fishes. I have obtained them from fish caught in the Great Lakes, but without feeding experiments to rear the adult worm from the larva it is impossible to determine the species of *Dibothriocephalus* and the probability is in favor of such larvae being of some species other than *latus*—the parasite of man."

Diphyllobothrium cordatum, another parasite of dogs, has a characteristic heart-shaped head, 2 mm. by 2 mm. in diameter, and it is certain that the species we have found is not *D. cordatum*.

D. fuscum was described from the dog in Iceland by Krabbe. According to Neveau-Lemaire (1912), this worm has a compressed, lanceolate head, a neck slightly narrower than the head, followed by segments which are at first indistinct. In our specimens there is no neck and the first segments, though small, are quite distinct. It is, however, difficult to make distinctions of this sort. We are frankly unable to ascertain with any certainty whether our specimens correspond to the meager description of *D. fuscum,* and we merely assume that since the agreement is not exact, it is fairly unlikely that rare material from such widely separated localities should be the same species.

D. serratum is named as a parasite of dogs by a number of writers, but is then disregarded and no description is available to us. Some writers list it with a question mark, indicating uncertainties in regard to it, and we are compelled to disregard it.

Bothriocephalus spiratus is listed by Neveau-Lemaire (1912) as found in the dog in Italy. Such a species is not listed by Gedoelst (1911) or Stiles and Hassall (1912), and it seems likely that this is a printer's error for *B. serratus,* which is not named in Neveau-Lemaire's list of dog parasites.

In order that the species found here by us may have some name to which it may be referred, we propose for it the name of *Diphyllobothrium americanum.* Should it develop later that this name is a synonym of some existing name, it will be easy to suppress the synonym. In the meantime, we believe it is more convenient to have a name and we are following the advice of Stiles in such matters—that it is better to give a new name which may be later suppressed than to confuse two species under one name. Of course, we do this in the belief that this species cannot be identified with *D. latum, D. cordatum* or *D. fuscum* and it is not feasible to make a comparison with *D. serratum.* Specimens will be deposited in the collection of the U. S. Bureau of Animal Industry where they will be available for future examination.

It might be noted here that the bothriocephalid larvae, or plerocercoids, found by Nickerson in fish from the Great Lakes may have been the larvae of this species, an idea which is in agreement with Nickerson's statements. The idea is of interest, as bothriocephalids parasitic in man are commonly capable of parasitizing dogs, and vice versa. It may be, therefore, that fish caught in the Great Lakes and consumed here in Detroit and elsewhere are parasitized by a plerocercoid other than that of *D. latum* but possibly capable, nevertheless, of parasitizing man.

The following key to the bothriocephalid worms of the dog makes use of such distinctions as can be drawn in view of the scarcity of detailed description:

1. No available description....................*Diphyllobothrium serratum*
   Descriptions available..2
2. Heart-shaped head, 2 mm. by 2 mm. in diameter............*D. cordatum*
   Head not heart-shaped, longer than wide............................3
3. No neck, the first segment following immediately behind head.......
   ....*D. americanum*
   Neck present..4
4. Neck slightly narrower than the head.....................*D. fuscum*
   Neck thin; strobila attains a length of 2 to 9 meters...........*D. latum*

It is possible, even probable, that *D. americanum* is normally a parasite of wild carnivores.

In this connection, it might be noted that the life history of the bothriocephalid tapeworms has just been ascertained by Janicki and Rosen (1917; 1918). It has long been known that the larval form occurred in fish and that the adult worm developed in suitable hosts when raw fish were ingested, but attempts to infect fish with the eggs or embryos of the adult tapeworm have always been unsuccessful. Janicki and Rosen met with no better success in feeding experiments of this sort than other investigators had achieved, so they began a search for an intermediate host capable of becoming infested by the embryos of the worm and in turn infesting the fish. In this search they were successful, the intermediate hosts found being small invertebrate animals known as copepods. Of these, *Cyclops strenuus* and *Diaptomus gracilis* were found to function as hosts. The ciliated embryo of the worm was found to be taken into the digestive tract of the copepod; from there it penetrated the wall of the intestine and transformed in the body cavity into an intermediate larval form, the procercoid, which is armed with hooks on a globular caudal appendix. Not more than two of these were found in one host. When these infested copepods were eaten by fish, they were digested and the larval worms set free. The procercoid loses its hooks and the caudal appendix, if these have not already been lost in the copepod, and the plerocercoid thus formed traverses the wall of the stomach, attains the body cavity and thence enters the musculature or the liver. The parasitized copepods lose their active movements and move slowly along at the bottom of the water. This admirable piece of work by Janicki and Rosen furnishes us the first case of a tapeworm having two intermediate hosts with two larval stages and will doubtless open a large field of investigation and theorizing.

We take this occasion to summarize briefly the status of the dog tapeworms as regards their occurrence on this continent, so

far as records are available to us. Most of the common species of
dog cestodes have been reported from the dog on this continent,
and some rare forms have been found. Other tapeworms, some of
which have only been reported as found once in the dog in Europe,
are not known on this continent.

Mesocestoides lineatus has been reported by Stiles and Hassall (1894) as represented in Leidy's collection by specimens collected from an Esquimaux dog by Kane.

Dipylidium caninum is a common parasite of dogs in the
United States. It has been reported from children at least three
times, in cases in Detroit, Mich., Ithaca, N. Y., and Norwich, Conn.

Dipylidium sexcoronatum has been reported from dogs in the
United States at Bethesda, Md., and Detroit, Mich., by Hall (1917).
We find it fairly often here at Detroit and our impression is that
it is as common here as *D. caninum*. The strobila is much narrower
than *D. caninum*. Some of the specimens with a narrow strobila
appear to have only 5 rows of hooks and should be studied with a
view to determining whether *D. sexcoronatum* has sometimes 5
rows of hooks, as well as 6 rows, or whether this material belongs
to a new species.

Of 200 dogs examined by us at Detroit, 46 per cent had *Dipylidium* but other investigations did not permit of taking time to
determine the species in all these cases. The average number of
worms present in a dog was 14.8; the largest number was 205 and
the next largest 100.

Taenia pisiformis (*Taenia serrata*) is probably the commonest
of the dog tapeworms belonging to the genus *Taenia*. Ward (1897)
found it present in 45 per cent of the dogs examined by him at
Lincoln, Neb. As long as dogs have access to our wild hares and
rabbits, the hosts of the larval tapeworm, this worm will probably
be common in dogs. It is naturally commoner in dogs in the country and in villages and small cities and less common in large cities
where the dogs seldom get outside the city and where the rabbits
and other game are killed off for some distance out from the city.
At Detroit we found this parasite in 6 dogs, 3 per cent of our 200
dogs, the largest number present being 7 and the next largest 5. A
dog not in this series of 200 had 20 *T. pisiformis*.

Taenia hydatigena (*Taenia marginata*) is still fairly common
in dogs in the United States, but it appears to be of less common
occurrence than was the case 10 or 20 years ago. The increased ap-

plication of adequate meat inspection to the abattoirs of the United States and the increased care in the disposal of slaughter-house refuse will make this worm increasingly scarcer and it will eventually, and perhaps very soon, disappear. We only found it in 2 dogs, 1 per cent, of our 200 dogs here, and suspect that these dogs probably acquired the infection in the country, where the primitive methods of disposing of viscera of slaughtered animals by feeding to the dogs still prevail in some sections. As more and more farmers learn the impropriety and danger of such practices, it is likely that this will be one of the first dog tapeworms to become extinct.

Taenia krabbei was reported from Alaska by Ransom (1915), the adult tapeworm being obtained by feeding the corresponding bladderworm from the reindeer to dogs. Ransom (1913) had previously reported the larva of this tapeworm from reindeer in Alaska.

Taenia ovis has been experimentally developed in dogs in this country by Ransom (1913), by feeding larvae collected from the muscles of sheep. Ransom reports the larvae from sheep in Montana, Idaho, Washington, Oregon, California, Colorado and Nevada.

Taenia balaniceps was described from the dog in Nevada and the lynx in New Mexico by Hall (1910).

Multiceps multiceps, the gid tapeworm, has been experimentally developed in dogs in this country by Hall (1909) and by Taylor and Boynton (1910). The larva, or gid bladderworm from the brain, has been reported from sheep in this country a number of times and has been enzootic for many years in northern Montana. Ransom (1913) reports gid as present in Arizona and occasioning the loss of a considerable number of sheep.

Multiceps serialis has been experimentally developed in the dog in this country by Hall (1910) and has been reported from dogs in natural infestations by Ward (1897), Stevenson (1904) and Ransom (1905). The bladderworm, or larval stage, is common in jack rabbits in many parts of the western United States, occurring in the subcutaneous and connective tissues.

Echinococcus granulosus (*Taenia echinococcus*) was reported from the dog in this country by Stiles and Hassall (1894), the specimens being collected by Curtice at Washington, D. C. This tapeworm has also been reported from the dog in Alaska by Ransom (1915).

REFERENCES

BRAUN, MAX. 1906. The Animal Parasites of Man. London. 453 pp., 290 figs.

FIEBIGER, JOSEF. 1912. Die tierischen Parasiten der Haus- und Nutztiere. Wien u. Leipzig. 424 pp., 303 figs.

GEDOELST, L. 1911. Synopsis de Parasitologie de l' Homme et des Animaux domestiques. Lierre et Bruxelles. 332 pp.

HALL, MAURICE C. 1909. A discussion of de Renzi's treatment of somatic taeniasis with male fern, and some tests of the treatment in gid. Amer. Vet. Rev., Vol. 36 (3), Dec., pp. 328-337.
1910. The gid parasite and allied species of the cestode genus Multiceps. I. Historical Review. U. S. Bu. Anim. Indust. Bull. 125, pt. 1, 68 pp.
1910. A new species of cestode parasite (Taenia balaniceps) of the dog and of the lynx, with a note on Proteocephalus punicus. Proc. U. S. Nat. Mus. (1870), Vol. 39, pp. 139-151, 9 figs.
1917. Parasites of the dog in Michigan. Jour. Amer. Vet. Med. Ass'n, N. S., Vol. 4 (3), June, pp. 383-396.

JANICKI, C., and ROSEN, F. 1917. Le cycle evolutif du Dibothriocephalus latus. Recherches expérimentales et observations. Bull. Soc. Neuchatel des Sci. Nat., Vol. 42, pp. 19-53. Not seen.
1917. Idem. Bull. Inst. Pasteur, Rev. et anal., Vol. 15 (24), 30 Déc., pp. 769-770. Rev. by Roubaud.

NEVÉAU-LEMAIRE, MAURICE. 1912. Parasitologie des Animaux domestiques: Maladies parasitaires non bacteriennes. Paris. 1257 pp., 770 figs.

NICKERSON, W. S. 1906. The broad tapeworm in Minnesota, with the report of a case of infection acquired in the state. Jour. Amer. Med. Ass'n, Vol. 46 (10), March 10, pp. 711-713.

RANSOM, BRAYTON H. 1905. The gid parasite (Coenurus cerebralis): Its presence in American sheep. U. S. Bu. Anim. Indust. Bull. 66, 23 pp., 12 figs.
1913. Cysticercus ovis, the cause of tapeworm cysts in mutton. Jour. Agri. Research, Vol. 1 (1), Oct. 10, pp. 15-58, pls. 2-4, 13 text figs.
1913. The Zoological Division. In Rep. of Chief of Bu. of Anim. Indust. for the year ending June 30, 1913; pp. 31-33.
1915. The Zoological Division. In Rep. of Chief of Bu. of Anim. Indust. for year ending June 30, 1915; pp. 58-60.

STEVENSON, EARLE C. 1904. Variations in the hooks of the dog tapeworms, Taenia serrata and Taenia serialis. Studies Zool. Lab., Univ. of Neb., (59), pp. 409-429, 6 pls.

STILES, CH. WARDELL, and HASSALL, ALBERT. 1894. A preliminary catalogue of the parasites contained in the collections of the United States Bureau of Animal Industry, United States Army Medical Museum, Biologic De. partment of the University of Pennsylvania (Coll. Leidy) and in Coll. Stiles and Coll. Hassall. Vet. Mag., Vol. 1 (4), Apr., pp. 245-253; (5), May, pp. 331-354.
1912. Index Catalogue of Medical and Veterinary Zoology. Subjects: Cestoda and Cestodaria. Hyg. Lab. Bull. 85, 467 pp.

TAYLOR, WALTER J., and BOYNTON, WM. H. 1910. Gid found in sheep in New York. Ann. Rep. N. Y. State Vet. Coll. for 1908-09, pp. 69-77, 3 pls.

VÁN ES, L., and SCHALK, A. F. 1917. Notes on parasitic anaphylaxis and allergy. N. D. Agri. Exp. Sta. Bull. 125, pp. 151-193, fig 1.

WARD, HENRY B. 1897. Animal parasites of Nebraska. Rep. Neb. State Bd. Agri. for 1896, pp. 173-189, 12 figs.

EXPERIMENTS IN THE TRANSMISSION OF TRICHINAE

H. B. RAFFENSPERGER
U. S. Bureau of Animal Industry, Chicago, Ill.

In the literature of trichinosis, statements' are occasionally seen that infection may be brought about by the ingestion of feces or the intestinal contents of animals harboring the intestinal stage of the parasite. From time to time the results of experiments have been recorded which it is claimed demonstrate the transmission of the parasite in this way. Höyberg (1907) for example concluded that infection may result from the swallowing of feces or intestinal contents of infested animals, and recently Salzer (1916) reported infection from feeding the feces of infested dogs. Various highly competent investigators, however, including such well-known authorities as Leuckart and Pagenstecher have reached the conclusion that infection cannot be brought about through the swallowing of intestinal trichinae or the newly born larvae which may occasionally be found in the feces of animals during the time when adult trichinae are present in the intestine. A few years ago, Stäubli (1909) reported a series of experiments in feeding to white rats the intestines of rats and guinea pigs containing trichinae in various stages of development and his results were consistently negative. Incidentally in the course of investigations upon trichinae in which the present writer has been engaged during the past two years under the direction of Dr. B. H. Ransom, Chief of the Zoological Division of the Bureau of Animal Industry, some experiments similar to those of Stäubli have been carried out. The results like those obtained by Stäubli were in all cases negative and like his tend to prove that infection through feces containing intestinal trichinae, if it occurs at all, must be a rare phenomenon.

Seven wild rats were fed trichinous pork February 14 and February 16, 1916. On the night of February 16, three rats died. These rats were examined the following day. Live trichinae were found in the intestine in each case. The contents of the duodenum and jejunum were placed in a gelatin capsule and fed to a guinea pig February 17. Two more of the seven rats died on the night of February 17, three days after the first feeding and one day after the second feeding. Many live trichinae were found in the intestines. The contents of the duodenum and a portion of the jejunum were fed to the guinea pig that had been similarly fed the day before. This guinea pig was killed and examined March 21, or 34 days after the first feeding. The diaphragm was cut into thin strips which were compressed between two pieces of glass and examined carefully under the microscope. No trichinae were found.

Rat No. 6 was killed February 18, four days after the first feeding. Post mortem examination revealed many adult trichinae in the intestine. The contents of the duodenum and a portion of the jejunum were fed to a guinea pig on the same day. This pig was killed April 4, or 46 days after feeding. Examination of the diaphragm gave negative results.

Rat No. 7 died on the night of February 21, seven days after the first feeding, and five days after the second feeding. Post mortem examination the following day showed many live adult trichinae; a number of the females were depositing their embryos. The duodenum and a portion of the jejunum were fed to a guinea pig. This pig was killed April 4, or 42 days after feeding. No trichinae were found on examination of the diaphragm.

A white mouse was fed trichinous meat on February 18, 1916. The mouse died February 23, five days after feeding. Post mortem examination the following day revealed many adult live trichinae in the intestine; full grown embryos were observed in the uteri of all the females examined. The entire alimentary tract, exclusive of the stomach, was fed to a guinea pig. This pig was killed April 13, or 49 days after feeding. Examination of the diaphragm gave negative results.

Another white mouse, fed trichinous meat February 18, 1916, was killed February 28, ten days after feeding. Many adult trichinae were found in the intestine. The females examined under the microscope showed the presence of many embryos in the uterus. Some of the females were expelling fully developed embryos. The entire alimentary tract of the mouse, exclusive of the stomach, was fed to a guinea pig. This pig was killed April 22, or 53 days after feeding. Examination of the diaphragm gave negative results.

Concerning the stage at which trichinae in the muscles become infectious it is usually stated in the literature that non-encysted trichinae are not infectious. Leuckart (1860) fed a dog with muscles of a young girl containing trichinae none of which so far as observed were yet encysted. After seven days the dog was killed and its intestine was found to contain trichinae. He therefore concluded that encystment is not a necessary condition for the further development of Trichinella. It is questionable, however, whether there might not have been also encysted trichinae present in the muscle fed. Pagenstecher's experiments (Pagenstecher, 1865) throw more light on the subject, since he gives definite information concerning the age of the trichinae which he fed. Trichinous rabbit meat seventeen days after artificial infestation of the animal from which it was taken was fed to rabbits which were killed within 24 days and found to be free from trichinae. Trichinous meat from a mouse 15 days after artificial infestation failed to produce intestinal trichinosis in a rabbit which was killed 4 days after feeding. Similarly, pigs escaped intestinal trichinosis after eating rabbit meat 14 days after artificial infestation. However, another pig was fed rabbit meat 18 days after artificial infestation and when killed 9 days after feeding was found to contain small intestinal trichinae, the males measuring 0.9 mm. and the females 1.75 mm. in length. In one experiment he reports a successful infestation of a rat as a result of feeding mouse meat 15 days after artificial infestation. The rat was killed 4 days after feeding and was found to contain in the intestine 3 females with a maximum length of 1.45 mm. and 2 males. He also observed that copulation had already taken place. This experiment is open to objection, however, since the same mouse had been fed trichinous meat about three weeks previous to the infestation on the basis of which the age of the infection was computed. Pagenstecher after killing the mouse concluded that the first infestation must have been unsuccessful since he found only unencapsuled trichinae in the muscles. It is not unlikely, however, that the muscles contained encysted trichinae from the first infection, which were overlooked, and that it was these which developed into the adults found in the rat.

Goujon (1867) states that as a result of feeding trichinous meat containing non-encysted trichinae he succeeded in producing light infestations in various animals. He admits the possibility that some of the trichinae may have been encysted and concludes that the infestations produced as a result of eating meat containing unencysted parasites are much lighter than those which follow the eating of meat containing encysted trichinae.

Though the present writer has not attempted to trace all the published records of experiments on the infectiousness of trichinae

at various stages of their development in the muscles it is evident
that the general opinion is that trichinae which have not yet become
encysted are not infectious, and the results of experiments which
he has made are in harmony with this opinion as shown by the following:

Rabbit No. 1, fed trichinous meat May 22, 1917. Killed June
6, or 15 days after feeding. Post mortem revealed the presence of
many unencysted larvae in the diaphragm. Diaphragm fed to another rabbit June 6. Killed July 5, or 29 days after feeding. Diaphragm negative.

Rabbit No. 2 was forced fed trichinous meat August 2, 1917.
Killed August 20, or 18 days after feeding. Post mortem revealed
many unencysted larvae in diaphragm. Diaphragm fed to another
rabbit August 20. Killed September 18, or 29 days after feeding.
Diaphragm negative.

Rabbit No. 3, fed trichinous meat August 2, 1917. Killed August 23, or 21 days after feeding. Post mortem revealed many
faintly encysted larvae in diaphragm. The cyst wall was not very
distinct in outline under the low power of the microscope. Diaphragm fed to another rabbit August 23. Killed September 24, or
32 days after feeding. Diaphragm showed many encysted larvae.

Guinea pig No. 1, fed trichinous meat September 26, 1917.
Killed October 11, or 15 days after feeding. Post mortem showed
many unencysted larvae in diaphragm. The entire diaphragm
and portions of muscles of the thigh were fed to another guinea pig
October 11. Killed December 7, or 27 days after feeding. Diaphragm negative.

Guinea pig No. 2, fed trichinous meat September 26, 1917.
Killed October 13, or 17 days after feeding. Post mortem showed
many unencysted larvae in diaphragm. Fed the entire diaphragm
and portion of thigh to another guinea pig October 13. Killed
December 7, or 55 days after feeding. Diaphragm negative.

CONCLUSIONS: The experiments failed to show that infection
with trichinae can be produced by feeding to experimental animals
the intestinal stage of the parasites.

No infection resulted from feeding meat containing unencysted trichinae taken from animals killed 15, 17, and 18 days
after infection, respectively, but infection resulted from meat containing newly encysted trichinae taken from an animal killed 21
days after infection.

The evidence obtained from the experiments supports the generally accepted opinions that trichinae are not transmissible through the feces, that unencysted trichinae are not capable of development when meat containing them is ingested, and finally that trichinae are spread from one host to another only as a result of the swallowing of meat containing the encysted larvae of the parasites.

(We are under obligations to Dr. B. H. Ransom, Chief of the Zoological Division, Washington, D. C., for assistance in literature cited, also to Dr. L. Enos Day, in charge of the local pathological laboratory, of Chicago, Illinois, where the work was done, for courtesies extended.)

LITERATURE CITED

GOUJON, L. 1867. Expériences sur la Trichina spiralis. J. de l'anat. et physiol. [etc.], Par., v. 4 (5), Sept.-Oct., pp. 529-533.

HÖYBERG, H. M. 1907. Beitrag zur Biologie der Trichine. Ztschr. f. Tiermed., Jena, v. 11 (3), pp. 209-235.

LEUCKART, K. G. F. R. 1860. Untersuchungen über Trichina spiralis. Zugleich ein Beitrag zur Kenntniss der Wurmkrankheiten. 57 pp., 11, 2 pls., 4°. Leipzig & Heidelberg.

PAGENSTECHER, H. A. 1865. Die Trichinen. Nach Versuchen im Auftrage des Grossherzoglich Badischen Handelsministeriums ausgeführt am zoologischen Institute in Heidelberg von Christ. Jos. Fuchs und H. Alex. Pagenstecher. 1 p. 1, 116 pp., 2 pls., 4°. Leipzig.

SALZER, BENJAMIN F. 1916. A study of an epidemic of fourteen cases of trichinosis with cures by serum therapy. Preliminary communication. [Read before Meet. of Staff, Path. Lab., Mount Sinai Hosp., N. Y., July 12.] J. Am. M. Ass., Chicago, v. 67 (8), Aug. 19, pp. 579-580.

STAEUBLI, CARL. 1909. Trichinosis. xii+295 pp., 12 1, charts, pls. A-B, 1-12. 4°. Wiesbaden.

—Dr. O. H. Davison, formerly at Cheyenne, Wyo., has been transferred to Denver, Colo.

—Dr. G. H. Bruns, formerly at Birmingham, Ala., is now located at Baton Rouge, La.

—The annual meeting of the Oklahoma State Veterinary Medical Association will be held at the Agricultural College, Stillwater, Okla., July 10 and 11, 1918.

—Dr. James G. Jervis has removed from Vancouver, B. C., to Strathmore, Alberta.

—Dr. H. E. States, formerly Chief Veterinarian for the Board of Health at Detroit, Mich., has been promoted to the directorship of the Dairy and Food Department.

THE SIGNIFICANCE OF THE SEVERAL KINDS OF INFLAMMATION

Samuel Howard Burnett, Ithaca, N. Y.

Inflammation is the local tissue-reaction to an injury. It is the record of the interaction of the injury and the resisting and healing forces of the body. The characters in which the record is written are pathological processes. It is possible for those understanding the language in which they are written to read them and understand their meaning. Some of the characters are large print; others are less easily seen. To get the full meaning of any inflammation the fine print as well as the coarse needs to be read.

The important factors that determine the tissue reaction are the cause of the injury and the resisting and healing forces of the body. Each of these may be complex. There are other factors also: the length of time the cause acts, the nature and the position of the tissue affected, and secondary tissue changes produced by or following preceding changes.

Sometimes the cause may be determined by the character of the lesion produced. Mechanical injuries produce different effects from those produced by chemicals or bacteria. Naturally occurring suppurative inflammation is due to certain bacteria, but may be produced by chemicals. There are, however, certain differences between chemically produced suppuration and that due to bacteria, though the difference may be mainly due to the length of time the cause acts. Different groups and different varieties of bacteria produce different effects. Though the differences may not be great, there is a marvelous variety in the effects produced by different causes. In general the nature of the cause can be detected from the lesion produced. The more definite knowledge one has of the reaction to different irritants the fewer exceptions will he find to the foregoing statement. It seems reasonable to expect the same cause acting on the same kind of tissue to produce the same result each time. So far as known, it is true qualitatively. The best apparent exceptions are found in inflammations due to infection. In general bacteria that produce suppuration do not produce fibrinous inflammation; those that produce diphtheritic inflammation do not produce suppuration. To be more definite, *Bact. tuberculosis* produces a reaction characterized by the multiplication and accumulation of cells resembling endothelial cells. Necrosis occurs soon afterwards in the center of the lesion. When suppuration occurs in a tuberculous lesion it is supposedly due to other organisms. The same thing is probably true of actinomycosis and botryomycosis. Some cases of glanders of lymph glands may prove to be an exception. It is a more reasonable view that suppurative glanders is to be classed as a quantitative change, because even in the small caseous glanders nodules, found in the lungs, polymorphonuclear leucocytes are present as a part of the reaction. Changes in the character of the reaction due to changes in the intensity of the irritant or the strength or weakness of the resistance are quantitative changes. For example, a certain irritant may produce death of tissue at the center of action while a little farther away degeneration and still farther proliferation of tissue are produced.

Another very important factor is the relative intensity of the irritant. Variation in the intensity or strength of the irritant, in the resisting powers of the body, or in both produces differences in the tissue-reaction. A moderate degree of heat may produce redness and swelling of the tissue affected. A greater degree may produce blisters and a still greater degree may produce death of tissue with a more intense reaction. Strong nitric acid produces a different effect from that produced by the same acid diluted. Different effects may be produced with pathogenic bacteria by inoculating virulent or attenuated cultures of the same organism. Inoculation of an attenuated culture of anthrax bacteria may produce some active hyperemia and a moderate infiltration of leucocytes with a small amount of fluid exudate. A somewhat more virulent culture of the same organism produces a more marked migration of leucocytes and death of tissue with abscess formation. The same kind of variation may be produced by using a virulent culture with individuals of lessened or increased resistance.

Variation is produced also by differences in the length of time the injurious agent acts. A cause acting continuously produces a different reaction from one that acts momentarily. An injury that acting once would produce little or no noticeable change may, when repeated several times, produce a marked tissue-reaction.

The nature of the tissue affected makes some difference in the reaction. A reaction in vascular tissue differs from one in nonvascular tissue. A blow on the eye produces a different result from one on the flank. Exudation from the skin tends to produce vesicles and blisters, but not from a mucous surface. Inflammation of a serous surface shows a greater tendency to spread than one of a cutaneous or mucous surface. Excretory organs sometimes are injured in removing irritating material.

Some variation is due to the position of the affected tissue. Suppuration in deep or superficial tissue presents differences in appearance. An abscess does not look like an ulcer though the process may be the same.

So much for the factors that produce variation in the appearance in different cases of inflammation. The meaning of the inflammation is not to be found in any process that may be present taken by itself. The meaning is to be discovered by a study of the entire reaction. There are, however, certain general indications given by the predominance of one process or general feature of the reaction.

There are certain conditions that require some time for their development, as the formation of any considerable amount of connective tissue. Certain other changes found indicate that the condition was too severe to have acted very long. Marked hyperemia or much fibrinous exudate indicates an early stage of a very severe reaction. Necrosis without a beginning even of an attempt at encapsulation is an earlier stage than a partially encapsulated necrosis. When encapsulation has begun it is an indication of the presence of considerable resisting power. A wide-spread process, as necrosis or production of tissue, means less resistance than a restricted or circumscribed process. Some specimens of tuberculosis of the omentum furnish an instructive example of this. Cases occur that begin as scattered, sharply defined, separate nodules, each surrounded by fibrous connective tissue. The patient at that time had considerable resistance. Later each nodule may be surrounded by young fibrous connective tissue that spreads out on the omentum. They are no longer sharply localized lesions. The condition has become more wide-spread which indicates that the animal's resistance is much lowered.

A parenchymatous inflammation may be present in an acute or a chronic disease. It may have been of short or longer duration. It is not difficult to determine which it is by the processes present. For example, if there is much hyperemia or there is recent hemorrhage it is of short duration. If there is proliferation of connective tissue as part of the same reaction it is a longer

· standing condition. Parenchymatous inflammations are due to chemical injury. They may be inorganic or organic poisons. The harmful substances may be elaborated by bacteria and even by the body itself.

Hemorrhagic inflammation is due to a severe injury, usually mechanical, or bacterial. It may be due to intoxication. The best examples of hemorrhagic inflammation due to infection are due to filterable viruses, as hog cholera. These may not be bacteria. Hemorrhagic inflammation occurs in acute disease. Slight hemorrhage may occur in chronic disease.

Fibrinous inflammation is also a severe condition. Much fibrinous exudate signifies a condition of short duration. A slight amount of fibrinous exudate may occur in a chronic condition. A healing fibrinous inflammation should not be mistaken for a chronic productive inflammation. Fibrinous inflammation indicates an infection.

Serous inflammation is usually of longer standing and of less severity than a fibrinous or hemorrhagic inflammation. It is usually due to infection.

A purulent inflammation may occur in an acute or a chronic disease. The naturally occurring cases are due to infection. Experimentally it may be produced by chemicals.

A catarrhal inflammation is generally due to infection. It may be due to intoxication, as inhalation of irritating gases. It may be acute or chronic.

A suppurative inflammation may be an acute or a chronic condition. The extent of the process, the presence of connective tissue, and its amount give valuable information as to the duration of the condition. Suppuration is practically always due to infection by bacteria. It may be produced by certain chemicals.

Diphtheritic inflammation occurs only in severe and recent conditions. It is due to infection.

Caseous inflammation is met with in long standing conditions. Caseation requires some time for its production. It occurs in certain infections.

Gangrenous inflammation shows a severe condition of short duration. It is due to infection.

Chronic productive inflammation indicates a mild injury. It is due to mild repeated mechanical injury, to the continued action of a low grade infection or a weak poison.

These observations on the general significance of different kinds of inflammation are not intended to be more than suggestive. Each case must be considered by itself and its meaning found after a study of all of the processes present. Apparently subordinate processes may convey a good deal of information. The condition needs to be studied as a whole, not as a collection of separate processes.

———◆———

HORSE MEAT

GEO. H. GLOVER, Fort Collins, Colo.

Recently there has been considerable agitation respecting the use of horseflesh as human food. Considering the fact that food in abundance is a dire necessity at this time and that there are already several horse markets legalized in this country, and more contemplated, the use of horse meat for food has become a real vital issue. There are four important considerations in connection with the use of horse meat for human food, none of which should be overlooked or treated as of trivial importance.

PALATABILITY. The objection to horse meat is purely esthetic. The meat of the whale and shark, once despised because of their cannibal existence, is now relished, indeed is considered a delicacy. Livers, brains, lymph glands, intestines, are all objected to esthetically but necessity forced the issue. The meat of the prairie dog is both palatable and wholesome. If this animal had fortunately been named the prairie squirrel, we would not now be devising ways and means to exterminate him, for we would be in the position of the Maori chief, who, being asked about his enemies, replied, "I have no enemies, I have eaten them all". Many things long neglected are now being utilized for food. I have before me a bulletin which advocates the growing of sunflowers for ensilage. The loveapple (tomato), now a staple food, was for a long time grown as an ornamental flower and as a curiosity. True, it belongs to a poison weed family, so does the wonderberry and the potato.

It is difficult to see wherein we can have a well-founded antipathy to horse meat if we stop to consider the cleanly habits of the horse and the food he eats. He lives entirely upon the richest and cleanest cereals, the most succulent grasses and will go for days until almost famished before he will drink stagnant water. France is one of the older civilizations and her people have developed the finer sensibilities, and in all that pertains to a high appreciation of the esthetic, they are surpassed by no other nation. We have been in the habit of going to Paris for our fashions. The French people have long eaten horse meat and by many it is preferred to all other meats.

HEALTH. The horse is healthier than the cow or pig and has fewer transmissible diseases than any of the flesh producing animals, barring possibly the sheep. The horse is practically immune to tuberculosis while 9 per cent of hogs and 4 per cent of our beef cattle under federal inspection are condemned as unfit for food. With a mortality from tuberculosis that is decimating the human race, and in this country where less than half of the meat consumed is subject to any sort of inspection, we are facing a problem that must eventually be met by drastic measures. Horse meat is easily digestible, is wholesome and safe.

COMPETITION IN MEAT PRODUCTION. If horseflesh is used for food, it will mean a decreased demand for, but not necessarily a decreased consumption of beef, pork and mutton. It will simply mean that our people at home and our allies abroad will be better fed. It will help win the war.

One conscientious objector, overlooking the importance of the "army behind the army" and forgetting that for the time being self interest must, during this crisis, be subservient to the one proposition of winning the war, expressed his sentiment in the following words: "Personally I feel that we are eating enough varieties of meat now and that our meat producers are having a hard enough time in keeping ahead of the game without being obliged to suffer new competition by the slaughter of discarded, undersized, and generally useless horses. Would you like to eat a pot roast with potato pancakes made from a rump of a $5 steed?" Necessity will not be balked by the self interests of the producer. There is a demand for meat and the producer must not, and should not expect, to revel in high prices while we are fighting to save the world from autocracy and millions are hungry or starving in Europe. There is no possibility of horse meat coming into general use in the near future. Cowmen, sheepmen and bogmen need have no fear that all of the old discarded, and generally useless horses are going to be rounded up, slaughtered, and thrown on the market in competition with their products, this year or next; the use of horse meat must come gradually, which it will. This thing will necessarily come slowly and as prejudice against horse meat subsides, the producer will have ample time to adjust his business to the end that he may find the growing of horses for food as profitable as any other, and he will be in on the ground floor.

A WAR NECESSITY. How long shall we continue to condone a moral wrong because it is an established precedent and because of a foolish and groundless sentiment? We have a penchant for following the "calf paths of the mind". The precedent thing is not necessarily the right thing. Our veneration for precedent is worthy of a better cause. This war is teaching us many useful lessons, not the least of which is economy. We are now paying the price of our past prodigality and wastefulness. The western plains bear silent testimony to the wholesale death of animals from starvation and neglect. With cattle under old range conditions, every summer was a feast and each winter meant a famine. Cows and even heifer calves have gone to the block and now we stand aghast at our food shortage.

In the war ridden countries food substitutes are saving the day. In this country we are now getting our first regular ration of food substitutes but they are in the main wholesome and palatable. Food substitution in the fighting countries of Europe means something very different and this thing may be in store for us in the very near future. In our large cities, even now, the high price of beef, pork and mutton has made their consumption almost prohibitive for the poor, while pneumonia, tuberculosis and other diseases stalk in the wake of the insufficiently nourished. A rump roast of horse meat and potato pancakes would not only look mighty good to many an American today, but it would be consumed with all of the mad relish and gluttony of a famished denizen of the jungle, by many a starving refugee in the war scourged districts of the Orient. Because we who are well fed decline a horse pot roast is there any sane argument why we should deny it to those who want it? Let us not forget that there are many foreigners in this country who must be fed and who from habit do not have a natural aversion to horse meat. Certainly we cannot consistently deny wholesome horse meat to these people, then why not legalize horse markets in our large cities at least?

It has been fully demonstrated that we Yankees dearly love hog and that is why we eat so many of them. The hog fed on garbage and offal, wallowing in the filth of contaminated pens, constitutes our favorite meat. From the hog we contract tuberculosis, tapeworms, trichina and other diseased conditions. Horse meat transmits none of these diseases to the human. There are thousands of horses living under the healthiest possible conditions on our western plains that might constitute no meager food supply were it not for the sickly, senseless sentiment against eating horse meat. "Consistency, thou art a jewel."

We have our wheatless days, our meatless days, and smokeless days seem imminent as an economic necessity, and other days are coming before this thing is over. We are sending up special petitions on high for more abundant harvests when at our very door is a possible food supply that our unwarranted prejudice has thoughtlessly eliminated.

The only argument presented is, that we are not in the habit of eating horse meat, we are not obliged to eat it, and by the eternal we are not going to eat it. This argument is in the first line trench and seemingly hard to dislodge, even though it has no weapons to defend it. The stories we read of "down and out" hack horses in Paris, finding their way to the horse markets have no doubt stimulated the prejudice in this country but we must remember that aged cows and bulls are not always consigned to the fertilizer tank, if they are healthy, even in cultured America. Horse markets should, of course, be subject to the same efficient meat inspection regulations that now prevail under federal supervision.

If we do not want to eat horse meat we should for the sake of suffering humanity, and winning the war, not object to those eating it who want it, and who are starving, remembering that before this thing is over we may be glad to eat potato pancakes with horse pot-roast gravy, for the stomach's sake.

—The North Carolina State Veterinary Examining Board will hold a meeting June 25 at High Point. The State Veterinary Medical Association will meet at the same place June 26 and 27.

—The Colorado Veterinary Medical Association will hold its next meeting at Fort Collins, June 27 and 28.

THE VALUE OF THE LABORATORY TO MEAT INSPECTION

R. H. Cook, V.S.

Veterinary Inspector, Health of Animals Branch, Dept. of Agriculture, Canada

The intimate association of meat inspection and the laboratory is very essential to the best understanding of all affections of meat food products—they go together—in fact, they are inseparable. This does not necessarily mean that every inspector must be an expert pathologist or bacteriologist, or on the other hand that every bacteriologist must be an artist on meat inspection. As a matter of fact the improvement of each in the other's line would be quite in keeping. Nevertheless we each have our special field of importance and each forms a very necessary cog in the wheel which spells efficiency.

These are the days of specialization and with the intensive analysis now necessary and exacted it is next to impossible for one individual to master all the specialties. We have, therefore, to content ourselves and confine ourselves more or less to our own particular line and work it to the best advantage.

To get the best results from our specialty we are compelled to call in consultation our pathologist on every occasion in which there is a doubt as to the character of the diseased affection. These calls should be in proportion to our knowledge. This does not necessarily follow that the inspector making the fewest calls is the best diagnostician. Human nature is so prone to let things go by default—it is the easy way—the line of least resistance, but it gets us nowhere worth while and eventually lands us in an abyss of ignorance.

I wish to show the relationship of post mortem inspection and the laboratory and emphasize the necessity of a knowledge of their interdependence.

In our own work how often do we hear the remark—this continual grind, the sameness, the monotony? These feelings are real and tangible. They are the bugbear of every line of work. They arise too often from lacking interest on the part of the supervisor. They are also on the other hand the natural product of the individual who confessedly knows all that he wants to know—in other words, the sealed book. To overcome such a condition a special effort is well worth while.

Our work, which carries with it the investigation of diseased conditions and their relation to the animal economy, is but in its infancy and the room for development and the newness which awaits us at every turn should make our work most interesting.

All abnormal conditions are due to a cause. An effort should be made to demonstrate or prove the causal agency and the actual tissue changes produced. Whatever condition arises which has not been personally noted previously should be laid aside for the pathologists' investigation and report. The laboratory is filled with appliances for all the finer pathological tissue changes and is also well equipped for bacterial examination, culture and isolation. We feel quite safe in their hands. Associated with this safeguard the macroscopic or gross appearance on our part must not be overlooked if we wish to benefit by our work and that of the pathologist. Again much interest and benefit may be derived by working out many of these problems and demonstrations for ourselves, aided of course by previous advice. Time and inclination are the absolutely necessary requisites for commencement. If we can only get a sufficient quantity of inclination gathered together, it is marvelous where the time comes from.

While our department does not furnish us locally with an oil immersion lens, microscope and a local outfit for specimen preparation and staining, they have provided us with a fully equipped laboratory at Ottawa, which is ours to use whenever we have the inclination. Locally the department has favored us with a good low power lens microscope and it is wonderful the field that can be covered with it. For all tissues and all tissue changes caused by bacterial or any other cause, this is the only medium for examination either here or at the laboratory. This includes the pathological tissue changes caused by the bacillus of tuberculosis, *Bacillus pyogenes,* actinomycosis, in fact, everything we meet—all parasites, tumor formations or abnormal conditions, even the *Streptothrix actinomyces,* the cause of actinomycosis. So much then for the low power.

While the oil immersion lens is indispensable for bacterial research we need not be discouraged because it is confined to the laboratory. We have a big field to work without it. The equipment for pathological research can quite readily be improvised when even access to a gas jet, wash basin, running water and freezer can be obtained. The same obtains if we wish to enter on a small scale the bacterial research—the only additional requisite being the necessity of purchasing an oil immersion lens. While the microscopic outlook is quite within our province and should afford a means of increasing the interest in our work, it also has the effect of raising the standard of education and efficiency for the profession. Nevertheless, we must lay special emphasis on the macroscopic and gross view and never lose sight of its importance to a quick and correct diagnosis. A correct diagnosis means very much. Our reports are compiled and are a reflex of our ability as diagnosticians. From these reports are collected the statistics of diseases for the state. How easy a matter it would be to alter those statistics and give a very injurious conception of the amount of certain contagious diseases in our country. This is very important—the tuberculosis and actinomycosis reports have been at times very badly mixed. We can recall from earlier days a time when every lesion found in the submaxillary gland in cattle was recorded as tuberculosis. The only actinomycotic affections noted were of the superior and inferior maxillary bone. The answer to this was, what difference does it make, the head was tanked? This filled the bill as far as the tank was concerned, but how does it look? It contributes nothing to thoroughness; it bungles our work; it makes misleading and injurious statistics; it discredits our knowledge before all those who may happen to examine our reports; as any critic worth while knows that tuberculosis in the submaxillary gland of cattle is a very rare occurrence and is usually, when it does occur, associated with a general glandular affection of the carcass.

A study of the gross or macroscopic appearances are of equal import to the study of microscopic appearances. A commonly recognized good practice with pathologists is to use the lowest power lens possible in order to view a specimen. First, necessarily, comes the naked eye and when properly trained its correctness is surprising. It is splendid practice to forward to the pathologist every specimen where the disease lesion varies from the known macroscopic characteristic.

Meat inspectors and the laboratory are so interdependent and inter-related that we cannot help venturing a hope that the barrier of time and space may at some early day be removed and that we may have a sister laboratory established here in our midst as it were. Meat is one of the most important constituents in our midst.

To be able to judge of its freshness and freedom from disease is of great practical value.

If this practicable value of individual judgment can be supplemented by laboratory methods that will tend to unify that judgment, then, so much the better. If by supplementary laboratory investigation the public can obtain fuller protection in the character of the food that comes to his table, he is justified in demanding this protection and authorities responsible for food surveillance must provide it. Again, many of our judgments are based upon preliminary laboratory research, for example, tuberculosis and tubercular processes had to be first demonstrated by laboratory workers before our judgment and disposition of tubercular animals could be even approximately formulated or before our knowledge of the infectivity of the bovine type of bacillus to man could be established. In short, systems of food control are based almost entirely upon the results of medical and veterinary laboratory research. If it be true then that the laboratory is the forerunner of scientific inspection of meat and food products, it follows logically that the laboratory will even bear an intimate and inseparable relationship to practical post mortem inspection upon the floor of the slaughter house. This dependence of all practical sanitary control upon laboratory methods is too often unrecognized by practical sanitarians. As a concrete argument let us consider what significance meat or milk inspection would have if it had not been demonstrated that the flesh of those animals on which we depend largely for our meat is structurally similar to our own bodies, that there is physiologically an intimate relationship between the lower animals and ourselves, and that the diseases to which food animals are subject are identical with or allied to our own, all of which evidence has been revealed by laboratory methods. The important relationship of the laboratory to practical meat inspection is fully recognized by many European countries, also in the United States where in the large packing house centers there is a chemical and bacteriological laboratory maintained in connection with each chain of houses. The function of these laboratories is to make bacteriological and pathological judgment in cases where the inspection is in doubt, or where an unusual case comes under observation. To assist in definitely outlined problems in connection with the basis of judgment and to secure the efficiency of processing in terms of bacteriology.

· These laboratories provide great educational features not only for the men actively concerned with the laboratory end of the work, but also for the inspectors who submit their specimens for examination. Having the advantage of comparing the macroscopic and the microscopic characters of their specimens, they are able to form a more intelligent opinion as to the nature of the lesion— a knowledge which usually serves them in subsequent experience.

The level headed packer, also, has seen the significance of laboratory investigation for controlling the processes of preservation and the treatment of their products, for in many establishments they now have fully equipped laboratories in charge of well paid laboratory workers whose sole concern is to keep tab on the products of the establishment with a view to uniformity and to experiment with newer and simpler methods of handling.

The preservation of food by sterilization is merely the practical and wide application of a laboratory method. This is a discovery of vital economic importance for it means the saving of a large amount of food, but like all laboratory methods adopted for commercial purposes, entrusted sometimes to employees who do not understand the fundamental principle involved, it may become a dangerous factor if uncontrolled; since too much may be expected from the process. It is not always recognized that changes may occur in the food owing to the development of poisonous properties from ptomaines or toxins that no amount of heating will render inert. It is within probability that systematic laboratory analysis of the constituents of canned food products and sausages would lessen the danger of food poisoning. Rapid methods of analysis could doubtless be evolved whereby a batch of canned goods or sausages would not be held too long to make such procedure impracticable.

After a little experimentation definite standards might be arrived at by quantitative bacterial examination, just as we have such standards for measuring the relative cleanliness of milk. It is just as offensive to preserve unclean meat products as it is to pasteurize dirty germ laden milk and say it is fit for human consumption. This latter practice would not be tolerated by milk sanitarians.

It is the tendency to consider many of the conditions met with in practical meat inspection as settled questions. Even conditions of common occurrence and wide distribution like tuberculosis present problems that have not been fully studied by experimental methods. It may be that when investigators go more deeply into the problems of tuberculosis that our judgment now based very much on empirical factors or because it is the custom to dispose of affected carcasses this or that way in other countries—may be completely revolutionized. May it not be possible that future experimental data will establish a safe and quick method of differentiating between active and inactive lesions, or in the case where we find active macroscopic lesions in a group of glands in one part of the body, are we sure that the invading organism is not at work in another group of glands in another part of the body but owing to insufficient activity or to increased resistance of the tissues no structural change is yet evident to the naked eye? Thus a case might well be classed as localized according to our standards of judgment, while in reality it is a generalized case potentially.

———•———

CLINICAL AND CASE REPORTS

STUDIES IN ABDOMINAL PURULENT CONDITIONS OF THE HEN AND SOME STUDIES IN THE RESISTANCE OF THE FOWL TO THE PUS PRODUCING ORGANISMS

B. F. KAUPP, Pathologist, N. C. Experiment Station, West Raleigh, N. C.

Purulent peritonitis of the fowl is frequently observed, especially in the heavy laying hen. In this article there are recorded some typical cases and also some studies in experimental inoculation of birds with the various common pus producing organisms. The first two cases, also case 5, are hens that died from purulent conditions. Cases 3 and 4, also case No. 6, were cases used in experimental inoculations.

CASE NO. 1. PROTOCOL. Date of death, November 11, 1916.

Subject.—A nine-months-old Single Comb Rhode Island Red hen.

Head.—The unfeathered regions were a purplish-pink in color.

Mouth.—There was some slimy mucous in the mouth.

General condition.—The general condition of the plumage was good. The carcass had a fair amount of fat. The crop contained a pultaceous mass.

The internal organs.—The liver appeared dark but was normal in size. The gall bladder was full of bile. The peritoneal surfaces were covered by a mildew-like material. The carcass was cold due to the fact that it had been in refrigeration over night. This condition may be, at least partially, due to this cause.

The spleen was normal in size. The intestines appeared normal except for the above described condition. The small intestines contained a small amount of ingesta and some gas. The large intestines and caeca were in a similar condition to the small intestines. The pancreas appeared normal.

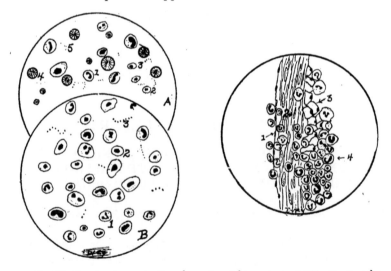

Fig. No. 1. A—A preparation from the right ureter and kidney. 1, polymorphonuclear leucocyte or pus cell; 2, mononuclear pus cell; 3, a cell somewhat the shape of a thrombocyte; 4, sodium urate crystal; 5, streptococci.

B—From the peritoneal fluid of the purulent peritonitis case No. 1. polymorphonuclear pus cell; 2, mononuclear pus cell; 3, streptococci. A composite drawing from purulent peritonitis.

Fig. No. 2. A section of the wall of the right ureter. 1, the epithelial cells lining the lumen; 2, the wall invaded with polymorphonuclear and mononuclear pus cells; 3, fat cells outside the wall; 4, pus cells.

The kidneys were a light mottled gray. The anterior lobe of each kidney appeared highly congested and the appearance of cloudy swelling was present. The collecting tubules were dammed up with urinary sediment. The ureters were distended by the same.

The ovary was inactive and of a pinkish color.

. MICROSCOPIC STUDY. The right kidney contained a thin slimy secretion which, upon a microscopic examination, was found to contain myriads of short chains of small cocci. The urinary sediment of the left ureter was somewhat thicker than that of the right. (See Fig. 1.)

There was present in the abdominal cavity about five cubic centimeters of a milky, thin purulent material containing myriads of short chained streptococci.

Abundant pus cells of both polymorphonuclear and mononuclear varieties were present. The urine was loaded with crystals of sodium urate among which are found masses of the streptococci. Smears made from the renal substance likewise contained myriads of streptococci.

Stained smears from the pleura, lung blood, and heart blood all were negative for streptococci.

Tissue studies:

The spleen appeared normal.

The pancreas appeared normal.

The ureter wall was thickened. At this point the inner wall was lined with squamous epithelium. Pus cells appeared in the lumen, outside the wall and scattered throughout the wall. Figure 2 shows a drawing from a section. 1 indicates the epithelial cells lining the lumen. At 2 may be seen the connective tissue making up the bulk of the walls together with their nuclei. 3 shows fat cells which are adherent to the outside of the ureter wall. A group of polymorphonuclear leucocytes were piled up against the outer wall.

The kidney showed both active and passive congestion. Cloudy swelling was present. The collecting tubules were packed with sodium urate crystals. Pus, blood cells and streptococci were found in the various sections of the renal tubules. Some contained blood indicating hemorrhage into the tubules.

The peritoneum.—Purulent peritonitis was present.

Focal areas of the renal tissue were invaded with polymorphonuclear and mononuclear cells.

The ovary was normal.

. The liver was congested, showing both active and passive congestion. Cloudy swelling and hemosiderosis were present.

SUMMARY. Purulent peritonitis was studied in a Single Comb Rhode Island Red hen.

The purulent peritonitis was generalized.

A quantity of thin liquid pus, containing streptococci and pus cells, was found in the peritoneal cavity.

The inflammatory processes involved the serous coverings, ureter and renal tissue. The liver also showed the results of irritating products absorbed from the abdominal cavity.

CASE NO. 2. PROTOCOL. Date of death, November 20th, 1916.

Subject.—An eight-months-old Silver Campine pullet. Leg band No. 254 N. C. E. S.

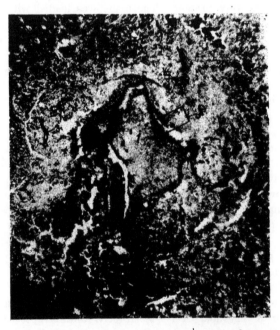

FIG. NO. 3. A photomicrograph of a section of the right kidney of case No. 2. Purulent inflammation of the right abdominal air sac. 1, focal area of necrosis; 2, fibroblastic area; 3, blood vessels; 4, area of tubules.

Head.—The unfeathered regions were a purplish red.

Mouth.—Normal.

General condition.—The bird was rather thin in flesh. Upon opening the abdominal cavity there appeared an unnatural sac-like body which occupied the posterior right abdominal quadrant and in the posterior region of the right abdominal air sac. The surface appeared pinkish and the blood vessels were congested.

This sac-like body was punctured by laboratory methods and smears made and stained. Myriads of pus cells were found in the smears and many fine, slender and rather short bacilli. Stained smears from the heart blood were negative for microorganisms.

This body proved to be an abscess, the walls of the right ab-

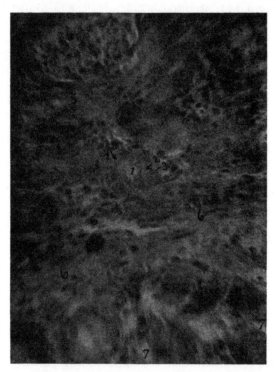

FIG. No. 4. A photomicrograph of higher magnification as indicated from Fig. No. 3. 1, lumen of convoluted tubule; 2, cell of tubule; 3, its nucleus showing nucleoli; 4, these cells are in a state of cloudy swelling and dissolution as indicated at 4; 5, collecting tubules filled with polymorphonuclear and mononuclear cells; 6, fibroblastic zone; 7, caseating mass.

dominal air sac forming its walls. To put it another way, there was a suppurative inflammation of the right abdominal air sac. The walls of the sac were greatly thickened and the cavity was distended with the purulent products.

This abscess measured 8x5 cm in two of its diameters. It contained a batter-like grainy pus of a whitish color.

The ureters, especially the right, was greatly distended with the urinary sediment.

The kidneys appeared mottled and were blocked with urinary sediment.

Cultures were made from the bacilli found so numerous in the pus and in pure cultures. 4 c.c. of a four-day-old bouillon culture was inoculated intraperitoneally into a 2-year-old Single Comb White Leghorn hen on November 28, 1916, and at the time of writing this report, December 8, 1916, the hen was apparently in good health.

MICROSCOPIC STUDY. Sections of the kidney were stained with hematoxylon and eosin and clarified in beechwood creosote and mounted in Canada balsam for study. Under low magnification (6x1½) there appeared areas of focal necrosis. These areas were irregular in outline and some appeared surrounded by new forming connective tissue.

Under high magnification (6x—95x) it was found that the central part consisted of débris, a few polymorphonuclear leucocytes, and many large disintegrating cells with rather large round nuclei —probably mostly disintegrating renal cells. (See Fig. 3.) Some of the nuclei were pyknotic and there was some evidence of karyorrhexis. There were many large mononuclear cells with acidophile granules.

Surrounding this caseating mass there is noted an area of fibro-blasts, indicating the commencement of capsule or limiting membrane formation. (See Fig. 4.) Just outside of this second zone there was noted an area in which the cells of the renal tubules were in a state of cloudy swelling and many, especially the collecting tubules, were filled with polymorphonuclear leucocytes. Many of these cells showed either pyknosis or karyorrhexis. Many cells were in a state of dissolution, the nuclei having partially or completely disappeared.

The kidney was in a state of passive and active congestion.

The liver showed passive congestion and hemosiderosis.

SUMMARY. Purulent inflammation of the right abdominal air sac was studied in a Silver Campine hen.

The abdominal air sac was greatly enlarged, walls thickened, and its cavity filled with a granular pasty pus.

A small slender bacillus was found in myriads in the pus, apparently in pure cultures, but one inoculation failed to prove it pathogenic.

The purulent inflammation was confined to the air sac.

CASE No. 3. HISTORY. A four-months-old Single Comb White Leghorn cockerel was used for experimental inoculations of the *Staphylococcus pyogenes aureus*. This bird had band No. 153.

The inoculations were made intraperitoneally.

The cultures were Aii and were obtained from the research laboratories of Parke, Davis and Co., Detroit, Mich.

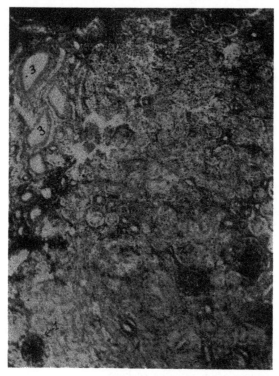

FIG. No. 5. A photomicrograph of the kidney from case No. 3. 1, the glomeruli which are apparently normal; 2, the convoluted tubules in a state of cloudy swelling, pyknotic and dying; 3, the collecting tubules.

The organism was *Staphylococcus pyogenes aureus* and was isolated from a case of furunculosis in a human subject, May 13, 1912. It had been kept growing on nutrient agar and about 70 transfers had been made up to the time the transfer was obtained by this laboratory.

This culture before being used in the fowl was inoculated subcutaneously into a rabbit weighing 430 grams. The rabbit died in 72 hours as a result of the inoculation. An abscess was found at the seat of inoculation which measured .5x2 cm. Smears showed pus and active phagocytosis. The heart blood contained the micro-organisms. The Staphylococci were reisolated and used for a second inoculation into a rabbit.

The second inoculation was made intraperitoneally into a rabbit weighing 450 grams. The rabbit died of generalized septicemia. The organism was reisolated from the peritoneal cavity, liver and heart blood.

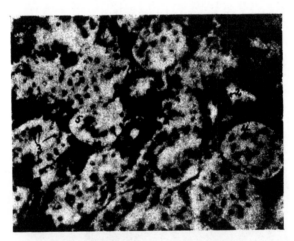

Fig. No. 6. A photomicrograph of a higher magnification of Fig. No. 5. 1, congested blood vessels; 2, tubules in the first stages of cloudy swelling; 3, cells of a convoluted tubule showing pyknosis and beginning karyorrhexis; 4, a tubule in which the cells have assumed a chaotic mass obliteratng the lumen; 5, a tubule in which the cells have begun to leave the periphery.

The organism from the rabbit dead of septicemia constituted the basis for inoculation into the cockerel.

The following inoculations were made:

Date	No. Inoculation	Kind of cult.	Wt. bird in lbs.	Remarks
11-11-1916	First	Agar slant	3.0	
11-14-1916	Second	Agar slant	2.7	
11-17-1916	Third	Agar slant	2.6	
11-21-1916	Fourth	Bouillon	2.5	Symptoms of
11-27-1916 Died				roup

This bird was kept in a comfortable coop but contracted roup on the 21st. The feed consisted of equal parts wheat, corn and oats with an occasional feed of dry mash. The bird had good water at all times. It will be noted that prior to the development of roup the bird gradually lost weight though it was on a fattening ration.

The cultures were all three days old when inoculated. The bouillon furnished products of growth as well as the microorganisms.

PROTOCOL. Pure cultures of *Staphylococcus pyogenes aureus* were isolated from the peritoneal cavity.

The head in the unfeathered regions was pale. The nostrils showed a mucopurulent discharge with characteristic odor of roup.

The carcass was emaciated. There were no visible lesions in the liver, kidneys or adrenal glands which could be attributed to the inoculations. The peritoneal cavity was quite moist. Smears from the peritoneal surfaces showed myriads of phagocyting polymorphonuclear leucocytes as well as free clusters of the inoculated bacteria.

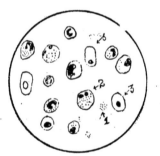

FIG. No. 7. A composite drawing of the peritoneal exudate. 1, cocci; 2, phagocytes; 3, mesothelial cells.

MICROSCOPIC STUDY. Sections of the kidneys were stained with hematoxylon and eosin and clarified in beechwood creosote and mounted in Canada balsam for study. There was noted passive congestion. Cloudy swelling with pyknosis and karyorrhexis were also present. Some portions of the sections were more badly affected than others. The cells of some of the convoluted tubules appeared swollen, occluding the lumen and in a state of cloudy swelling with some nuclei in a pyknotic and exploding condition, others in a state of lysis and faintly visible. Many of the convoluted tubules therefore were in a state of dissolution or necrosis. Many of the convoluted tubules showed their cells slightly dislodged from the periphery with occluded lumen. Some of the cells of the convoluted cells were vacuolated. The glomeruli were apparently normal. In some areas polymorphonuclear leucocytes were numerous. In still other areas hemosiderosis was noted.

The liver was in a state of congestion and cloudy swelling.

SUMMARY. The results of experimental intraperitoneal inoculations of the *Staphylococcus pyogenes aureus* were studied in a Single Comb White Leghorn cockerel.

In the later stages of the inoculation period the bird developed roup as a complicating factor.

The intraperitoneal inoculations were made from transfers of *Staphylococcus pyogenes aureus* originally isolated from a case of furunculosis of a human patient.

The organism had been passed through about 70 subcultures after isolation from the case of human furunculosis.

The organism had been passed through two rabbits, in the latter producing septicemia, to increase its virulency.

Pure cultures of the organism were isolated from the peritoneal cavity.

The kidneys showed cloudy swelling, pyknosis, karyorrhexis and passive congestion.

Hemosiderosis and leucocytic invasion were present in certain portions.

The liver was in a state of cloudy swelling and congestion.

CASE No. 4. HISTORY. A two-year-old Single Comb White Leghorn hen. This hen was a member of an egg producing flock on a Leghorn farm near Raleigh. She had been suffering for some weeks with edema of the comb and face and had been used as one of the experimental hens in intraperitoneal injections with pus producing organisms.

This hen had received several inoculations intraperitoneally of the pure cultures of Aii. The transfers were from the same culture as in case No. 3.

This hen received the following inoculations:

Date	No. Inoculation	Kind of culture	Wt. of bird in lbs.
11--11-1916	First	Agar slant	3.4
11-14-1916	Second	Agar slant	3.3
11-17-1916	Third	Agar slant	3.2
11-21-1916	Fourth	Bouillon	3.1
11-27-1916	Fifth	Bouillon	2.8
12- 4-1916	Sixth	Bouillon	2.3

The agar slant cultures were washed off in sterile physiologic salt solution. At the time of each inoculation other transfers were made, thus the age of the first culture was 3 days; the second, 3 days; the third, 3 days; the fourth, 4 days; the fifth. 6 days. and the sixth, 6 days. The bird died December 4, 1916.

PROTOCOL. Head.—The unfeathered portion of the head was very pale and edematous.

Mouth.—The mouth was normal. Eyes normal.

General condition.—The carcass was very thin in flesh. The feathers appeared in an unkempt condition.

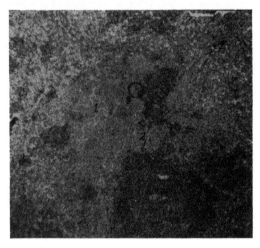

FIG. No. 8. Photomicrograph, lower power (6X-16mm), liver of case No. 4. 1, liver tissue in a state of cloudy swelling; 2, area of round cell infiltration.

The internal organs.—The liver was enlarged and was of a mottled mahogany-gray. The liver weighed 70 grams (the average weight of a normal liver of this sized hen is approximately 35 grams).

The spleen was very large and was pale grayish in color. It weighed 18 grams and measured 35 mm. x 45 mm. (the weight of a normal spleen of this sized hen should be approximately 1 gram).

Both kidneys appeared a mottled gray. The two kidneys weighed 17 grams (the two kidneys should normally weigh approximately 12 grams).

Cultures made from the splenic substance and incubated at 38° C. were negative; from the peritoneum, positive; heart blood, one colony; kidney substance, positive; liver, negative. In each case pure cultures of the organism inoculated were obtained.

MICROSCOPIC STUDY. Sections were made of the liver, spleen and kidney. These were stained with hematoxylon-eosin and clarified in beechwood creosote and mounted in natural balsam for study.

Kidney.—The cells of the convoluted tubules were in a state of cloudy swelling. Some of the cells showed pyknosis and others were in a state of karyorrhexis.

. As in case No. 3, some of the cells of the convoluted tubules were in a state of dissolution, lysis of the nuclei gradually taking place, while others showed cells separating from the periphery, forming a mass toward the center or lumen.

Areas of the renal tissue were infiltrated with small round cells. In fact, in some areas these cells were packed so closely together that only a portion of the normal arrangement of the kidney could be seen. Some of these areas showed, also, some polymorphonuclear leucocytes mixed with the round cell type.

Spleen.—The capsule was infiltrated with round cells of a similar type as observed in the sections of the kidney. (See Fig. 10.) This infiltration was in only a part of the splenic capsule area.

Islands of amyloid infiltration were found throughout the splenic pulp. (See Figs. 10 and 11.) This had, no doubt, added to make the waxy appearance of the spleen on gross examination. The amyloid material in the newer infiltrated areas was laid down in strings or columns, finally these coalesced and made large islands.

The splenic pulp was packed with small round cells as noted in the capsule. There were noted among these, many polymorphonuclear cells.

Frisch[2], in 1877, was the first to announce the experimental production of an amyloid-substance. He produced keratitis in rabbits by injection into the cornea of fresh blood from a case of anthrax. He reports positive results in 4 out of 300 cases injected. The resulting lesions gave characteristic reactions with iodine and with iodine and sulphuric acid. The reaction with aniline dyes was lacking and the material was doubly refracting. It seems doubtful, therefore, whether the substance was amyloid.

Birch-Hirschfeld[3] observed amyloid in the spleen of a rabbit that died after six weeks of chronic subcutaneous suppuration produced by the injection of pus from a case of osteomyelitis of the tibia. Other similar experiments gave negative results.   •

Bouchard[4] observed amyloid in two rabbits. One had been

injected subcutaneously with *Bacillus pyocyaneus* and subsequently four times intravenously at intervals of several months. The animal lived for about a year. Amyloid was found in the kidneys and also in the vessels of the heart and in the heart muscles. The second rabbit lived 34 days after injection with material from a human tubercular area and with a culture of tubercle bacilli. Amyloid was present in the kidneys. There was none in the heart, spleen or liver.

Czerny[5] reports that he produced amyloid in the spleen and a few vessels of the kidneys of dogs. These dogs were injected subcutaneously with turpentine. The cutaneous suppurations thus produced lasted ten to sixteen weeks. The material deposited gave the iodine-sulphuric and methyl violet reactions. Czerny believes that the iodophilic granules of leucocytes result in the formation of amyloid.

Krawkow[6] was the first to study systematically the question in a large series of different animals. He produced chronic suppuration by subcutaneous injection of broth cultures of *Staphylococcus pyogenes aureus* into dogs, rabbits, frogs, doves and hens. In eight of the twelve rabbits he produced amyloid, mainly in the spleen, in certain instances also in the gastro-intestinal tract, kidneys, liver and in the salivary glands. In dogs the results were negative after subcutaneous suppuration lasting 2 to 3 months. The results in pigeons were also negative. He found amyloid much easier of production and more extensive in hens than in other animals, three of the four hens and each of four cocks giving positive results in 1½ to 2 months.

Nowak[7] experimented on rabbits and hens and found it much easier to produce amyloid in the latter. He used staphylococcus, streptococci, *Bacillus pyocyaneus*, *Bacillus coli communis* and their sterile filtrates. He also used tuberculin, fresh and sterile pus, croton oil, and turpentine. Of seven rabbits injected with living *Staphylococcus aureus*, two, of 10 and 102 days' duration, showed amyloid in the spleen only. All hens so injected showed amyloid. Two rabbits injected with living *Bacillus pyocyaneus* were negative; two hens were positive. Two rabbits injected with living *Bacillus coli* and also two hens showed no pus and no amyloid. Rabbits injected with putrefied bouillon gave negative results, while each of two hens were positive. Of the rabbits injected with sterile filtrates of cultures of various organisms, one rabbit only, which had been injected with a filtrate of a culture of *Bacillus pyocyaneus* for 60 days, showed a few nodular deposits in the spleen which gave the amyloid reaction with aniline colors. Of nine hens injected with sterile filtrates, three were positive; two hens of these had been treated with filtrates of *Staphylococcus pyogenes aureus* cultures, and one with a filtrate of cultures of *Bacillus coli*. Of two rabbits and two hens injected for long periods with large doses of tuberculin, one of each showed nodules in the spleen which gave doubtful reactions. Of three rabbits injected with

FIG. No. 9. Photomicrograph (10X-3mm) through the edge of an area of round cell infiltration of liver as indicated at 3 Fig. No. 8. 1, liver cells; 2, round cells infiltrating this area.

fresh pus, one, in 8 days, showed amyloid in the spleen and liver; of two hens similarly injected, one showed amyloid in the spleen and liver. Rabbits injected with sterile pus were negative; two hens were both positive. Croton oil gave negative results. Of two rabbits injected with turpentine, one showed amyloid in the spleen and liver in 201 days; each of five hens so injected showed amyloid in the spleen and liver, and two of these also in the kidneys.

Bailey[8] reports repeated injections of rabbits with living *Bacillus coli communis* over long periods has resulted in the formation of amyloid deposits in the spleen, liver and kidneys. Suppurative lesions were not present in most cases and therefore not a factor in its production. The results were constant in that amyloid was found in all rabbits, eight in number, which were injected over a period of 88 days or more. Eight rabbits showed amyloid in the spleen, six of these in the kidneys, and three in the liver.

The kidneys of these eight rabbits also showed as a result of the injections a subacute and chronic glomerulitis, parenchymatous degeneration, some interstitial infiltration with round cells, and a slight cellular proliferation of connective tissue, thus resembling the chronic parenchymatous nephritis of man which is so commonly associated with amyloid disease.

In all of our intraperitoneal inoculations pure cultures of virulent microorganisms were used. In our later experiments we used bouillon cultures for the purpose of using the products of the organisms in growth as well as the organisms themselves.

Klotz[9] in his review and work in lipo-amyloid degeneration refers to the statement of Krawkow that amyloid is a homogeneous, semisolid substance deposited as a product of altered metabolism. It is said, by this investigator, to be composed of chondrotin sulphuric acid and a protein body. It is therefore a compound. The protein base which was isolated had the characters of histon. The product he worked with was from the thymus gland. It is agreed, however, that amyloid is not a true chemical entity, but that a variety of amyloid-like substances occurs which may account for the variation in the microchemical reactions frequently reported (Schmidt). Nevertheless, it would appear from Raubitscheck that the amyloid materials from different sources are similar in the biological reactions as determined by precipitin reaction after the inoculation into animals. The chondrotin sulphuric acid radical being a normal constituent of the body, being found in cartilage, elastic tissues, spleen, ligamentum nuchae, and interstitial tissues of glandular organs, is readily available and perhaps accounts for the deposition in so many tissues of the amyloid substance in general amyloidosis. The protein derivatives becoming available under the circumstances of chronic bacterial infections as well as other processes of protein decomposition, and by the interaction of a ferment the combination to form amyloid results.

In dealing with the amyloid infiltrated tissue[10] it is found to be insoluble in water, alcohol, ether, and dilute acids, and is not digested by pepsin and hydrochloric acid. It is distinguished from other homogeneous substances, except glycogen, by the fact that it is stained mahogany brown by iodin in solution. If the section containing amyloid be quickly and lightly stained in iodin solution and then transferred to sulphuric acid, the color of the amyloid will usually change at once or in a few minutes from red, through violet, to blue. Sometimes the color turns simply of a deeper brown. The hematoxylon-eosin and Van Gieson methods of staining are also used.

A microscopic study of the liver of case No. 4 showed the cells in a state of cloudy swelling. There was noted throughout the liver substance areas of round cell infiltration. A few of the vessels showed perivascular infiltration with round cells and was considered the commencement of such infiltrations. There was a few small areas of amyloid infiltration.

SUMMARY. Experimental purulent peritonitis was studied in a Single Comb White Leghorn hen. The cells of the renal tubules were in a state of cloudy swelling and many in a state of pyknosis and karyorrhexis. The kidney was infiltrated by round cells and many of the tubules were in a state of dissolution.

Islands of the splenic pulp were packed with round cells.

There were areas of amyloid infiltration in the splenic pulp.

The hepatic cells were in a state of cloudy swelling. Areas of the liver substance were packed with round cells similar to those of the kidney and spleen.

Amyloidosis was present in this case, in the spleen and to a slight degree in the liver.

From the microscopic study in this case it will be seen that the renal conditions are similar to the studies of Bailey in chronic experimental nephritis. There is a round cell infiltration in the kidneys, spleen and liver. Chronic tubular degenerative changes. That the glomerular changes were not advanced may be explained by the fact that the case was not of long standing and the intraperitoneal injections of virulent *Staphylococcus pyogenes aureus* were large and frequent.

CASE No. 5. HISTORY. A nine-months-old White Plymouth Rock pullet. This pullet was raised on the plant and was a member of a flock used for cotton seed meal experiments. She died December 15th, 1916.

PROTOCOL. The plumage appeared in a somewhat unkempt condition.

There was some evidence of a slight diarrhea.

The unfeathered portions of the head appeared in a normal condition.

The carcass was fat.

Upon opening the abdominal cavity a purulent peritonitis was observed. The intestines were adherent on their serous surfaces. The exudate was apparently fibroplastic with several cubic centimeters of thin purulent milky appearing fluid.

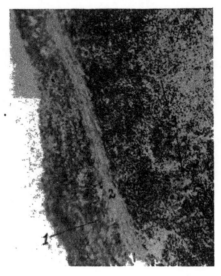

Fig. No. 10. Photomicrograph (16mm-10X) of spleen of case No. 4. 1, infiltration of superficial layer of capsule of the spleen; 2, connective tissue of lower portion of splenic capsule; 3, areas of amyloid infiltration.

Smears from the peritoneal fluid showed myriads of polymorphonuclear leucocytes. Cocci were present. The polymorphonuclear leucocytes were particularly phagocytic for these microorganisms.

Pure cultures were obtained from the peritoneal fluids indicating that this organism was the only one present.

The liver and spleen appeared normal in size. The kidneys appeared hyperemic.

MICROSCOPIC STUDY. Liver.—Both active and passive congestion is present. There was a generalized fatty degeneration with pressure atrophy of the hepatic cells.

Kidney.—Both active and passive congestion as well as cloudy swelling.

SUMMARY. One case, in a White Plymouth Rock hen, of fibro-purulent peritonitis was studied.

Smears from the peritoneal exudate showed phagocytes and a coccus, which cocci were being phagocyted.

The liver showed both active and passive congestion with generalized fatty degeneration. Pressure atrophy of the hepatic cells was present.

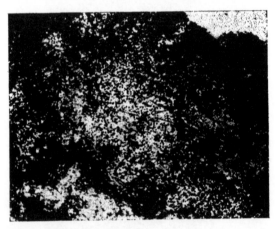

FIG. No. 11. Photomicrograph of a section through the splenic pulp of case No. 4. 1, amyloid infiltration.

The kidneys showed both active and passive congestion, and cloudy swelling with pyknosis.

CASE No. 6. HISTORY. A Single Comb Rhode Island Red hen, three years old, and a member of a breeding flock suffered with ulceration of the anus. This hen had been kept by the laboratory for twelve months previous to its death. It received enemas of a warm sulphate of iron solution after which it temporarily made an apparent recovery. It was then placed in a station breeding flock but has not laid during the year. A recurrence of the ulceration followed from which effects the hen died. There was a very offensive odor present.

PROTOCOL. The condition of the general plumage was normal.

The unfeathered portion of the head was normal.

The mouth was normal.

The carcass was emaciated.

There was noted an ulceration of the anus.

Upon opening the abdominal cavity the ovary was noted to be in a quiescent state. There were six tumor-like bodies in the oviduct though the wall of the oviduct did not appear to be thickened. Three of these tumefactions measured 1 centimeter in diameter and two measured 1 by 3 centimeters, and one 2 by 5 centimeters. Upon opening these tumor-like masses it was found that they were masses of inspissated egg material. These eggs had

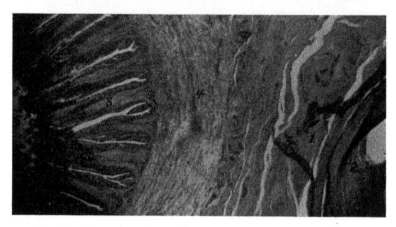

Fig. No. 12. Photomicrograph (16mm-6X) of a transverse section through the rectum and oviduct of a S. C. Rhode Island Red hen affected by ulceration. 1, musculature of the wall of the oviduct; 2, caseous products of inflammation from the ulcerated portion; 3, glands of the lower rectum; 4, the rectal musculature; 5, the ulceration.

been arrested in the oviduct owing to the involvement of the lower part of the duct by ulceration. This later resulted in the cessation of the activity of the ovary. There was no apparent fibrosis in the region of these tumefactions. The ulceration involved the anus and a portion of the rectum as well as the lower portion of the oviduct. The walls of the rectum and oviduct in the ulcerated areas were greatly thickened. There was an apparent productive inflammation.

The kidneys were greatly enlarged and of a mottled gray. Some peritonitis was present, especially in the region of the ovary and oviduct.

The liver, spleen and pancreas were apparently normal.

MICROSCOPIC STUDY. A section was made through the oviduct and rectum, including the structures that lie between. In a gross study it was noted there was a mass of material in the lumen of each with evidence of a possible inflammation and necrosis of the mucosa of both the lower portion of the oviduct and rectum.

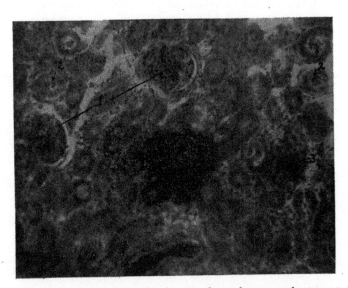

FIG. No. 13. 1, two glomerules showing glomerulitis; 2, collecting tubules containing pus cells; 3, an area infiltrated by polymorphonuclear leucocytes.

Upon examining specimens, stained with hematoxylon and eosin and clarified in beechwood creosote, it was found that the glandular cells were in a state of cloudy swelling and many in a state of necrosis. Denuded areas were noted, leaving the glandular connective tissue core exposed. (See Fig. 12.) This subepithelial layer was invaded to a more or less extent by polymorphonuclear and round cells. Ulceration of the involved mucous areas then was evident. The material in the lumen of both the rectum and oviduct consisted of material similar to that found in caseation necrosis being mostly necrosing cells, some fibrin and myriads of pus cells of both mononuclear and polymorphonuclear cell types.

A microscopic study of the kidney showed that in the medullary portion the convoluted tubules were in a state of cloudy swelling and necrosis. Some of the cells appeared granular, the nuclei

pale and finally there were cells in which the nuclei have entirely
disappeared. In some of the convoluted tubules masses of these
swollen cells filled the lumen of the tubules, the bases of many of
the cells had separated from their normal position. Some cells
were pyknotic. Finally other areas of focal necrosis were observed.

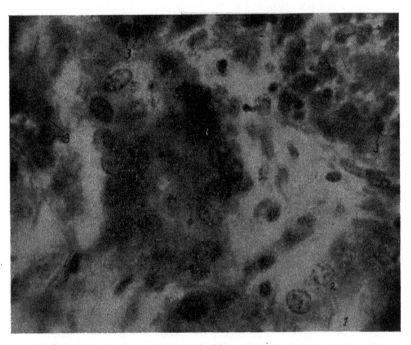

FIG. No. 14. An area of kidney highly magnified, showing cloudy swelling, cellular disintegration with light cellular invasion (first stages of necrosis). 1, lumen of tubule in which cells are in a state of cloudy swelling; 2,
a nucleus undergoing lysis; 3, cellular invasion; 4, a longitudinal section of a
tubule showing swollen and disintegrating cells obliterating the lumen.

In some areas of the medullary portion of the lobules the cells
of the collecting tubules were in all stages of albuminoid degeneration, from the early stages of cloudy swelling to complete cellular
necrosis. The collecting tubules contained from a few cells, mostly
polymorphonuclear leucocytes, to many. In fact some of the
tubules were packed with the products of inflammation. (Figures
13 and 14). There was an occasional area of cellular infiltration,
consisting mostly of polymorphonuclear with some mononuclear
leucocytes. In some areas fibrin was noted.

SUMMARY. A study was made of a S. C. Rhode Island· Red hen with ulceration of the anus and oviduct and surrounding structures involving to a more or less extent the peritoneal structures.

The case was of more than twelve months' standing. It did not yield to enemas.

The condition resulted in the cessation of the function of the ovary early in the disease.

The ulceration involved the mucosa of both the rectum and the oviduct.

A gross study of the kidneys showed them to be a mottled gray. Upon a microscopic examination of the kidney there was found cloudy swelling, cellular necrosis, glomerulitis and cellular infiltrated areas.

RESISTANCE TO INOCULATIONS. In all, 17 fowls were inoculated subcutaneously, and in the pectoral muscles. Ten of these birds were inoculated with the *Staphylococcus pyogenes aureus,* four with the *Staphylococcus pyogenes albus* and three with the *Streptococcus pyogenes.* All cultures were isolated from abscesses of either human or animal source. Three cultures were proved to possess powers of producing septicemia in rabbits. In none of these cases were abscesses produced. The quantity of organisms injected varied from one to fifty billions. In some cases the inoculations were made from bouillon cultures and in others from cultures of agar slants washed off with sterile physiological salt solution. In one case, receiving ten billions in the pectoral muscles, there followed a slight swelling which subsided in three days. In one case, a two-year-old hen, receiving fifty billions subcutaneously, and in the pectoral muscles, death ensued in about twelve hours. At autopsy there was found great edema at the seat of inoculation and pure cultures were obtained from the heart blood and from the liver. This hen and the one just previously described were inoculated by cultures of the *Staphylococcus pyogenes aureus* which had six days previously been isolated from a carbuncle from the neck of a man. These cultures were the second transfers. Thus we have in one case, receiving an unusually large injection of virulent *Staphylococcus pyogenes aureus,* septicemia, in two edema at the point of injection, and in fifteen no reaction, and in all a total absence of abscess formation.

From these tests we note that the ordinary pus producing organisms ordinarily do not produce pus in the domestic fowl.

That, so far, we have failed to produce an abscess from Staphylococci and Streptococci isolated from abscesses of human and animal sources. That birds will succumb to sufficiently large doses is rather indicated by the production of amyloidosis by repeated inoculations of Staphylococci and their products and by the production of septicemia in one case. Birds in their evolutionary ascent have come to the reptilian line and not the mammalian. In our work with drugs in making tests to determine the physiologic and the therapeutic dosages we found that birds have a great resistance to drugs, that is, it required larger doses in proportion to the weight to produce the desired result than with mammals. Thus with pus producing organisms we find great resistance. The statement has been made that the reason why pus producing organisms as well as some others did not prove to be pathogenic for the domestic fowl was because of the high temperature of the bird. To determine the normal temperature of the domestic fowl data was gathered on 50 birds of different ages and breeds. The data is as follows:

Class	Breed	Variety	Age	Sex	Temperature
American	Plymouth Rock	Barred	2½ yrs.	Hen	107.7
American	Plymouth Rock	Barred	2½ yrs.	Hen	106.4
American	Plymouth Rock	Barred	2½ yrs.	Hen	107.0
American	Wyandotte	Columbian	2½ yrs.	Hen	106.6
American	Wyandotte	Golden	2½ yrs.	Hen	108.0
American	Wyandotte	Golden	2½ yrs.	Hen	106.4
American	Rhode Island Red	Single Comb	8 mos.	Pullet	106.3
American	Rhode Island Red	Single Comb	8 mos.	Pullet	107.0
American	Rhode Island Red	Single Comb	8 mos.	Ckl.	106.6
American	Rhode Island Red	Single Comb	8 mos.	Pullet	106.6
American	Rhode Island Red	Single Comb	8 mos.	Pullet	105.2
English	Orpington	Buff	2½ yrs.	Hen	106.8
American	Plymouth Rock	Partridge	2½ yrs.	Hen	108.4
American	Plymouth Rock	White	2½ yrs.	Hen	107.4
French	Houdan	Mottled	2½ yrs.	Hen	107.0
Continental	Campine	Golden	2½ yrs.	Hen	107.4
Continental	Campine	Silver	2½ yrs.	Hen	107.6
Continental	Campine	Silver	8 mos.	Ckl.	107.0
Mediterranean	Black Spanish	White-Face	2½ yrs.	Hen	105.3
Mediterranean	Black Spanish	White-Face	2½ yrs.	Hen	105.8
Mediterranean	Leghorn	S. C. White	1½ yrs.	Hen	106.0
Mediterranean	Leghorn	S. C. White	1½ yrs.	Hen	106.2
Mediterranean	Leghorn	S. C. White	1½ yrs.	Hen	106.2
Mediterranean	Leghorn	S. C. White	1½ yrs.	Hen	107.5
Mediterranean	Leghorn	S. C. White	1½ yrs.	Hen	106.4
Mediterranean	Leghorn	S. C. White	1½ yrs.	Hen	106.6
Mediterranean	Leghorn	S. C. White	1½ yrs.	Hen	105.2
Mediterranean	Leghorn	S. C. White	1½ yrs.	Hen	107.2
Mediterranean	Leghorn	S. C. White	1½ yrs.	Hen	106.2
Mediterranean	Leghorn	S. C. White	1½ yrs.	Hen	106.6
Mediterranean	Leghorn	S. C. White	1½ yrs.	Cock	107.3

Class	Breed	Variety	Age	Sex	Temperature
Mediterranean	Leghorn	S. C. White	1½ yrs.	Hen	106.4
Mediterranean	Leghorn	S. C. White	1½ yrs.	Hen	106.8
Mediterranean	Leghorn	S. C. White	1½ yrs.	Hen	105.9
Mediterranean	Leghorn	S. C. White	8 mos.	Pullet	105.4
Mediterranean	Leghorn	S. C. White	8 mos.	Pullet	105.8
Mediterranean	Leghorn	S. C. White	8 mos.	Pullet	106.7
Mediterranean	Leghorn	S. C. White	8 mos.	Pullet	106.3
Mediterranean	Leghorn	S. C. White	8 mos.	Pullet	106.2
Mediterranean	Leghorn	S. C. White	8 mos.	Pullet	107.5
Mediterranean	Leghorn	S. C. White	8 mos.	Pullet	107.1
Mediterranean	Leghorn	S. C. White	8 mos.	Pullet	107.6
Mediterranean	Leghorn	S. C. White	8 mos.	Pullet	107.1
Mediterranean	Leghorn	S. C. White	8 mos.	Pullet	107.2
Mediterranean	Leghorn	S. C. White	8 mos.	Pullet	107.2
Mediterranean	Leghorn	S. C. White	8 mos.	Pullet	107.7
Mediterranean	Leghorn	S. C. White	8 mos.	Pullet	107.0
Mediterranean	Leghorn	S. C. White	8 mos.	Pullet	106.7

Total, 5334.3; average, 106.6

As a summary of this tabulation we find that the average temperature of the domestic fowl is 106.6° F. In this tabulation five classes, eight breeds, and eleven varieties were used. As the usefulness of a bird is considered approximately three years, birds over that age were not used. There is no great range of difference between the birds 8 months old and those 2½ years old. Only three males were included in this list but the temperature of these were the same as those for hens. The range of temperatures of the different classes, breeds and varieties are similar.

To test the influence of temperature on growth, eight cultures were grown at different temperatures. These results are tabulated below.

TEMPERATURE TESTS IN GROWTH OF PUS PRODUCING MICROORGANISMS

	Test				Control		
No.	Kind of cult.	Temp.	Growth	No.	Kind of cult.	Temp.	Growth
1a	S. p. aureus	110°F.	+	1a	S. p. aureus	38°C.	+
2a	S. p. aureus	110°F.	+	2a	S. p. aureus	38°C.	+
1b	S. p. albus	110°F.	+	1b	S. p. albus	38°C.	+
3a	S. p. aureus	110°F.	+	3a	S. p. aureus	38°C.	+
1a	S. p. aureus	107°F.	+	1a	S. p. aureus	38°C.	+
2a	S. p. aureus	107°F.	+	2a	S. p. aureus	38°C.	+
1h	S. p. albus	107°F.	+	1b	S. p. albus	38°C.	+
3a	S. p. aureus	107°F.	+	3a	S. p. aureus	38°C.	+

We have here three strains of *S. p. aureus* and one strain of *S. p. albus* all of which grew at 107° F., and also at 110° F., or more than three degrees higher than the average rectal temperature of the domestic fowl. The growth at 110° F. was not so luxuriant as that at 107° F., nor was that at 107° F. as luxuriant as that at 38° C. However, all growths were decidedly marked and in none could the growth even be considered veil-like, but rather luxuriant. We do not think that the temperature of the fowl has anything to do with the resistance of the fowl to the pus producing organisms but that the fowl has a natural resistance and will not under ordinary, or normal, conditions develop abscess as a result of natural infection with the Staphylococci.

GENERAL SUMMARY. That the domestic fowl has great resistance to certain common pus producing organisms is shown by the fact that to one young cockerel of three pounds weight there was given 29 c.c. of a 3-day-old bouillon culture of *Staphylococcus pyogenes aureus* and *Staphylococcus pyogenes albus* with no noticeable ill effects. The *S. p. aureus* was originally isolated from a furuncle of human origin and had been passed through two rabbits producing septicemia in each case. The *S. p. albus* was isolated from an abscess of a horse and likewise was passed through two rabbits causing septicemia in each case. Subsequently two hens were given subcutaneously 10 c.c. each of a three-day-old bouillon culture of the same organisms without any noticeable ill effect. The great resistance is also shown by the way fowls uniformly stand up under repeated intraperitoneal injections of bouillon cultures of these organisms. It is only after a prolonged course of injections of this nature that changes in the internal organs are produced and local purulent inflammation of the peritoneum results. Following these injections there is noted a very active phagocytosis. In the scrapings from the peritoneum may be found both polymorphonuclear neutrophiles and some mononuclear and mesothelial cells, all engulfing masses of the cocci, the former being especially the more active.

Amyloidosis can be produced in the domestic fowl by repeated injections of large doses of Staphylococci and extending over long periods. The amyloid deposits appear in the liver, spleen and kidneys.

Products of suppuration produce acute parenchymatous nephritis in the hen.

BIBLIOGRAPHY

1—KAUPP, B. F. Anatomy of the Domestic Fowl. W. B. Saunders Co., Philadelphia.

2—FRISCH, A. Ueber eigentheimlich Produkte mykotischer mit der Reaction des Amyloides, *d. k. Akad. d. Wissensch. Math naturw.*, Cl., 36 Abt., 1877, LXXVI, 109.

3—BIRCH-HIRSHFELD, F. V. Lehrbuch der pathologischen Anatomie, Leipsig, 1882, I, 45.
4—BOUCHARD. Degenerescence Amyloide Experimentale, *Compt. rend. Soc. de biol.*, 1888-v, 688.
5—CZERNY, A. Zur Kenntniss der glycogen und Amyloiden Eutartung, *Arch. f. Exper. Path. u Pharm.*, 1893, XXXI, 190.
6—KRAWKOW, N. P. Ueber bei Thieren experimentale hervorgerufeues Amyloid, *Centralbl. f. allg. Path. u. path. Anat.*, 1895, VI, 337.
7—NOWAK, J. Experimentale untersuchungen über die Aetiologie des Amyloidosis, *Virchows Arch. f. Path. Anat.*, 1898, CIII, 162.
8—BAILEY. *The Journal of Experimental Medicine*, Vol. XXIII, No. 6.
9—KLOTZ. *The Journal of Medical Research*, Vol. XXX, No. 3.
10—MALLORY and WRIGHT. Pathological Technique.

OBSERVATIONS REGARDING THE TOPOGRAPHY OF THE ESOPHAGUS

JAS. D. GROSSMAN, D.V.M., and T. S. LEITH, D.V.M.
Iowa State College, Ames, Iowa

Since using the apparatus, for fixing the head in nearly the normal position, described in the JOURNAL OF THE AMERICAN VETERINARY MEDICAL ASSOCIATION, Vol. LI., N. S. Vol. IV, No. 2, pp. 237-

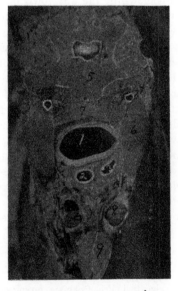

FIGURE 1. 1, Trachea; 2, Bi-carotid trunk; 3, Esophagus; 4, Vertebral vessels; 5, Seventh cervical vertebra; 6, Scalenus; 7, Longus coli; 8, Jugular veins; 9, Sterno-cephalicus.

239, May, 1917, we find the following position of the esophagus existing; ventral to the sixth cervical vertebra the trachea is on the medial side, the esophagus inclining obliquely downward and backward to a position ventral to the trachea beneath the seventh

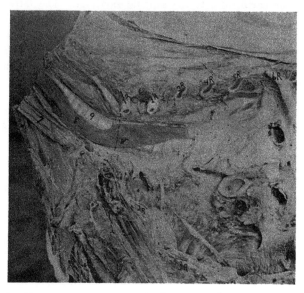

FIGURE 2. 1R-6R, Stumps of first six ribs; 7, Jugular Vein drawn down; 8, Esophagus; 9, Trachea; V indicates course of Vagus Nerve. Dotted line indicates anterior border of first rib. Vessels, and nerves held down by a hook in thoracic cavity.

cervical vertebra (see Fig. 1) after which it again crosses the lateral surface of the trachea upward and backward between it and the first rib (see Fig. 2) gaining the dorsal surface opposite the third rib.

A MALFORMATION
(Ectopia Cordis)

F. M. HAYES, Davis, Calif.

SUBJECT: Pure-bred Toggenburg kid born Feb. 26th, at end of normal period of pregnancy and in a state of good general health, but with a malformation of the heart and sternum.

OBJECTIVE SYMPTOMS: The ventricular area of the heart appeared externally through a ring 4 c.m. in diameter just anterior to the xiphoid cartilage. The ventricle could be seen and felt pulsating within a thin transparent membrane (pleura). This membrane was adherent to the edges of the ring completely closing the thoracic cavity. The sternum was found divided from and including the cariniform to the xiphoid cartilage. The latter cartilage and skin was the only tissue communicating with the right and left ribs. Respirations were 45 and pulse 70. Repelling the heart to the thoracic cavity and any manipulation cause dyspnea and marked decrease in the rate and force of the contractions. Complete collapse and death occurred 5 hours after birth. The death, no doubt, was hastened by handling the heart.

AUTOPSY: The heart was about 10 cm. long and hourglass shaped. The dimensions were, one auricle of a diameter of 4 cm.

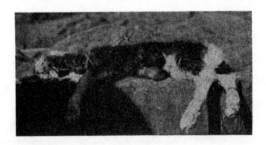

and one ventricle of a diameter of 3.5 cm. with an imperfectly formed auriculo-ventricular valve. Only one vessel (aorta) left the base of the ventricle and 2 cm. after emergence gave off right and left branches to the lungs. 1 cm. farther this vessel divided into posterior and anterior aorta, the latter then apparently into right and left carotids after giving off one branch (brachial). Externally the auricle looked normal but no septum divided them internally. Venous sinuses appeared to take care of the blood returning from the lungs and only one vena cava entered the auricle. Whether this description makes it clear or not, the course of the circulation appeared as follows: venous blood from the common vena cava and aerated blood from the lungs entered the common auricle. Through the one auriculo-ventricular valve to the common ventricle, out of the ventricle through one vessel which gave off two branches to the lungs, this dividing into anterior and posterior aorta which appeared to continue normally.

ABSTRACTS FROM RECENT LITERATURE

PYEMIA. Capt. Ralph Bennett, F.R.C.V.S., A.V.C. *Veterinary Record.*—Under this name, among several cases recorded by the author, is one of an eight-year-old bay mare which had received a shell wound in the lumbar region on the right side and from which escaped a prolific discharge with a most offensive odor. On examination nothing of the shell was found but a very extensive burrowing of pus was discovered. The burrow being followed, it was found necessary to make six incisions for drainage, one below the original injury, one over the 12th rib, one just behind the scapula, another half way down the ribs, one just above the spur vein and one under the sternum. The panniculus carnosus was extensively gangrenous and removed almost entirely. An enormous quantity of pus was liberated and all the above mentioned openings found connected. The cavities were cleaned out, packed with wool soaked in permanganate of potash solution and the wound flushed with a solution of chloride of sodium and was plugged with carbolized tow. Stimulants and tonics were administered internally. Recovery was rapid. The case is illustrated with a plate showing the location of the incisions made.

A. L.

MORPHINE SULPHATE IN DOG PRACTICE. Georges Yatt, F.R.C.V.S. *Veterinary Record.*—An interesting report of the effects observed in two dogs by the administration, in hypodermic injections, of ¾ of a grain of morphine sulphate.

A Dachshund, the subject of an operation for a discharging fistula over the left orbit, received the above injection and for 8 days afterward remained in a lethargic condition. "Placed with difficulty upon his feet, he remained in this position for a few moments only, his legs crossed, there was marked incoordination and he fell to the ground. After several attempts he maintained himself erect, moved slowly and sought the support of a near object. He took food and had difficulty in picking up small pieces of meat, he drank with difficulty."

The prognosis was gloomy notwithstanding the treatment. In a second case of an Irish terrier, the effects were similar but less severe. Recovery took place after a few days.

A. L.

UTILIZATION OF SEAWEED FOR FEEDING OF HORSES. (Translation of a report by Mr. Adrian, of French Ministry of War, forwarded by Consul General A. M. Thackara, Paris, March 11.)— For a long time I have been interested in finding a substitute for normal alimentary products, especially as relates to the horse, in case of a shortage of oats which might be the consequences of a war.

Last May, when I had again taken up the study of this question, an industrial chemist came to propose to me for the waterproofing of materials a product derived from seaweed of the laminary class from which the salt had previously been extracted by a special treatment.

Knowing the centesimal composition of seaweeds thus treated, I was immediately struck by its analogy to that of oats of Brie, which is shown by the analysis of Mons. Balland, head pharmacist, as follows:

ANALYSIS	Seaweed per cent.	Oats per cent.
Water	14.40	12.55
Hydrocarbonic matter	52.90	68.80
Nitrogenous matter	17.30	9.10
Cellulose	11.50	8.45
Mineral matter	3.90	3.10

HAS HIGH PERCENTAGE OF NITROGEN. From this comparison it is seen that if the treated seaweed contains less hydrocarbonated matter, on the other hand it contains a much higher percentage of nitrogen, which should make it a first-rate rebuilding product if it is digestible and assimilating.

On account of urgency, I made, as early as June, 1917, a series of direct experiments on six horses placed at my disposal by a manufacturer at Aubervilliers, M. Verdier-Dufour. These animals were all in a bad state and affected with lymphangitis. They were divided into two lots. Three were submitted to the ordinary diet of oats, hay, and straw, and the other three were placed on a diet of alimentary seaweed. These six horses were submitted to normal work. In the ration of the three animals of the second lot, alimentary seaweeds were substituted during the first eight days for half the quantity of oats at a rate of about 0.35 kilo for 0.45 of oats. During the rest of the experiment, which lasted 24 days, seaweed was substituted entirely for oats. On the 24th day it was noticed that, taken as a whole, the horses fed on alimentary seaweed had increased 6 per cent in weight and that their general condition had greatly improved, while the lymphangitis had disappeared.

This affection, on the other hand, still existed in the animals of the first lot.

SEEMS WORTHY OF BEING RETAINED. General conclusions cannot, of course, be drawn from such a small experiment as regards the therapeutic action of alimentary seaweed on lymphangitis, but there is an indication which is worthy of being retained in view of later studies. This action may be due, according to Prof. Lapicque and Dr. Legendre of the Museum, to traces of organic iodine existing in the seaweed after washing and extracting the salts. At any rate, a result was obtained—the animals had accepted, digested, and assimilated the new aliment in place of oats.

In view of such an encouraging result, it was decided to make a new series of experiments on the horses of a regiment of cavalry. On August 8, two lots of 20 horses were made up in the First Cuirassiers, at the Dupleix Quartier, in the same squadron. One lot was placed on a normal diet; the other received 1 kilo of alimentary seaweed in place of 1 kilo of oats. This experiment, made with the greatest care, was watched by Mons. Jacoulet, director of the veterinary service of the retrenched camp of Paris, under the high control of Mons. Fray, veterinary inspector. The experiment lasted two months, and on weighing the horses on October 8 it was found that those fed on alimentary seaweed had gained individually 13 kilos in two months, while the others had scarcely gained 2 kilos.

GROWS ABUNDANTLY ON BRITTANY COAST. The first experiment was thus entirely confirmed. Following these tests, I estimate that 0.75 kilo of alimentary seaweed is equal to 1 kilo of oats, but this is a point which it will be necessary to verify. As this sort of seaweed grows abundantly on the coast of Brittany, alimentary seaweed seems destined to play an important role as a substitute for oats.

In ordinary times we import yearly 2,000,000 quintals of oats, representing an expenditure of 35,000,000 francs, an amount which has quadrupled today. This money will remain at home the day we realize that the sea can supply the supplementary crop that our fields have not been able to furnish.

I foresee the employment of seaweed in human alimentation, and very interesting results have already been obtained in this order of ideas. Other experiments are being made.

N. S. MAYO.

INTERESTING CASES.—A number of these are recorded in the numbers of the *Veterinary News*. Mr. Robinson, M.R.C.V.S., mentions first a case of *high temperature* in a horse where he found the thermometer registering 109.8° F. This gradually decreased until the third day when it was normal. The elevation of temperature was observed after a chill.

The same writer mentions a case of a pony which was *twice affected with tetanus*. He recovered from an attack following a wound in the head; he had a second several months afterward following an injury of the foot. Bromide of potassium and phenic acid were used in treatment.

Captain E. Brayley Reynolds, M.R.C.V.S., recorded a case of *placental strangulation of a foal's foot,* which was observed after an abortion from the mother and where it was found that the allantoid membrane had become twisted round the pastern and strangulation had taken place. From the small size of the foot compared with the rest of the leg and also the appearance of the os suffraginis it was concluded that the strangulation must have taken place some considerable time before the abortion.

A. L.

ALOPECIA. G. Mayall, M.R.C.V.S. *Veterinary Journal.* Under this heading the author calls attention to this trouble said to be due to disturbance of the nutrition of the skin, and which on examination of the scrapings, under the microscope, can be distinguished from acariasis. In a cart horse, which he attended, he has observed it on five annual occasions. The place most regularly attacked was the hollow of the near flank. Little spots arose, which widened and coalesced. There was a fair amount of dry scales and eventually an oval patch arose about a foot and half long and one foot wide. Carbolized oil or lead and potash oils soon brought about complete recovery. Occasionally the same trouble occurred in the neck. The subject was of a nervous temperament, a good worker and had never suffered from any general disease.

· A. L.

NOTE ON THE FEEDING OF CATTLE DURING A PERIOD OF DEFICIENCY. M. Viollette. *Recueil de Médecine Vétérinaire*, Vol. 93, pp. 443-445, 1917. Office of the General Food Administrator. Circular to Chiefs of Departments. Paris, July 18, 1917.

The feeding of our cattle should particularly retain our attention. It is advisable that during 1917-1918, not a single method of feeding be misunderstood. We have consulted the Director of the Veterinary School at Alfort on this important question. The response which we have received reveals the possibility of utilizing resources that our cultivators have not been in the habit of utilizing, but which, under the present circumstances, may become absolutely precious. Following is the text of the note:

Note on the feeding of cattle during a period of deficiency.

Many feeds that are habitually little used or even totally neglected may enter into the feeds of domestic animals: horses, bovines, sheep, hogs and poultry.

To replace the deficiency in the stock of grains and press cakes, various leguminous grains not suitable to human use are employed: beans and horse beans, buckwheat, rice and especially rice bran, millet and sorghum, the chestnuts not suitable to human use, carob beans (St. John's bread), etc.

Feeds that are voluminous and watery and entirely suited to cattle are: the marcs of raisins, apples, mistletoe, furze, heath, the leaves and twigs of trees, vine leaves and twigs, cucurbitaceous fruits, etc. In the feed of hogs one should also include reeds that grow along rivers and streams. They might even be made to consume the hide trimmings coming from tanneries; a hog can consume 750 grams per day without inconvenience; fish meal obtained by drying and treating unsold and spoiled fish; the contents of the rumen of slaughtered cattle.

The specialists in feeding have studied all these feeds; the amounts and methods of feeding are known. The general use of the horse chestnut and acorn is possible. Horse chestnuts are especially good for sheep; bovines eat them also, but with less satisfactory results; they may be fed to horses. Hogs refuse them in every form and in spite of every artifice; horse chestnuts are poisonous for poultry, ducks and geese.

They are used as follows: Sheep: 500 grams of the fresh horse chestnuts are equivalent to 1500 grams of beet trimmings (betteraves fourragères). One may go up to a maximum of 1 kilogram. (Per day? author does not state.)

Cattle: 2-3 kilograms; for fattening, preferably cooked.

Fresh or dried horse chestnuts, when not cooked, are mashed and mixed with other feeds.

All animals can consume acorns, but they must not be permitted to consume more than the maximum doses given below, if one is to avoid enteritis and albuminuria.

	Fresh acorns	Dried acorns
Horse, of 500 kilograms	4 kilos.	2.5 kilos.
Beef, 600-700 kilos	6 kilos.	3.5 kilos.
Milk cow, 500-600 kilos	4 kilos.	2.5 kilos.
Sheep	0.8 kilos.	0.5 kilos.
Hogs	1.3-1.5 kilos.	0.8-1.0 kilos.

For the horse, 4 liters (or quarts) are equivalent to 2 liters (or quarts) of oats. After using this feed for a month, discontinue it for a week. Horses and cattle are fed the acorns raw, broken and freed from the shells.

For hogs, the acorns are broken and coarsely ground, and mixed with boiled potatoes, or better, boiled with them.

There can be no doubt that quantities of feed materials of real value remain unused or poorly utilized. Certain feeds known in some sections are not known in others. It is therefore an economic interest of the first order to propagate practical knowledge of this nature among the great masses of owners and raisers of animals.

We pray you to communicate this information to your department, and to use it, by every means you possibly can, to spread among the rural population in your province, the practical points it contains. For us, at the present hour, it is a prime necessity to permit nothing to be lost from the totality of our resources.

The Minister of Agriculture: Fernand David.

The General Food Administrator: Maurice Viollette.

BERG.

———•———

ADENOMA OF THE KIDNEY IN A HORSE. Lieut. J. J. Aveston, M.R.C.V.S., A.V.C. *Veterinary Journal.*—A seven-year-old draught gelding entered the hospital on account of general debility. He had bloody urine, which contained an extreme quantity of albumin. His pulse and temperature were normal. His visible mucous membranes were very pale and anemic in appearance. Rectal examination revealed nothing abnormal. A mallein test proved negative. The appetite was good all the time he was under observation. For a whole month he showed no sign of pain or discomfort. The urine remained blood stained all the time. He was finally destroyed; his post mortem revealed an enormously enlarged kidney, the right, which weighed 60¾ pounds. It had actually extended over to the left side and enveloped the normal kidney of that side. Notwithstanding the size of the tumor an elliptical portion of the organ remained apparently normal in structure. Examination by the microscope revealed the adenomatous nature of the lesion.   A. L.

EQUINE MANGE TRANSMITTED TO MAN. Major Perot. *Rev. de Pathol. Comp.*—From numerous observations the writer comes to the following conclusions: 1st, Sarcoptic mange of horses is transmissible to man and probably not to woman; 2nd, the Acarus does not take so strong a hold in man as it does in horses, but yet it gives rise to pimples and characteristic itching; 3rd, the treatment does not require more than two antisporic baths and two frictions of Helmric ointment, altogether 48 hours.   A. L.

NATIONAL ACADEMY OF SCIENCES. Annual Meeting, April 22, 23, 1918, Washington, D. C.—The writer attended these meetings; several of the papers may be of interest. Drs. Benedict, Miles and Smith presented the results of their work on ''The Effects of a Prolonged Reduced Diet on Twenty-Five College Men''. This number of men received a daily diet which furnished but 2/3 of the usual food amounts for men of their weight, etc., for four months. At the end of this time numerous physical and psychological tests showed that the men had not suffered in any way as the result of the restricted diet.

Dr. Simon Flexner spoke on ''The War and Medical Research''. He stated that many of the problems of military medicine had been solved. These were the problems pertaining to the prevention of such diseases as typhoid fever, dysentery, etc. The greatest menaces at present are pneumonia and meningitis. The recent outbreak of pneumonia in the various camps was caused, not by the usual *Diplococcus pneumoniae,* but by an entirely different and hitherto unknown streptococcus which causes a pneumonia having a different pathological picture entirely.

Dr. Flexner spoke of the recent investigations of Bull and Pritchett, who have prepared the toxin of the gas gangrene bacillus, and who have injected horses with the toxin with the expectation of obtaining a serum that would be useful in the treatment of gas gangrene. Large quantities of the serum are being tried.

Dr Flexner spoke of the *Bacillus welchii* (also called *B. perfringens, B. aerogenes capsulatus* and still other names) as if it were the only etiological agent of gas gangrene.

Dr. H. F. Osborn spoke of the new "Liberty Field Hospitals". These are designed on the unit construction plan, can be easily assembled and transported. When the war is over these hospitals will be taken apart and used for building homes, into which they can be easily and quickly transformed.   BERG.

———

A REBELLIOUS SUB ORBITAL FISTULA IN A DOG. A. Guillaume. *Rev. Generale.*—Although probably not frequently used in dogs, this case is presented as strong evidence of the benefit the polyvalent serum of Leclainche and Vallée can give. By its use complete recovery was obtained in this case in eight days, while a whole year of more varied applications had failed.

The case was simply an old lacrymal fistula following a wound of the cornea which had given rise to a suppurative inflammation of the lacrymal sac (phlegmonous dacryocystitis).

A small Teneriffe bitch had some trouble with a cat and received a scratch of the cornea of the right eye. The keratitis following was treated and recovery resulted. Sometime later, however, a small abscess formed below the eye. This closed and returned leaving a small fistulous tract. Examination of the mouth showed all the teeth normal and sound. A treatment was instituted for the fistula which several times closed and reopened, single or multiple, notwithstanding the free incisions and treatments with oxygenated water, boric acid, salol, camphorated naphtol, permanganate of potash, iodoformed ether, iodine, methylen blue, tannoform, etc. Even the extraction of a premolar tooth covered with tartar was useless. Finally the polyvalent serum was resorted to. Each day after a free washing with tepid physiologic solution the fistula was injected with serum and a cotton plug moistened with the same introduced in the tract. In eight days the recovery was perfect and has remained without any further indication of trouble.   A. L.

———

—Dr. F. L. Skrable has removed from Waterloo to Sioux City, Ia.

—Dr. H. O. Mantor has removed from Beaufort, N. C., to Tucson, Arizona.

ARMY VETERINARY SERVICE

REPORT ON THE BRITISH ARMY VETERINARY SERVICE

MAJORS L. A. KLEIN AND A. L. MASON, V.C., N.A.

1. As directed by Special Orders No. 23, Paragraph 25 (G.H.Q., A. E. F., January 23, 1918), we proceeded to ———, France, to study the organization, operation, administration and equipment of the veterinary service of the British Army. On arriving there on January 29th, we reported to ———, Director of the Veterinary Service, who afforded us every opportunity possible for making our investigation. To him and to his officers we feel under the deepest obligation for the courtesies extended. We were conducted to four groups of veterinary hospitals on the L. of C., each group consisting of a reception hospital, a mange hospital and one or two general hospitals; three convalescent horse depots; one base veterinary supply depot; two advance veterinary supply depots; and five divisional areas in two different corps.

2. The British veterinary service is organized to detect communicable disease as soon as it appears in a unit and to immediately institute measures to prevent its extension; to call attention to unsanitary conditions and unhygienic practices and to make recommendations regarding their correction; to relieve the mobile units of sick or inefficient animals, and to transfer such animals as promptly as possible to veterinary hospitals on the L. of C. in order to reduce the period of treatment to the minimum and to afford opportunity for disposing of incurable or unserviceable animals while they are still in a condition to permit of such disposition. Prompt institution of treatment has the effect of not only diminishing the period of inefficiency but it very often makes it possible to cure a condition which would not respond to treatment begun later. The salvage of incurable or unserviceable animals is of great economic importance. The receipts from sales of animals to farmers and butchers and of the products of economizer plants amounted to $3,500,000 in one year, much of which would have been lost if the animals had not been promptly evacuated from the units at the front.

ORGANIZATION. 3. The organization of the British veterinary service is very simple. Veterinary officers and enlisted personnel are attached to divisional units to keep the animals under close

observation for symptoms of communicable diseases and for unsanitary and unhygienic conditions, to report animals for, evacuation to hospital, to treat trivial conditions and to apply such
treatment as may be immediately required by animals to be
evacuated. A mobile veterinary section is attached to each division to evacuate animals from the units and transfer them to a
veterinary hospital. Each division has a Deputy Assistant Director of Veterinary Service, who is a major of the Veterinary Corps,
to administer the veterinary service of the division.

4. An Assistant Director of Veterinary Service, who is a
Lieut. Colonel of the Veterinary Corps, administers the veterinary service of each corps, and a Deputy Director of Veterinary .
Service, who is a Colonel of the Veterinary Corps, administers
the veterinary service of each army.

5. Each veterinary hospital on the L. of C. is commanded
by a Major of the Veterinary Corps who has six to eight veterinary
officers to assist him, the number depending on the size of the hospital. The veterinary supply depots are also in charge of veterinary officers or of non-commissioned officers of the Veterinary
Corps. The L. of C. is divided into two areas and the veterinary
formation in each area is under the supervision of a Colonel of
the Veterinary Corps. Over the whole organization is an officer
of the Veterinary Corps who formerly had the rank of Brigadier
General but who was recently promoted to Major General.

OPERATION. 6. The principal functions of the veterinary offi--
cer attached to a unit is to look out for communicable disease and
conditions which may affect the health or efficiency of the animals,
and to see that animals requiring hospital treatment or those which
are unserviceable are promptly evacuated. He also treats minor
ailments and injuries and applies any treatment which may be immediately required by animals to be evacuated. Animals to be
evacuated are conducted to the mobile veterinary section by a
non-commissioned officer or enlisted man of the Veterinary Corps,
but when many are to be evacuated the commanding officer of the
unit details a sufficient number of men to assist. The veterinary
officer makes out a statement which is sent with the animal, giving
the designation of the unit, the age, color, markings and sex of the
animal, and the reason for evacuation. A linen tag bearing the
same information is also attached to the halter; a red tag for mange
or other communicable disease, a blue tag for surgical cases and a
white tag for medical cases.

7. The mobile veterinary section is situated back of the wagon line, near a wood and a watering place, within one to three miles of the railhead. Its location is indicated by the flag of the Veterinary Corps. When a division takes a new position during active operations, similar flags are put up along the roads leading from the front to the mobile section to direct men bringing horses back.

8. When an animal arrives at the mobile section, a receipt is issued for it and the information on the accompanying statement is entered in a book and the case is numbered. This number and the number of the mobile section is stenciled with white paint on a clipped area on the left croup. The animal is then examined, any treatment required is applied and it is then stabled.

9. The officer commanding the mobile veterinary section communicates with the railway transportation officer at the railhead regarding the number of animals to be transferred to hospitals and is notified when to send them to the railhead. When there is not much activity at the front, the mobile veterinary sections in a given area send their cases on certain specified days to a particular reception hospital. This plan was adopted so that the railroads could make up special trains. They objected to taking a car or two of animals in their regular trains. The special trains make the run to the hospital in such good time that they are now used whenever possible. When a big push is on, the mobile sections report to the Assistant Director of Veterinary Service (Corps Veterinarian), through the D.A.D.V.S. (Division Veterinarian), the number of animals to be transferred to hospital and the A.D.V.S. arranges with the railway transportation officer for the necessary trains. The destination of the animals at such times depends upon the state of the hospitals and information on this point is furnished to the A.D.V.S. through the Deputy Director of Veterinary Service (Army Veterinarian) by the Director of the Veterinary Service.

10. When animals are transferred to a hospital, the officer commanding the mobile veterinary section prepares a statement which gives the designation of the unit from which each animal came, the reasons for evacuation and the number given to the case by the mobile section. Until a short time ago, the age, color, markings and sex of each animal were also given but at present an experiment is being made to see if this data cannot be omitted and thus save clerical labor. This statement is made in triplicate,

one copy is retained, one is forwarded to the A. D. V. S. (Corps Veterinarian) through the D.A.D.V.S. (Division Veterinarian), and the other is forwarded with the animals. Mange cases are shipped in special cars, which are plainly marked.

11. Up to the present time, it has been the practice to send one man with each car of horses, with a non-commissioned officer in charge of the party, but the plan is to be changed to send one man with each two cars, as this number is believed to be sufficient. Each man is provided with a bucket to water the animals and sufficient forage for the journey is also sent.

12. When the train arrives at the railroad station near the reception hospital, it is met by a veterinary officer from the hospital, to whom the non-commissioned officer from each mobile section delivers his descriptive statement. The animals are then taken out of the cars and examined, those showing symptoms of mange, catarrhal disease, periodic opthalmia, ulcerative cellulitis, or other communicable disease, being placed in separate groups from the others. The mange cases are sent directly to the mange hospital and the others are taken to the reception hospital.

13. On arriving at the reception hospital, the animals are checked off on the descriptive statements and each animal is given a hospital number, which is entered on the descriptive statement in the proper place. This number is stamped on a strip of biscuit tin 1x3 inches, together with the date, and the piece of tin is then wrapped around the left cheek strap of the halter. Another tag stamped with the number of the mobile section and the date is fastened to the hair of the tail. A receipt is given for the animals which is returned by the non-commissioned officer to the officer commanding the mobile section. Each case is entered in the hospital book; a hospital card is made out for each animal and accompanies it wherever it goes until the case is terminated.

14. The several groups of animals are then stabled separately and the palpebral mallein test is applied, the animals from each mobile section being kept separate until the test is completed. If an animal reacts and shows open lesions of glanders, it is traced by means of the tags, the hospital records, descriptive statement, etc., to the unit from which it was evacuated and the D.A.D.V.S. (Division Veterinarian) is directed to have the other animals of the unit tested for glanders. Cases of other varieties of communicable diseases are reported back in the same manner so that the

necessary action can be taken to prevent the spread of infection. In any event, all animals are given a second mallein test two weeks after their arrival at the hospital in order to detect any case of glanders which may have been in the period of incubation when the first test was made.

15. When the mallein test is completed the animals are classified according to their condition and stabled accordingly in the reception hospital or are transferred to a general hospital, depending upon the state of the hospitals. The animals taken to the mange hospital are handled in a similar manner. When animals have recovered they are sent to a remount depot if ready for service; if not, they are sent to a convalescent horse depot to recuperate.

16. A close check is kept on the time animals are in hospitals and convalescent horse depots. As a general rule, it is not economical to keep an animal under treatment more than three months, including the time in hospital and convalescent horse depot. The officers in charge of subdivisions of veterinary hospitals and convalescent horse depots are required to report each week to the commanding officer the time by months the animals in their charge have been under treatment and the commanding officer then inspects those which have been under treatment over three months and decides which shall remain under treatment and which shall be sold. Whenever it appears at the time of the arrival of an animal at a hospital that its treatment will not be profitable it is disposed of at once.

17. The cars which carry the animals to the hospitals from the mobile sections are cleaned and disinfected before they leave the station at which they were unloaded. It is also the policy to disinfect all hospital stables every two weeks. Disinfection is usually carried out by painting the wood surfaces, except the floors, with tar and then flaming this and all metallic surfaces with a blow lamp after which all surfaces, including the floors, are washed down with cresol solution. The blankets and other equipment of animals affected with mange are also disinfected, the former by steam and the harness with chloride of lime. Grooming kits are disinfected by soaking in soda solution and then immersing in cresol solution, the brushes being subsequently soaked in salt solution to stiffen the bristles.

18. At all of the veterinary hospitals and convalescent horse

depots, the oats fed to the animals are either crushed or steamed
and are mixed with bran and cut hay. ——— is of the opinion
that it is very good practice to mix the grain with cut hay for
horses with weak digestive powers and he thinks it pays to crush
or steam the oats because their digestibility is greatly increased
thereby.

19. Casualty Clearing Stations are now being organized to
relieve the mobile sections of a part of their duties and to reduce
the possibility of their being congested with cases during a big
push. There will be one for each corps but they will be army
troops and their stations will be determined by the D.V.S. (Army
Veterinarian).

20. The Casualty Clearing Station will receive animals from
the mobile veterinary sections operating in the vicinity and care
for them until they can be placed on railroad cars to be transferred
to a reception hospital. The first mallein test will be applied at
the casualty clearing station, thus providing for the earlier detection of animals affected with glanders and consequently reducing
the danger of spreading the infection. Facilities will also be provided for performing surgical operations so that the treatment of
many of the animals requiring surgical interference can be begun
earlier than under the present arrangements, thus reducing the
time of hospital residence.

21. At some of the stations, if not all of them, a dipping vat
will be constructed for the immersion of animals in the corps area
which have been exposed to infection with mange. There will also
be facilities for disinfecting blankets and horse equipment. One
such plant is under construction and nearly completed. Animals
affected with mange will be evacuated to mange hospitals on the
L. of C. and dipped there, as heretofore.

22. The dipping vats and disinfection facilities at the casualty clearing stations are being introduced as an additional means
of controlling the disease by dipping animals which have been exposed to infection and thus subjecting to treatment animals which
may be infected but which do not as yet show visible signs of the
disease. The treatment of animals affected with mange by hand
applications in the units to which they belong is strongly discouraged and anyone persisting in this method is sharply rebuked.
This is because it has been found by experience that hand applications for the cure of mange may frequently produce considerable

irritation to the skin, with swelling and cracking of the same. This occurs usually when the mixtures applied contain a drying oil, but it has also occurred when a bland fat like lard was used. Another serious objection to this method of treatment is that diseased areas are likely to be overlooked for a time, the period of treatment thus being extended and the cure of the animal sometimes being made impracticable. Experience has taught that the best method of treating the disease is by immersing the infected animals in a bath containing calcium sulphide.

23. Near each group of hospitals on the L. of C. a rendering plant will be installed to dispose of the carcasses of animals which die or which are destroyed in the hospitals. During a big push, the disposition of dead animals is an almost insurmountable difficulty. Local knackers are not to be depended on and burial is slow and occupies large numbers of men. For several months, a small rendering plant has been in operation near the ———— group of hospitals and it has proven so profitable that it has been decided to erect similar plants near the other hospital groups. This plant is unique in that it is operated by gas obtained from a chalk pit in which animals and manure were deposited last year, the gas being generated by the decomposition of the carcasses and manure. An experiment to determine if gas could be obtained from manure dumps for fuel purposes demonstrated that the inflammable gases were not produced in sufficient quantity in manure alone to be of practical value.

ADMINISTRATION. 24. The veterinary officers attached to divisional units prepare a report every Thursday of the number of animals evacuated during the week preceding, the number treated in the unit, the conditions affecting them, the number of animals on duty, the sanitary condition of the horse lines, etc., and on Friday morning they meet the D.A.D.V.S. (Division Veterinarian) in conference, when the report is presented and questions pertaining to the veterinary service of the division and to the health and efficiency of the animals are discussed. If an officer cannot attend the conference he sends his report by special orderly. These reports and the report from the mobile veterinary section of the division are consolidated by the D.A.D.V.S., who presents his report to the A.D.V.S. (Corps Veterinarian) on Saturday morning at a conference at which the veterinary affairs of the corps are discussed. The A.D.V.S.'s meet the D.D.V.S. (Army Veterinarian) in conference on Sunday morning and present their own reports and those from the divisions in their corps. All of the reports are then forwarded by the D.D.V.S. to the Director of the Veterinary Service. This system causes reports to be delivered promptly, makes it unnecessary to send them back for correction, and provides an opportunity for the discussion of difficult problems and for an interchange of views regarding various phases of the work. When the reports are received in the office of the Director of the Veterinary Service the information they contain is tabulated and from these tables one is able to see almost at a glance the conditions existing in any division, corps or army.

25. Requisitions for veterinary supplies made by veterinary officers attached to the units are presented to the D.A.D.V.S. (Division Veterinarian) and after approval or modification are forwarded by him to an Advance Veterinary Supply Depot, from which the articles called for are issued to the officer direct. The advance depots receive their supplies from Base Veterinary Supply Depots, which in turn receive their supplies from the Principal Veterinary Depot at ———, England. The advance depots supply the field units, the base depots supply the advance depots and the veterinary hospitals on the L. of C.

26. The veterinary hospitals on the L. of C. are of three kinds: Reception, general and mange hospitals, but the administration is the same in all cases. Each hospital is in command of a major of the Veterinary Corps, with a staff consisting of six to eight officers, depending upon the capacity of the hospital. The organization is divided into a headquarters and five to eight subdivisions, each subdivision having charge of two hundred and fifty animals. Each subdivision is entirely self-sustaining but the headquarters personnel is distributed among the different subdivisions for quarters and messing. The headquarters personnel consists of the commanding officer, a quartermaster, who also acts as adjutant, a sergeant-major, and the necessary men for the orderly room, quartermaster's store, pharmacy, laboratory, operating room, saddler's shop, hauling and preparing forage, and police. The personnel of each subdivision consists of the veterinary officer in charge, the men necessary for feeding, grooming, stable police, dressing, etc., and cooks. The veterinary officers in command of subdivisions are responsible to the commanding officer for the care and treatment of the animals in the subdivision and for the personnel.

27. At the end of each day a report is prepared by the officer in charge of the subdivision and turned in to the orderly room giving the number of animals received for treatment, conditions affecting them, the number evacuated, number died or destroyed, and the number remaining under treatment; also the number of men on duty, number sick, etc. These reports are consolidated in the orderly room and an abstract showing the state of the hospital is telephoned each evening to the Deputy Director of Veterinary Service in charge of the L. of C. area in which the hospital is located. On the basis of this information, the D.D.V.S. directs the transfer of animals from the front on the succeeding day.

28. A weekly report is prepared from the daily reports and forwarded through the D.D.V.S., to the Director of Veterinary Service, in whose office the information contained therein is tabulated for convenient study and reference. A weekly report of the period of residence of animals in the hospital is also sent through the same channel. Similar reports are made by the officers commanding convalescent horse depots.

EQUIPMENT. 29. Each veterinary officer in the field is provided with a veterinary officer's wallet, which contains the medicines, instruments and materials necessary for emergency treatment, and a veterinary officer's field chest containing the instruments, medicines, etc., required for general treatment. A farrier's wallet is furnished to each sergeant of the veterinary corps on duty with troops and to each noncommissioned officer in a mobile veterinary section, while a unit veterinary chest, containing the supplies necessary for first aid treatment, is supplied to all organizations having a representative of the veterinary corps attached.

30. In addition to the above, each mobile veterinary section is provided with picket lines, stable equipment, one wagon, one ambulance, four draft horses and fifteen riding horses. This is sufficient to provide mounts for all but six of the men and this number is usually engaged in conducting horses to a hospital. When a mobile section remains stationary for any time, shelters for the personnel and horses are erected from any material at hand and great ingenuity has been exhibited in this respect.

31. At the veterinary hospitals on the L. of C. tents were used at first as shelters for the animals but these have been almost entirely replaced by iron and wood buildings. Beech plank, beech and pine blocks, stone and cement are used for floors. A noticeable

feature of hospital construction is the extensive use made of the wire from baled hay. Hay racks, fences, hay baskets, holders for grooming kits and many other useful contrivances were made from this material.

32. All of the hospitals are very neatly kept. No manure is allowed to collect and the vacant spaces are sown in grass or planted with flowers. They are all supplied with a simple but complete veterinary equipment.

33. The horses in the first wagon line of the divisional areas which we visited had shelters and standings similar to those provided for the veterinary hospitals and the animals were all in excellent condition. They were well shod, apparently well fed and thoroughly groomed and in their appearance they would compare favorably with the horses in very well conducted city stables in peace times.

RESULTS. 34. The excellence of the veterinary service of the British Army is attested by the results. Of the animals treated in the hospitals from August 18, 1914, to December 27, 1917, only three per cent died; seventy-seven per cent were cured and twenty per cent were sold to farmers and butchers or destroyed on account of incurable conditions. These results would be considered very creditable if obtained under peace conditions; under war conditions they are remarkable.

35. The incidence of disease has also been held down to a very low point, compared with other wars and other armies. During the week ending January 24, the animals in the hospitals and those in convalescent depots represented 10.6 per cent of the animals in the British Expeditionary Force. But this percentage is in excess of the actual proportion of animals requiring treatment in hospitals or convalescent horse depots because it includes animals which are ready to be transferred to remount depots but which the latter cannot receive for lack of room. At times, the percentage of animals in hospitals and convalescent horse depots has been as low as seven.

36. Glanders, which has always prevailed to an extensive degree in every large army previously mobilized, is under complete control and practically does not exist. During the week ending January 24, not a single case was reported.

37. Mange, another disease which always appears and, unless preventive measures are instituted, spreads rapidly in armies, is

not only being held in check but is being repressed. At the present time there are fewer cases than at any time since March, 1916, when the greatest number of cases occurred, and it is expected that the methods now in operation will further reduce the prevalence of this disease. A difficulty in the control of this disease is that private stables in the zone of the armies are very generally infected with mange mites.

38. In the beginning of the war, all but a very small percentage of the mange cases were of the psoroptic variety but now this variety is quite rare and most of the cases are sarcoptic mange. A considerable proportion of the animals reported as affected with mange are found to be infested with forage acarini.

39. The disease which is of most concern at the present time is periodic ophthalmia. This disease appeared only a few months ago and its source is at present unknown. The institution of preventive measures is a difficult problem because neither the cause nor the method of transmission is known. During the week ending January 24, the incidence of this disease was 421 to the 100,000.

40. Epizootic lymphangitis is another serious disease which has required attention. The first case did not appear until last October and since then, although a sharp lookout has been maintained only a comparatively small number of cases have been discovered and those have been promptly destroyed and the exposed animals placed under observation. On account of the insidious character of the disease, contagious character, and its tendency to progress until the animal is rendered useless or dies, its appearance is a matter of grave concern and considerable attention is being devoted to its control and repression.

41. Ulcerative cellulitis has decreased, the incidence for the week ending January 24 being 43 to the 100,000. For the same week the incidence of necrotic dermatitis was 12 to 100,000; quittor, 12 to the 100,000. Those conditions being prevented to a large extent by the dry standings provided for the animals at the front. Wounds from gun fire are surprisingly few, only 14 to the 100,000 being reported for the week ending January 24. The other diseases and conditions reported are such as usually met with in an ordinary general veterinary practice.

42. The British Army is to be congratulated on the efficiency of its veterinary corps and the officers of that corps have every reason to be proud of the service they have rendered.

—Lieut. P. E. Johnson, formerly of Sioux Falls, S. D., is now stationed at Camp Greenleaf, Ga.

—Lieut. Melvin R. Sebright, formerly of Crofton, Neb., is stationed at Camp Greenleaf, Ga.

—Lieut. C. J. Cook, formerly at Fort Keogh, Mont., has been transferred to Camp Cody, Deming, N. M.

—2d Lieut. O. A. Longley, formerly of Oakland, Calif., is now at Camp Greenleaf, Chickamauga Park, Ga.

—Captain Emlen Wood, formerly at Camp Hancock, Ga., is now with the American Expeditionary Forces.

—2d Lieut. J. E. Reedy, formerly of Tillimook, Ore., is now at Camp Greenleaf, Chickamauga Park, Ga.

—Lieut. G. L. Richards, formerly of Ordway, Colo., is now stationed with the 78th Field Artillery at Camp Doniphan, Okla.

—First Lieut. R. C. Smith, formerly at Marfa, Texas, is now with the 6th Cavalry at Fort Sam Houston, Texas.

—Lieut. H. B. F. Jervis is with the American Expeditionary Forces.

—Captain James R. Mahaffy, formerly at Front Royal, Va., is now Senior Veterinarian, Eastern Purchasing Zone, at Washington, D. C.

—Lieut. Walter E. Campbell, formerly of Berwyn, Pa., is stationed at Camp Shelby, Hattiesburg, Miss.

—Lieut. J. M. Twitchell has been transferred from Camp Greenleaf, Ga., to Camp Lee, Virginia.

—Applications for A. V. M. A. membership have recently been received from 1st Lieut. Robert S. Tillie, 2d Lieut. Geo. W. Moon, 2d Lieut. Leon M. Getz, 2d Lieut. Jas. B. McNamara, 2d Lieut. Roy H. Tesdell, of the V. R. C., U. S. Army. It is pleasing to the members of the association to see the number of applications coming in from the young men in the service, and we hope before many months to see them all in the fold.

—Captain Raymond M. Hofferd, V. C., N. A., 88th Division, Camp Dodge, Iowa, was called home for a few days in the middle of May on account of the serious illness of his father. He lives at Norway, Iowa.

—Letters from Lieuts. Floyd S. Sharp and Homer S. Perdue, formerly of the 88th Division, but now with the Expeditionary Forces in France, have been received, telling of the safe journey across and the rather strenuous duties of the troops overseas.

—Lieut. Fred Middleton, V. R. C., of the 88th Division, Camp Dodge, Iowa, was called to his home at Cedar Rapids, Iowa, by the illness of his wife, about May 1st, 1918.

—Major W. J. Stokes has been transferred from Schofield Barracks, Hawaii, to Camp Greenleaf, Chickamaugua Park, Ga.

—Lieut. E. B. Parker, formerly of Newton, Ill., is stationed at Del Rio, Texas.

—Lieut. David E. Sisk, formerly at Gibson City, Ill., is Brigade Veterinarian at Camp Custer, Mich.

ASSOCIATION MEETINGS

DOMINION VETERINARY MEAT INSPECTORS' ASSOCIATION OF CANADA

The annual meeting of the D. V. M. I. Association of Canada was held Saturday evening, March 16th, Occident Hall, Toronto.

The meeting was called to order and Dr. F. L. Wingate was requested to conduct the proceedings in the absence of the president and vice president, who were, unfortunately, absent from the city.

The auditor's report of the yearly statement of the secretary-treasurer showed a membership list of 83; the receipts for the year were $154.00 and disbursements $132.00, showing the association to be in a very fair financial condition.

In the absence of Dr. Bone, the president, the account of his stewardship for the past year was read by the secretary and met with the hearty approval of the members present, who frequently caused interruptions with their applause, which showed in no unmistakable manner that they agreed with the sentiments as expressed by Dr. Bone in his report, a copy of which follows:

To the Officers and Members of the Dominion Veterinary Meat Inspectors' Association of Canada—"Greetings":

While our constitution does not ask for a written annual report from your president of his official acts during his term of office, I believe it to be a step in the right direction and is embodied in the revised constitution. It is to be doubted whether a report showing merely my activities as your president would prove either interesting or instructive. As president of your association, I have endeavored at all times without fear or favor, to do the things which have seemed to me to be for the best interests of the association as a whole.

In the first place, allow me to thank you one and all for the very great honor you have reposed in me in electing me for three succeeding terms to the most honorable position in your association. I wish especially to thank the members who have held office during my term as president. Especially do I wish to mention the committee who have had charge of the drafting and completion of our two memorials to the Honorable Minister of Agriculture, Ottawa.

Also do I wish to mention our worthy secretary-treasurer for the very able manner in which he has carried out the duties of his office. I would not be honest to my trust if I did not at this time especially mention our executive committee. Members of this association owe a debt of gratiude to them for their zeal in furthering our interests and also the assistance they have rendered to the special committee who have had charge of the formation of our Memorial No. 1, "Pay for Overtime". It is to those gentlemen that all Meat Inspectors whether or not members of this association are so deeply indebted for the very able manner in which they carried to its satisfactory completion this memorial as the result of which we all receive alike the same benefit.

I do not purpose at this time to go into a detailed account of the business done for the past year or two. Toronto members by their attendance at meetings and other members through the medium of the mail, have a fair knowledge of the business transacted. Let me briefly mention some items of interest to all members.

(1) The reading of papers, which were of timely interest and instructive, received adequate discussion.

(2) The drafting of our Memorial No. 1 dealing with "Pay for Overtime".

(3) The appeal by resolution of the members of this association to the Veterinary Director General, to uphold the dignity of the profession by the use of veterinarians only to do ante mortem and post mortem inspection.

(4) The equalization of salary of eastern and western Veterinary Meat Inspectors, which is still under consideration by the Honorable, the Minister of Agriculture.

PREAMBLE. Our object is to unite fraternally all veterinary

Meat Inspectors employed by the Department of Agriculture. To secure by discussion of topics pertaining to meat inspection a uniform interpretation of the departmental rules and regulations and thus promote the efficiency of the service—to secure through cooperation with the Department of Agriculture more equitable salary rates and regulation of hours of labor. To obtain for its members full benefit of all laws existing and which may be hereafter enacted, and by the upholding of all civil laws.

A fact much to be regretted is that we have not at all times been able to satisfy all members of our organization and have been unable to have their support when most needed. Among the discouraging features with which we have had to contend is that some inspectors have been content to remain outside the organization; some Toronto members to make themselves conspicuous by their absence from the meetings. It is as if they would say that if any good comes from our efforts, they will receive the same benefit as if they had given us their moral as well as their financial support, (as indeed they will and have) and it would appear that this very fact ought to suggest that in all fairness to their fellow inspectors, they should come into the organization, attend the meetings and thus bear a fair share of its burdens. It gives me great pleasure to say, however, that men of this character have constituted a very small minority. It is my contention that our chiefs or heads should recognize this fact, that organization improves the service, that honest membership makes a meat inspector the better and more efficient. The spirit of unity makes for harmony at a plant—and besides the product of good fellowship is cooperative and results in better performances of duty.

Since our association has become purely a veterinary association the executive officers and special committee have been very busy. It is not my purpose to claim that these members are infallible. We are but human, and are, therefore, liable to make mistakes, but I am firm in the belief that when our actions have been subjected to the closest scrutiny, as I have no doubt they will be, it will be found that the business of this association has been conducted along purely business lines, and in keeping with our preamble, to at all times "uphold the dignity of the profession—as well as an equitable salary in exchange for an honest efficient service".

Some of our superior officers have seemed to be somewhat cold or opposed to the association's actions along certain lines. We would like to impress upon the minds of any such officers (if there be any) that the Dominion Veterinary Meat Inspectors Association was not formed for the purpose of creating a militant power with which to overthrow their authority and retard their progress, but to assist them in the promulgation of those fundamental principles of progress, efficiency and justice, which must exist in order to promote the welfare of the meat inspection system in this Canada of ours, and raise it to a higher standard of efficiency. To accomplish this, greater inducements in the way of salary and working conditions must be held out to those entering our service in order to make it attractive.

I wish here to quote to you from the Honorable Dr. Roche, Chairman of the Civil Service Commission, in his address of welcome to the delegates to the convention of the Civil Service Federation in Ottawa, November 27th, 1917. He says: "I extend a most hearty greeting to you on your assembling here in Ottawa for conference on the subject of the Civil Service Act, and especially on the proposal of the government to bring under the operation of that act several branches of the outside service. That is a step for which I am sure public opinion is ripe, for both press and parliament are ready for it. I was, until recently, a member of the government and I assure you that if I were a member, I would welcome such a proposition. When all parties interested are of much the same mind on this most important question, I do not think it will be so very difficult to work out a practical plan, one that will be accepted by all concerned.

"The particular form of the change to be made is a matter, of course, for the government to decide. However, their object is to do away with patronage and to have appointments made on merit, the same as is intended in the case of the inside service. Legislation will be required, of course, to work it out finally and embrace the whole of the public service. In the matter of promotion, for instance, the object to be kept in view is not merely the raising of a man's salary, but keeping true to the principle that promotion shall be given for merit alone."

A question by a member of the federation to Dr. Roche—re recommendations to the commission if they would be received, or if they would have to go through the proper deputy heads—Dr. Roche replied: the great question, as I see it, is whether the commission would welcome suggestions from this federation not made by the deputy head in his report. Be sure we will welcome all information that will help us to arrive at a settlement of any question over which we have jurisdiction; let it be as to salaries or anything else, for we may be consulted later on that matter, and your suggestions may be of value to us.

You ask me, how may all this be attained? The most potent factor in the industrial and commercial world today is organization. To it may be credited most, if not all, that has been accomplished in the last three decades and to it we must look for the realization of our hopes for the future. Canada was not the first to recognize this fact, but although late in starting, particularly in comparison with European countries, she has made rapid strides in this direction. Already every progressive and successful manufacturer belongs to Canadian Manufacturers' Association. Every miner of any standing, in this industry, is a member of the Canadian Mining Institute. Pulp and paper makers are members of the Pulp and Paper Association. Publishers, large and small, are members of the Canadian Press Association. For agriculture, there is the Dominion Grange, the Grain Growers' Association, the Dominion Sheep Breeders' Association, the Dominion Swine Breeders' Association, and some eighteen branch associations among the breeders of the various classes of horses and cattle, as well as other associations for horticulture, fruit growing, bee keeping, etc. In insurance and banking there are such organizations as the Life and Fire Underwriters' Association and the Canadian Bankers' Association. In the professions there are: Teachers' Institutes, to which all teachers belong; the Dominion and Provincial Medical Association, to which all doctors belong; the various Provincial Bar Associations, to which all lawyers belong; the Canadian Society of Civil Engineers; the Society of Chemical Industry, etc.; the Civil Service Federation of Canada, and last but by no means least, Dominion Veterinary Meat Inspectors Association, to which belong almost every veterinary meat inspector, east of Fort William. To the individual inspector the advantages to be derived from this association cannot be estimated, any more than can the schools which offered him the facilities of acquiring his education, as in the case of the school, the benefit any inspector may derive from this association is directly proportionate to the interest he takes in it. In the past, the Dominion Veterinary Meat Inspectors Association has not been able to do all that was expected of it, but considering the limited resources it has it has done a good service and every inspector, whether a member of it or not, has shared alike in what has been accomplished. This coming year especially will bring new ideas for members to consider. Let me briefly outline a few of them:

(1) Persistently keeping our memorial before the attention of the Honorable, the Minister of Agriculture for an equalization of salary between eastern and western inspectors.

(2) The safeguarding our interests, and the upholding of the dignity of our profession in asking that only veterinary inspectors perform ante or post mortem inspection.

(3) To inquire into the advantages to be derived by bringing under the civil service act this branch of the outside service.

(4) The advisability of approaching our chiefs with the view of securing a fifty-hour-a-week service.

(5) The including of Dominion holidays as overtime, etc.

(6) The proposition of soliciting the cooperation of the veterinary meat inspectors west of Fort William. Our association, as its name indicates, is open for membership from any part of Canada. I hope in the near future to see our western inspectors, members, when we can say that our association extends from ocean to ocean; when every veterinary meat inspector in Canada will be united to assist our superior officers to promote the welfare of the meat inspection system, and raise its present high standard to a yet higher plane of efficiency.

In conclusion, words fail me to express my gratitude for the great honor you have conferred upon me in electing me, by acclamation, to a fourth term as your president. I want to take this opportunity of assuring you that I appreciate the honor. I shall endeavor to transact the business connected with the office to the best of my knowledge and ability. I ask you to assist the officers of this association by your regular attendance at meetings. We are now at a critical stage, before you cast your vote, consider, then I hope you will cast your vote for the man who will do the best and most good for the organization. Again, gentlemen, I thank you.   D. R. BONE.

The election of officers for the ensuing year was then proceeded with. The ballot showed that the members have implicit faith in Dr. Bone by electing him unanimously as president for a fourth term. Dr. R. H. Cook was unanimously chosen to fill the office of vice president in Toronto, while Dr. W. H. James will fill the same position and conduct the Montreal meetings.

The three members elected for the executive committee from Toronto were Drs. T. M. Pine, C. Brind and Wm. Tennent; Dr. C. J. Johannes will represent the Hamilton and Western Ontario members and Dr. G. W. Starnaman the members in Montreal and Eastern Canada.

The duties of secretary-treasurer again fall upon Dr. T. E. H. Fisher.

A suggestion was brought forward as to the possibility of securing accommodation in the Ontario Veterinary College for the holding of meetings and a committee was appointed to interview Dr. E. A. A. Grange in this regard.

The secretary was directed to write the president-elect, Dr. Bone, and convey to him the thanks of the association for his unflagging zeal and endeavors to uplift the standard of inspection and to smooth out the rough places in the road which every veterinary inspector has to travel.

During the month the secretary, as instructed, wrote Dr. Torrance, the V. D. G., inviting him to meet the association and take up subjects of interest to inspectors and inspection. Dr. Torrance's reply, in which he stated that it was inconvenient for him to meet the association, was read and laid over to be dealt with at the next meeting.

A letter from Dr. R. Barnes, Chief Meat Inspector, was also read and laid over for consideration later.

A communication was read from Mr. O'Halloran, Deputy Minister of Agriculture, stating that the Minister, upon consultation with Dr. Torrance and in consideration of our letter of January 24th, urging our petition of August 22nd, 1917, had decided upon a readjustment of salaries in April.

The communication elicited most favorable comment and the members are now living in hope that the financial strain under which they have been laboring for some years past will be to some considerable extent lightened.

No further business being to hand the meeting was adjourned.

On March 4th, Dr. Bone was transferred from Toronto to Edmonton and before leaving the members of the association held a smoker and progressive euchre in his honor. During the even-

ing the assembly was called to order by Dr. Irvine, who, in a few
well chosen words, explained the reason for the assembling of the
members, commented upon the esteem in which Dr. Bone is held
by his associates, upon the work of the association, expressed the
opinion that in the near future the association would receive the
benefits of the transfer of Dr. Bone in the form of application for
membership from prospective members in Western Canada, and
asked Dr. Cook and Dr. Bone to come to the dias. Dr. Cook then
read the following address to Dr. Bone:

It is with a great many regrets that we learn that our department has concluded that your services are required in another and
quite distant part of the Dominion. In our work we know that
transference is an inherent, and quite frequently, a very necessary
part of the institution.

Nevertheless, in the face of the known inevitable, our regrets
will come to the surface. In this particular instance our regrets
are of the selfish nature, they emanate from the knowledge of a
distinct loss on our part, we are the losers. They present themselves
as the hydra-headed monster of old, from almost every conceivable
angle.

We keenly feel the loss of a congenial companion, a courteous
and whole-souled friend, one we feel the better to have known and
one whom to know is to like.

As president of our association we will the more greatly miss
your guiding hand. We have noted your splendid and successful
efforts to build up a strong and useful organization and to raise
the professional standard wherever opportunity presented itself.
We know it has been no easy task, the bringing together of the dis-
cordant elements and welding them into one harmonious whole, to
be known as the Dominion Veterinary Meat Inspectors Association
of Canada. We feel that your untiring energy has been the force
behind, or the *vis a tergo,* if you will, that has given our organization the tone and vigor of youth and strength.

We hope you will take with you a consciousness of a task well
done, a work of monumental effort. The development of a solid
foundation which can, with safety, be built upon. We note with
pride your tact and diplomacy in the handling of the many important problems that have from time to time approached us for settlement, and the results of your zeal we are daily reaping the
benefit from.

We have met this evening, soliciting a kind permission to tender you a slight token of our esteem and respect, and to thank you for your indefatigible efforts in our behalf. We desire to convey to you our whole-hearted impression, you gave us the very best you had and it was good. We anticipate that your new field will be considerably as your old one has been. We expect the work of organization will exist in plenty and be awaiting an organizer. We are prepared to state that they will ere long have one.

In parting we extend to you our hearty congratulations. We sincerely hope the parting will not be for long. The best wishes for your prosperity is the permanent thought of every veterinary meat inspector east of the Great Lakes.

Dr. Cook then presented him, on behalf of his Toronto associates, with a beautiful leather traveling bag, handsomely fitted with the little necessities which make traveling more comfortable. Dr. Bone, who was taken entirely by surprise, thanked the assembly for their thoughtfulness, appreciation and good wishes. Laudatory speeches were made to Dr. Bone by Drs. C. Brind, J. H. George, A. R. Torrie, T. W. R. MacFarlane, D. C. Tennent, T. M. Pine and others.

T. E. Hartman Fisher, Secretary.

CONNECTICUT VETERINARY MEDICAL ASSOCIATION

The annual meeting of the Connecticut Veterinary Medical Association was held at the Hotel Garde, in Hartford, on February 5, 1918. There were twenty-one members present.

The treasurer reported that he had bought a one hundred dollar liberty bond as a patriotic investment for the association. This was endorsed and accepted by vote of the association.

Dr. J. R. Morin and Dr. A. M. McHugh were elected to membership.

Mr. J. M. Whittlesey, Commissioner on Domestic Animals for the State of Connecticut, was elected to honorary membership.

The following officers were elected:

President, Dr. Chas. L. Colton; 1st vice president, Dr. E. F. Schofield; 2nd vice president, Dr. A. W. Sutherland; secretary, Dr. A. T. Gilyard; treasurer, Dr. Thos. Bland.

Board of Censors—Dr. G. W. Loveland, Dr. P. T. Keeley, Dr. Harrison Whitney, Dr. L. B. Judson, Dr. H. E. Bates.

It was voted that the president appoint a legislative committee of five members.

The matter of the Allied Veterinary Relief fund was taken up and the association voted to contribute one hundred dollars from its treasury and individual pledges amounting to one hundred and twenty dollars were secured. Up to the present the individual paid subscriptions amounting to one hundred and seventy dollars and a check for two hundred and seventy dollars has been sent to Dr. Thomas E. Smith, treasurer of the fund. Contributions are still being sought and we hope to make the amount at least three hundred dollars.   A. T. GILYARD, Secretary.

CAMP DODGE VETERINARY MEDICAL ASSOCIATION

The veterinarians at Camp Dodge, Des Moines, Iowa, have organized the Camp Dodge Veterinary Society and held their first meeting May 20th, 1918. We take great pleasure in welcoming this new veterinary society, as practically all of its members belong to the A. V. M. A. and we are sure that the training and experience the members will gain in presenting papers before their local society will give them confidence as well as a desire to participate in the activities of the National Association.

Report of the secretary, Camp Dodge Veterinary Society:
May 20th, 1918.

Meeting called to order at 7 p. m.

Major John H. Gould, temporary chairman.

First order of business, election of officers. The ballots were cast with the following result:

President, Major John H. Gould; vice president, Lieut. Lawrence A. Mosher; secretary and treasurer, Lieut. Robert C. Moore.

Motion made by Lieut. Mosher, seconded by Captain O'Hara, "That meetings be held weekly, for the present". Motion carried.

Paper read by Major John H. Gould, "Treatment of Mange in Army Horses". Discussed freely by Capt. O'Hara, Lieut. Moore, Lieut. Pine, Lieut. Mosher, Lieut. Dawson, Lieut. Jones and Lieut. Moye.

Membership roster of the Camp Dodge Veterinary Society:

Major John H. Gould, Captain Raymond M. Hofferd, Captain Edw. J. O'Hara, Lieut. Joseph F. Derivan, Lieut. Russell E. Elson, Lieut. Alverda J. Dawson, Lieut. Fred Middleton, Lieut. George

W. Moon, Lieut. David B. Pine, Lieut. James B. McNamara, Lieut. Robert S. Tillie, Lieut. Ralph A. Moye, Lieut. Lawrence A. Mosher, Lieut. Lester L. Jones, Lieut. Roy H. Tesdell, Lieut. Spencer K. Nelson, Lieut. Guy M. Parrish, Lieut. Leon M. Getz, Lieut. Robert C. Moore, Lieut. Wilbur C. Smith.

BUREAU OF ANIMAL INDUSTRY VETERINARY ASSOCIATION OF MICHIGAN

At a meeting of Bureau of Animal Industry Veterinarians in Detroit, Friday evening, May 17th, the Bureau of Animal Industry Veterinary Association of Michigan was organized. The meeting was well attended and during the preliminary discussion every Bureau veterinarian present expressed himself as being heartily in favor of such an organization. It was the concensus of opinion that the organization will make for the advancement of the interests of the Bureau veterinarians, increase professional efficiency, and greatly aid the Bureau work within the state. Also, that combination and cooperation with the A. V. M. A. could be but for mutual advancement.

The following officers were elected: Dr. E. P. Schaffter, Detroit, president; Dr. H. M. Newton, Lansing, vice president; and Dr. B. J. Killham, Adrian, secretary-treasurer.

B. J. KILLHAM, Secretary-Treasurer.

BUREAU OF ANIMAL INDUSTRY VETERINARY ASSOCIATION, NEW YORK

ORGANIZATION OF THE BUREAU OF ANIMAL INDUSTRY VETERINARIANS. Under a strong appeal following a long period of advocacy of Dr. John D. DeRonde, the Bureau of Animal Industry Veterinarians of New York, Brooklyn, Jersey City, Newark and Paterson convened at the New York State Veterinary College at New York University in March and discussed the advisability of forming an organization for alignment with the American Veterinary Medical Association.

A temporary organization followed with the selection of Dr. L. D. Ives as chairman, and Dr. J. D. DeRonde as temporary secretary. A committee on form of organization was selected consisting of five members representing New York, Brooklyn, Jersey City, Newark and Paterson, groups of the service.

At a subsequent meeting, in April, it was decided to form a permanent organization under the name of "Bureau of Animal Industry Veterinary Association. Metropolitan Division".

PURPOSES. 1st. The advancement of the professional and material interests of the veterinarians of the Bureau of Animal Industry.

2nd. To combine and cooperate with the American Veterinary Medical Association for mutual advancement and the bettering of our condition in the service.

3rd. To secure legislation that will promote the veterinary service of the B. A. I. and make this service more attractive to those now attached to the Bureau, and to give encouragement to those contemplating entering the same.

Election of officers followed with the following being elected:

Dr. J. D. DeRonde, president, 48 East 89th St., New York City; Dr. F. C. Wilson, vice president; Dr. J. A. Eadie, secretary, 104 West 42nd St., New York City; Dr. C. W. Humphrey, treasurer.

At the May meeting some twenty-five applications for membership were forwarded to Acting Secretary Day of the American Veterinary Medical Association. This number will be doubled at the June meeting.

At the April meeting, Dean W. Horace Hoskins was elected an honorary member, and it is through him as chairman of the legislative committee this association expects to cooperate for the best interests of the association.

The announcement of the death of Prof. A. F. Liautard was feelingly referred to and a committee appointed to draft suitable resolutions in recognition of his distinguished services. The committee submitted the following minute for their records:

In the fullness of time—great length of years—there has passed from our midst a great leader of men

PROFESSOR ALEXANDRE FRANCOIS LIAUTARD.

Richness of purpose, unselfish devotion in a life time service for a world's progress in veterinary medicine. He has given to us an honored name, an unsullied career, an exemplary life.

How deeply grateful we should all feel that he was given to us for such a length of years.

Four score and three years—more than sixty of these given to the advancement of veterinary science.

A soldier veterinarian in his native land of France. A distinguished surgeon and practitioner in America. A profound and true teacher of more than fifteen hundreds of veterinarians in America. A maker of American veterinary journalism. A rich giver to veterinary literature, a liberal contributor at home and abroad to veterinary journalism.

He was given to us for this great service. He fulfilled in the greatest measure his accepted task. Let us in recording this tribute of loving admiration, renew our fealty to the cause he served so well, bowing our heads in profound thankfulness for the exemplary life he has given to us.

COMMUNICATIONS

DR. A. F. LIAUTARD

New York, N. Y., May 15, 1918.

Editor Journal of the American Veterinary Medical Association,
Ithaca, N. Y.:

Dear Sir: When I sent the notice of the death of Dr. Liautard for publication in your May issue, the only information I had was that contained in a cablegram from his daughter which contained the simple announcement, "Father died yesterday"; and from the date of its receipt I assumed that he had died on April 20th. But I am now in receipt of a letter from his son-in-law, Mr. O. Boyer, dated Bois Jerome, France, April 21st, giving the details in connection with Dr. Liautard's death, which I know the profession is awaiting as anxiously for as I have been.

Mr. Boyer writes: "Mrs. Boyer and I confirm our cablegram announcing the death of our dear father, Dr. Liautard, which occurred on April 18th, at 8:10 o'clock in the evening. He had a heart attack on Tuesday, the 16th, during the night, from which he suffered for forty hours. He called for me and I arrived from Paris on Thursday, the 18th, in the afternoon. He was bright and conscious to the last minute. The doctor came to see him half an hour before he died, and he asked him what was his prognosis and whether he should take some digitalis? The doctor explained to him that as he had already taken spartein he could not give him digitalis at that time. After the doctor had gone he asked me what I thought of him, as he was not his regular attendant, he being himself sick.

"I thought, owing to his strong constitution that he would

get over it; but the heart was too weak and used up, and he went peacefully, after having asked me to put his watch to the hour. 'But the old hour,' he said, as on account of the war we have advanced the time one hour.

For months, evidently, he had known of his condition; as we found a little diary in which he was marking his condition day by day.''

Further along in his letter Mr. Boyer says: ''Mrs. Boyer leaves it to you to make any communications to the profession through its press. You know he loved his profession and his ''boys'', as he was always calling you. He worked for the *Review* to the last day of his life, as it had always been his wish to do. So communicate to the societies, as you must know them all. He was a very modest man, of few words, and left us no papers concerning communications to the veterinary press.''

This beautiful letter of Mr. Boyer's brings us to the bedside of our dear departed friend in the very last hours of his life, which we find filled with the same devotion to his profession as has been all the long years since he had embarked upon it. It seems that he had worked all through the day of April 16th, preparing copy for our JOURNAL—which seems to have been still the *Review* to him—and in writing letters to many of his correspondents in the ''States'', and retired that evening—although unconsciously so—with his lifework finished. A lifework that will remain a monument to his memory and an example that should be an inspiration to future generations of our profession. And, oh, how those letters bearing that date on which this great man, with all his faculties at his rich old age, prepared his last contribution for the JOURNAL which he founded, will be cherished by the recipients of them!

How they will cause them to reflect when they see the clear firm hand and the beautiful signature, that to the last moment he. was still at his post doing his part for veterinary education on the very day that he wrote them that letter, and that then he lay down and went to sleep. His profession and his correspondents were his last thought.

Very truly yours,
ROBERT W. ELLIS.

CORRECTION

Editor Journal of the American Veterinary Medical Association:
  Ithaca, N. Y.

Dear Sir: If it will not inconvenience you too greatly I should like to have a correction made on page 295 of the review made by S. H. B. He claims to quote: ''The statement is made that in cases of digestive disorders the autopsy should be performed with the horse lying on its back so that a possible twist of the intestines might be discovered." I have positively not made any such statement in that book. I have been very particular to advocate the right side position as opposed to the dorsal position for autopsy of the horse at all times. S. H. B. comments on this statement which is not in the book: "I must confess that I have never seen a case where having the horse lying on its back made the slightest difference. By the time an autopsy on a horse is made the intestines are under sufficient pressure to change their *position* when the abdominal cavity is opened." Allow me to suggest that more careful perusal of the text will show that I make it quite clear that determination of the *position* of the intestines, while an important item, is not all that constitutes an autopsy. I claim that the right side position as opposed to the dorsal position better facilitates the location of the points of intestinal ligation, for subsequent incision and ablation, that they may be later opened and carefully examined. Post mortem pathology with systematic post mortem technic is a pioneer on the veterinary curricula of this country and it will take time and much experience at the autopsy table before many will be able to appreciate the difference of post mortem technical methods. I am very grateful for S. H. B.'s comment, however, as it so forcefully corroborates his last statement in referring to the book. "It is much needed."

Very truly yours,

W. J. Crocker, Professor of Pathology.

LOOKING FORWARD

Editor, Journal of the American Veterinary Medical Association:
Ithaca, N. Y.

There are many reasons for becoming a member of the American Veterinary Medical Association. By your membership it becomes powerful and has more influence. This is due the A. V. M. A. for the good it has done the profession. It has been instrumental in securing army legislation, giving us the Army Veterinary Service. The War Department recognizes the value of well-trained veterinarians, and this recognition by the War Department has been of inestimable value to us and the profession in placing it on a plane with the other professions.

Membership secures for you the Journal of the A. V. M. A. and the Journal is not only for members, but for the profession. We might have secured the meeting place for our State if we had shown strength. Let the Ohio veterinarians wake up to the fact and become members, attending the next meeting in Philadelphia.

Ohio veterinarians have accepted the fruits of the A. V. M. A. by entering Army Veterinary Service. This reflects credit on the individual and the association. Let us give our best efforts to our country and profession. Become a member of the association which looks to good legislation for the betterment and protection of the veterinarian and his profession.

Blanks may be obtained and filled out. Mail dues to L. A. Merillat, 1827 S. Wabash Ave., Chicago, Ill. (Enos Day, acting secretary). See to this at once. This will be the act that counts. Enjoy the privilege and acquaintance membership will give you. Attend the meetings—you will be pleased. Enlarge your vision of the profession chosen, by your contact with the best men in the profession. Make a supreme effort—you need to do it. You will get value received. Follow instructions carefully found on blank. Hope to meet you in Philadelphia.

A. S. COOLEY, State Secretary.

CONSERVATION

Winona, Minn., May 7, 1918.

Editor Journal of the American Veterinary Medical Association:
Ithaca, N. Y.

Dear Sir: Owing to the fact that the question of conservation is being recommended in all departments by our Government, and in order to be able to fulfill this suggestion at the time when conservation is most needed, it has been decided by vote of the Board of Directors of the Minnesota State Veterinary Medical Association not to hold a summer meeting as usual in July, 1918, thereby conserving to the society and its members the expense necessary for its upkeep.

Very truly yours,

DR. G. ED. LEECH, Secretary.

REVIEW

BALLADS OF THE REGIMENT

MAJOR GERALD E. GRIFFIN, U. S. A.
Published by George U. Harvey Publishing Company, Inc.,
New York, N. Y. Price $1.00.

The Ballads of the Regiment, as the title indicates, deals with life in the Army. The poems cover a wide range of interest. Some are descriptive, sentimental, patriotic, and all have the true poetical rhythm. References to various localities indicate that the author has travelled extensively and that the muse has inspired him in Cuba, the Mexican border, the plains of the West, and in the Philippine Islands. His long connection with the Army has made him familiar with the details of Army life with which a number of his poems deal.

The style is free and incisive and in some instances suggests that of Kipling, as, for instance, in "Baldy":

> "Come! you bunch of loafing cripples,
>   Hit the breeze! Get down and nip!
> Snake her out! Get in the collar!"
>   Then he'd crack his black snake whip.
> " 'Winkie', lad! You're playing 'possum;
>   Git! You pop-eyed, lop-eared fool!
> 'Spinkey'! Darn your lazy carcass! ·
>   You're not fit to be a mule."

Some of the patriotic poems lend themselves to a musical setting, one of which is "Come Along":

> We have heard the foolish gabble
>   Of the Kaiser and his band,
> We have seen the desolation
>   Of his bloody withered hand;
> Now we answer in a manner
>   That they soon will understand;
> , We're marching on the road to Germany.

Major Griffin, with his years of service as an Army Veterinarian, may justly be expected to have a great affection for the horse. His sentiment is expressed in "Inspected and Condemned":

> 'Tis but a horse, a small brown horse,
>   Why should I grieve or care?
> He served with me for twelve long years
>   That flag you see up there.
> Companion of the camp and trail,
>   True friend who knew no fear;
> To save him from an unkind hand
>   I'd die for "Carbineer".

So far as we know Major Griffin is the first poet to appear in the veterinary profession. His collection of verse evidently represents the result of intervals of inspiration spread over a number of years and are now presented in available form for the public. We recommend the book to veterinarians as well as others who have any poetry in their nature and hope it will meet with the success it deserves.   P. A. F.

NECROLOGY

M. VINCENT DEGIVE

The death of M. Vincent Degive occurred at Ixelles, Belgium, on February 3rd. He was a well-known veterinary surgeon, and as director and the organizer of the veterinary school and of the Central State office for the production of calf lymph for vaccination, he has rendered most important service to science. He was also so eminent a "savant" that he was elected on several occasions President of the Royal Academy of Medicine, and was an Associate of the Central Society of Veterinary Medicine of France.

M. Degive received numerous decorations and distinctions, among which we may especially mention "Commandeur de l'Ordre de Léopold et Officier de l'Ordre de la Couronne".

He was born at Horion-Hozimont on January 31, 1844.— *L'Independence Belge*, Jeudi, Mars 7.

CHARLES ARTHUR RAPP

Dr. Charles Arthur Rapp died at Great Falls, Montana, April 6. Dr. Rapp was born in Nebraska January 10, 1876, and graduated from the Iowa State College at Ames with the degree of D.V.M. in June, 1904. He had been a resident of Montana since 1913, and at the time of his death was Veterinarian in Charge for the Bureau of Animal Industry for the State of Montana.

RUFUS E. THOMSON

Dr. Rufus E. Thomson, inspector in charge of meat inspection at Tacoma, Washington, met with an accident April 13, 1918, which resulted in his death twenty-four hours later. He was driving his new Reo car to the government office about seven o'clock in the morning. On the way to the office it is necessary to pass over a bridge which spans a deep ravine. There are two street car tracks that cross this bridge, and he was running his car along one of these lines. Midway on the bridge he tried to steer his car from one side of the bridge to the other, and in attempting to do so, his car skidded and turned crosswise, and, breaking the railing of the bridge, backed off and dropped forty feet to the ground below. In the descent the car turned and landed on the front end. Eye witnesses went to the rescue of the doctor and found him lying forward in the car with his face against the wind shield. He was immediately taken to the hospital and on examination it was found that both his legs and back were broken, and that he had sustained severe contusions of the head and face, and also internal injuries. As already stated, he lived about twenty-four hours after the accident, and was conscious to within a short period of his death. On learning the seriousness of his injuries, he did not expect to recover, and gave instructions to his wife concerning the disposition of his body, and also planned the funeral arrangements.

Dr. Thomson was born in the State of Ohio and graduated from the Ohio State University in 1908 with the degree of D.V.M. Shortly after graduating, he married Miss Mae Morgan of Frankfort, Ohio. To this union two children were born, Mary Virginia and Ruth, ages seven and three years, respectively, who, with his wife and mother, survive him. In the same year of his graduation he was appointed a veterinary inspector in the Bureau of Animal Industry, U. S. Department of Agriculture, and was assigned to Chicago. With the exception of one year with the Bureau in Columbus, Ohio, his entire services to the time of his transfer to Tacoma, Washington, were rendered at Chicago, at which station he was one of the supervising veterinarians.

Dr. Thomson possessed a splendid physique and was of athletic stature and bearing. During his college career in the O. S. U. he did track work; played on the football team, and won the much coveted "O". He was a member of the Alpha Psi fraternity; of the Veterinary Association of the O. S. U.; A. V. M. A., and of the Veterinary Inspectors' Association of Chicago. He was also a member of Banner Blue Lodge of A. F. & A. M. of Illinois. He met his untimely death at the early age in life of 35 years. During the short time that he resided in Tacoma, he made many friends. He was an active member of the Methodist church of Chicago, and also took an active interest in church work at Tacoma, as is shown by the fact that at the time of his death he was a teacher in a Methodist Sunday school. He was respected and held in high esteem by the men under his supervision at his official station. This was evidenced by the kindly assistance rendered to Mrs. Thomson and the two little girls after the doctor's death. Nothing that human hands could do was left undone by those who stood by him in life in his official duties, and who in the sad hour of death dropped tears of sympathy with Mrs. Thomson, and rendered every help possible to make the bereavement lighter.

His many friends at the Chicago station desire to extend to Mrs. Thomson and the children their deepest sympathies. We can use no more fitting words than those of Fitz Green Halleck:

"Green be the turf above thee,
Friend of my better days!
None knew thee but to love thee,
None named thee but to praise."

He was laid to rest at Frankfort, Ohio, where Masonic burial was accorded him.   H. B. RAFFENSPERGER.

TIMOTHY DELANEY

Doctor Timothy Delaney of New York City, for many years a member of the New York County Veterinary Medical Association, passed away after a long period of illness on May 17th, 1918, at the age of 62 years. Doctor Delaney enjoyed for a long period of years an extensive practice among the pleasure horses of the Metropolitan district.

CHARLES H. PERRY

Dr. Charles H. Perry died May 3 at his home, 82 Park Ave., Worcester, Mass., in his 49th year. After graduating from the public schools at Worcester, Dr. Perry entered upon his veterinary course at the Veterinary College at Harvard University, from which he graduated in 1897. Later he attended the Chicago Veterinary College. He was a member of the Worcester Harvard Club, Indian Lake Driving Club, Speedway Club, Massachusetts Veterinary Association and the American Veterinary Medical Association.

Surviving him are his wife and son and two sisters.

BERT BRENETTE STROUD

Dr. Bert B. Stroud died suddenly from dilatation of the heart at Somerville, Mass., about May 12. Dr. Stroud graduated from the N. Y. State Veterinary College at Ithaca, N. Y., with the class of 1903. For a number of years he was pathologist at the Long Island State Hospital at Brooklyn. He left this position in 1917 and received a commission as Second Lieutenant in the Veterinary Reserve Corps and was stationed at Camp Upton until December, when, on account of physical disability, he was honorably discharged. At the time of his illness he was about to enter the service of the Bureau of Animal Industry at Boston, Mass.

He is survived by his mother. Burial services under Masonic auspices were held at Dryden, N. Y.

MISCELLANEOUS

—Dr. B. L. Cook has removed from Red Wing to Farmington, Minn.

—Dr. W. M. Pendergast has purchased the property at 620 Court St., Syracuse, for his veterinary practice.

—Dr. H. A. Smith has removed from Jacksonville, Fla., to Kentland, Indiana.

—Dr. S. H. Burnett has resigned his position in Pathology at New York State Veterinary College at Cornell University.

—Dr. Lee C. Hoover, formerly at Richmond, has located at Spiceland, Ind.

—Dr. G. W. Lobach has removed from Columbus, O., to Bethlehem, Pa.

—SEIZES SO-CALLED HOG-CHOLERA REMEDY. .ATTEMPT TO SELL PRODUCT IN IOWA AND OTHER STATES LEADS TO IMMEDIATE ACTION TO PROTECT PORK SUPPLY. Seizures of sixty-two cases of a so-called hog-cholera remedy in Iowa and North Carolina upon order of the Federal Courts mark a determined effort on the part of the United States Department of Agriculture to stop interstate traffic in so-called hog-cholera remedies which do not cure, prevent nor control this disease which has such an important bearing on the Nation's pork supply. The seized goods are now in custody of United States Marshals pending action under the Food and Drugs Act. The Government charges that this remedy will not prevent or cure hog cholera, as claimed on the labels of the seized products.

The Bureau of Animal Industry, through its veterinarians and experts in animal diseases, is cooperating actively with the Bureau of Chemistry in this campaign to control interstate traffic in fraudulent stock remedies.

—Swine Mortality from Disease at Lowest Mark. The death rate in swine from all diseases for the year ending March, 1918, announced by the United States Department of Agriculture as 42.1 per 1,000, is the lowest in thirty-five years, according to the records kept during that period.

This unprecedentedly low rate of mortality presents a great contrast with those of earlier periods, particularly with the losses of 133.8 per 1,000 in 1887, 144 per 1,000 in 1897, and 118.9 per 1,000 in 1914, years marked by severe outbreaks of hog cholera. This is even a remarkable reduction from the normal low rate of losses which has remained slightly above 50 per 1,000 when the disease was least prevalent.

The approximate number of hogs on hand January 1, 1918, was 71,374,000. The loss of 42.1 per 1,000 for the year ending March, 1918, therefore represented approximately 3,000,000 of these animals, equivalent to the consumption of pork and pork products by the entire population of the United States for 1917 for 25 days.

These recent losses should be compared with that of 7,000,000 hogs in 1914, which curtailed production to the extent of the national consumption for that year for 37 days.

The marked reduction in the losses of swine in 1918 over preceding periods, in view of the fact that 90 per cent of these losses are due to hog cholera, indicates clearly the benefit from the combined efforts of State and Federal agencies in protecting the farmers against the ravages of this exceedingly fatal disease.

THE LITTLE GRAY MULE

No one asked what he thought of war,
How his conscience stood, or anything more,
But they took him to France, to stand his chance,
It's all right, only a mule.
He pulled his load to the top of the hill,
A shot rang out and he lay quite still,
"Anyone hit?" "No, we're fit,"
It's all right, only a mule.

—The Rider and Driver.

JOURNAL
OF THE
American Veterinary Medical Association
Formerly American Veterinary Review
(Original Official Organ U. S. Vet. Med. Ass'n)

PIERRE A. FISH, Editor · ITHACA, N. Y.

Executive Board
GEORGE HILTON, 1st District; W. HORACE HOSKINS, 2d District; J. R. MOHLER,
3d District; C. H. STANGE, 4th District; R. A. ARCHIBALD, 5th
District; A. T. KINSLEY, Member at large.

Sub-Committee on Journal
J. R. MOHLER R. A. ARCHIBALD

The American Veterinary Medical Association is not responsible for views or statements
published in the JOURNAL, outside of its own authorized actions.
Reprints should be ordered in advance. A circular of prices will be sent upon application.

VOL. LIII., N. S. VOL. VI. JULY, 1918. No. 4.

Communications relating to membership and matters pertaining to the American Veterinary Medical Association should be addressed to Acting Secretary L. Enos Day, 1827 S.
Wabash Ave., Chicago, Ill. Matters pertaining to the Journal should be sent to Ithaca, N. Y.

CONSERVING HEALTH

Many factors have at various times been enumerated as essential to the winning of the war. Man-power, food, ships, air-
planes, labor, munitions and morale are concerned. Not one of
these factors as a separate entity is sufficient. They must be properly coordinated and directed. The power concerned in the production of each factor is health.

Facing us is an implacable, relentless and intriguing foe by
no means subdued, or likely to be, until much fresh blood from the
armies of this country is mingled with that of the allies upon the
shell-torn soil of France, Belgium and Italy. America has the
privilege of *helping* to win this war, which for nearly four long
and bitter years the allies have so gloriously and so patiently en-
dured. If America is to *help* win freedom for the world, to *help*
take the Germ out of Germany—the germ of the hellish heresy
that she is divinely appointed to dominate the world, that murder,
rape, enslavement, extermination, thievery and hypocrisy are jus-
tifiable when committed in the service of the State; then our country must be prepared for the sacrifice involved in the depreciation
of our man-power and submit as cheerfully as have the allies to the

necessary restrictions upon our usual method of life. The horror of today will give way to the peace of tomorrow. The present is in our hands; the future is in the hands of our children. In fighting for their freedom, it is a correlative duty to conserve their lives under healthy conditions in order to conserve the strength of the Nation.

War does not take its toll from casualties alone. Disease and pestilence have stalked through the ranks and in former wars have caused even greater havoc than have bullets and shells. The strategy of sanitation, immunology and correlated branches is as important as military strategy. The discoveries of Pasteur, Lister and Koch have made possible the restoration of a larger percentage of the wounded than ever before. Quite as favorable results have been obtained in the prevention of disease.

In the light of the present day efficiency, it is difficult to believe that only twenty years ago, in the Spanish-American campaign, 86 per cent of all deaths were due to typhoid fever which attacked and weakened practically 20 per cent of the small army employed for a few months. In 1911, anti-typhoid inoculation was made compulsory in the United States Army. For a slightly longer period than the Spanish-American conflict there was an average of over 742,000 men in American cantonments and camps, and only 114 cases of typhoid fever occurred—a signal triumph over former conditions. The deaths from wounds among the American overseas forces have been approximately only about five per cent.

In the Civil War, the federal forces lost 110,000 men as the result of wounds, and 249,000 who perished because of disease. Contrast with this the statement of German casualties up to January 31, 1917, in which 929,116 were reported to have been killed in action or to have died from wounds, while only 59,230 died from disease. According to Surgeon-General Gorgas, the death rate of our American forces of over 1,000,000 men on March 11, 1918, was at the rate of ten per thousand, while a few years ago the Japanese mortality rate of 20 per thousand was hailed as a remarkable achievement.

Linked with human health is animal health. Veterinary science has progressed with medical science. In the Boer war there was a loss of over 50 per cent among the army horses. In the present war the loss has been reduced to somewhat less than 10 per cent. Laboratory research is assuming a definite and permanent place in military quarters. Vaccines, sera, antitoxins are becoming as vital to the health and welfare of the military forces as the daily rations.

Because of the intimate relation of the domesticated animals and their products to the food problem, the veterinarian has a high function to perform in conserving their health. In Belgium, Serbia and Roumania there is now a practical exhaustion of these animals. Germany has acquired these animals in her characteristic way and has therefore been able to conserve her own stock for a longer period. According to the Food Administration, the allies have reduced their herds and flocks 45,787,000 head, while Germany has reduced her supply about 18,000,000 head. Neutral nations show a total net reduction of 1,412,000 head. There is thus represented a loss of about 65,000,000 livestock in Europe, without taking into consideration Austria, Turkey and Russia, which, if included, would doubtless bring the total to over 100,000,000. The total number of cattle, sheep and swine now in the United States is estimated at about 187,000,000. This makes a striking comparison with the depletion of 100,000,000 animals in Europe with its larger human population. When it is considered that the animals still alive are doubtless in poor condition involving a reduction in live weight and a limitation in their products, it is obvious that the animal resources of Europe have been very considerably diminished.

The result is obvious, an ill-nourished population, human and animal, induces ill-health. In the long run the strength of a nation and its armies depends upon Health.   P. A. F.

OUR DUTIES

At no time in the history of our country has the veterinary profession been confronted with more serious problems than at present. All conditions, especially those affecting the food supply, have changed since the outbreak of the present great world conflict and since our participation in the war the conservation of the food supply became the key note of the leaders. It is rightly said that food will win the war and while this slogan is used in a figurative way, nevertheless the outcome of this great struggle is greatly dependent on our ability to provide food for our army and the armies of the allies. At the same time the preservation of our resources and especially of our livestock industry must not be lost sight of.

For many years to come after the conclusion of peace the depletion of livestock in all countries in Europe will continue to make them dependent upon outside sources for their meat food. From the present outlook the United States and Argentina will be especially called upon to make up the deficiency created in European countries. The great demand for foreign shipment resulting in a marked increase in value of all livestock brought about a natural tendency among the breeders and stockmen to immediately realize the profits and disregard to some extent the future as far as the supply of livestock is concerned.

For this and many other reasons it is obvious that it is the duty of the veterinarians to enlighten stock owners of the necessity to maintain their breeding stock at a maximum and to conserve the health and quality of the animals. All means and precautions should be taken to guard against losses from diseases and the authorities should conscientiously enforce all measures by which it is possible to guard against the spread of diseases.

In this regard the occurrence of sporadic diseases among the livestock is of minor importance when compared with those scourges which are responsible for the death of thousands, yes, hundreds of thousands of animals. It must also be considered that the veterinary profession has been considerably depleted from calls to active service with our armies and from the present outlook this will continue for some time to come so that those remaining at home will be called upon to cover larger areas and increase their activity accordingly.

There should be no slacking on the veterinarian's part and unless he realizes that it is his patriotic duty to assist with all his ability in the conservation of livestock he fails to do his bit.

                                                        A. E.

—The semi-annual meeting of the Veterinary Medical Association of New Jersey will be held July 11 and 12 at the Hotel Marlborough, Asbury Park, N. J. Visiting veterinarians will be welcome and a very successful meeting is anticipated.

—Dr. M. H. Rhoades, formerly stationed at Oklahoma City, has resigned from the Bureau of Animal Industry service to engage in farming and the production of livestock near Fort Collins, Colo.

*SERUM TREATMENT OF CANINE DISTEMPER

A. SLAWSON, New York, N. Y.

Canine distemper has long been held in great respect by those whose dogs have been brought into contact with it, but its ravages have not dampened the ardor with which dog lovers have gone on developing the various breeds in which they are interested. Also, most individuals who have lost their pets from this disease have come back within a short time to give dogs another trial. In fact, the breeding of dogs has gone on apace so that in spite of the large mortality annually from the dog plague, there are today in this country more dogs of the various breeds developed to a higher de- gree than ever before: Such is the effect which losses from distem- per have had upon the lovers of dogs. It is no wonder then that those whose dogs have suffered from this scourge should look for- ward with relief to any treatment which offers a greater measure of success than any used heretofore.

It was my fortune first to become familiar with dog diseases in October, 1901, while in the employ of the late Dr. Thomas G. Sherwood of New York City, and my interest in dogs has been in- tensified yearly up to the present time. The treatment of dog dis- temper from my own knowledge, namely from 1901 to 1912, was principally along general medicinal lines, combined with pains- taking nursing. Everyone here knows what that means. No prog- nosis was certain. After laborious days and nights, especially with toy breeds, and highly inbred dogs, the majority of cases termi- nated fatally. In my opinion, a conservative estimate of recover- ies, counting all breeds, would be 40%. When a case was diag- nosed, even in the early stages, it was obliged to run a fairly con- stant course, becoming gradually worse until the third or fourth week, when a convalescent period of two weeks, more or less, would take place. It was quite safe to say, if the dogs survived the se- verest stages, during the third or fourth week, they would recover, provided no complications or sequelae resulted. The gist of this summary is that the treatment of canine distemper was unsatis- factory alike to veterinarian, client and patient, for I am sure could the latter have spoken, he would have told us so. This ap-

*Presented at the 54th Annual Meeting of the American Veterinary Medi- cal Association, Kansas City, Mo., August, 1917.

plies also in the present tense where the old line treatment is still
followed.

In 1911, I first met Dr. John C. Torrey, and from that time
on have consistently applied vaccine and serum in the treatment
of canine distemper. This has led to my using serum for curative
purposes, and as a prophylactic only when exposure to the disease
has taken place. As in the treatment of all disease the earlier a
case is diagnosed, and the right treatment applied, the greater the
chance of recovery. For this reason it is important to recognize
canine distemper in its earliest stages, for it is then that the use of
serum rapidly aborts the disease. Some objection may be raised
to this, as it could be said that resistant dogs might recover anyway. Having kept this point in mind I will cite some cases later
to prove that it is a mistake not to treat all dogs just as soon as a
diagnosis has been made.

ETIOLOGY. Although some veterinarians and others still believe the cause of canine distemper has not yet definitely been
fixed, from my work with vaccine and serum prepared from *B.
bronchisepticus*, in the early stages of the disease before much secondary infection has taken place, I believe *B. bronchisepticus*,
named by Ferry of Detroit, but found independently also about
the same time by Torrey of New York and by McGowan of Edinburgh, Scotland, to be the causative agent of this disease.

SYMPTOMS. The early symptoms should easily be recognized.
One of the first signs is a hacking, dry cough which is very characteristic. This is caused by the development of the organism,
first in the upper air passages, and then in the bronchial tubes.
The owner will state either that his dog has swallowed something,
which has lodged in his throat, and is trying to "bring it up", or
that his dog has a "cold". Sometimes sneezing is noticed. The
animal sleeps a good part of the time. Varying appetite and loss
of weight usually occur. Skin eruptions may also be present,
but they are not a constant symptom. The sclerotics are congested,
at first very slightly, showing a pinkish tint. The bowels are costive or loose, rarely normal. The temperature varies considerably,
from 101° to 106°, although the high temperatures in the beginning are not dangerous as they usually drop several degrees after
the first reaction to infection has taken place. The pulse is rapid
and wiry, varying from 120 to 160 according to the extent to which
the dog is affected by the toxins in his system. The respiration is

quickened. Nervous dogs must be taken into consideration as their pulse rate and temperature may be slightly above normal. As the disease progresses the nostrils become dry and discharge a serous, then muco-purulent exudate. The conjunctivae and sclerotics become more congested and a muco-purulent discharge appears. This condition usually becomes so severe that corneal ulcers develop unless the eyes receive careful treatment. Even then the ulcers may occur. The bowel evacuations become soft, then watery, and often blood is passed with the stool, which has a characteristic offensive odor. The cough is still present, and the bronchial condition varies from a severe bronchitis to a bronchial pneumonia. Streptococcic stomatitis or streptococcic pneumonia occasionally complicates the disease. Chorea or partial or complete paralysis may appear at any time during the course of the disease. Occasionally in dogs, as is usual with cats, the disease is confined to the head, that is to the upper air passages, the nose being dry and the eyes affected, but no loose bowels occurring; constipation being the order. Sneezing and snuffling is noticeable. However, most times the toxins of *B. bronchisepticus,* and secondary invaders, eventually break down the resistance of the body, and the disease becomes generalized.

When I first began the treatment of distemper with biologics, I pursued the old line methods in conjunction with the vaccine and serum. If the temperature was high febrifuges were given from the beginning, and for dysentery the usual medicines were prescribed. The vaccine treatment meant repeated injections and visits but with the advent of Dr. Torrey's serum the treatment became simpler and the results were better. Large or small dogs received 5 c.c. of the serum every other day for three doses. Occasionally four doses were given. In the three years—1913 to 1916 —outside of the cases in my practice I treated one hundred cases of various breeds of dogs, of which I have no full records. They were dogs belonging to several dog exchanges in New York City. The results were not satisfactory because little care was given the dogs in spite of repeated cautioning. These cases I have thrown out because a record of them would not be fair to the serum. If in mid-winter a man is told to put a jacket on a dog, and this is not done, if a dog is allowed to run about with a beginning of bronchial pneumonia when the owner has been warned to keep the animal quiet, if a dog is allowed to remain on a wooden or stone floor

without protection, exposed to constant drafts when he should be
kept off the floor, and if the right kind of nourishment has not been
given regularly, then the man and not the serum is to blame if the
dog does not recover. The best results are obtained when the animal is taken care of, and instructions followed implicitly.

As stated before, I had been accustomed to the old line treatment of distemper, on which account it took some time to adjust
my treatment to the use of serum. From 1912 to the summer of
1916, I used first vaccine, and shortly after the serum prepared by
Dr. Torrey. While the serum was efficacious from the start, toward
the end of the period mentioned the best results were obtained.
In "Studies in Canine Distemper", by J. C. Torrey, Ph.D., and
Alfred H. Rehe, published in January, 1913, in the *Journal of
Medical Research*, the way in which Dr. Torrey began his researches is discussed. The work was first undertaken in 1908 by
Dr. Oscar Teague on a fund raised by the late Dr. T. G. Sherwood,
but due to Dr. Teague's departure for the Philippines the work
was soon interrupted and discontinued until 1910, when as a result of the cooperation and financial assistance of the Continental
Field Trial Club and others, a systematic investigation of canine
distemper was begun. Dr. Torrey carried on his work until the
summer of 1916. As other matters in the department of experimental pathology at the Cornell Medical College in New York were
occupying his time, and as he had completed the work he had in
mind when the investigation was first undertaken, he discontinued
the preparation of the serum. Dr. Torrey's serum was then taken
over and prepared by E. R. Squibb & Sons, 80 Beekman Street,
New York City. The serum having become indispensable to me in
the treatment of distemper I continued using their serum with
better results than before, the two reasons for this being the higher
potency of this serum and a better understanding of how to use it.

After making a diagnosis I inject from 3 to 7 c.c. of serum
according to age and breed of the dog. Only puppies from two to
four months old are given 3 c.c. All small breeds over six months
of age, such as Pomeranians, Pekingese, Japanese spaniels, French
bull dogs, Boston terriers, etc., are given 5 c.c., larger dogs are
given 7 c.c. Three doses of serum are given two days apart. More
than three doses are rarely necessary. No more than four doses
should be given. The serum cannot safely be given *ad libitum*.
It is important not to lose sight of this point. It takes strength to

absorb the serum and care must be taken not to weaken the animal. Moreover, if antibodies enough have not been introduced into the system by three or four doses of serum, sufficient, together with those produced by the body itself, to effect a favorable change in the condition of the animal, then it may be said that the blood has reached a state of negative phase, in which case nursing and medicinal treatment should be followed. Occasionally in these cases leucocyte extract is of value. Except in very high temperatures, 107° and over, I give no antipyretics in beginning the treatment. If the temperature remains 105° the day following the second dose of serum, febrifuges may be given. If the bowels are loose and remain in this condition after the third dose of serum has been given, which is rare, anti-diarrhetics may be prescribed. With the first dose of serum strychnine sulphate is prescribed in doses of 1/500 to 1/200 gr. two to three times daily, according to the age and size of the dog, in order to keep up arterial tension. In these doses this drug may be given to dogs for several weeks without danger of a cumulative action. This is very important as the heart muscle is weakened as a result of the action of the combined toxins of the various organisms and over-stimulation from too large doses of strychnine might result in collapse of the heart. With proper attention this can be avoided.

The best diet in cases that refuse nourishment is raw eggs and milk, the quantity given depending on the size of the dog and the condition of his stomach. Much of this food is absorbed through the lacteals. The pouring of a constant stream of chyle through the receptaculum chyli, and as lymph through the lymphatic glands and vessels aids in keeping up a supply of lymphocytes, which are constantly needed to replace the rapidly worn out polymorphonuclear types. Of course, other foods may be given according to appetite and habit of feeding the animal, but the importance of a raw egg and milk diet should not be forgotten. The dog should be kept as quiet as possible, and the owner warned not to play with him, especially during the treatment even though the animal appears brighter, as exercise of any kind taxes the heart, and keeps the temperature up. After the third injection of serum these precautions should be carried out for fully two weeks, and the animal should not be bathed during that time in order to prevent chilling. In the fall, winter and spring a flannel jacket should be kept on the dog from the beginning of the treatment, and care taken not to let him get wet from rain or snow, and to keep him dry and warm, so that the danger from bronchial pneumonia may be minimized.

If the serum treatment is carried out according to the foregoing directions, canine distemper becomes a disease easy to treat with corresponding satisfaction as stated before alike to veterinarian, client and patient. In most cases the symptoms begin to disappear after the second injection of serum, in a less number after the third injection. This is seen in the disappearance of fever and a clearing or whitening of the sclerotics. Within a week the dog is on the road to recovery, and at the end of two weeks is practically well. A temperature of one or two degrees may go on for two or three weeks after this, but it is unimportant. Thus the disease, instead of running its course of six weeks, is shortened to two weeks. With ordinary care the eyes come out beautifully, corneal ulcers being conspicuous by their absence. Nervous lesions are prevented, nervous symptoms seldom developing. From forty per cent of recoveries under old treatment, eighty to ninety per cent may be expected under the new. Occasionally, several days after the serum treatment has been completed, the owner will state that although his dog appears brighter and eats well, the cough is still present. In those cases in which deep-seated bronchitis or bronchial pneumonia exists, when the animal is first presented for treatment, the cough is apt to continue, with varying degrees of severity, for two or three weeks, and it should be remembered and explained to the owner that although the serum treatment destroys the organisms in the bronchial tubes, deep-seated congestions do not clear up at once. The fact that good has been done is shown by the improvement in the dog. In such cases expectorants may be given, but I wish to warn against the use of these until three days after the last dose of serum has been injected. My reason for this is that shortly after the first dose of serum is injected a marked destructive action takes place in the mucous membranes of, and the lung tissues bordering on, the bronchial tubes, due to the action of the phagocytes on *B. bronchisepticus*. While this is going on resolution of the congested areas takes place rapidly and any drug eliminated through the bronchial tubes may act as an irritant and check the activity of these leucocytes, thereby increasing the congestion and the danger of its spreading to contiguous lung tissue. By waiting a few days, until after the last dose of serum has been injected, expectorants may be given without interfering with the specific action of the serum, and the best results from the use of this class of drugs may then be expected. The reason attributed by me to the satisfactory action of the serum is first its specific action on *B. bronchisepticus*, and, second, the inherent bactericidal power of all serum, which is of the greatest aid in overcoming secondary infection.

The following cases have been treated with serum under my personal care, eighty-four of this number during the year just closed:

Breed	Number Treated	Recoveries	Deaths	Percentage of Recoveries
American foxhound.............	1	1		
Boston terrier...................	10	9	1	
German shepherd (police dogs)....	15	10	5	
Airdale	3	3		
Maltese terrier..................	7	5	2	
White Spitz....................	3	3		
Irish terrier....................	2	2		
Pointer	11	11		
Setter	15	14		
French bull....................	1	1		
Fox terrier.....................	5	4	1	
Japanese spaniel................	5	2	3	
Dachshund	2	2		
Pekingese spaniel................	24	22	2	
Water spaniel..................	2	1	1	
Poodle (French)................	3	3		
Pomeranian	2	2		
Chow Chow....................	2	2		
Russian wolfhound..............	4	3		
Bull terrier....................	1	1		
Mongrel terrier.................	2	2		
Collie	1	1		
Angora Cat....................	1	1		
Total.......................	122	105	17	83.6%

All deaths except in the Japanese spaniels occurred in cases neglected by their owners in the beginning. The wolfhound that died had a temperature of 107.4 with a bronchial pneumonia when first treated, and lived for three days while the treatment was being given, his temperature dropping to 105°, but rising to 108.4 when death occurred. The case of the Angora cat is interesting. He was ten months old, and had been snuffling and sneezing for one month when first seen. He had not been altered. He was affected with sarcoptic mange about the head, ears and neck. The treatment for mange was begun, and three days later the cat was given ether and altered. A Boston terrier puppy was in a cage next to the cat and had been well for four weeks when the cat was admitted. In five days the puppy began to snuffle and cough, showing unmistakable signs of distemper. He was at once given 3 c.c. of serum, followed by the same amount in two days, and 5 c.c. two days after that. The cat was given two doses of 3 c.c. each. Both cases made uneventful recoveries.

Not wishing to be hasty in administering the serum I have occasionally had people return with their pets two to three days after having made an examination. In doubtful cases this is the best method to pursue, and in these very early cases the delay can work no harm to the patient. Two doubtful cases in point are two fox terriers. One case had a normal temperature and no cough, but the sclerotics were pink and the pulse 130. The dog was sleepy and refused food, but the bowels were open as castor oil had been given. The treatment was explained to the owner, and he was advised to call again in two days' time. However, he did not have time to do this, so the treatment was begun at once. All symptoms had begun to disappear when the dog was presented for the second injection of serum two days later. The dog made an uneventful recovery. The other fox terrier brought in the same day was a doubtful case. He had been costive a week and had had several doses of castor oil, and had varied in spirit and appetite. The sclerotics were pink. Temperature 101, pulse 120; he had had a slight cough a few days before this, but this had disappeared. The serum treatment was explained to the owner, some tablets given for the dog, and the owner advised to return the dog in three days. This was on June 2nd, but the dog was not brought back until June 20th, eighteen days later, when he showed unmistakable, but not severe symptoms of distemper. The owner explained the dog had shown improvement from the medicinal treatment, and that he thought recovery would take place. The serum was then given, and the dog made a rapid, uneventful recovery. In this case the animal showed great resistance to the disease. Another resistant case occurred in a Boston terrier. He was first seen December 16th and 17th, temperature 102, pulse 140, varying appetite and spirits, and loss of weight noticed. Serum not desired by owner at that time. Called again on January 29th, over five weeks later. Condition of the dog the same as before. The serum treatment was given and the dog made a rapid uneventful recovery.

Another fox terrier had all the symptoms of a case in the early stages of distemper, the bronchial symptoms being especially severe. Tablets given and serum treatment advised. This was on December 7th and 8th. Serum not desired by owner. Called again on December 25th. Dog no better and serum treatment given. He seemed to make an uneventful recovery as the owner told me so over the telephone. However, I was again called to see this dog on March 12th. The dog showed marked dyspnea, but his general condition seemed fair, the distemper symptoms having disappeared. The owner stated that the dog had begun the labored breathing five weeks earlier, and it had gradually grown worse. Pulse 160 and wiry, temperature 101. It was difficult to make a diagnosis on auscultation and percussion in this restless dog. The sound of the heart action was so dull, however, and the mucous membrane so anemic, that I ventured a diagnosis of hydroperi-cardium, with danger of collapse of the heart, and advised at the same time that the animal be destroyed. An autopsy was performed. All organs with the exception of the lungs were normal. Both lungs showed numerous areas of firm caseation, varying in size from a pea to a hazelnut. The mediastinal and bronchial lymph glands were normal, as were the lymph glands throughout the body. This was not a case of tuberculosis, but very likely a case of streptococcic infection. In this case had the serum treatment been given when the dog was first seen it is probable that he would have overcome this secondary infection. This shows with the other cases mentioned that it is best not to count on the resistance of a dog to combat the disease, but to give the serum treatment at once. One point more, when the serum treatment is once begun it should be completed, as one dose of serum is not enough to effect a cure. In only two cases, a Dachshund and Maltese terrier, were two doses given as the heart action of these dogs was so weak that I stopped the serum and continued the treatment along general lines. However, these dogs also made rapid recoveries.

From the foregoing results it seems to me that the serum treatment of canine distemper has come to stay. It appears to be only a matter of a short time before it will be more generally used than at present. To me it has meant an ever widening circle of satisfied clients. I shall continue to urge the use of the serum whenever a case of canine distemper is presented to me for treatment.

DISCUSSION

DR. QUITMAN: Is the Torrey serum a prophylactic serum?

DR. SLAWSON: It is a curative serum.

DR. QUITMAN: Doesn't he get out a prophylactic serum?

DR. SLAWSON: No. I think that was said at first. I said I gave it for curative purposes, and as a prophylactic only when exposure has taken place. 1 do not think any serum I have heard of is prophylactic. I mean it will protect them if they have been exposed, but then they should be removed so that they do not undergo further exposure, say after a period of a couple of weeks. I think the immunity wears off then. In other words the serum confers a passive and not an active immunity.

DR. QUITMAN: I wish to compliment Dr. Slawson on his excellent paper and the great thoroughness of it. It is one of the best papers I have ever heard on this disease. As to this prophylactic serum, it is probably an early label that was gotten out, because I know I have a package marked for prophylactic purposes, and I thought when the package was sent me I was to receive an inactive serum, and consequently never used it. In a floating city practice one does not commonly have use for the prophylactic serum. With Dr. Slawson's explanation of this serum, I am now anxious to try it.

DR. PIERCE: What fee do you charge for this treatment?

DR. SLAWSON: I charge my fee according to the client. A poor person needs treatment for his dog as well as a rich man. Whatever may be my fee I charge that plus one dollar for each injection of serum. I cannot afford to open a package of serum, because it is expensive, and charge less than that. I make them understand my fee is so much, plus three dollars for three injections of serum. Sometimes where there is a little more profit one way or another, you can give a poor person a lower rate. I think you have to charge three dollars for the serum to come out even in all cases.

A MEMBER: There are a number of people who have serums on the market for canine distemper. Do you know anything about them?

DR. SLAWSON: I know nothing about them. The only reason I have been using this serum is because I had worked on it before I knew it was going to be taken up. Dr. Torrey worked without any thought of compensation. It was purely scientific work and work in the laboratory for the purpose of helping people. There is a division of the Cornell Medical College in New York City and I got to know Dr. Torrey there. It was only because in his earlier work he wanted somebody to use his vaccine and serum in the treatment of distemper that I got to work with him.

A Member: How is it put up?

Dr. Slawson: It is put out as a serum in bottles of 20 c.c. each.

A Member: How much of an injection do you give?

Dr. Slawson: Three injections, 5 c.c. each, sometimes four injections.

Dr. Pierce: We very often have dogs brought in which are suffering from chorea or paralysis to a greater or less extent, and I would like to ask what success has been had in those cases that had already developed?

Dr. Slawson: The treatment is unsatisfactory. I had several cases that cleared up, but that has not been true of all of them. In those cases, you can be pretty sure, unless the dog is nearly well when these symptoms appear they will not do well. Most of them die. I have used a preparation of Inula and Echinacea put up by Lloyd Brothers of Cincinnati in these cases. I have used that intramuscularly. I had one case in which I felt I did not wish to use the serum. It was pretty well recovered and seemed more rheumatic than paralyzed. I gave this dog three injections of five c.c. each, two days apart, intramuscularly. I gave it in the group of muscles behind the scapula instead of the gluteal muscles as recommended. This dog showed no particular response to this treatment. I gave it in this manner because I gave it once to a dog in the gluteal muscles. This was in a case of autointoxication which had convulsions, which stopped, but when the dog got home he was paralyzed. I thought perhaps it was due to pressure on the sciatic nerves, and then an abscess developed. After treating this dog one month he had to be destroyed. After that I have always injected it in the muscles back of the shoulder. Another case was a little Pekingese with chorea. I gave it to him in three c.c. doses for three injections, and he seemed to do very well, but I did not follow it up.*

Another severe case of chorea I had was in a Boston terrier to which I gave the same preparation (Inula and Echinacea) and he did very well. It was a case where the head would strike the ground, he was so bad; the woman was delighted with the treatment, but a month later she came back and said the dog was the same as before. I felt there was nothing specific about that treatment and I was sorry I had not used the serum.

---

*A year later, April, 1918, I learned this little dog did not recover.

—Dr. Don McMahan has removed from Calvin to Fargo, N. D.

—Dr. J. H. Webster has removed from San Francisco to Coalinga, Calif.

INVESTIGATIONS ON BLACKLEG IMMUNIZATION*

Prof. Naoshi Nitta
Laboratory of Vet. Pathology and Bacteriology,
Agric. Coll., Tokyo Imperial University

INTRODUCTION. For a long time there has been prevalent among the cattle in the western part of Japan an acute enzoötic disease commonly known as "Tachi". No attempt had been made to describe the disease until 1893, when the "Tachi" disease in Yamaguchi Prefecture was first referred to by K. Shiraishi, who claimed to have found, on microscopic examination of muscles from an affected cow, together with a variety of organisms, a spore-bearing bacillus morphologically similar to that of blackleg and who suggested that the "Tachi" disease might be identical with the blackleg prevalent in Europe and America. I was also informed personally by Professor G. Suto, who was for a few years Professor in the Agricultural College at Sapporo, that he had seen a case of blackleg in sheep during his tenure of office there.

It was only in the year 1897 that systematic investigations of the "Tachi" disease were first undertaken by the writer. The material used for that purpose was some pieces of dried flesh from an affected animal sent from the above-mentioned prefecture.. Besides these, pieces of dried blackleg flesh sent from Germany in 1899 by Professor H. Tokishige, who was then studying in Professor Kitt's Laboratory at the Royal Veterinary College in Munich, served as the basis of our investigations. The following is the résumé of my investigations (1905).

1. It may be safely stated that the "Tachi" disease is identical with the blackleg prevalent in foreign countries.

2. The experiments with guinea pigs and with cattle in some infected districts show that the "Tachi" vaccines prepared according to Arloing, Cornevin, and Thomas may be successfully used in practice.

3. The "Tachi" immune-serum prepared by hyperimmunization of cattle has a protective, and to a certain extent also a curative action when used in time, as stated by Kitt, Leclainche-Vallée, and Arloing.

*Bulletin of the Central Veterinary Medical Association, April, 1918, Tokyo, Japan.

Official statistics of blackleg in this country for recent ten years (1907-1916) are given below:

Years	1907	1908	1909	1910	1911	1912	1913	1914	1915	1916
Total	120	171	159	128	181	191	209	172	186	165

A BRIEF REVIEW OF EXISTING METHODS OF IMMUNIZATION AGAINST BLACKLEG. It was Arloing, Cornevin, and Thomas, who, in 1880, first discovered that animals could be protected against blackleg by a subcutaneous injection of minimal doses of fluid from a blackleg tumor and also by an intravenous or intratracheal injection of the virus. These methods, however, were abandoned as being too dangerous or too complicated to be of practical value. In 1883, the French scientists recorded a method of vaccination which has ever since been practised largely in France, Switzerland, and other countries. In this method two vaccines of different virulence are employed: the first or weaker vaccine is prepared by exposing the dried juice obtained from a blackleg tumor to a temperature of 100°-104° C. for six hours, and the second or stronger vaccine by exposing it for the same length of time to a temperature of 85°-90° C. The under surface of the tail is the seat of inoculation, the operation being attended with some difficulty owing to the density of the subcutaneous tissue of the part.

Kitt, in 1888, published a simplified method of vaccination in which a single vaccine is prepared by heating virulent muscle powder at a temperature of 100° C. for six hours in a steam sterilizer. The vaccine is injected in the shoulder region where the skin is loose. This vaccine has been used largely in Bavaria.

Nörgaard, of the Bureau of Animal Industry, U. S. Department of Agriculture, 1896-1897, also prepared a vaccine, which, by a single inoculation, will produce practical immunity, and which since then has been used extensively in the United States of America. Like Kitt's vaccine, this is also muscle-powder heated in an oil bath having a temperature of 93°-94° C., the site of injection being the side of the neck or chest.

In Thomas' method, a bundle of threads impregnated with virulent muscle-juice from an infected animal—*fils virulents* in French, or *blacklegine* in English—is introduced with a special inoculation-harpoon under the skin of the tail where a local culture of blackleg organism will result. It is reported that he later adopted two kinds of attenuated virus for the preparation of *fils virulents*.

Detre prepared from Lyons vaccine a liquid vaccine by separating spores and toxin from muscle-fibers and coagula of albuminous matters and then by mixing them in hypertonic saline solution.

Since all the vaccines mentioned above, except that of Thomas, consist of dried muscle-juice or muscle-powder from an infected animal attenuated by heating, they all have the following common disadvantages. First, there is a considerable variation of the amount, virulence, and resistance to external influences, especially to heat, of the virus (spores) in the blackleg material from which the vaccines are prepared; second, the effect of attenuation upon the virus accordingly varies greatly in different lots of the material, which is the principal cause of irregularities in the immunizing action of the vaccines prepared; third, an accurate standardization of the vaccines is very difficult; fourth, contamination of the vaccines, as will be seen from the various methods of preparation in vogue, is unavoidable, and this may result in the occurrence of complications; finally, losses from vaccination and insufficient immunity are occasionally observable.

For the reasons just described, several investigators have made attempts to obtain a pure and uniform vaccine from artificial cultures of the blackleg organism. Kitasato (1889) was the first to experimentally immunize animals with a pure culture. He stated that guinea pigs could be immunized by an injection of a broth culture, over two weeks old, or of a fresh virulent broth culture heated for 30 to 40 minutes at a temperature of 80° C.

In 1894, Kitt demonstrated that sheep and cattle also could be immunized by an injection of a less virulent broth culture. In Bavaria and Austria this method was for a time practised. Kitt later found that this method was not dependable, because by leaving the culture to stand for several weeks, or by making frequent transfers the blackleg organism gradually loses its virulence, which itself varies considerably with different strains, an accurate dosage being thus quite impossible. The same author also stated that an old blood-broth culture, left for several weeks, is inoffensive so that sheep could be immunized by an injection of 1-2 c.c., while an injection of 0.2 c.c. of a fresh culture kills sheep; and, an accurate dosage being impossible, this is also impracticable. Furthermore, Kitt immunized sheep by an injection of minimal doses of a dried blood-broth culture from which was prepared a vaccine in tablet

form by mixing starch soluble in water. He had also observed
that vaccines prepared by heating the dried culture in glass tubes
in a steam sterilizer at 97° or 100° C. for five to six hours confer
immunity on sheep.

Leclainche-Vallée used a direct blood culture from an affected
cow, and also a pure culture in horse blood, for the preparation of
vaccines; that is to say, they dried the culture in an incubator, divided it into two portions, heating one at 102° C. for seven hours,
and the other at 92° C. for the same length of time: they were
able to immunize guinea pigs by successive injections of these two
vaccines. The French authors later employed a five to eight days
old Martin broth culture (spores) heated at 70° C. for two hours,
which by a single injection of 2 c.c. confers solid immunity on
calves.

A few years ago the same scientists mentioned a new method
of single vaccination in which is used a pure culture of the blackleg organism attenuated by long cultivation at a high temperature
(42°-43° C.). This method has since been practised largely in
France.

In 1911, Foth recorded the preparation of new vaccines. The
powder vaccine ("A" type) is prepared by heating, at 93° C. for
seven hours, blackleg spores grown in a peptone-liver-broth with
addition of minced meat, and by precipitating it with absolute
alcohol; this vaccine is rich in spores. The alcohol precipitate of
the filtrate, obtained by passing through a thick layer of stamped
filter-paper pulp of a virulent culture, may also be used as a vaccine; it contains a small number of spores ("F" type). A single
injection of the powder vaccine or of the filtrate-precipitate confers on guinea pigs, sheep, and cattle solid immunity. Repetition
of the injection—twelve days later—of larger doses increases the
immunity. With cattle and sheep the ear is the seat of the first
inoculation and behind the shoulder for the second. A subcutaneous injection of small doses of a filtrate-powder solution on the ear,
and at the same time the introduction of threads impregnated with
spore-powder solution under the skin of the tail, also confer on
sheep and cattle solid immunity. The alcohol precipitate of the
germ-free filtrate obtained by passing through a bacterial filter of
a virulent culture again confers immunity on guinea pigs ("F'"
type). Foth immunized ten sheep by inoculation with "A" type
vaccine alone, or by a combination of threads and "F" type vaccine, and one cow by the latter method,

In Poel's method, cotton-wool soaked in a virulent pure culture and dessicated afterwards, is introduced under the skin of the tail. In Holland, 1904-1906, 21,329 calves were inoculated, with an inoculation loss of 1%-1¼%.

In addition to the foregoing, attempts have been made to immunize animals by an injection of metabolic products of the blackleg organism. As early as 1888 Roux demonstrated that an intraperitoneal injection of a broth culture, over two weeks old, heated at 115° C., or of the filtrate of the culture, or of a subcutaneous injection of the filtrate of the blackleg exudate, confer immunity on guinea pigs.

A few years later, in 1894, Dünshmann also stated that an injection of the filtrate of the tissue-juice from an affected animal confers immunity on guinea pigs.

Grassberger and Schattenfroh made a study of the blackleg toxin and stated that while it was difficult to immunize guinea pigs with the toxin, rabbits, cattle, and sheep could be easily immunized in this manner; the result in practical use, however, was unsatisfactory, since out of 306 inoculated cattle 23 died of intoxication, while 40-50 were severely affected. The same authors then demonstrated that an injection of a mixture of toxin and antitoxin serum conferred immunity on rabbits, sheep, and cattle: in 1903, 206 cattle in a blackleg district were inoculated with the mixture (12-20 c.c.), with no effect on the animals except a very slight local reaction; the report on natural losses was lacking.

Foth's germ-free filtrate has been already mentioned.

Schöbl (1910-1911) studied the aggressin immunity in blackleg and demonstrated that a subcutaneous, intraperitoneal, or intravenous injection of 0.5-1.5 c.c. of germ-free aggressin, obtained by centrifugalization of the edematous fluid from an affected part of guinea pigs which had died of blackleg, confers immunity on guinea pigs. He then proved that the aggressin obtained from cattle in doses of 5-10 c.c. also confers immunity on calves when used subcutaneously or intravenously.

That the serum taken from the hyperimmunized animals has a protective and even curative action had already been demonstrated by Kitt, Arloing, and Leclainche-Vallée. The latter authors stated that an injection of the immune serum and virus, mixed or separately at the same time, did not confer immunity on animals but that successive applications of the serum and virus proved a practicable method of immunization (10-20 c.c. of horse serum injected in the shoulder region, 5-8 days later 0.5-1.0 c.c. of pure culture attenuated by heating at 70° C. for three hours subcutaneously at the same place, neck, ear, or tail).

Grassberger and Schattenfroh employed for immunization the serum of cattle hyperimmunized first with toxin and then with virulent material, with unsatisfactory results. They also used a neutralized mixture of toxin and antitoxic serum (5-10 c.c.) : in 1904 over 4500 cattle, in Austria, were inoculated without direct loss; of these 78 died of natural blackleg.

AËROBIC CULTIVATION OF THE BLACKLEG ORGANISM. For the preparation of blackleg vaccines on a large scale from pure cultures it is essential to consider how to obtain, in the simplest way possible, as much virulent culture as may be needed. Nothing but an aërobic culture of the organism will properly serve this purpose. So let us first review the methods of aërobic cultivation of strict anaërobes to which the blackleg organism belongs, as worked out by many investigators up to the present time.

Kitt was the first to grow aërobically the blackleg organism; for this purpose he used a ½-1 liter flask filled with broth, inoculating a comparatively large quantity (0.5-1.0 c.c.) of a fresh broth culture or a small mass of an agar culture, but this method is not always successful.

I also proved that the organisms of blackleg, malignant edema, and tetanus could be grown in a tube, with a neck in the middle part, up to the neck filled with broth. In his work on immunization experiments against braxy, Prof. Tokishige recorded that my method was also successful for the cultivation of the braxy organism.

Kitt later stated that the blackleg organism develops luxuriantly in broth with the addition of sterile blood or fresh muscle (a pigeon's breast muscle) and the culture thus obtained is highly virulent.

Recently many other investigators were able to grow strictly anaërobic organisms in broth by simply adding pieces of animal or vegetable tissues. Smith published a method of aërobic cultivation of anaërobes which consists of pouring broth into fermentation tubes and adding sterile pieces of an animal organ. Hibler cultivated the organisms of tetanus, malignant edema, and blackleg in culture-media with sterile blood or sterilized minced brain.

Leclainche-Vallée used pure blood for the cultivation of the blackleg organism. Elers employed serum coagulated by heat for the same purpose. Tarrozzi demonstrated that the organisms of tetanus, pseudotetanus, and blackleg grow well in ordinary broth with sterile pieces of an organ or a tissue. Wrzosek confirmed Tarrozzi's experiment, furthermore stating that vegetable tissues, potato for example, and sterilized animal tissues could also be used. Harrass mentioned that *Bac. butyricum, Bac. botulinus, Bac. chauvaei* and *Bac. edematis maligni* grow aërobically in media prepared from finely minced calf's liver or brain. Pfuhl also recommended the broth made from liver. Hata not only confirmed the investigations of Smith and Wrzosek but also proved an ordinary broth with certain reducing agents, especially sodium sulphite, to be fit for the aërobic cultivation of anaërobes, addition of a small quantity of serum favoring the production of toxin, for instance in the case of tetanus.

After trying all the various methods mentioned above I found an ordinary peptone-beef-broth containing plentiful small pieces of boiled meat or liver to be one of the most suitable and simple media for aërobic cultivation of the blackleg organism, and in our laboratory it is called "meat-piece or liver-piece broth". The preparation of the broth is as follows: as may be required by the quantity of culture obtainable, use test tubes, or flasks of ½ or 1 liter; first put a number of small pieces of previously boiled lean beef or calf's liver into each vessel, so that a layer a few centimeters thick of the pieces is formed. Next pour the usual quantity, or better, a little more than the usual quantity, of the ordinary broth into the vessels, plug them with cotton-wool, and then sterilize the vessels and their contents in a steam sterilizer. It is advisable to heat them again in a steamer immediately before use and then to cool them quickly. Usually a large loopful of blackleg exudate or culture (broth or agar) is inoculated into each tube or flask. After incubating for about 24 hours at 37° C. there occurs a general cloudiness of the medium, a considerable amount of gas being produced. On microscopic examination of the culture the growth of the blackleg organism is demonstrated. After a few days flocculi form, which fall to the bottom, and the medium gradually becomes clearer, and a luxuriant spore formation is observed which will be complete after five to ten days' incubation. The culture thus obtained is as highly virulent as anaërobic culture, so that 0.1-0.2 c.c. of the culture generally kills guinea pigs in 10-24 hours and 0.1-0.5 c.c. calves within three days. To preserve a culture rich in spores it is advisable to add an equal part of 60-80 per cent glycerine, which proved excellent for the purpose, since no alteration in the virulence of the preserved culture was observable even after lapse of 10 months. The following are the results of inoculation tests on guinea pigs:

Guinea pig No.	Weight (grams)	Date of Innoculation	Culture-Media	Age of Culture (hours)	Dose (c.c.)	Result (died in)
23	215	Sept. 25, 1911	Beef p. b.	36	0.2	10 hours
34	375	Oct. 8, 1911	G. p. liver p. b.	15	0.1	26 hours
38	305	Oct. 16, 1911	Pork p. b.	22	0.2	23 hours
39	215	Oct. 25, 1911	Pork p. b.	20	0.1	10 hours
41	415	Nov. 6, 1911	Beef p. b.	36	0.1	27 hours
45	430	Nov. 10, 1911	Beef p. b.	36	0.1	10 hours
56	310	Dec. 4, 1911	Beef p. b.	40	0.1	34 hours
59	350	Dec. 7, 1911	Beef p. b.	24	0.1	48 hours
68	475	Dec. 12, 1911	Beef p. b.	24	0.1	48 hours
74	545	Jan. 13, 1912	C. liver p. b.	18	0.2	55 hours
75	485	Jan. 13, 1912	C. liver p. b.	18	0.1	34 hours
91	255	March 6, 1912	Beef p. b.	17	0.1	18 hours
96	565	March 7, 1912	Beef p. b.	17	0.1	20 hours
98	515	March 25, 1912	Beef p. b.	16 days	0.25	21 hours
99	375	March 25, 1912	Beef p. b.	16 days	0.1	22 hours
143	510	May 24, 1912	Beef p. b.	14 days	0.1	24 hours
159	555	June 14, 1912	Beef p. b.	23 days	0.1	35 hours

IMMUNIZING EXPERIMENTS WITH PURE CULTURES ATTENUATED BY HEAT. To ascertain if practicable vaccines could be obtained from a pure culture of the blackleg organism by heating it, as done by Leclainche-Vallée, I used for this purpose pure cultures rich in spores, preserved with an addition of glycerine, as previously stated, exposing it in bottles to a temperature of 75° C. for 1 to 5 hours in a water bath; the inoculation experiments with guinea pigs proved that the cultures heated even for as long as 5 hours showed no expected alteration in virulence. The temperature was then raised to 85° C., the time of heating being for 1-3 hours, and the result of animal experiments was nearly the same as in the previous case.. The culture heated at a temperature of 90°-92° C. for 1 to 3 hours, however, was so attenuated, that 0.1-0.5 c.c. and even 1-3 c.c. of the heated culture no more killed the guinea pigs inoculated, and in the majority of the animals that were treated twice with the attenuated culture the production of immunity was proved, since guinea pigs resisted against control-inoculation, a single inoculation being insufficient.

As it was proved that two successive inoculations with the attenuated culture conferred solid immunity on guinea pigs, I have tried to immunize three calves by inoculations with the same material, with satisfactory results. No. 1 received two inoculations (10 and 20 c.c.), and No. 2 one inoculation (2 c.c.), both showing a slight local reaction and a slight increase in temperature. No. 3 was inoculated once with a larger dose (10 c.c.), the reaction also being slight; these three calves were proved to be immune against control-inoculation made after about 2-4 weeks.

In the summer of 1912, 157 cattle in Okayama Prefecture were inoculated with the heated culture with satisfactory results: 59 were inoculated twice with 1 and 3 c.c. and 98 once with 2-3 c.c., but later it was found that the uniform attenuation by heating at a temperature of 90°-92° C. of the preserved culture could not be always expected in all different bottles, so that this method has since had to be abandoned.

IMMUNIZATION WITH A MIXTURE OF IMMUNE SERUM AND VIRUS. Leclainche-Vallée stated that injections of immune serum, and, a few days later, of virus confer immunity on animals treated; injections of both at the same time or of a mixture of both, however, not doing so. The truth of the first part of the statements of the French authors was confirmed in our laboratory; but contrary to the results obtained by them I found that a mixture of immune serum and virus in a proper proportion could produce solid immunity in the animals treated, reactions in the vaccination being slight.

As it was proved that an injection of a mixture of immune serum and virus conferred immunity on guinea pigs, I have tried to immunize three calves with the mixture (1-2 c.c. of serum and 0.5-1 c.c. of virus), all animals being proved to be immune against control-inoculation, as will be seen in the following:

No. 1.—Black and red bull-calf weighing 135 kilos.

April 30, 1912. Morning 38.7°; Evening—.
May 1, 1912. Morning 38.8°; Evening 39.4°.
2 p. m. injected subcutaneously into the right side of the thorax a mixture of 1 c.c. of serum and 1 c.c. of a strong preserved virus, incubated for one hour.
May 2, 1912. Morning 38.1°; Evening 38.7°.
A swelling the size of a hen's egg at the point of injection.
May 3, 1912 Morning 38.5°; Evening 38.8°.
May 4, 1912. Morning 38.7°; Evening 38.6°.
The swelling disappeared.
June 5, 1912. Morning 38.5°; Evening 38.8°.
12 noon, injected subcutaneously into the left side of the thorax 0.2 c.c, of a strong preserved virus.
June 6, 1912. Morning 39.1°; Evening 38.7°.

A slight swelling at the point of injection, and slight edema at the under-breast.

June 7, 1912. Morning 38.0°; Evening 38.9°.
The local swelling decreased, the edema at the underbreast disappeared.

June 8, 1912. Morning 37.9°; Evening 38.5°.
June 9, 1912. Morning 37.5°; Evening 38.6°.
The swelling nearly disappeared.

June 19, 1912. Morning 37.8°; Evening 38.6°.
11 a. m. injected subcutaneously into the right side of the thorax 0.5 c.c. of a strong preserved virus.

June 20, 1912. Morning 38.1°; Evening 38.7°.
No local reaction.

June 21, 1912. Morning 38.3°; Evening 38.5°.
June 22, 1912. Morning 38.3°; Evening 38.1°.
June 23, 1912. Morning 38.6°; Evening 38.2°.

No. 2.—Red and White bull-calf. Weight, 160 kilos.

April 30, 1912. Morning 38.7°; Evening—.
May 1, 1912. Morning 38.8°; Evening 39.2°.
2 p. m. injected subcutaneously into the right side of the thorax a mixture of 2 c.c. of serum and 1 c.c. of a strong preserved virus, incubated for one hour.

May 2, 1912. Morning 38.1°; Evening 38.3°.
A trace of swelling at the point of injection.

May 3, 1912. Morning 38.4°; Evening 38.7°.
No swelling.

May 4, 1912. Morning 38.6°; Evening 38.9°.
May 5, 1912. Morning 38.2°; Evening 38.8°.
June 8, 1912. Morning 38.8°; Evening 39.4°.
4 p. m. injected subcutaneously into the left side of the thorax 0.2 c.c. of a strong preserved virus.

June 9, 1912. Morning 39.0°; Evening 40.3°.
A slight swelling at the point of injection, and edema at the underbreast.

June 10, 1912. Morning 39.2°; Evening 39.1°.
The edema somewhat increased.

June 11, 1912. Morning 38.9°; Evening 39.1°.
The edema decreased.

June 12, 1912. Morning 39.6°; Evening 38.8°.
June 13, 1912. Morning 38.7°; Evening 38.9°.
June 14, 1912. Morning 38.9°; Evening 39.2°.
The local reaction entirely disappeared.

June 19, 1912. Morning 38.6°; Evening 39.6°.
11 a. m. injected subcutaneously into the right side of the thorax 0.5 c.c. of a strong preserved virus.

June 20, 1912. Morning 38.7°; Evening 39.0°.
No reaction.

June 21, 1912. Morning 38.6°; Evening 38.7°.
June 22, 1912. Morning 38.8°; Evening 38.7°.

No. 3.—Red bull-calf weighing 300 kilos.

May 14, 1912. Morning 38.6°; Evening—.
May 15, 1912. Morning 38.4°; Evening 38.6°.
12 noon injected subcutaneously into the right side of the thorax a mixture of 1 c.c. of serum and 0.5 c.c. of a strong preserved virus, incubated for one hour.

May 16, 1912. Morning 38.7°; Evening 38.3°.
A goose's egg sized swelling at the point of injection.

May 17, 1912. Morning 38.0°; Evening 38.7°.
May 18, 1912. Morning 38.2°; Evening 38.4°.
May 19, 1912. Morning 38.2°; Evening 38.2°.
The local swelling disappeared.

June 12, 1912. Morning 38.6°; Evening 38.9°.

12 noon injected subcutaneously into the right side of the thorax 0.2 c.c. of a strong preserved virus.

June 13, 1912.　Morning 39.3°; Evening 38.6°.

A swelling the size of a hen's egg at the point of injection.

June 14, 1912.　Morning 38.6°; Evening 39.0°.

June 15, 1912.　Morning 38.6°; Evening 38.9°.

June 16, 1912.　Morning 38.5°; Evening 38.4°.

The swelling disappeared.

June 26, 1912.　Morning 38.7°; Evening 39.0°.

11 a. m. injected subcutaneously into the right side of the thorax 0.5 c.c. of a strong preserved virus.

June 27, 1912.　Morning 38.6°; Evening 38.7°.

A slight swelling at the point of injection.

June 28, 1912.　Morning 38.4°; Evening 38.9°.

The swelling decreased.

June 29, 1912.　Morning 38.9°; Evening 39.6°.

June 30, 1912.　Morning 38.6°; Evening 38.6°.

The swelling disappeared.

IMMUNIZATION WITH AGGRESSIN. Schöbl (1910-1911) first published aggressin immunity in blackleg. He collected edematous fluid from the affected parts of guinea pigs which had died of inoculation blackleg and injected into guinea pigs subcutaneously (intraperitoneally or intravenously) the fluid after making it free of the blackleg organism by centrifugalization in doses of 0.5-1.5 c.c., the animals being proved to be immune against subsequent injection of blackleg virus. He then demonstrated that calves also could be immunized by an injection of the aggressin obtained from a calf in the same way as in the case of guinea pigs.

In our laboratory the truth of Schöbl's statement was confirmed. Edematous fluid was collected from subcutis and muscles of a calf dead of inoculation blackleg and passed through a Chamberland filter, and the filtrate was injected subcutaneously into two guinea pigs. As a result of control-inoculation made three weeks later the production of immunity against blackleg in the animals treated was proved. Experiments were then made to ascertain if the same result could be obtained by treatment of animals with the filtrate of a broth culture of the blackleg organism. For this purpose I used a meat-piece or liver-piece broth culture, 2-3 weeks old, and obtained from it a filtrate free of the organism by passing through a Chamberland filter. The majority of guinea pigs injected subcutaneously with 0.5-2 c.c. of the filtrate proved to be immune against the control-inoculation made after 2-6 weeks. However, a mixture of the filtrate and well-washed blackleg spores was highly virulent, while the spores alone were avirulent. The table on the next page shows the results of immunization of guinea pigs with the filtrate.

Since satisfactory results were obtained with guinea pigs, the filtrate was injected into four calves to prove if immunity could be produced also in cattle by treatment with the filtrate. One of them received 5 c.c. and the other three 10 c.c., reaction being slight. One calf died of pneumonia before control-inoculation. Three remaining calves proved to be immune against subsequent control-inoculation made 9 or 10 days later. The details will be seen in the following:

Guinea pig		First Injection		Second Injection		Control Inoculation		
No.	Weight (grams)	Date (1912)	Dose of Filtrate (c.c.)	Date (1912)	Dose of Filtrate (c.c.)	Date (1912)	Dose of Preserved virus (c.c.)	Result (local swelling the size of)
146	300	May 29	0.5	—	—	June 2	0.2	Little finger's end
147	315	May 29	1	—	—	June 2	0.2	Thumb's end
148	410	May 29	2	—	—	June 19	0.2	Trace
149	460	May 29	4	—	—	June 19	0.2	Bean
165	420	June 22	0.5	—	—	July 9	0.2	Died in 24 hours
172	715	July 11	2	—	—	Aug. 5	0.2	Thumb's end
173	685	July 11	2	—	—	July 29	0.2	Trace
174	600	July 11	1	—	—	Aug. 5	0.2	Thumb's end
175	590	July 11	1	—	—	Aug. 5	0.2	Little finger's end
176	638	July 11	0.5	Aug. 5	2.0	Aug. 20	0.2	No swelling
177	495	July 11	0.5	—	—	Aug. 5	0.2	Died in 36 hours
185	465	Aug. 6	2.5	—	—	Aug. 20	0.2	Little finger's end
186	455	Aug. 6	2.5	—	—	Aug. 20	0.2	Died in 24 hours
187	615	Aug. 6	2	—	—	Aug. 20	0.2	Trace
188	575	Aug. 6	2	—	—	Aug. 20	0.2	No swelling

No. 1.—Red and white calf weighing about 77 kilos.

June 25, 1912. Morning 38.5°; Evening 38.7°.
June 26, 1912. Morning 38.6°; Evening 39.6°.
11 a. m. injected subcutaneously into the right side of the thorax 5 c.c. of the filtrate.
June 27, 1912. Morning 39.4°; Evening 39.6°.
A slight local swelling.
June 28, 1912. Morning 38.5°; Evening 39.2°.
A decrease in the swelling.
June 29, 1912. Morning 39.1°; Evening 38.9°.
June 30, 1912. Morning 38.6°; Evening 38.5°.
No swelling remaining.
July 15, 1912. Morning 38.7°; Evening—.
July 16, 1912. Morning 38.7°; Evening 39.4°.
11 a. m. injected subcutaneously into the left side of the thorax 0.2 c.c. of a strong preserved Virus.
July 17, 1912. Morning 39.3°; Evening 39.5°.
A hen's egg sized swelling at the point of injection.

July 18, 1912. Morning 39.5°; Evening 39.6°.
The swelling same as on the previous day, appetite somewhat poor.
July 19, 1912. Morning 39.2°; Evening 39.4°.
The swelling disappeared.
On July 29 this animal was again injected subcutaneously into the right side of the thorax with 0.5 c.c. of a strong preserved virus, showing a very slight local reaction only.

No. 2.—White and black bull-calf. Weight, about 211 kilos.

June 25, 1912. Morning 38.1°; Evening 38.1°.
June 26, 1912. Morning 38.5°; Evening 39.1°.
11·a. m. injected subcutaneously into the right side of the thorax 10 c.c. of the filtrate.
June 27, 1912. Morning 39.7°; Evening 38.8°.
A slight local swelling.
June 28, 1912. Morning 38.3°; Evening 38.8°.
June 29, 1912. Morning 38.4°; Evening 39.4°.
June 30, 1912. Morning 38.6°; Evening 38.4°.
The swelling disappeared.
This animal later suffered from acute pneumonia and died on July 22 before control-inoculation.

No. 3.—Black and white bull-calf weighing about 77 kilos.

August 19, 1912. Morning 39.0°; Evening—.
August 20, 1912. Morning 38.7°; Evening 39.0°.
1 p. m. injected subcutaneously into the right side of the thorax 10 c.c. of the filtrate.
August 21, 1912. Morning 38.5°; Evening 40.0°.
A goose's egg sized swelling at the point of injection.
August 22, 1912. Morning 38.9°; Evening 39.2°.
August 23, 1912. Morning 38.4°; Evening 39.7°.
August 24, 1912. Morning 39.3°; Evening 40.1°.
August 25, 1912. Morning 38.7°; Evening 38.7°.
The swelling disappeared.
September 18, 1912. Morning 38.4°; Evening 38.9°.
11 a. m. injected subcutaneously into the left side of the thorax 0.2 c.c. of a strong preserved virus.
September 19, 1912. Morning 38.1°; Evening 38.8°.
A fist-sized swelling at the point of injection.
September 20, 1912. Morning 38.6°; Evening 38.7°.
September 21, 1912. Morning 38.4°; Evening 38.6°.
The swelling disappeared.
October 2, 1912. Morning 39.1°; Evening 39.2°.
3 p. m. injected subcutaneously into the right side of the thorax 0.1 c.c. of a virulent liver-piece broth culture, 18 hours old.
October 3, 1912. Morning 39.4°; Evening 39.5°.
A hand-sized swelling at the point of injection, appetite somewhat poor.
October 4, 1912. Morning 38.8°; Evening 39.3°.
Appetite normal.
October 5, 1912. Morning 38.6°; Evening 39.1°.
Reduction of the swelling.
October 6, 1912. Morning 38.5°; Evening 38.7°.
October 7, 1912. Morning 38.9°; Evening 39.3°.
Increase in the swelling to the size of a hen's egg.
On October 11 the local swelling nearly disappeared.
No. 4.—Red cow. Weight, 318 kilos.
October 13, 1912. Morning 38.2°; Evening—.
October 14 1912. Morning 38.2°; Evening 38.5°.
12 noon injected subcutaneously into the right side of the thorax 10 c.c. of the filtrate.

October 15, 1912. Morning 38.4°; Evening 38.6°.
A swelling as large as two hands at the point of injection.
October 16, 1912. Morning 38.3°; Evening 38.8°.
Enlargement of the swelling.
October 17, 1912. Morning 38.2°; Evening 38.2°.
Decrease in the swelling.
October 18, 1912. Morning 38.5°; Evening 38.5°.
The swelling nearly gone.
October 30, 1912. Morning 38.5°; Evening 38.5°.
12 noon injected subcutaneously into the left side of the thorax 0.2 c.c. of a strong preserved virus.
October 31, 1912. Morning 38.3°; Evening 38.6°.
A hand-sized swelling at the point of injection, appetite somewhat poor.
November 1, 1912. Morning 38.5°; Evening 38.6°.
Decrease in the swelling.
November 2, 1912. Morning 38.6°; Evening 38.5°.
November 3, 1912. Morning 38.1°; Evening 38.3°.
The swelling nearly gone.

In the summer of 1912 I had an opportunity to make a further inoculation experiment of the filtrate with nine cattle, the results proving satisfactory. Since that time this method of immunization of animals against blackleg alone has been practised in this country; the statistics are as follows:

	1913	1914	1915	1916	1917
No. of cattle treated...	1,226	1,514	2,041	1,119	1,145

In addition to the above the amounts of the filtrate used in Corea are: 1,000 c.c. in 1913, 2,000 c.c. in 1914, 33,000 c.c. in 1915, 46,000 c.c. in 1916, and 100,000 c.c. in 1917.

While visiting the United States of America, on the way home from Europe the year before last, I gave Dr. A. Eichhorn, then Chief of the Pathological Division, Bureau of Animal Industry, .U. S. Department of Agriculture, in Washington, an outline of my method and mentioned the good results obtained through it during a few years in this country. In the June, 1917, number of JOURNAL OF THE AMERICAN VETERINARY MEDICAL ASSOCIATION, Dr. Eichhorn, now of Lederle Antitoxin Laboratories, published an article on "Blackleg Filtrate" in which the fact that my method of immunization against blackleg produced solid immunity and was totally unaccompanied by danger was well confirmed. In April last I was asked indirectly by Dr. Haslam, Purity Biological Laboratory, U. S. A., how to prepare the filtrate, so that some information relating to its preparation was made indirectly.

RÉSUMÉ. In conclusion I will here summarize the results of my investigations concerning immunization of animals against blackleg.

1. A virulent aërobic blackleg culture, rich in spores, can be readily obtained by using meat-piece or liver-piece broth as the culture medium and it can be preserved for a year or more with the addition of glycerine.

2. Efficacious blackleg vaccines can be made by heating the aërobic culture rich in spores, but uniform attenuation of the virus

is not always expected, so that the practical use of these vaccines should be abolished, owing to possible losses from injection.

3. A mixture of immune serum and virus in proper proportion confers an active immunity on animals treated. To determine its practical value, however, further experiments are necessary.

4. An injection of the germ-free filtrate of blackleg exudate also produces an active immunity in animals treated. To prepare the amount sufficient enough for its practical use it is very expensive, because it is necesary to use living calves in order to obtain blackleg exudate.

5. The filtrate of a pure culture of the blackleg organism confers a solid immunity on animals treated and it has been already successfully used in thousands of cattle in infected districts. It is inexpensive, the material for the preparation being aërobic cultures of the organism in meat-piece broth, and its injection is not accompanied by the least danger, because the filtrate is quite germ-free. The filtrate can be preserved for several months with the addition of toluol.

[Work done in the Institute for Infectious Animal Diseases, Nishigahara, the principal part of which was published, in 1914, in the Sixth Report of the Institute (Japanese).]

BIBLIOGRAPHY

1. ARLOING, CORNEVIN et THOMAS. Méchanisme de l'infection dans les différents modes d'inoculation du charbon symptomatique. Application á l'interprétation des faits cliniques et á la méthode des inoculations préventives. *Comptes rendus des séances de l' Académie des Sciences,* Vol. XCII, p. 1246.

2. ARLOING, CORNEVIN et THOMAS. Moyen de conférer artificiellement l'immunité contre le charbon symptomatique ou bactérien avec du virus atténué, *Ibid,* Vol. XCV, p. 189.

3. ARLOING, CORNEVIN et THOMAS. Détermination des causes qui déterminent la réceptivité de certaines régions de l'organisme pour le virus du charbon bactérien ou symptomatique et transforment une inoculation mortelle en inoculation préventive. *Ibid,* Vol. XCVIII, p. 1071.

4. ARLOING. Sérothérapie du Charbon symptomatique. *Ibid,* Vo. CXXX.

5. DUENSCHMANN. Etude experimentale sur le charbon symptomatique et ses relations avec l'oedeme malin. *Annales de l' Institut Pasteur,* Vol. VIII (1894), p. 403.

6. FOTH, H. Neue Rauschbrandimpfstoffe. *Zeitschrift für Infektionskrankheiten der Haustiere,* Vol. X (1911), p. 1.

7. GRASSBERGER u. SCHATTENFROH. Ueber das Rauschbrandgift und ein antitoxisches Serum. *Monographie,* 1904.

8. GRASSBERGER u. SCHATTENFROH. Das Rauschbrandgift. *Kraus u. Levaditi, Handbuch der Technik und Methodik der Immunitätsforschung,* Vol. I (1908), pp. 161-175.

9. GRASSBERGER u. SCHATTENFROH. Das Rauschbrand-Antitoxin. *Ibid,* Vol. II (1907), pp. 186-203.

10. HARRASS, P. Zur Frage der aëroben Züchtung sogenannter obligatanaërober Bakterein. *Münchener Med. Wochenschrift,* 1906, p. 2237.

11. HATA, S. Ueber eine einfache Methode zur aërobischen Kultivierung der Anaëroben, mit besonderer Berücksichtigung ihrer Toxinproduction. *Centralblatt für Bakteriologie* 1, Abt., Orig., Vol. XLVI (1908), p. 539.

12. V. HIBLER, E. Beitràge zur Kenntnis der durch anaërobe Spaltpilze erzeug-ten Infektionserkrankungen der Tiere und des Menschen, sowie zur Begründung einer genauen bakteriologischen und pathologisch-anato-mischen Differentialdiagnose dieser Prozesse. *Ibid*, 1. Abt., Vol. XXV (1899), p. 603.

13. HUTYRA, F. Rauschbrand. *Hutyra u. Marek, Spezielle Pathologie u. Therapie der Haustiere.* 3. Edit., Vol. I (1910), pp. 39-58.

14. KITASATO, S. Ueber den Rauschbrandbacillus und sein Culturverfahren. *Zeitschrift für Hygiene*, Vol. VI (1889), p. 115.

15. KITT, TH. Ueber Abschwächung des Rauschbrandvirus durch strömende Wasserdämpfe. *Centralblatt für Bakteriologie*, 1. Abt., Vol. III (1888), p. 572.

16. KITT, TH. Ueber Rauschbrandschutzimpfung mit Reinkulturen. *Monat-shefte für prakt. Tierheilkunde*, Vol. V (1894), p. 19.

17. KITT, TH. Die Züchtung des Rauschbrandbacillus bei Luftzutritt. *Cen-tralblatt für Bakteriologie*, 1. Abt., Vol. XXVII (1895), p. 168.

18. KITT, TH. Serumimpfung gegen Rauschbrand. *Monatshefte für, prakt. Tierheilkunde*, Vol. XI (1900).

19. KITT, TH. Neues über Rauschbrand. *Ibid*, Vol. XIII (1892), p. 181.

20. KITT, TH. Immunität u. Schutzimpfungen bei Rauschbrand des Rindes. *Kolle u. Wassermann, Handbuch der pathogenen Mikroorganismen*, 2. Edit., Vol. IV (1912), pp. 819-836.

21. LECLAINCHE-VALLÉE. La pratique des vaccinations contre le charbon symp-tomatique. *Revue générale de Médecine Vétérinaire*, 1908, No. 131.

22. LECLAINCHE-VALLÉE. Sur la vaccination contre le charbon symptoma-tique. *Comptes rendus des séances de l' Académie des Sciences*, Vol. CLVI (1913), p. 989.

23. NITTA, N. A Method of Aërobic Cultivation of Anaërobic Bacteria. *Tokyo-Igakukai-Zasshi*, Vol. XII (1899), p. 393.

24. NITTA, N. Investigations on Tachi disease in Cattle in Japan. *First Re-port of the Institute for Infectious Animal Diseases* (Japanese), 1905, p. 84.

25. NITTA, N., and OKUDA, K. Investigations on Blackleg Immunization. *Sixth Report of the Institute for Infectious Animal Diseases* (Japan-ese), 1914, p. 43.

26. NÖRGAARD, V. A. Blackleg in the United States and the Distribution of Vaccine by the Bureau of Animal Industry. *Fifteenth Annual Report of the Bureau of Animal Industry, U. S. Dept. of Agric.*, 1898, p. 171.

27. NÖRGAARD, V. A. Blackleg. Its Nature, Cause and Prevention. *Circular No. 31. U. S. Bureau of Animal Industry*, 1915.

28. PFUHL, E. Die Züchtung anaërober Bakterien in Leberbouillon, sowie in Zuckerbouillon und in gewöhnlicher Bouillon mit einem Zusatz von Platinschwamm oder Hapin unter Luftzutritt. *Centralblatt für Bak-teriologie*, 1. Abt., Orig., Vol. XLIV (1907), p. 378.

29. ROUX. Immunité contre le charbon symptomatique conféré par des sub-stances solubles. *Annales de l'Institut Pasteur*, Vol. II (1888), p. 49.

30. SCHÖBL, O. Ueber Aggressinimmunisierung gegen Rauschbrand. *Cen-tralblatt für Bakteriologie*, 1. Abt., Orig., Bd. LVI (1910), p. 395.

31. SCHÖBL, O. Weitere Versuche über Aggressinimmunisierung gegen Rausch-brand. *Ibid*, Vol. LXII (1912), p. 296.

32. SHIRAISHI, K. Rauschbrand in Yamaguchi Prefecture. *Chuo-Juikai-Zas-shi*, Vol. VI (1893), No. 3, p. 55.

33. SMITH, TH Die Gährungskölbchen in der Bakteriologie. *Centralblatt fur Bakteriologie*, 1. Abt., Vol. VII (1890), p. 502.

34. SMITH, TH., BROWN, H. R., WALKER, E. L. The fermentation tube in the study of anaërobic bacteria with special reference to gas production

and the use of milk as a culture medium. *Journal of Medical Research*, Vol. XV (1915), No. 1.

35. SMITH, . TH. Ueber einige Kulturmerkmale des Rauschbrandbacillus. *Zeitschrift für Infektionskrankheiten der Haustiere*, Vol. I, No. 1.
36. SCHÜTZ-ELLENBERGER. *Jahresbericht uber die Veterinar-Medicin.*
37. TARROZZI, G. Ueber ein leicht in aërober Weise ausführbares Kulturmittel von einigen bis jetzt für strenge Anaëroben gehaltenen Keimen. *Centralblatt für Bakteriologie*, 1. Abt., Orig., Vol. XXXVIII (1905), p. 619.
38. THOMAS. La vaccination d.l. charbon symptomatique. *Répertoire de police sanitaire vétérinaire et d'hygiène publique*, 1900, No. 1, p. 31.
39. TOKISHIGE, H. Immunisierungsversuche gegen Bradsot. *Monatshefte für prakt. Tierheilkunde*, Vol. XII (1901), p. 6.
40. WRZOSEK, A. Beobachtungen über die Bedingungen des Wachstums der obligatorischen Anaëroben in aërober Weise. *Centralblatt für Bakteriologie*, 1. Abt., Orig., Vol. XLIII (1907), p. 17.
41. WRZOSEK, A. Weitere Untersuchungen über die Züchtung von obligatorischen Anaëroben in aërober Weise. *Ibid*, Vol. XLIV (1907), p. 607.

HEMORRHAGIC SEPTICEMIA AND ITS CONTROL IN PENNSYLVANIA*

J. B. HARDENBERGH and FRED. BOERNER, JR.

Division of Laboratories, Pennsylvania State Livestock Sanitary Board

In presenting data gathered during our three years' experimental work with vaccine in the control of hemorrhagic septicemia, we intend to dwell but briefly upon the occurrence, etiology, anatomical changes, symptoms, etc., of the disease. For these details the reader is referred to some of the recent works in veterinary medicine regarding pathology and therapeutics or pathology and diagnosis. It is our purpose to show from statistics gathered in vaccinating over 2,000 animals on various farms throughout the state, why we feel that this method of control is valuable, and that sanitarians can only lend all possible aid when it is employed.

In 1895, in his annual report, Pearson mentioned sudden deaths of cattle due to some unknown cause, and concluded that while many were due to known diseases not recognized, others were no doubt due to diseases of which but little was known, or that certain poisons had operated to destroy the animals.

In 1896 his report cited the occurrence of an outbreak in Lancaster County in November. Twelve animals were found ill, eleven unable to stand; all had a low fever and a slightly accelerated

---

*Read at the Pennsylvania Medical Association, Harrisburg, Pa., Jan. 22nd, 1918.

pulse. The appetites were gone, and there were indications of abdominal pain, while weakness seemed to be more noticeable in the hind quarters than in the front. Some animals showed considerable excitement, and all but two were constipated. Necropsy on two that died revealed only slight changes in most of the parechymatous organs, but there were some changes of the digestive tract, also a yellowish serum around the kidneys, and congestion of the lungs. There was a history of their having been kept in a corn stalk field for five days prior to the time when it was noticed that they staggered in walking, rapidly lost strength, became unable to stand, and exhibited the other symptoms already mentioned.

In 1897 reference is made to an outbreak in Huntingdon County, following the purchase of seven yearlings in Center County, which, shortly after reaching their destination developed a severe cough, lost condition, and became emaciated, four of the animals dying. Subsequently some other cattle on this farm developed similar symptoms, leading to the belief that the infection was contagious. The owner, suspecting tuberculosis, had the animals tested with entirely negative results. A post-mortem examination on one of the heifers showed that the anterior lobes of the lungs were solidified, dark red in color, upon cross examination revealing numerous small cavities, containing a yellowish cheesy pus. The bronchial tubes contained frothy mucus, and the lining membrane was thickened. The connective tissue septa between the lobules were infiltrated with serum and thickened; pleura and lymphatic glands normal, and other organs normal in appearance, although somewhat pale.

In 1898 the same writer made quite a lengthy reference to "Corn Stalk Disease", which had occasioned enormous losses in some of the principal corn growing states of the West, and referred to the outbreak mentioned in the 1896 report as being of the same nature. This disease was not supposed to be contagious, although its cause had not been fully ascertained. On account of the length of this report, we cannot quote from it fully. Outbreaks were reported from several farms in different counties, and the symptoms and autopsy findings seemed to warrant a diagnosis of "Corn Stalk Disease".

In this 1898 record a part of the report on investigation of an outbreak in Franklin County in December 9, 1898, reads as follows: "All the animals that died recently had a history of having been fed from a few days to several weeks on corn fodder. *However, a number of animals had died on farms south of St. Thomas during the months of October and November of a disease having somewhat similar symptoms, were at pasture when they died, and had not received any corn fodder."* This report also mentioned that while under certain conditions of moldiness and fermentation, corn stalks and corn fodder become exceedingly poisonous to many cattle, it was noted that all cattle exposed in the same way did not become affected and that the symptoms varied.

In 1900 he reported a disease, prevailing in the spring and summer, among cattle in wild mountainous regions, that failed of identification during the year, but which destroyed several hundred cattle annually, and was so prevalent as to make large areas of land useless for pasturing purposes.

In 1902 investigations were conducted as to the etiology of the so-called "Mountain Disease" and as the result Pearson and Gilliland proved it to be identical with "Rinderseuche" of Germany, and with *hemorrhagic septicemia* that had been recognized among cattle in Minnesota and Wisconsin, stating that this discovery removed a cloud of doubt as to the cause of the loss of great numbers of cattle. In this same report, Pearson stated that "hemorrhagic septicemia or spotted fever" of cattle has also been known in Pennsylvania as "Carbon County Disease" or "Mountain Disease of Cattle", and that it was believed to have occurred during that year in the counties of Cameron, Carbon, Center, Clearfield, Franklin, Forrest, Huntingdon, Lackawanna, Lycoming, Perry, Potter, Somerset, Wayne, and Warren.

Following is a description of the symptoms and pathological changes noted by him: "Fever, loss of appetite, dullness, diminution of milk flow, groaning, discharge of bloody mucus from the nose, staring coat, red mucous membranes, swelling about the throat; which is hot, rather tense and painful and is sometimes accompanied by harsh or difficult breathing. There is usually a little discharge of blood from the anus. Sometimes there is a little leakage of blood through the skin at various points as though the animal had been stung by large flies or pricked with needles. In other cases the disease seems to affect the intestinal tract chiefly and in this case there is a diffuse hemorrhagic gastro-enteritis, causing much depression, accumulation of gas, evidence of pain in the abdominal cavity and the feces are covered with blood, shreds of fibrin or mucus. The course of the disease is usually short, varying from twelve hours to a week, and it terminates in death in nearly all cases.

· On post mortem examination it is observed that the tissues beneath the skin in the region of the throat are infiltrated with serum and that scattered through this infiltrated area there are many points of hemorrhage; sometimes the hemorrhage is extensive, causing the entire infiltrated area to be of a red color. This swelling about the throat usually involves the walls of the pharynx and larynx. The root of the tongue is often swollen and infiltrated with yellow serum. Points of hemorrhage may be observed beneath the skin on any part of the body. Sometimes the lungs show evidence of hemorrhage into them and there is an accumulation of blood in the chest cavity. If the intestines are involved there is hemorrhage into large or small areas of the wall, causing it to be of dark red color and considerably thickened. The appearance of the blood is not materially altered; it coagulates in the usual way. The most characteristic alterations are the points of hemorrhage indicating an escape of blood from the vessels into the subcutaneous connective tissues, into the lining membranes of the abdominal and thoracic cavities and into the swollen areas about the throat and at the root of the tongue. Young or old cattle may be afflicted by this disease.''

In the foregoing reference to the various named diseases, it is not claimed that those outbreaks of ''Corn Stalk Disease'' and catarrhal or broncho-pneumonia were what we now know as hemorrhagic septicemia, nor that they were due to an organism belonging to the hemorrhagic septicemia group. There are distinct pneumonias and certain distinct cases of forage poisoning, but from the fact that we do not have reports of these two diseases sent in from counties where they previously existed, and as we are and have been for several years receiving reports of hemorrhagic septicemia outbreaks in these same and additional counties, we are strongly inclined to the belief that many of the outbreaks previously reported under other names were in all probability due to organisms belonging to the hemorrhagic septicemia group. Investigations by Billings, Gamgee, Mayo, Moore, and others, tend to confirm this belief.

Hemorrhagic septicemia of cattle is usually an acute, less frequently a subacute, infectious disease, in the course of which the febrile symptoms are often accompanied by manifestations of an acute gastro-enteritis, inflammatory edema of the skin, or frequently a necrotic-pneumonia associated with edema of the interalveolar connective tissue. The causative agent is *B. bovisepticus.*

OCCURRENCE. The disease occurs practically everywhere, either sporadically or enzootically, especially during the late summer and fall months. *In Pennsylvania, by far the greatest number (90%) of the outbreaks during the past three years, have been reported in August, September, and October.* There is a mistaken idea held by some veterinarians that hemorrhagic septicemia does not occur in successive years on the same farm, but this has no foundation. We have repeatedly seen it recur in different herds. Since 1878, when described by Bollinger as occurring near Munich among deer and wild boars, it has been observed in cattle, sheep, hogs, and occasionally in horses and mules. Among the latter cases may be mentioned an outbreak in Lancaster County, Pa., August, 1916, in young mules, resulting in five deaths and the subsequent positive necropsy and bacteriological findings in the two cases seen. To date we have not diagnosed the disease in sheep in this state. The outbreaks are confined to the mountains or to those sections in which the land is wild, broken in contour, wooded, and covered with rank vegetation. Seldom has it occurred in the southeastern part of the state where the land is flat, rolling, and farmed extensively, except in steers (feeders) intended for fattening for the spring markets and introduced on farms in the fall after passage through various stockyards. Our records show that animals of all ages are affected, cases having been reported in calves, young heifers, and aged cows up to and including twelve years of age during the year 1917.

SYMPTOMS. The period of incubation in natural infections is probably in the majority of cases from twelve to seventy-two hours, but this is variable, and, except in the chronic cases, may run from six hours to eight days. At first there is a rapid rise in the body temperature to over 40° C. (104° F.) accompanied by a quickened pulse, dullness, rough coat, and muscular tremblings. In some cases the surface of the body feels alternately hot and cold, while the muzzle is cold and dry. There is also cessation of the appetite, rumination and milk secretion. Peristalsis is often retarded; constipation at this stage may be noticed. Later there are symptoms of colic with much straining, when the animal passes, instead of the usual dry, dark brown feces, a mushy and finally a thin fetid fluid which is frequently mixed with fibrin and mucus flakes, as well as with blood. Often blood exudes from the nose, and sometimes may be passed in the urine. Some animals show affections of the throat and are unable to swallow except with difficulty. Others show disinclination to move, exhibit stiffness, and in some instances actual lameness. Occasionally painfully edematous swellings are seen about the legs and shoulders as well as in the throat. Animals have been observed to drop to the ground and die in a short time, apparently without pain. Others live for several hours in great pain, as indicated by groans and muscular spasms. Animals sick for any length of time rapidly lose flesh. In the edematous (exanthemous) form the head and neck swell, especially in the region of the throat and develop, as a result of the rapidly increasing inflammatory edema of the subcutaneous connective tissue, causing a deformity of these parts. In such cases swelling of the legs or inflammatory enlargements of the different joints may be observed. The skin over the swollen parts of the body is very tense, warm, and sensitive. An acute conjunctivitis, and the yellowish colorization of this membrane, frequently develops with profuse lachrymation. The buccal mucous membrane is bright red, warm, dry, and swollen. Deglutition may be difficult or impossible, causing saliva to accumulate in the mouth and drivel from the corners in long tenacious strings. The tongue may swell to such an extent that it entirely fills the mouth cavity, or it even may protrude, appearing bluish red or dirty reddish brown in color.

Respiration is difficult and the animal breathes heavily. Some die of asphyxiation, or asthenia, which is caused by a marked enteritis. The "sweating of blood" mentioned by Pearson has been observed in a number of cases.

The pectoral form is characterized by an acute pleuro-pneumonia and the animal stands immovable with back arched, has a dry painful cough and a colorless or reddish foamy discharge from the nose. One or both sides of the thorax may show a dullness over different areas with bronchial breathing and vesicular rales, or there may be a total absence of respiratory sounds. Respiration is greatly accelerated and labored. Rumination ceases, peristalsis of the rumen and intestines is frequently suppressed. Constipation is followed by bloody diarrhea, after which the weakened animal rapidly succumbs. The pectoral and abdominal forms of the disease are the ones seen in Pennsylvania and we can recall no instance of having observed the edematous (exanthemous) form reported by some writers.

ANATOMICAL CHANGES. *The characteristic lesions of the disease are widely distributed areas of hemorrhage varying in size from a pin-point to several centimeters in diameter, in color from light red to almost black and frequently accompanied with a serofibrinous exudate, usually yellow but occasionally dark red in color.* These serous hemorrhages, petechiae and ecchymoses, when extensive, give the entire abdominal or pectoral viscera the appearance of having been splashed with blood. All cases show some hemorrhagic areas in the subcutaneous connective tissue, the number and size of these varying in different individuals. Gas is not present in the subcutaneous connective tissue except as a post mortem change. The edematous cases show gelatinous infiltrations of the tissues. The abdominal and thoracic cavities may contain several liters of yellow or reddish colored serous fluid.

Acute hemorrhagic inflammations of the intestinal tract are frequent—with thin fluid contents, gray in color or blood-stained, and having a very fetid odor. The blood is usually of a normal color and clots readily. The surface of the lungs is often petechiated or even ecchymotic. Pneumonia of the lobular type is a very constant complication. On section this organ often presents areas of red and gray hepatization having the marbled appearance seen in contagious pleuro-pneumonia and when squeezed, exudes a yellow serum. The heart shows petechiae, ecchymoses or more extensive hemorrhages of the pericardium, epicardium or endocardium. The spleen is usually normal in appearance or at most may be swollen in localized areas presenting a few spleen tumors or petechiae. The liver in a small number of cases shows hemorrhagic infarcts, and is rich in blood. The kidneys are slightly if at all affected, and sometimes show a few petechiae macroscopically.

Reynolds reports an outbreak in which meningitis was invariably present. Wilson and Brimhall report an animal four months pregnant which showed small hemorrhages in the placental membranes.

DIAGNOSIS. Primarily this must depend upon the history and symptoms and can be verified by necropsy and bacteriological findings. Care should be taken not to mistake anthrax for hemorrhagic septicemia. A few of the most constant symptoms are repeated.

Animals show marked dullness and depression. They segregate themselves, stand with arched back, the coat is lusterless and staring. The feces are blood-stained and in some instances appear as almost pure blood. Some show bloody nasal discharge, others petechiae of nasal mucous membranes and conjunctiva. Temperatures run very high and "sweating of blood" is frequently observed. Edemas, particularly of the throat, are fairly constant.

Hemorrhagic septicemia may be differentiated from blackleg and malignant edema by the absence of gas in the subcutaneous tissue—from anthrax by the fact that on autopsy the spleen is not swollen and the blood is normal in appearance and clots readily. In anthrax the spleen is almost without exception uniformly swollen, the blood is dark and tarry and does not coagulate.

Decomposition changes on a carcass dead for some time, alter the lesions, and render diagnosis more difficult; therefore it is essential that carcasses should be examined shortly after death.

The pectoral form may readily be mistaken for pleuro-pneumonia, therefore in calves and shipped animals care should be taken not to confuse it with this disease. The history should be of help in such cases.

CONTROL. Because most investigators believe that hemorrhagic septicemia is a disease of the soil, and the fact that the organism dies rapidly under adverse conditions, traffic restrictions have not been rigid. Originally it was thought best to separate the sick from the well animals, removing them to other pastures, dividing them into small lots, and paying strict attention to the burning of carcasses, cleaning and disinfection of stables, etc. Hutyra and Marek state that in India they aim to control the disease with the aid of protective vaccination, but give no results. Holmes found the simultaneous vaccination with serum (which he produced through the subcutaneous inoculation of cattle and buffaloes) and with virulent cultures most effective, though it is claimed that such vaccination is not without danger for the animals. It is stated that the employment of cultures killed by heat, and also sterilized pleuritic exudate, has given good results. Baldrey employed a vaccine prepared with cultures sensitized to immune serum and subsequently killed at 60° C., reducing his losses from 100% among nonvaccinated cattle to 22% to 28% in the vaccinated animals.

In 1912 Mohler and Eichhorn reported on some work done in immunizing the buffalo herd in Yellowstone Park the previous year, and had no losses during the following twelve months. At this time they demonstrated by means of the complement fixation test that vaccinated animals responded with the production of immune bodies, and reactions were noted even three months following the vaccinations.

Having experienced very unsatisfactory results with the isola-. tion methods and internal medication recommended, we decided to do a small amount of experimental work with vaccines. The method employed in the production of this vaccine, and the reasons for its use in preference to other preparations have already been set forth in two publications.

During the year 1915, the laboratory of the State Livestock Sanitary Board prepared and sent out vaccine which was used on 434 animals in eight different herds. Three hundred and sixty-six (366) sick and healthy animals in six herds were vaccinated. As a result of outbreaks in these herds 42 deaths had occurred prior to vaccination and six were sick when vaccinated. Three of the sick and two apparently healthy animals in one herd died within one week. In other words in 1915 the disease was immediately checked in five of the infected herds, and there was not a single loss in any of the herds after one week from the date of vaccination. In addition to this we vaccinated 166 other animals, on pastures adjoining those showing infection, with not a single loss.

In 1916, following the satisfactory results of the 1915 work, vaccine was used on 366 animals in seventeen infected native herds. Fifty-three deaths had occurred prior to vaccination. Nineteen were sick when reported and were vaccinated along with the 347 remaining healthy animals. Ten of the sick and four apparently healthy animals died within one week and seven healthy after one week following the administration of the vaccine. These losses all occurred in six herds. In summarizing we find that during that year the disease was immediately checked in eleven of the seventeen herds, and that fifteen of the seventeen herds showed no losses one week after vaccination. In addition to these, eighty-eight animals on farms adjoining those having outbreaks were vaccinated prophylactically with no losses. The above figures for 1916 refer to outbreaks in native herds on pasture. Two hundred and fifty-eight (258) animals in herds exposed to the "Shipping Pneumonia" or so-called "Stockyard's Pneumonia" occurring in steers brought to the state as feeders were treated prophylactically and our records show a total of twenty-three sick steers distributed through eleven herds with twenty-two recoveries, and but one death following the vaccination, while none of the vaccinated cattle developed the disease.

Continuing in 1917, we vaccinated 895 animals in 38 herds on farms where the records showed 109 deaths prior to the receipt of the reports and administration of the vaccine. At the time of vaccination 18 animals were sick. Nine of these and eleven apparently healthy animals died following the vaccination. Eleven of those twenty deaths, including the nine sick, occurred within one week. In twenty-five of the thirty-eight infected herds the disease was immediately checked without a single further loss and in thirty-four of the thirty-eight (38) herds not a single loss was reported after one week from the date of vaccination. In other words there were but nine deaths from a total of 895 animals after one week following the vaccination and these deaths include everything reported as being lost by the owner, between the time of vaccination and the rendering of the report which was received from six weeks to four months later. One hundred and sixty-three (163) animals, on which the vaccine was used as a prophylactic, showed not a single outbreak.

In summarizing our work of vaccination for the control of hemorrhagic septicemia during the three years 1915 to 1917 inclusive, we find a total of sixty-one infected herds, containing 1831 animals, showing 204 deaths, or 11.1% prior to vaccination. Fifteen hundred and eighty-four (1584) healthy animals and forty-six (46) sick animals received vaccine. Twenty-two of the sick animals or 51.1% died. Twenty-four apparently healthy animals among the 1584 vaccinated, or 1.5%, died following the vaccination, eight of these within one week. Approximately one per cent (1.0%) of losses only was recorded in treated stock and as previously mentioned this includes all deaths, some of which were no doubt not due to hemorrhagic septicemia. In forty-one of the total sixty-one herds, the disease was immediately checked without further losses, and in fifty-five of these sixty-one herds not a single loss was recorded after one week from the date of vaccination, during which time we have figured the animal should have developed some immunity. The mortality prior to vaccination, including the sick animals which died, has been 12.3%. The mortality following vaccination, including deaths within one week, has been 1.5%. The mortality following what we term the completion of the vaccination at the end of one week has been less than 1%.

Furthermore, there has been but one reported case of hemorrhagic septicemia in the twenty-three\ (23) vaccinated herds of 1915 and 1916. This herd was vaccinated in 1916, and showed a recurrence in August, 1917. Of the four unvaccinated control herds from 1915, two have shown the reappearance of the disease. Other strong evidence in favor of the vaccine may be added from the prophylactic vaccination of several hundred animals on pastures adjoining those having outbreaks, and on which not a single case of the disease was reported.

We have frequently heard the remark that even though not vaccinated the remaining animals in infected herds might have shown no further losses. This may have been true of a few herds but it is reasonable to presume that the disease would immediately stop in forty-one herds and not a single loss would be recorded in fifty-five out of sixty-one herds over a period of three years with merely a visit and diagnosis by the local veterinarian without the aid of some prophylactic.

The method employed in the production of the vaccine used in the foregoing work and the reasons for its use in preference to other preparations have already been set forth in two publications. The only standard which we have been able to fix upon is that the cultures must be virulent for rabbits and that five (5) c.cms. injected intravenously shall be innoxious for young cattle.

We have no knowledge as to the efficiency of bacterins or other preparations. as the results following the work done by us were obtained with the exclusive use of this living vaccine,

SUMMARY

	Total herds	Total animals in herds	Deaths prior to vaccination	Sick prior to vaccination	Healthy vaccinated	Sick vaccinated	Deaths of sick following vaccination	Deaths of following vac.	Death after 1 week from vaccination	Herds showing no deaths following vac.	Herds O. K. 1 week after vaccination
1915	6	408	42	6	350	6	3	2	0	5	6
1916	17	419	53	19	347	19	10	11	7	11	15
1917	38	1004	109	18	877	18	9	11	9	25	34
Total.....	61	1831	204	43	1584	43	22	24	16	41	55
Percentage			11.1	2.3+			51—	1.5+	1%	67+	90+

LITERATURE

1895 Penna. Report of the Dept. of Agriculture, p. 57.
1896 Penna. Report of the Dept. of Agriculture, p. 117.

1897 Penna. Report of the Dept. of Agriculture, p. 135.
1898 Penna. Report of the Dept. of Agriculture, pp. 162-165.
1900 Penna. Report of the Dept. of Agriculture, pp. 119-120.
1902 Penna. Report of the Dept. of Agriculture, p. 100.
1902 Penna. Report of the Dept. of Agriculture, p. 156.
BILLINGS. The Corn Stalk Disease in Cattle. *Bulletins Nos. 7, 8, 9 and 10, Neb. Agr. Exp. Station*, 1886-88.
BILLINGS. The Corn Fodder Disease in Cattle and other farm animals, with a special relation to contagious pleuro-pneumonia in American beeves in England. *Bulletins Nos. 22 and 23, University of Nebraska Agricultural Experiment Station*, 1892.
GAMGEE. Diseases of Cattle in the United States. *U. S. Dept. of Agriculture,* 1896.
MAYO. Corn Stalk Diseases in Cattle. *Bulletin Kansas Agricultural Experiment Station*, 1896.
MOORE. Investigation into the nature, cause and means of preventing the Corn Stalk Disease of Cattle. *Bulletin No. 10, U. S. Bureau of Animal Industry,* 1896.

———◆———

NOTES ON THE ACANTHOCEPHALID AND ARTHROPOD PARASITES OF THE DOG IN NORTH AMERICA

MAURICE C. HALL, Ph.D., D.V.M., and MEYER WIGDOR, M.A.
Research Laboratory, Parke, Davis & Co., Detroit, Mich.

This paper is primarily intended to cover additional information regarding the rare thorny-headed worm of the dog, but in view of the fact that the writers are summarizing in other papers, published (Hall and Wigdor, 1918) and in manuscript, the available data as to the occurrence of protozoan, cestode, trematode and nematode parasites of the dog in North America, in connection with some new findings, a summary of our knowledge of arthropod parasites is included in this paper in order to complete a series covering the parasites of dogs in North America. These summaries are intended to be comprehensive, but not exhaustive. Not all records of a given parasite are cited and by no means all the literature possibly involved has been examined.

ACANTHOCEPHALA. *Echinorhynchus canis* was described from this country by Kaupp (1909) on 4 specimens collected from a dog at San Antonio, Texas. No subsequent writers have reported this species. Dr. Clifford C. Whitney collected one specimen of what is evidently this species from a young, black and white, male, mongrel dog at College Station, Texas, on March 8, 1917, and sent it to one of us (Hall) at Detroit. It appears, therefore, that this rather rare parasite is established in Texas, at least.

Through the courtesy of Dr. Whitney, we were allowed to retain his specimen for study. A brief description is as follows:

The worm is a female, 14 mm. long. The proboscis is armed with 6 rows of hooks, the largest set anteriorly. The hooks in the 4 anterior rows have anterior and posterior roots resembling the handle and guard of the taenioid cestode hook; those in the 2 posterior rows are rosethorn-shaped (see figs). The proboscis shows 33 hooks, of which 18 are large and 15 small. It is likely that 3 of the small hooks have been lost and that the total number present should be 36. The proboscis is 2 mm. long. The mounted specimen shows that the body is distinctly annulated. The body form and out-

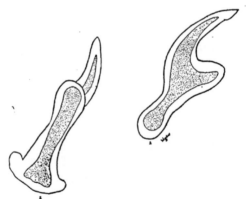

FIG. 1. *Gigantorhynchus canis*
Large hooks from first and second rows as numbered x180

line is substantially that figured by Kaupp (1909). There are eggs present, but apparently these have not been fertilized (this was the only specimen present in the host animal) and segmentation has not begun.

The cuticular annulation, the proboscis structure and the hooks indicate that this worm belongs in the family Gigantorhynchidae. As regards its generic position, it is difficult to ascertain this accurately by an examination of the one immature female specimen in our possession, but it appears to have the essential characters and appearance of the genus *Oncicola*, Travassos, 1916, and it is accordingly designated *Oncicola canis* (Kaupp, 1909) Hall and Wigdor, 1918.

In view of the fact that Acanthocephala forms have been reported from the dog in Europe, the question naturally comes up
as to whether the European and American forms are identical.
The European species is listed by Railliet (1893), Neveau-Lemaire
(1912) and other recent writers as *Echinorhynchus grassii* Deffke,
1891. An examination of Deffke's (1891) paper, shows that he has
in his list of dog parasites "*Echinorhynchus grassi,* 1888". This
is evidently not an attempt to name an *Echinorhynchus* species
after Grassi, as the date after Grassi's name shows, but is a reference to Grassi's paper of that date regarding this parasite. So
far as we can ascertain, Grassi and Calandruccio (1888) listed an
Echinorhynchus from the dog in Sicily; they state that Sicily is
an exception to the rule that in general *Echinorhynchus* is rare in
mammals other than swine, and that not infrequently they found

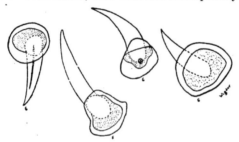

FIG. 2.   *Gigantorhynchus canis*
Small hooks from fifth and sixth rows as numbered x240

an *Echinorhynchus,* probably a new species, in the small intestine
of the dog. Travossos (1917) makes *Echinorhynchus grassii* a
synonym of *Moniliformis moniliformis,* which eliminates the possibility that the European and American forms are identical. Granting the accuracy of the Brazilian authority's synonymy, it follows
that the dog is parasitized at times by at least 2 echinorhynchs,
Moniliformis moniliformis and *Oncicola canis.* The latter is probably a customary parasite of some Texan carnivore other than the
dog. *O. canis* is very similar to *O. oncicola* (v. Ihering, 1892).
Both species show asymmetrical hook bases in some hooks and re-
curved projections on hook tips, but the hook measurements are
so dissimilar as to make it quite unlikely that the species are identical. Travassos gives measurements for 4 types of hooks in *O.
oncicola,* the first type being the hooks of the first and second (or
anterior) rows, the second type the hooks of the third row, the

third type the hooks of the fourth row, and the fourth type the hooks of the fifth and sixth (or posterior) rows. His measurements and ours are as follows:

Species	Hook type	Distance, tip of blade to tip of apical root (microns)	Distance between root extremities (microns)
O. oncicola	First.................	348	177
O. canis	First.................	200	148 to 160
O. oncicola	Second...............	268	149
O. canis	Second...............	140	50
O. oncicola	Third.................	227	130
O. canis	Third.................	166	116
O. oncicola	Fourth...............	120	—
O. canis	Fourth...............	130	—

In the measurements of hooks of the third type, we have measured from the tip of the asymmetrical process on the root, as Travassos appears to have done. Without this projection, the distance from the tip of the blade to the tip of the apical root is 130 μ; that between the root extremities is 60 to 64 μ. *O. oncicola* occurs in *Felis (Leopardus) onca* and *Felis (Catopuma) jaguarundi*, and it is quite likely that *O. canis* is normally parasitic in some of the Felidae.

ARTHROPODA. *Otobius megnini (Ornithodoros megnini)* has been reported from dogs in the southern United States by Hooker, Bishopp and Wood (1912).

Ixodes ricinus is reported from dogs in Canada by Hewitt (1915).

Ixodes scapularis is reported from dogs in the southern United States by Hooker, Bishopp and Wood (1912).

Ixodes cookei is reported from dogs in Canada by Hewitt (1915) and in the United States by Banks (1908).

Ixodes kingi is reported from dogs in the western United States by Hooker, Bishopp and Wood (1912).

Ixodes pratti is reported from the dog in Canada by Hadwen according to Hewitt (1915).

Rhipicephalus sanguineus, the brown dog tick, has been collected from the dog in Texas and in Mexico, according to Hooker, Bishopp and Wood (1912). Specimens of this tick from a dog on one of our battleships have been sent to this laboratory for identification, with the statement that the dog apparently became infested in New Orleans.

Margaropus annulatus, the cattle tick, has been reported from dogs in the southern United States by Hooker, Bishopp and Wood

(1912) and other writers, but it is very rare on this host.

Amblyomma maculatum has been reported from dogs in Texas and Louisiana by Hooker, Bishopp and Wood (1912).

Amblyomma americanum has been reported from dogs in Texas by Hooker, Bishopp and Wood (1912).

Amblyomma cajennense has been reported from the dog at Panama by Hooker, Bishopp and Wood (1912).

Dermacentor andersoni (*D. venustus*) has been reported from dogs in the western United States by Hooker, Bishopp and Wood (1912), by Stiles (1910) and by others.

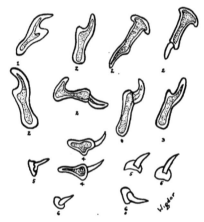

FIG. 3. *Gigantorhynchus canis*
Hooks from different rows as numbered x75

Dermacentor occidentalis is reported from the dog in the Pacific coast region of the United States by Hooker, Bishopp and Wood (1912).

Dermacentor variabilis is a common and widely distributed parasite in the United States, the dog being the usual host, and has been reported from the dog in Canada by Hadwen (1912).

Sarcoptes scabiei canis is the cause of sarcoptic mange in the dog. It appears to be much less common in the United States than demodectic mange.

Demodex folliculorum canis, the cause of demodectic mange in dogs, is common in the United States. We have had a number of cases here at Detroit.

Linognathus piliferus, the sucking louse of the dog, appears to be more common on the west coast of the United States than in the East. We have found a few cases here at Detroit.

Trichodectes latus, the biting louse of the dog, is fairly common in the United States. In connection with tests of the efficacy of sodium fluoride against biting lice, proposed by Bishopp and Wood (1917) for use against biting lice of poultry and reported by Hall (1917) as effective against biting lice of the horse, we have made some tests in this laboratory of its efficacy against the biting louse of the dog and find it effective. We have seen no bad results from it, but the possibility of trouble from poisons ingested through licking the hair and skin must be kept in mind in treating dogs. In a test to determine the toxicity of sodium fluoride, we gave a 9-kilo dog 1 gram of sodium fluoride in a gelatine capsule, followed by a small amount of water. The dog seemed in fairly good health for 3 days, but was found dead on the fourth day; there was a severe gastro-enteritis, with some hemorrhage, and an acute nephritis.

Ctenocephalus canis, the dog flea, is common on dogs in the United States.

Pulex irritans, the human flea, is not an uncommon parasite of dogs, especially on the west coast of the United States.

Echidnophaga gallinacea, the stick-tight flea, is often found on the ears of dogs in the southern and southwestern part of the United States, according to Bishopp (1915).

Gastrophilus intestinalis (*G. equi*), *G. nasalis* and *G. hemorhoidalis* have been reported from the dog in experimental infestations in the United States by Hall (1917). *G. intestinalis* functions readily as an incidental parasite of the dog; *G. nasalis* did not adapt itself to the dog so readily; *G. hemorrhoidalis* apparently had little or no capacity for parasitism in the digestive tract of the dog.

Cochliomyia macellaria (*Chrysomyia macellaria*), the screwworm, is a common parasite of domesticated animals in the southern United States. Dunn (1918) has recently recorded a case of infestation in the dog at Ancon, Panama.

Cuterebra emasculator, the rabbit bot, has been collected from the scrotum of the dog, apparently in North America, according to Gedoelst (1911).

Dermatobia cyaniventris (*D. hominis*) is reported as parasitic in dogs in tropical America by Verrill, according to Osborn (1896), and others.

Myiasis, due to infestation with various dipterous larvae, is not uncommon among dogs in the United States. We have several times seen cases of rectal myiasis in the dog, especially dogs that were sick and weak, and more particularly those that had diarrhea or blood in the feces. Fish (1910) records an interesting case of cutaneous myiasis, where a collie pup was found to have hundreds of maggots in the dense hairs along the spine from the neck to the scrotum, many of the maggots being imbedded in the skin. The species of fly responsible for these infestations is commonly not ascertained.

Simulium molestum is reported by Packard, according to Osborn (1896), as attacking the Newfoundland dogs of Labrador and driving them to take to the river for protection.

' *Simulium pecuarum* is recorded in reports of the U. S. Department of Agriculture, according to Osborn (1896), as attacking dogs in the United States.

Stomoxys calcitrans is reported by Hewitt (1917) as attacking dogs in Canada.

Tabanus lineola and *T.trijunctus* are reported by Snyder (1917) as annoying dogs in southern Florida.

There are numerous other biting flies that attack dogs on occasions, but the records are frequently indefinite and uncertain.

BIBLIOGRAPHY

BANKS, NATHAN. 1908. A revision of the Ixodoidea, or ticks, of the United States. *U. S. Bu. Entom.,* Tech. ser., (15), June 6, 61 pp., 10 pls.

BISHOPP, F. C. 1917. Fleas and their control. *U. S. Farm Bull.* (897), 15 pp., 5 figs.

COLE, LEON J., and PHILLIP B. HADLEY. 1910. Blackhead in turkeys: A study in avian coccidiosis. *R. I. Agric. Exp. Sta. Bull.* (141), pp. 137-271, 11 pls.

DEFFKE, O. 1891. Die Entozoen des Hundes. *Arch. f. wissensch. u. prakt. Thierh,* Berl., v. 17 (1-2), pp. 1-60; (4-5), pp. 253-289, pls. 1-2, figs. 1-11.

DUNN, L. H. 1918. Studies on the screw worm fly, *Chrysomyia macellaria* Fabricius, in Panama. *J. Parasitol.,* v. 4 (3), March, pp. 111-121.

FISH, P. A. 1910. A fly-blown and distempered dog. *Rept. N. Y. St. Vet. Coll. for yr.* 1908-1909, pp. 48-49.

GEDOELST, L. 1911. Synopsis de parasitologie de l'homme et des animaux domestiques. Lierre et Bruxelles. xx+332 pp., 327 figs.

GRASSI, GIOVANNI BATTISTA and SALVATORE CALANDRUCCIO. 1888. Ueber einen Echinorhynchus, welcher auch in Menschen parasitirt und dessen Zwischen. wirth ein Blaps ist. *Centralbl. f. Bakteriol. u. Parasitenk.,* Jena, 2. J., v. 3 (17), pp. 521-525, figs. 1-7.

HALL, MAURICE C. 1917. Parasites of the dog in Michigan. *J. Am. Vet. Med. Assn.*, v. 4 (3), June, pp. 383-396.
1917. Notes in regard to horse lice, *Trichodectes* and *Haematopinus*. *J. Am. Vet. Med. Assn.*, v. 4 (4), July, pp. 494-504.
1917. Notes in regard to bots, *Gastrophilus spp.* *J. Am. Vet. Med. Assn.*, v. 5 (2), Nov., pp. 177-184.

HALL, MAURICE C., and MEYER WIGDOR. 1918. Canine coccidiosis, with a note regarding other protozoan parasites from the dog. *J. Am. Vet. Med. Assn.*, v. 6 (1), Apr., pp. 64-76, 1 fig.
1918. A bothriocephalid tapeworm from the dog in North America, with notes on cestode parasites of dogs. *J. Am. Vet. Med. Assn.*, v. 6 (3), June, pp. 355-362, 1 fig.

HEWITT, C. GORDON. 1915. A contribution to a knowledge of Canadian ticks. *Trans. Roy. Soc.*, Canada, ser. 3, v. 9, sec. 4, pp. 225-239, 3 pls., 1 map.
1917. Report of the Dominion Entomologist, C. Gordon Hewitt, D.Sc., F.R.S.C., for the year ending March 31, 1916. 73 pp., 9 figs.

HOOKER, W. A., F. C. BISHOPP and H. P. WOOD. 1912. The life history and bionomics of some North American ticks. *U. S. Bu. Entom. Bull.* (106), Sept. 7, 239 pp., 15 pls., 17 text figs.

KAUPP, B. F. 1909. *Echinorhynchus canis.* *Am. Vet. Rev.*, v. 35 (2), May, pp. 154-155, 3 figs.

NEVEAU-LEMAIRE, MAURICE. 1912. Parasitologie des animaux domestiques. Paris. 1257 pp., 770 figs.

OSBORN, HERBERT. 1896. Insects affecting domestic animals: An account of the species of importance in North America, with mention of related forms occurring on other animals. *Div. Entom. Bull.* (5), n. s., 302 pp. 170 figs.

RAILLIET, A. 1893. Traité de zoologie médicale et agricole. 2 éd. (fasc. 1), 736 pp., 494 figs, Paris.

SNYDER, T. E. 1917. Notes on horse flies as a pest in southern Florida. *Proc. Entom. Soc.*, Washington, v. 18 (4), pp. 208-210. Dated Dec., 1916; actually published June 11, 1917.

STILES, CH. WARDELL. 1910. The taxonomic value of the microscopic structure of the stigmal plates in the tick genus *Dermacentor.* *Hyg. Lab. Bull.* (62). 72 pp., 43 pls.

TRAVASSOS, LAURO. 1917. Contribuçoes para o conhecimento da fauna helmintolojica brazileira. vi. Revisao dos acantocefalos brazileiros. Pt. I. Fam. Gigantorhynchidae Hamann, 1892. *Mem. d. Inst. Oswaldo Cruz*, v. 9 (1), pp. 5-62, pls. 1-24A.

—The New York State Veterinary Medical Society will hold its annual meeting at Ithaca, N. Y., July 24, 25 and 26.

—The Oklahoma State Veterinary Medical Association has changed its time of meeting from July 10th and 11th to July 31st and August 1st.

—The South Carolina Association of Veterinarians will hold its ninth annual meeting at Columbia, S. C., September 4th and 5th.

—The Virginia State Veterinary Medical Association will hold its next meeting at Ocean View, Va., July 11 and 12.

AN ANALYSIS OF TUBERCULIN TESTS AND POST MORTEM RESULTS—ACCESSORIES TO THE TUBERCULIN TEST

Burton R. Rogers, D.V.M.
118 East 43rd Street, Chicago, Illinois

Progress in medicine, and in any branch of science, is based upon a careful study and observation and modification of past experiences, practices and methods, and the *application* of new ideas that are perpetually evolved from new and old facts, discoveries and theories.

With this in mind, much good ought to come from a review of the use and results of tuberculin tests from the very beginning.

The U. S. Bureau of Animal Industry at one time reported the records of 23,869 positive reactors out of which 23,585 or 98.81% showed "lesions" on post mortem.

Unfortunately post mortem records do not exist to show the extent, degree and distribution of the lesions, so they can be grouped on a basis of the post mortem lesions, nor is this information available in the larger number of tests by practitioners and others not included in the Bureau figures. The "alpha" and the "omega" lesions are the same.

In some recent extensive and intensive research reading, I ran across Bulletin 102 of the University of Illinois, published in 1913, and showing in detail the results of the tuberculin test of the college herd, and the lesions and disposition of the slaughtered on post mortem. This herd, therefore, may well be taken as a type. Veterinarians might advantageously at this point try to recall and gather together into one composite herd every animal and herd they may recall testing and posting.

Let us consider all the *facts* now known and discovered that have a bearing and might be *applied* today for the improvement of the past. Of these the most important are that healthy cattle and closed tuberculin-reacting cattle *do not* give off tubercle bacilli, but that both reacting and non-reacting *open* tuberculous cows cough up, swallow and pass out tubercle germs in their feces, in numbers proportionate to how open and dangerous each case is; and the additional fact is that hogs will eat the feces and become proportionately tuberculous. Therefore, the hog *test*, and on post mortem will positively show the degree in the cattle.

Let us carefully view and study Table I of the University of Illinois in the light of present knowledge, and ascertain if it might not be possible to modify and improve the same with more science, less cost, and more conservation, by assuming to interject between the conclusion of the tuberculin test and the *ruthless slaughter* as an accessory and adjunct to the tuberculin, the pig recheck test.

TUBERCULOSIS IN THE ILLINOIS UNIVERSITY DAIRY HERD.
BULLETIN No. 162.

TABLE I—RESULTS OF SLAUGHTER

Herd No.	Test	Post mortem	Herd No.	Test	Post mortem	Herd No.	Test	Post mortem
1	+	±	71	++	±	Lad	—?	±
10	++	±	72	++	±	90	No test	±
12	+	±	76	+	±	85	—	±C
16	++	±	77	+	±	34	—	±C
19	+	±	80	+	±	13	+	?
20	+	±	83	+	±C	21	+	?
27	+	±	84	+	±	29	+?	?
28	+	±	86	+	±	23	+	?
30	+	±	87	+	±	17	+	0
31	++	±	88	+	±	33	?++	0
36	++	±	92	+	±	61	?+	0
37	++	±	95	+	±	67	++	0
39	++	±	97	+	±	69	+—	0
41	++	±	129	+	±	79	+	0
42	+—	±	1002	+	±	Heifer	+—	0
44	+	±	1004	+	±	Heifer	+	0
45	++	±	1005	++	±	Joe	+	0
46	+	±	1007	+	±	65	+	Not s'l't'd
47	++?	±	1008	+	±	14	No test	0
49	++	±	1017	+	±	68	— — —	0
51	+++	±C	Bull	+	±	104	—	0
52	+	±C	Grade	+	±	106	—	0
53	+	±	Heifer	+	±	109	—	0
54	++	±	Heifer	+	±	Heifer	—	0
56	++	±	Grade	+	±	1027	—	0
57	++	±C	Heifer	+	±	120	—	0
58	+++	±C	Heifer	+	±	100	—	0
59	++	±	Heifer	+	±	106	—	0
60	++	±	Heifer	+	±	122	+	0
64	++	±	15	—?	±	124	+	0
66	++	±C						

+ = a reaction; — = test without reaction; ± = disease found; ? = questionable; 0 = nothing found; C = carcass condemned.

There were 91 cattle in the Illinois herd. All but two (Nos. 14 and 19) were tuberculin tested. 90 of the cattle were slaughtered and one not. 76 of the tested cattle reacted to the tuberculin test. 19 of the reactors alone were worth over $3000. The whole herd of 76 must have thus been worth not far from $10,000. Such an amount demands and requires the very best caution, judgment and conservatism consistent with sanitary safety possible, as to their final disposition. Error or fault in this regard might financially ruin a single individual owner.

It will be noted that out of the 76 reactors, eleven showed no lesions at all on post mortem. Four others had lesions so slight as to be doubtful. Of the 61 reactors showing lesions, *only* six were bad enough to condemn, and these, no doubt, represented the *open* reactors. This leaves a total of 55 so slightly affected that they were not even condemned after slaughter, and no doubt were the closed cases. A little later effort will be made to show a possible way to have found out the condition of the six *before* slaughter, instead of only *after* slaughter, and similarly for the 55 which need not have been slaughtered.

But more serious than the above is the fact that of the 13 which did *not* react, four or 32% showed lesions. Of these, two (Cows 34 and 85), were so *badly* diseased they were condemned. One of these two was the *worst* case the writer of the bulletin had ever seen. Therefore the *worst* one was left back in the healthy herd unconsciously. Of the eight animals condemned, two or 25% of the eight did *not* react, nor did they show physical signs of the disease. This is unfortunate, because it *defeats* the very object and high ideal of the test—and in addition created a false confidence. How many multiples and variations of this have occurred in the common herds of the country and state, where trained experts were not constantly with the herd? A little later, effort will be made to show a possible way the existence of such *unsuspected* non-reacting open spreaders might be ascertained, and regain confidence.

At this point it may be well to quote in fine type three paragraphs from the bulletin referring to Cows 34, 85 and 68. Study and analyze these carefully, accepting the *facts*, but exercising caution and care in accepting or making conclusions and "deductions". Science is classified knowledge, and consists of known facts that may be fewer, but always sound. "Deductions" from facts are many, and sometimes wrong, and therefore dangerous and in many instances thus more important than facts. Imagine the effects of the following on the farmer. Does the bulletin tend to encourage or discourage the use of the tuberculin test, when no qualifying hope is offered? Is there any to offer? There is.

"*Cow 34 failed* to react when tested in May, 1906. At that time she was not milking and failed to breed; hence she was in excellent condition. About a year later she began to go down in flesh, and would have died in July had she not been killed.

"When examined she proved to be the *worst* case the writer (of bulletin) had ever seen; the abdominal cavity was one mass of tubercles, and other parts of the body were badly diseased.

"It is probable that she was too far advanced and her system was already too full of the poison at the time tested to react. However, it was entirely possible for her to have become infected after the test. (Rogers cannot agree with such a deduction, and if so, the *only* cow that possibly could have infected Cow 34 was Cow 85 described below.) The writer (of the bulletin) believes that this cow was responsible for spreading much of the infection revealed by the test made in May, 1908. A large percentage of the two-year-old heifers which were with her in the pasture reacted. (Rogers feels Cow 34 *could* be responsible for *every one* of the 70 uncondemned reactors, together with the condemned ones [7]; it would be interesting to know if they were bought out of the same original herd.)

"*Cow 85* passed through *three* tests *without* reacting. She was a small cow and a heavy milker and feeder. Up to the time slaughtered, she was in very good flesh and physical condition. The only thing which would indicate the disease was a *cough*. She failed to breed readily and was sold for *beef* subject to inspection. *She was found to be very badly diseased.*

"In general, cows in which the disease is too far advanced to react to tuberculin, show external symptoms, but the writer (of bulletin) does not believe that *even an experienced veterinarian would have detected the disease* in Cows 34 or 85 by a physical examination. These two cases emphasize the fact that mature animals in a herd which is badly infected should be looked upon with much suspicion, even if they do not react. (Rogers thinks the original herd source of the bad or light animals should help determine this.)

"*Cow 68* passed several tests successfully, but had a *cough* for two or three years. Since she was one of the animals in the badly infected herd, it was *thought* that possibly she might have the disease in the *advanced* stage. She was *not* in as good condition *as Cow 85*. She was *slaughtered* but proved to be *free* from disease, the *cough* being due to some *other* cause."

Would the unqualified facts and lack of hope of the above tend to encourage or *discourage* tuberculin testing? Would not confirmed experiments and facts concerning the "pig-recheck" overcome this? Further on in the bulletin it is stated that the *only* means and method we have of detecting, reducing and checking the disease is with *tuberculin*. Is this wholly true to justify its admitted errors?

All of us have sometimes heard veterinarians in groups or in meetings say in substance and in variation: "I tested a herd of 75 cattle and (in hysterical tone) *twenty-five reacted*—and 24 showed *lesions*" (more hysteria). Let us have intelligence and hysteria in the right places, but the teachers and leaders are largely responsible, some and most of them unconsciously. Many veterinarians have conscientiously tested a herd, based on the advice and articles of teachers and authorities, and advised the owner to dispose of the reactors, and to thoroughly disinfect the premises, and assured the owner he "would be all right thereafter". But has time proved the carrying out of this advice true? Would such advice have proved true in the Illinois herd? No! Can we modify it? Let us see.

First, let us recognize not only the *value*, but also the *limitations* of *tuberculin*, and seek and supply accessories and adjuncts to its limitations. Let us assume we were to re-handle the Illinois herd.

In the Illinois herd, for example, after the tuberculin test, is to *clean* and disinfect the quarters in which both the reacting and the non-reacting herds are to be placed. *Cleaning* is as essential as efforts at disinfection, for in conjunction with direct and diffuse sunlight, the former will accomplish the latter.

The next thing to do is to put a regular unseparated herd or bunch of pigs behind the non-reacting herd unit. About one pig per each cow should be sufficient, but no separate pens for the pigs or the cows are necessary at first, if at all. This is to be done to find out if there are, or are not, one or more *open* unsuspected spreader cases like Cows 34 and 85 left back in the non-reacting herd. If on regular slaughter *all* the pigs are *free* of tuberculosis, it is positively a clean herd, and probably will always remain so. However, this could be annually easily confirmed by allowing hogs to associate with the cattle as in ordinary farm practice until the generation of animals in the original tuberculous herd were disposed of, and tagging and tracing to slaughter.

However, if tuberculosis *is* found in the hogs following the non-reactors, as would have been the case in the Illinois herd, it means there is "dynamite" (Cows 34 and 85) left back in the herd.

If the herd is worth it, the individual *cow* or *cows* (like 34 and 85) *must* be found out by individual pig tests in isolated pens, in the same manner as will be described in the reacting herd below.

The 76 *reacting* herd of cattle should be handled in the following way: all animals which are not and never will be worth much more than beef value, should be sent for immediate slaughter for obvious reasons.

A physical examination of the remainder should be made, and, if possible, the cattle should be arranged in stalls in an order of their apparent degree. This arrangement might be made within a week, by collecting samples of tracheal, esophageal, mammary and rectal secretions and feces, and making microscopical and cultural bacteriological tests, but this is not necessary.

Have the 76 reacting cattle come to the same stalls at night. Provide 76 separate shovels or pails or other conveyors for the manure of each cow, so that possible contamination will not interfere with the test.

Build one large temporary pen, divided into 76 compartments, each large enough for one pig or two. Gates are not needed. If possible have each of these pig compartments directly behind the stall of each cow.

The pen can be wholly or partially inside or outside the barn, and if convenient, boards can be temporarily removed or holes cut for manure to be thrown out for each cow to each pig. Or by wheelbarrows, pailfuls of manure can be hauled through an alley to the pens.

Two months should be a sufficient length of time to conduct the feeding test, but of course the longer, the better.

The question of expense might come up here. One man should be able to do this alone and have some spare time for other duties. It is a question of $100 versus $10,000 tied up in a reacting herd and it is worth it.

Hogs for a two-month period after weaning, and then tagged and put together for the possible development of the disease until regular slaughter, would be one way. Or take hogs within two months of market weight or age should be satisfactory.

Mix most of the grain foods for the hogs with the night manure of the cattle. A little potassium iodide might increase the number of tubercle bacilli excreted as occurs in the human. Only the night and early morning manure need be fed, thus leaving the cattle out during the day.

About once a week, wash the mangers with clean water and feed the washwater to the corresponding pig. A little first milk from the same cow might be added.

At the end of 30 days tuberculin-test the pigs. Regroup the cattle of the corresponding reactor pigs.

Tag each hog by name and record number, and market the 76 hogs separately or with enough others to make a car-load. Ship to nearest market, other things being equal. Request that the load be slaughtered and inspected separately.

Get records of hogs having lesions in any degree, and not more than ten of the 76 hogs should show lesions. Get full reports upon the degree and extent of lesions of these ten tuberculous hogs.

If the whole 76 would have been allowed to follow the 76 cattle, the ten cattle would have infected *all* of the 76 hogs in some degree.

Back at the farm immediately separate the cattle that caused the tuberculous hogs from the others.

Determine the value of each and use judgment as to which of these it might pay to slaughter or which to keep under the Bang system.

This would leave three herds—1st, the non-reactor; 2nd, the open reactors; 3rd, the closed reactors, which I feel could be safely put with the non-reacting herd, but possibly not wise.

Such a plan would have discovered *Cows 51, 52, 57, 58, 66* and *83*, and also *Cows 34* and *85*, and possibly one or two others. These would be the only ones slaughtered. The other 81 or 83 cattle of the herd would be saved, or 66 of the 76 reactors be saved.

The "assumption" that all the reactors would get worse is entirely theoretical.

Cattle, out in the open, that will not produce tuberculosis in susceptible pigs within two months' intensive exposure, are not likely to become seriously tuberculous within a year at least.

This could be automatically checked and overcome by simply allowing succeeding crops of herds of hogs to naturally associate with the cattle, and if any of the hogs are found appreciably tuberculous, or as soon as they do, reconduct the intensive two-month individual hog test.

I do not feel that cattle with closed tuberculosis so often become progressively worse from the development and re-infection from their own lesions, as they do by being constantly re-infected day after day from *open* cases like Cow 34, and in the same way the first lesion was implanted. When *cows* like 34 are removed, the *cause* is removed. Owing to their outdoor life, most cows will be able to take care of and arrest further development of their own lesions, unless they are to a stage where they will infect hogs, and thus auto-infect themselves. The cow, with her "tracheal cud", is the queen of all auto-infectors, and I believe this explains why she is so often so extensively and badly infected. The beauty of the hog is, that it not only gets the spreader, but the auto-infector also.

Cow 34, and possibly also one or more of the seven other condemned or open cases, *infected* those with light lesions *before* the test. *After* the test, *Cows 34* and *85* infected the other that *reacted after* the first test, and showed only light lesions.

A herd that will not infect associating hogs has no open spreaders or auto-infectors in it.

A herd that will infect associating hogs, has one or more *open* spreaders and auto-infectors in it.

To find the open spreader and auto-infector as early as possible, and as fast as they may develop, is the *duty* and the *only* duty of the veterinarian.

Hysteria toward *all* reactors should be toned down, and the hysteria concentrated on the *open* cases.

Some of this can be reduced to an almost mathematical basis. This depends on the numbers of cattle; the numbers of germs passed per herd of cattle; the number of hogs sharing the germs; and the number of days or length of time exposed or sharing the germs, and innumerable combinations of these.

Ten cattle passing 30 lbs. feces each will pass 300 lbs. feces daily. Ten hogs will probably eat 30 lbs. moist feces daily each or a total of 300 lbs. 50 hogs would average 6 lbs. each, or in every case a fraction of the total feces available and eaten. One or five hogs would eat their share of the total eaten.

One cow passing one million tuberculous germs daily would give each of 10 unselfish hogs an average of 1/10th, or 100,000 germs. 5 hogs would get 200,000 each, and 50 hogs 20,000 and 100 hogs only 10,000 each,

Thus a large herd of hogs lightly infected might, in fact, point to a bad herd with one or more *bad* cases.

The unit degree of dangerousness in a herd, is equal to the average total number of virulent tubercle bacilli passed by the herd.

They may all be passed by *one* cow, or several cows may pass their proportion to make the same total.

That is, one cow only, in a herd of any size, may pass 1,000,000 tubercle bacilli daily.

In another herd of 100 cows, 10 cows may pass a daily average of only 100,000 each, yet the ten equal 1,000,000 germs, or an average of 10,000 per each 100 cows.

A herd of 100 hogs may be exposed *accidentally* or otherwise for *one* day only, to a herd daily passing 100,000,000,000 germs, and be lightly affected. In another case, one hog following for 200 days a cow passing only 1000 germs daily, would give the hog a total of 200,000 germs or twice as many, and show twice as severe lesions. This might apparently point to a herd of cattle twice as badly infected, which, in fact, would be only 1/1000th as bad.

That is why the author is always interested in, and has always shown the *total* number of hogs infected with lesions no matter in what degree. The dilution and length of exposure is unknown, in any case to the packing house inspector.

It seems plausible, in view of these apparent *facts,* that after a series of sufficient experiments of hog-association tests, almost absolute ante mortem accuracy can be predicted as to the condition of the cattle.

With the greatly increased value of cattle, some selling as high as $31,000.00, it behooves the veterinarian to give the matter serious thought so as to render the client and the country the maximum of service, with corresponding increased self-remuneration.

(An After-thought.) The hog will separate the acid-fast and hay bacilli from the tubercle formers—and the virulent from the non-virulent—and make a quantitative test also.

It is hoped all these facts will be carefully studied and weighed, as an accessory and adjunct to the tuberculin test, and that it will be used in connection with the accredited herd system, and thus assist in making it a real and lasting success, minus such mistakes as over-enthusiasm and over-confidence in tuberculin caused.

This should lead the way to putting tuberculosis location,

control and eradication, on a true scientific, conservative, intelligent basis.

And after 1918, it is hoped no more will valuable reacting herds be handled as inefficiently and wastefully as was the Illinois University herd and thousands of other herds, because of the pardonable limited and unapplied knowledge of that time.

SUPPLEMENT

Pounds Feces Passed				Number Tubercle Bacilli Open Cows Pass			
No. Cows	Daily	30 Days	100 Days	Daily	30 Days	100 Days	200 Days
1	30	900	3,000	1,000	30,000	100,000	200,000
1	30	900	3,000	1,000,000	30,000,000	100,000,000	200,000,000
5	150	4,500	15,000	5,000,000	150,000,000	500,000,000	1,000,000,000
10	300	9,000	30,000	10,000,000	300,000,000	1,000,000,000	2,000,000,000
50	1,500	45,000	150,000	50,000,000	1,500,000,000	5,000,000,000	10,000,000,000
100	3,000	90,000	300,000	100,000,000	3,000,000,000	10,000,000,000	20,000,000,000

Share of Number of Tubercle Bacilli per Hog					
Number Germs Daily	No. Hogs	One Day	30 Days	100 Days	200 Days
1,000	1	1,000	30,000	100,000	200,000
	5	200	6,000	20,000	40,000
	10	100	3,000	10,000	20,000
	50	20	600	2,000	4,000
	100	10	300	1,000	2,000
1,000,000	1	1,000,000	30,000,000	100,000,000	200,000,000
	5	200,000	6,000,000	20,000,000	40,000,000
	10	100,000	3,000,000	10,000,000	20,000,000
	50	20,000	600,000	2,000,000	4,000,000
	100	10,000	300,000	1,000,000	2,000,000
5,000,000	1	5,000,000	150,000,000	500,000,000	1,000,000,000
	5	1,000,000	30,000,000	100,000,000	200,000,000
	10	500,000	15,000,000	50,000,000	100,000,000
	50	100,000	3,000,000	10,000,000	20,000,000
	100	50,000	1,500,000	5,000,000	10,000,000
10,000,000	1	10,000,000	300,000,000	1,000,000,000	2,000,000,000
	5	2,000,000	60,000,000	200,000,000	400,000,000
	10	1,000,000	30,000,000	100,000,000	200,000,000
	50	200,000	6,000,000	20,000,000	40,000,000
	100	100,000	3,000,000	10,000,000	20,000,000
50,000,000	1	50,000,000	1,500,000,000	5,000,000,000	10,000,000,000
	5	10,000,000	300,000,000	1,000,000,000	5,000,000,000
	10	5,000,000	150,000,000	500,000,000	1,000,000,000
	50	1,000,000	30,000,000	100,000,000	200,000,000
	100	500,000	15,000,000	50,000,000	100,000,000
100,000,000	1	100,000,000	3,000,000,000	10,000,000,000	20,000,000,000
	5	20,000,000	600,000,000	2,000,000,000	4,000,000,000
	10	10,000,000	300,000,000	1,000,000,000	2,000,000,000
	50	2,000,000	60,000,000	200,000,000	400,000,000
	100	1,000,000	30,000,000	100,000,000	200,000,000

AN INFECTIOUS DISEASE OF GUINEA PIGS

A. K. GOMEZ, D.V.M.

(Fellowship student from the University of the Philippines)
Department of Pathology and Bacteriology, New York State Veterinary
College at Cornell University

INTRODUCTION. On July 12th, 1917, five guinea pigs were sent to this laboratory for the diagnosis of the disease which was causing a daily loss in a breeder's flock of 200 pigs. This loss amounted to two or three a day which continued until August 8th, after sanitary measures were instituted. Upon autopsy of the guinea pigs, lesions very similar to those of tuberculosis were observed, consisting of pearl-like nodules in the lungs, liver and spleen. They were not as prominent and numerous in the lungs as they were in the other affected organs. Some of the cervical lymph glands were caseous and encapsulated. On section through one of these nodules, it was found to contain yellowish, semi-dry caseated pus. No calcification was present. Smear preparations from this pus stained after the Ziehl-Neelsen method did not reveal the presence of *Bact. tuberculosis* or other acid fast bacteria.

Dr. Pickens isolated an organism from the lesions which appeared to be the cause of the disease. The present paper purports to give the observations made on a series of inoculation and feeding experiments conducted on twenty guinea pigs. A description of the morphological and biological characters of the organism is also given.

PROPOSED NAME. As far as the writer has been able to refer to bacteriological literature, the organism herein described is not identical with any of the heretofore known organisms. It is therefore considered as a new species and the name *Bacterium pickensi*, is therefore proposed.

The writer's attention was attracted to the descriptions given by different investigators on the Preisz organism causing caseous-lymphadenitis in sheep. In many respects their descriptions of this organism appears to be similar to that observed in *Bact. pickensi*. It was found, however, that *Bact. pickensi* is distinctly Gram negative and that in bouillon medium it presents a slight turbidity and a distinct ring formation, while with the Preisz organism these characteristics were not present. A strain of the Preisz organism was obtained from the American Museum of Natural History and when grown in the different media, its biological reactions coincided with the usual description given for it in textbooks and articles. Repeated tests on *Bact. pickensi* after the Gram's method using a 24 hours' growth invariably showed that it did not retain the stain. Smear preparations were made on the same slide with both organisms and were stained simultaneously following closely the directions given in the text. (Moore and Fitch's Bact. Diag.)

The descriptions of the gross appearance of lesions produced by the Preisz organism as described by different writers in guinea pigs appeared also to be strikingly similar to those produced by *Bact. pickensi.*

MORPHOLOGY AND STAINING. *Bacterium pickensi,* appears as minute slender rods and as cocco-bacilloid forms. In the hanging-drop, active brownian movements were observed but motility was not noticed, although repeated examinations were made. Diplo-bacilloid forms were also noticed. Short chains consisting of four or five organisms with their long axes parallel to each other were present. They measure from $.5\mu$x$.9\mu$ to $.5\mu$x1.5μ. The ends are rounded and no spores are formed. They stain readily with the ordinary aniline dyes but give the best staining reaction with $1:10$ aqueous dilution of carbol-fuchsin. They do not retain the stain when treated after the Gram method.

CULTURAL CHARACTERS. *Agar-Agar.* In twenty-four hours, an abundant growth is obtained when the organism had been growing on this medium for some time. When first isolated from the tissues, they do not readily grow; growth, however, may then be seen after forty-eight hours. The growth on agar-slant is abundant, filiform, raised, smooth and contoured. Along the stroke it spreads at the bottom of the tube covering almost the whole surface of the agar at this point. The water of condensation becomes turbid and a whitish sediment is formed. The upper part of the stroke reaches its limit of width in 72 hours, the width being 2 to 3 mm. The surface of the growth appears glistening and in very old cultures, a peculiar metallic lustre is observed on reflected light. On transmitted light the growth is opaque and of a greyish-white color. An odor resembling that of boiled shrimp is produced within the tube. When touched with the platinum needle, the consistency seems butyrous.

In stab cultures, the surface growth is restricted and that along the needle tract is scanty and filiform. The colonies on agar plates are punctiform and develop slowly. Under the low power of the microscope, they appear raised with smooth surfaces and entire borders. They are amorphous and present a brownish translucent appearance.

POTATO. No growth was detected on this medium.

NUTRIENT-BROTH. The growth in this medium is characteristic. The liquid becomes moderately turbid in 24 hours and remains so for a long time. A thin pellicle forms on the surface which is easily broken on slight agitation. It sinks to the bottom of the tube where a yellowish-white, flocculent sediment rapidly forms. A distinct heavy growth adhering to the wall of the tube forms a white ring at the level of the surface of the broth. The reaction remains neutral even after 48 hours.

GLUCOSE-BOUILLON. Gas is not produced in this medium. A viscid sediment collects at the bottom of the tube and no ring-formation takes place. The reaction is distinctly acid after 24 hours and remains so for at least two weeks.

LACTOSE-BOUILLON. Gas formation is not present. A heavy ring is formed on the wall of the tube. A flocculent sediment forms at the bottom. The reaction is distinctly alkaline after 24 hours and remains so for at least two weeks.

SACCHAROSE-BOUILLON. Gas is not formed. A distinct ring forms on the wall of the tube and a flocculent sediment collects at the bottom. The reaction is distinctly alkaline after 24 hours and remains so for at least two weeks.

MILK. A clearing without coagulation of the casein takes place very slowly in this medium. The reaction becomes faintly acid after 2 or 3 days.

LITMUS-MILK. No reduction occurs, the color remaining practically unchanged.

GELATIN. Growth is very slow and the medium is not liquified.

TEMPERATURE. The optimum temperature for growth is 37° C., the maximum is 50° C., and the minimum is 20° C.

RESISTANCE. A 1% carbolic acid solution kills the organism in five minutes. A temperature of 60° C. for five minutes is sufficient to destroy it. Exposures to direct sunlight in the month of March from 10 a. m. for three hours failed to kill the organisms while at four hours' exposure, no growth was obtained. This was done by smearing a 24 hours' bouillon growth on sterile cover-slips contained in a sterile petri-dish and after the exposures the cover-slips were immersed in sterile bouillon. The tubes were then examined daily for turbidity up to four days' incubation at 37° C. Agar cultures kept in the incubator at 37° C. were found to contain virulent organisms after 48 days. Cultures 135 days old were found to be dead.

Anërobiosis. The organism is strictly aërobic.

Indol is not produced in Dunham's peptone medium. The organism was grown in bouillon for about 10 days and then subjected to filtration through a Berkefeld candle. Two mils of the filtrate when injected intraperitoneally into a few weeks' old guinea pig proved to be non-toxic. A 4 mils dose of a shake extract of a killed culture, injected intraperitoneally into another young pig, proved also to be without effect. Two-tenths of a mil of a 24 hours' bouillon culture injected subcutaneously was fatal for an adult guinea pig.

SYMPTOMS. No opportunity was available for observation of the disease in the natural condition as it did not recur after sanitary measures were established. The writer came to Cornell for graduate work in October, 1917, and these experiments were undertaken in November. All the observations were therefore made in artificially infected animals.

The period of incubation was found to be three to four days. At the onset of the disease the animal becomes dull and the luster of the fur is lost. The coat becomes ruffled and has an unthrifty appearance. The animal "rounds itself up" and stands in a corner of the cage with half-closed eyes for intervals of time. A slight lacrymation is observed. The animal would perform masticatory actions, it would go to its food, take up a few kernels of maize, throw away half of the masticated amount and then it would drink with apparent thirst. In the feeding experiments, a majority of the pigs developed a submaxillary abscess which in some cases broke through the skin. Caseated pus could then be squeezed out. The cervical lymph glands become swollen and some undergo caseation. The animal sometimes elicits a cough and frequently a spasmodic trembling of the body has been observed. It soon loses its appetite, runs down in condition rapidly and becomes emaciated. The eyes are then sunken, the protuberances of the back and pelvis become salient, the animal when taken in the hand feels light and the bones of the skeleton can be easily traced with the fingers.

The two appended cases illustrate the clinical picture of the disease.

CASE 17. MARKINGS. Male, adult, white pig.

Jan. 15th, 1918. About 5 mils of a 24 hours' bouillon culture of the organism were mixed with the food and left in the cage so that the animal had free access to it.

Jan. 18th. A swelling the size of a hazel nut was noticed in the submaxillary region. The pig is dull and has a ruffled coat. It stands in a corner of the cage with half-closed eyes. Slight amount of lacrymation is observed. Every now and then it would mop its mouth with its two front feet.

Jan. 21st. Animal is very dull; "rounded up" in a corner of the cage. A small ulcer covered with dried pus is present at the left commissure of the lips. The submaxillary swelling is still hard. The respiration is labored and the temperature is 100.2° F. The leucocyte count is 44,000 per c. mm. Differential count revealed 34% of polymorphonuclears and 41.9% of lymphocytes.

Jan. 22nd. The animal is dull, with half-closed sunken eyes. It is losing flesh rapidly, has ruffled coat, would not eat and has a difficult respiration. The pellets of feces are hard and dry.

Jan. 23rd. It lies down flat on the abdomen practically all the time. A strong audible rattling sound is heard from its difficult respiration. Very weak. Is unable to stand up and when forced to move it slowly raises itself up, trembles in the act and walks for only a short distance with a wabbling motion. The thorax is "rounded".

Jan. 30th. Found dead and lying on its abdomen.

AUTOPSY. Typical nodules were present in the lungs, liver and spleen.

CASE 19. MARKINGS. White and tan, adult pig.

Jan. 15th, 1918. About 4 mils of a 24 hours' bouillon culture of the organism were mixed with the food, and left in the cage.

Jan. 16th. Ruffled coat; "rounds itself up" in a corner of the cage.

Jan. 22nd. Weak; dull; eyes are sunken and half closed. Stands isolated in a corner. The voice is weak and harsh; the respiration is difficult; shakes the body every now and then; emaciated. The leucocyte count is 35,000 per c. mm. Differential count shows 57% polymorphonuclears and 36% lymphocytes. Lies down on its abdomen most of the time.

Jan. 23rd. Found dead and lying on its abdomen.

AUTOPSY. Typical nodules were found in the lungs, liver and spleen.

In the course of the experiments, it was found that the leucocytes were increased to an average of 41,000 per c. mm. The red count was not materially increased. Differential counts revealed an average increase to 45% for the polymorphonuclears and to 43% for the lymphocytes.

The temperature rises to 102° F. at the height of the disease and falls to 95° F. just before death occurs. The average duration of the disease in feeding experiments is 10 days.

MORBID ANATOMY. The characteristic lesions consist of minute pearl-like nodules ranging from a pin-point to a large pin-head. Some may be conglomerate while others may be confluent, forming a large necrotic area, encapsulated by connective tissue. These nodules appear very similar to those of tuberculosis often produced in guinea pigs for diagnostic purposes. These characteristic nodules are found in the lungs, liver, and spleen. In one case (No. 11) the pancreas presented similar nodules grouped like clusters of grapes throughout the organ.

LUNGS. Multiple pearl-like nodules may be present in all the lobes. The majority of these nodules are raised while some appear only as white minute spots on the surface. They are not easily crushed with the knife, being quite resistant to pressure. On section through one of them, it is found to contain a yellowish-white, semi-dry pus. Calcification is never present. Several of these nodules may be fused to form a large necrotic area having a diameter of 5 mm. or more. In case No. 15, the whole mediastinal lobe became necrotic and a large white necrotic area of about 2 cm. in diameter was present in the right diaphragmatic lobe. The bronchial lymph glands are often enlarged and some are transformed into encapsulated abscesses containing semi-dry, thick, yellowish-white pus.

Microscopically, these nodules show a deeply stained necrotic center which is surrounded by a zone of leucocytes undergoing different stages of necrobiosis. Many large endothelial cells are also present which, with the leucocytes, fill up the lumina of the neighboring alveoli. A zone of connective tissue separates this necrotic area from the adjacent apparently healthy tissue. Many such areas may be confluent, forming a large one. In this instance, the zone of connective tissue is not very distinct. The microscopical picture is very much like that of a miliary tubercle with the exception that giant cells are not observed. Calcification is not present. The neighboring blood vessels are distended with blood. Their walls are thickened and a zone of emigrating leucocytes is observed around them.

In some cases in which a severe infection was produced, a fibrinous exudate was found in the thoracic cavity; the pleura was reddened and nodules 2 mm. in diameter were observed attached to the thoracic wall.

LIVER. This organ is enlarged to twice its normal size and presents multiple pearl-like nodules the size of a pin-point to that of a large pin-head. In some cases a fibrino-purulent exudate is present in the peritoneal cavity, causing the liver, stomach, spleen and the anterior coils of the intestines to become adherent to each other. The color of the liver is dark-brown and its edges are thick. On section, the lobules are indistinct and the surface of the incision is covered with blood. The cut surfaces are convex. Histological sections through these nodules show them to consist of a necrotic center in which the cells have disappeared, the area being deeply stained throughout. Surrounding this necrotic center is a relatively wide zone of leucocytes, the ones toward the center undergoing necrobiosis. Some of the young endothelial cells show vesicular nuclei. Surrounding the zone of leucocytes is a zone of connective tissue, forming a distinct capsule. Giant cells are not present and calcification was not noticed. The surrounding liver cells show distinct cell-wall, granular cytoplasm and evidences of fatty degeneration. The central veins are engorged with blood and show a surrounding zone of emigrating leucocytes.

SPLEEN. This organ is swollen and is of a dark-brown color. The edges are rounded and on section the pulp can be easily scraped off with the knife.. On its surface, it presents multiple pearl-like nodules varying in size from that of a pin-point to that of a large pin-head. Some are raised while others, especially the small ones, are not. On section they are seen to contain caseated pus. Some of the nodules are conglomerate while others are confluent. Microscopically, they show the same picture as that described for those of the liver.

PANCREAS. Only in case No. 11 in which the infection was very severe, were numerous nodules present.

HEART. The epicardial blood vessels are injected, otherwise no morbid changes are discernible.

KIDNEYS. These are reddened and swollen; the renal capsule peels off easily. On section the cortex is lighter in color than the medulla. The incision is bloody, the blood vessels are prominent and the cut surfaces are convex.

ADRENALS. These are yellowish in color; are enlarged to twice their normal size and on section the cortex is light yellow while the medulla is brown. The cut surfaces are convex.

BRAIN AND MENINGES. The blood vessels of the meninges show arborization. The brain shows no discernible morbid changes.

EPICRISIS. The disease is easily reproduced by feeding cultures of the organism with the food. In one experiment, Case No. 13*, a culture of the organism was rubbed on the nose and the disease was not produced. Others at the same time were fed with the material from the same culture and they all died showing typical lesions. This seems to show that the most effective channel of infection is by means of the food. A submaxillary abscess frequently develops as a result of the organisms being filtered into this gland. The gland undergoes inflammatory reaction by the irritation subsequently set up by the organisms; the lymphoid cells are destroyed by the toxin produced; leucocytic infiltration occurs and the abscess may break through the skin or become encapsulated. The organisms may also be carried through the lymph channels into the succeeding cervical glands which subsequently become swollen. From here they may be carried into the thoracic duct from which they gain entrance into the circulation. They are then circulated throughout the body. They finally localize in the minute capillaries of the lungs, liver, and spleen. The neighboring cells undergo necrobiosis and the product of the degenerative changes act as an irritant which brings about an inflammatory reaction. The surrounding blood vessels become engorged with blood; the leucocytes marginate, after blood stasis has taken place; they pass through the blood vessel wall and invade the necrotic area in immense numbers. They are subsequently destroyed by the toxins produced and the necrotic area enlarges. Soon the endothelial cells of the blood vessels proliferate and give rise to the large phagocytic cells with vesicular nuclei often seen in histological sections. The sur-

*See appended tables,

rounding connective tissue also proliferates and forms a capsule around this necrotic spot, forming the characteristic nodules seen in the gross specimens. The functions of the lungs, liver, and spleen are greatly impaired. The nutrition becomes very poor, the animal becomes weak and dies of inanition.

The organisms when taken in large numbers may survive the action of the digestive juices. They then may pass through the mucous membrane of the intestines and gain access into the lacteals from where they may either be taken into the mesenteric glands or directly into the blood stream. Once in the circulation they are then distributed throughout the body and finally localize in the lungs, liver, and spleen.

TREATMENT. Thorough disinfection of the premises should be immediately instituted. Proper disposal of the dead and the killing of the affected are indicated. The ease with which the organism is killed by disinfectants and the institution of proper sanitary measures should promptly control any great loss to the breeder.

CONCLUSIONS. 1. A new infectious disease of guinea pigs the lesions of which are very similar to those of tuberculosis has been described.

2. The causative agent of this disease is given the proposed name of *Bacterium pickensi.*

ACKNOWLEDGMENT. Acknowledgment and thanks are due Dr. Pickens for his invaluable help and suggestions and also for the culture of the organism. To Dr. V. A. Moore my gratitude is also expressed for his wise advice and the use of the laboratory.

REFERENCES

KROEBER, M. A. 1917. Guinea Pigs for Profit. *Jour. Lab. and Clin. Med.,* 2, pp. 381-382.

TYZZER, E. E. 1917. A Fatal Disease of the Japanese Waltzing Mouse Caused by a Spore-bearing Bacillus.

HOLMAN, W. L. 1916. Spontaneous Infection in the Guinea Pig. *Jour. of Med. Research,* N. S. 30, pp. 151-182.

BOXMEYER, CHAS. H. 1907. Epizootic Lymphadenitis. A New Disease of Guinea Pigs. *Jour. Infect. Dis.,* 4, pp. 657-664.

GILRUTH, J. A. 1903. Pseudo-tuberculosis in Sheep. *New Zealand Dept. Agri. Bul.* No. 1.

1902. Pseudo-tuberculosis in Sheep. *Jour. Comp. Path. and Therap.,* 10, p. 324.

GELSTON, S. M. 1901. The Study of an Epidemic Among Guinea Pigs. *Rep. Mich. Academy Sc..* Abt., pp. 86-87.

NORGAARD and MOHLER. 1899. The Nature, Cause and Economic Importance of Ovine Caseous Lymphadenitis, *B. A. I. 10th Annual Report,* pp. 639-660.

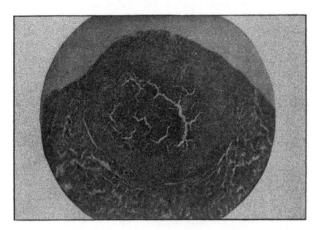

FIGURE I. Photomicrograph of a nodule in the spleen. This lesion is typical of those observed in this as well as the other organs. The necrotic centre and the contiguous zone of round cells may be distinguished. The reactionary zone is not well marked here. Mag. 55 diam.

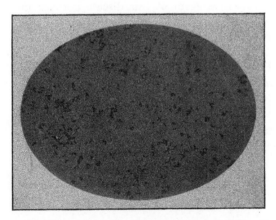

FIG. II. Photomicrograph of the causative agent of this disease, *Bact. pickensi.* The preparation was made from a 24-hour bouillon culture of the organism and was stained with a 1 to 10 aqueous dilution of carbol fuchsin, slightly decolorized with 95% alcohol. Mag. 750 diam,

INOCULATION EXPERIMENTS

No.	Color	Method	Amt. injected	Date of Inoculation	Date of Death	No. of days	Remarks
1	Tan, black stripes	Inj. subcutaneously	1 c.c.	Oct. 23, 1917	Nov.12, 1917	11 days	Nodules present in the spleen and liver
2	Tan, white on face	Inj. intraperitoneally	¼ c.c.	Oct. 23, 1917	Oct. 27, 1917	4 days	Nodules present in mesenteric lymph gland
3	Black	Inj. intraperitoneally	½ c.c.	Nov. 1, 1917	Nov. 4, 1917	3 days	Nodules present in spleen, liver, lungs and peritoneum
4	Tan, white on right side of face	Inj. intraperitoneally	¾ c.c.	Nov. 1, 1917	Nov. 4, 1917	3 days	Nodules present in spleen, liver and lungs
5	Black and White	Inj. intraperitoneally	½ c.c.	Nov. 1, 1917	Nov. 2, 1917	1 day	Died of fibrinous peritonitis. No nodules
6	Tan, large	Inj. subcutaneously	½ c.c.	Nov.15, 1917	....	......	Recovered
7	Black and White	Inj. subcutaneously	½ c.c.	Nov.15, 1917	Nov.18, 1917	3 days	Nodules present in lungs; microscopically foeal necrosis found in the liver and spleen
8	Tan and White	Inj. subcutaneously	½ c.c.	Nov.15, 1917	Nov.16, 1917	1 day	Nodules absent. Organisms recovered from liver and spleen
9	Tan small	Inj. subcutaneously	.2 c.c.	Dec. 5, 1917	Dec. 15, 1917	10 days	Nodules present in liver, spleen, lungs and peritoneum
10	Squirrel, white nose	Inj. subcutaneously	.3 c.c.	Dec. 5, 1917	Dec. 6, 1917	1 day	Died of pneumonia
11	Tan and White	Inj. subcutaneously	.2 c.c.	Dec. 12, 1917	Dec. 15, 1917	5 days	Nodules present in lungs, pleura, spleen, pancreas, liver and peritoneum

FEEDING EXPERIMENTS

No.	Color	Method	Amt.	Date of Experiment	Date of Death	No. of days	Remarks
12	Tan, small	Introduced into mouth with pipette	1 c.c.	Dec. 12, 1917	Jan. 2, 1918	21 days	Nodules present in lungs, liver and spleen
13	Mouse color	Rubber on nose	....	Dec. 12, 1917	....	....	Still alive
14	Mouse small	Mixed in food	4 c.c.*	Dec. 12, 1917	Jan. 2, 1918	21 days	Nodules present in liver, spleen and lungs
15	Black and White	Mixed in food	2 c.c.*	Dec. 12, 1917	Dec. 31, 1917	19 days	Nodules present in liver, spleen and lungs
16	Tan small	Mixed in food	4 c.c.*	Dec. 12, 1917	Dec. 21, 1917	9 days	Submaxillary abscess noticed. Killed and no nodules found in the organs
17	White	Mixed in food	4 c.c.*	Jan. 15, 1918	Jan. 30, 1918	18 days	Nodules present in liver, spleen, lungs and cervical lymph glands
18	Black	Mixed in food	4 c.c.*	Jan. 15, 1918	Jan. 23, 1918	8 days	Nodules absent, organism recovered from submaxillary abscess
19	White and Tan	Mixed in food	4 c.c.*	Jan. 15, 1918	Jan. 23, 1918	8 days	Nodules present in liver, spleen and lungs
20	Mouse color	Mixed in drinking water	4 c.c.*	Feb. 25, 1918	Mar. 6, 1918	9 days	Nodules present in mesenteric gland

*About 4 c.c. of 24 hours' growth suspended in bouillon was mixed with a handful of maize. This was left in the cage so that the animal had free access to it.

CLINICAL AND CASE REPORTS

FURTHER NOTES ON CONTROL OF GOITER IN THE NEW-BORN

HOWARD WELCH, Bozeman, Mont.

Certain sections in the northwest have for years been seriously hampered in their efforts at livestock production by the fact that a large percentage of the new-born domestic animals every year were goitered and otherwise so defective that they died. Pigs were hairless, showed extreme myxedema, and were born dead or

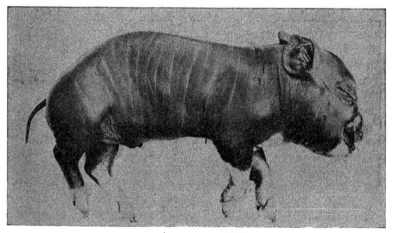

FIG. 1. Hairless Pig (Berkshire)
(*Bull. 119*, Agl. Exp. Sta., Bozeman, Mont.)

died in a few hours. Lambs and calves were similarly affected, though to a less degree. Foals, while seldom hairless, were weak, unable to stand, and soon died. It was not recognized that all these losses were due to the same cause until investigation at about the same time, by the Washington Experiment Station at Pullman and the Montana Station at Bozeman, showed that goiter and its allied conditions were responsible for the trouble.

Since we could easily demonstrate a deficiency of iodine in the defective young, we began feeding iodine to the pregnant females as an attempt at correcting the condition. We attempted to demonstrate a shortage of iodine in the agricultural products of the affected areas, but failed to do so. Nevertheless, the iodine feeding was a huge success from the first.

Our first experimental feeding was with sows and ewes, and the results, with less than a thousand females fed iodine, were so striking that we published a bulletin in the fall of 1917.

At the same time we inaugurated a campaign for a wider use of iodine in the affected areas, and by midwinter we distributed iodine to about 1600 sows, 1200 ewes, and a hundred mares and cows. These were located in Washington, Montana, North and South Dakota, Wyoming, and Canada, and were all on ranches where had occurred goiter for several years previous. The iodine was administered as potassium iodide in widely differing doses.

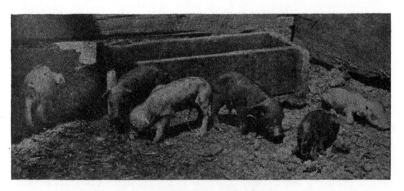

Fig. 2. Typical litter of hairless pigs
(*Bull. 119*, Agl. Exp. Sta., Bozeman, Mont.)

Some animals were fed 2 grains daily, some 1, and some ½ grain daily. Some received 2 grains twice a week, some 2 grains once a week. The females fed have all produced vigorous, normal young, and in no case has any tendency toward goiter been observed. There were no check experiments run, as we were reasonably certain of results, and the present great need for livestock production was greater than the need for additional proof of the efficacy of the iodine.

Though beyond a doubt a small amount of iodine will prevent the occurrence of goiter in the new-born, the cause of the trouble is still hazy. In Montana we have two distinct types of the malady; one in definite districts which we call "affected areas", where hairless pigs and goitered lambs and calves occur every year; and the other, or sporadic type, which occurs irregularly here and there, and is without doubt due to a poorly balanced ration. .

Dr. E. B. Hart, in the February number of the *Journal of Biological Chemistry*, throws light on this phase of the trouble. He has produced the identical condition in pigs by feeding a ration with a high protein content, with insufficient roughage. Curiously enough, iodine fed to a sow on this ration served to produce normal pigs, which apparently indicates that this type of ration in some

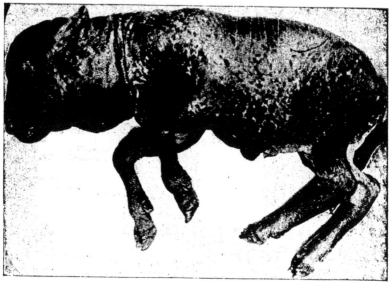

FIG. 3. New-born Lamb showing goiter and very little wool
(*Bull. 119*, Agl. Exp. Sta., Bozeman, Mont.)

manner interferes with thyroid metabolism and proper iodine assimilation.

But a faulty system of feeding cannot be the cause in the so-called affected areas. It is inconceivable that in an area like the Yellowstone Valley, about 400 miles long and from 5 to 50 miles wide, the ranchers every year should so mismanage their feeding that nearly one-half of the new-born animals would be defective. More than that, several feeding experiments in this valley, using carefully balanced rations, failed to correct the trouble. Further investigation will be necessary to definitely establish the cause of the endemic goiters.

Meanwhile, the method of control should be developed. Without doubt we have been feeding more iodine than was necessary. The cost of the treatment we estimated at about 50 cents per head, feeding 2 grains of potassium iodide daily for 90 to 100 days. This included a sugar of milk vehicle, 1 dram daily; and packing and mailing to the stockman. This cost can doubtless be much reduced, though the present figure seems low enough when compared with the results obtained. We do not know what the lowest advisable dose of iodine may be, though we have shown that anything over two grains daily is wasted. We have proved that the iodine must be supplied to the female during the early part of the gestation period, for in several instances even large doses of iodine failed to produce results when fed for the last 25 to 30 days of the period. We believe that potassium iodide, with some sort of dry diluent, is the most satisfactory way to feed iodine. A solution of the iodide was the most obvious method, but breakage of bottles in transit, by freezing, etc., made it inadvisable to use this method. It may be possible to find a cheaper iodine bearing feed than the rather expensive potassium iodide, or better yet, a system of feeding, even in the affected areas, that will render unnecessary the use of iodine in any form.

LAMENESS

J. E. NANCE, Stillwater, Okla.

Some months ago, a brown mare weighing about 900 pounds was brought to the veterinary hospital of the Agricultural and Mechanical College at Stillwater. The owner stated that this animal had been found lame in the right hind leg one morning and he had supposed that she had been kicked by a mule, but no swelling or injured place was noticed by him.

No positive diagnosis was made at the time the mare was brought.

Being very lame and the case a chronic one (at least of two years' standing) the owner was advised that treatment was useless. He consented to leave the animal to be used as a dissecting subject.

The writer first saw this case in August of last year. At that time the following symptoms were noted: no swelling or external lesion visible. No difficulty in extending the leg but marked lameness when weight was thrown on that limb. At times the leg was carried and when standing was always rested. Some adduction.

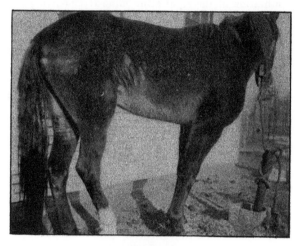

FIGURE I

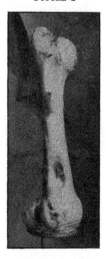

FIGURE II Femur from Fig. 1

No noticeable soreness on palpation but when the leg was flexed, as in the spavin test, pain was evidenced. Some atrophy of the gluteal and crural muscles. Mare in very good flesh. This subject was destroyed about January first of this year and used as a dissecting subject.

On examination of the right stifle joint after cutting away the tissues, a diseased condition of the lateral condyle of the femur was found to exist. With the exception of the inferior surface of this structure, the affected bone had a spongy, rough, uneven appearance and was studded in places with small exostoses.

The striking features of this case, to me, were the marked lameness shown, and the absence of any lesions or symptoms upon which a positive diagnosis could be made·ante mortem.

PERVERSE DIGESTION IN YOUNG RUMINANTS*

GEORGE B. JONES, Sidell, Ill.

The incentive by which we were prompted in the attempt to write a paper on this subject was the lack of any knowledge except that obtained by our own observations, but we hope by bringing the subject before this association to get the opinion and the experiences of those present and from this information form a nucleus for further investigations.

In searching veterinary literature from Genesis to Revelations we have as yet been unable to find a word of enlightenment on the subject, therefore, what we shall attempt to say will be mainly a record of our personal observations.

The title of this subject may be a misnomer, but it was given because of the lack of knowledge for a better name, but we hope to be able to describe the ailment so that you then can give it any name that may suit your individual idea.

This trouble is observed in young calves and lambs ranging in ages from three to twelve weeks, or at the time these young animals cease to depend wholly upon a milk diet but are beginning to partake of a solid diet such as grass, hay, straw, etc.

The time the trouble may occur depends upon the opportunities these animals may have had for obtaining solid food. Some calves are restrained in a dry lot with nothing but a milk diet until they are two or three months of age, while others may have access

*Read at the Ohio Valley Veterinary Medical Association, Terre Haute, Ind., Feb. 26, 1918.

to all kinds of food from birth. As a result of these different environments we can attribute the great range of time or age at which this trouble may occur.

It might be further stated that the tender green grass is not so liable to bring about the trouble as matured grass, hay or straw. My observations have been that over-ripened blue-grass tops is a very potent factor in producing the trouble and more especially in lambs.

In calves that are confined for the first few weeks in dry lots, with only a liquid diet, and are afterwards turned out to pasture it seems that most any kind of forage will produce the trouble. In one instance we recall where five calves had been confined in a dry lot for six weeks then turned to grass and shortly afterwards all became afflicted, although not all on the same day.

As a general rule in calves we see this ailment only in solitary cases while in lambs we may find several afflicted at the same time. This difference no doubt can be accounted for by the greater number of lambs of the same age compared to the number of calves of one age.

It might also be stated that more of this trouble is seen in dry seasons, and this, no doubt, is caused by the tough and woody condition of the grass.

While there are only a small percentage of the calves born during the winter months, a greater percentage of them become afflicted than those born during the spring and summer months.

In the breeding districts this trouble is far more prevalent than is supposed, but on account of it not being contagious and there usually being only an isolated case now and then the average farmer takes but little cognizance of the trouble.

We have never tried to get exact data on the cases but it is my belief that at least five per cent of the calf crop become afflicted, and without treatment nearly all afflicted ones die.

In order to get a better understanding of the cause of this trouble we will consider a few theoretical ideas, on digestion and rumination. Physiologically speaking the rumen is very small and poorly developed in the young animal while living wholly upon a liquid diet; in fact, it might be said that the rumen is dormant and inconsequential as far as the welfare of the animal is concerned for the first few days of its life.

If true, as claimed, that there are no alkaline secretions while

.the young animal is living on a milk diet, these alkaline glands are also dormant until the animal begins to partake of solid food. The act of rumination is wholly unknown while the animal is living only on a liquid diet, and in no wise aids digestion.

When the time comes and the animal is permitted to partake of solid food three radical changes are brought about.

First, the small and inactive rumen must expand and begin its peristaltic action; second, the dormant alkaline glands must begin secreting their juices in order to assist the digestion of these new solid foods; third, the act of regurgitation and remasticating of these solid foods must begin.

These three things are all now of vital importance to the well being of the young animal, and if any one of them should fail in its function a derangement of digestion would follow.

That we have a derangement of some of these functions is certain and as a result we have grassy or woody concretions resembling hair balls in the stomachs and bowels. These concretions are not egagropiles but balls formed from whatever solid foods the animal may have partaken. These balls may range in size from that of a small marble up to that of a hen's egg.

SYMPTOMS. As stated before, the ailment is usually seen in the animal that is from three to twelve weeks of age. The animal is gaunt, weak, eyes staring, grinds its teeth, and is more or less delirious. These symptoms are usually preceded by constipation, although some cases may show a slight or profuse diarrhoea.

As a typical case we will consider one where the calf is nursing its mother each night and morning. He may nurse all right this morning, but tonight when he is turned to his mother he walks up to her, gives the udder two or three hunches, grinds his teeth, but refuses to nurse. Later he will muss around the udder as though unable to nurse, saliva may drip from his mouth, looks wild out of his eyes, staggers away from his mother, falls down apparently in a fit, gets up and walks or runs into the fence only to fall again, then have a few more fits when death closes the scene. In prolonged cases the animal may stand in a secluded corner and bellow as though it were actually starving.

A very peculiar thing, in the more severe and protracted cases that recover, is that they will absolutely refuse again to nurse the mother.

In lambs we notice similar symptoms although they succumb more quickly than the calf.

TREATMENT. Oil and stimulants given in small doses three or four times a day and continued until the bowels are thoroughly cleared. In severe cases it may require this treatment for three or four days in order to obtain the desired effect.

My experience has been that it is beneficial to follow up with a few doses of lime water during convalescence.

In those cases where recovery is slow the calf should be given a quart of fresh milk three times a day as a drench because they sometimes die of sheer starvation on account of the deranged brain being slow to return to a normal condition.

AMAUROSIS AND AMBLYOPIA IN DOG AND CAT

OSCAR SCHRECK, New Haven, Conn.

There is so little written in our veterinary journals or text books, about this very important, but fairly uncommon, ailment, that it prompts me to report my success with the treatment of the disease. By amaurosis we understand blindness, occurring without apparent lesion of the eye, and its inability is dependent upon certain material changes. After considerable study and observation I have come to believe the condition, seen in the dog and cat is more of an atony or paresis of the optic nerve. Keeping this in mind the following treatment was given in five cases with the best results, but I wish to impress upon the minds of those who have a case of this kind not to expect to work wonders over night, as it generally takes a few weeks of treatment, and I believe this treatment will cure nearly all curable cases. It has proved in my hands the most satisfactory prescription in the above disease. The dose may seem large to some, but I claim we must give large doses in this disease to get results, and results are what count. The two prescriptions given below were given to a full grown English setter, in smaller animals you must reduce the dose to suit the animal in hand, and watch the action of your drugs.

I always begin my treatment by freeing the bowels well at the start with the following:

℞ Resin Podophylli....................Grains X
Aloin Powd........................Grains X

        Ipecac Powd.........................Grains V
    ·   Fel. Bovis Insp.....................Grains L
        Misce. et. Fiat. Capsules No. X
        Sig. One capsule T. I. D. after feeding

After the bowels have acted good and strong the following is
used:

    ℞ Strychnine Sulph.
        Acidi Arsenosi, aa..................Grain SS
        Ext. Sumbul......................Grains XXX
        Ferri Subcarbonatis................Grains L
        Quinine Valeriate
        Assafetida, aa...........................dr. I
        Misce. et. Fiat. Caps. No. XXIV
        Sig. One Capsule T. I. D.

The food should be nutritious, generous, and easy of digestion,
as constipation often depends on the first stage of digestion being
imperfect.

———◆———

ABSTRACTS FROM RECENT LITERATURE

SWINE PLAGUE IN MAN. M. Thomsen. Abstracted from "Hos-
pitalstidende", Copenhagen, February 13, 1918. Copied from *The
Journal of the American Medical Association,* Volume 70, No. 17,
April 27, 1918.—Thomsen has encountered three cases of a lesion on
the hand, resembling erysipelas, with lymphangitis running up the
arm, nausea and fever.

The first patient was a veterinarian and the diagnosis of swine
plague was followed by injection of 10 c.c. of the antiserum. In
less than an hour the malaise had subsided and in four days recovery was complete except for a little stiffness in the arm. The man
had been giving the antiserum to a sick hog four days before his
own sickness.

The farmer's wife who had helped to hold the hog during the
injection got some blood on her hand and a small lesion developed.
After failure of other measures, an injection of 10 c.c. of the anti-
serum cured the lesion in three days.

In another family a hog taken suddenly sick was slaughtered,
and the farmer's wife developed the same clinical picture as in the
first two cases. It dragged along untreated for two months and

then subsided. One meal was made from the pork but all eating it were taken with severe diarrhea and the rest of the carcass was buried. **M. J. HARKINS.**

PRELIMINARY REPORT ON THE VIRULENCE OF CERTAIN BODY ORGANS IN RINDERPEST. William Hutchins Boynton. *The Philippine Agricultural Review.* Volume X, No. 4.—The tissues used in the experimental work were liver, spleen, lymph glands, heart, intestines, thymus, skeletal muscle, larynx, pharynx and back of tongue. They came from animals dead from rinderpest either having been bled to death for virulent blood or having died in the regular course of the disease. The tissues were extracted with a 0.5%, 0.75%, 1% and 2% phenol solution. The extraction was made under sterile conditions.

The animals into which the extracts were injected to test their virulence were chosen for their high degree of susceptibility. They were closely watched in order to be sure that the disease did not develop from any source other than the injection of the extracted material.

The extracts worked as readily on animals outside of the laboratory as they did in the author's research work. It is most advisable to use a 0.75% phenol extract not over 15 days old.

From the results obtained in working with rinderpest the author suggests that similar or even better results may be obtained with the virus of hog cholera along similar lines. The liver, spleen, lymph glands, heart, fourth stomach, cecum and colon were found to be the organs best adapted to the work. **HAYDEN.**

GLANDERS IN FELINES. M. Carpano. Abstracted from "*Annali d'Igiene*", Rome. Copied from *The Journal of the American Medical Association*, Volume 70, No. 17, April 27, 1918.—Carpano found signs of acute glanders in the lungs of a tiger dying in captivity at Rome, and others have reported similar findings in lions and cats. The zoological gardens at Rome recently had an epizootic of acute glanders among the lions and tigers but the other animals escaped. Twelve of the large felines were affected and a number died. Cats inoculated from them developed the same set of symptoms in from three to five days, while other cats infected naturally from these cats showed an incubation period of six or seven days. The temperature, however, ran up the end of the fourth day. **M. J. HARKINS.**

ABORTION DISEASE IN CATTLE. L. Van Es. *Circular 18,* North Dakota Agricultural Experiment Station.—Abortion due to disease of the uterine mucous membrane and of the fetal membranes is much more common than other forms. The organism is found in the udder, vaginal discharges and in the infected uterus from which abortion has taken place. Animals may be infected through the genital organs, the digestive tract, and by means of the infective material carried by unclean attendants. The infected cow as well as the bull may serve as carriers of the disease. There is a possibility of reinfection. A calf that survives when born of an infected dam may be a carrier of the disease. The lesions produced by abortion infection are quite constant and aid greatly in the diagnosis of the disease. A certain degree of immunity is developed. The symptoms of an approaching abortion are very much like those of normal parturition. The complement fixation and agglutination tests are used to determine the disease. There is no notable degree of mortality in aborting animals. There is often a serious loss in production. There are no remedies that can be depended upon to eradicate the infection from the body. Isolation, comfortable quarters, removal of the afterbirth if necessary, and thorough disinfection of the parts are attentions that should be given the aborting animal. A frequent cleansing and disinfection of animals and premises will help to keep down the disease.   HAYDEN.

THE CULTURE OF THE PARASITE OF EPIZOOTIC LYMPHANGITIS AND THE EXPERIMENTAL PRODUCTION OF THE DISEASE IN THE HORSE IN FRANCE. Boquet, A., and Negre, L. *Comptes rendus des Séances de l'Academie des Sciences,* Year CLXVI, No. 7, pp. 308-311. (Abstract in *Internat. Rev. Sci. and Pract. of Agriculture,* April, 1918.)—Epizootic lymphangitis, "African farcy", is caused by a specific parasite discovered by Rivolta and placed by him in the Blastomyces—*cryptococcus farciniosus.* In spite of the researches of Tokishige, Marcone and Sanfelice the nature of the parasite was still doubted as, of late, certain authors considered it to be a protozoon.

The authors have shown, by their researches, the nature of Rivolta's cryptococcus by the growth of the parasite as mycelium in cultures which could be propagated and by the experimental production of the disease by inoculating these cultures into the horse. The experiments are fully described. Further work on vaccination and bacteriotherapy by means of heated cultures is in progress.   FISH.

A NOTE ON JHOOLING IN CAMELS. II. E. Cross. *Bulletin No. 72, 1917. Agricultural Research Institute, Pusa, India.*—Jhooling is a contagious disease of camels. It is manifested by the formation of local tumors which are hot and painful and terminate in suppuration and raw patches. The cause is probably a fungus. In the main it is a cold weather disease. Lesions occur as a rule on the neck, hindquarters or testicle. Several lesions appear and the camel loses condition. As the wounds heal small white patches persist for several months. In the treatment of the lesions a red iodide of mercury blister left on for three days is recommended. This is washed off with soap and water and then the diseased area is excised. Three dressings of permanganate of potash, well rubbed in, are applied at intervals of four days. Prevention is brought about by the isolation of the diseased camels.   HAYDEN.

PYOTHERAPY IN EPIZOOTIC LYMPHANGITIS: RESEARCHES IN ITALY. Lanfranchi, A., and Bardelli, P. *Il Moderno Zooiatro,* Series V, Year VI, No. 12, pp. 261-275. (Abstract in *Internat. Rev. Sci. and Pract. of Agriculture,* March, 1918.)—After summarizing the work carried out by Mangan, Belin and Velu on pyotherapy, the authors give a detailed description of their treatment of epizootic lymphangitis by means of pyotherapy, which has given completely negative results. "In all the animals treated, whether the lesions were slight, of moderate severity, or severe, the two series of six injections (each of 2 c.c. of pyovaccine) with an interval of eight days, caused no diminution of the progress of the disease," even with subjects used as controls, during the experiment, it was found that the injections of pyovaccine "have accelerated and aggravated the disease". Therefore, according to the authors, at the present state of our knowledge, autotherapy and pyotherapy are not methods of treatment the use of which could be advised in epizootic lymphangitis.   FISH.

—Dr. J. H. Bux has been transferred from Topeka, Kans., to Little Rock, Ark,

ARMY VETERINARY SERVICE

TRANSPORT SERVICE*
(The Innocent Abroad)

D. A. McAuslin, Brooklyn, N. Y.

Of all the component parts of the armies in this, the greatest of wars, no part is, to my mind, so absolutely innocent of having in any way played a part in bringing it about; none so essential in anything other than the actual fighting; none which has had so little voice as to whether he goes or stays and none so willing in the performance of his work, no matter how hazardous, as that of our equine friends, the army horse and mule. They are called upon to do the work when power machines fail, and it is due to the fact that they perform this work so creditably that they are retained in the face of all statistics compiled by the alert efficiency expert and salesman. It is not this work that I wish to bring to your attention but the lack of appreciation shown them for performances done or to be done. In seven voyages to Italy I have often wondered if it would be possible to destroy some horses that have gone through the ministrations of some of the so-called ocean-going veterinarians.

My first departure from New York was on the Italian Steamship *Taormina*—a large passenger-carrying ship before the war. The upper portions, reserved for horses, were fairly good, being the third-class passenger sections, but the lower decks could have been greatly improved so far as ventilation and drainage were concerned. The consignment consisted of 1076 horses and 150 mules, the latter rejects from former consignments. For four days previous to sailing these mules had been under my charge and treatment at the railway stockyards, and I was able to get a good line as to what was in store for me. They certainly were a sorry collection and were well styled "rejects"; but as they were a source of expense it was decided that I should endeavor to make the best of things and they were placed in a well ventilated part of the ship before the horses came alongside. The horses were transferred from the railway to the ship in the regulation double-decked cattle barge and loaded directly from its upper deck to the main deck of the ship and taken to the spaces allotted them in the holds,

---

*Read at the December, 1917, Meeting of the Veterinary Medical Association of New York City.

which on this vessel, numbered six, each three decks down. They were led singly from the barge by the crew who were to go over with them. They were given the halter-shank by the barge man and inasmuch as some of these men had never handled a horse before, it took considerable watching to prevent their being injured. We were fortunate in not having anyone injured. About 40% of the horsemen came on board intoxicated. It has been my experience since that it is these men who invariably make the best workers, as others, in a great many cases, are out for a joy ride, and when compelled to do their share have to be watched carefully or they would neglect to feed and water properly; while the "rummy", when sobered up, will invariably attend to his charges without being told and in the majority of cases is willing to do little things outside of his duties, and he is more easily handled. Especially is this true if you expend a little money on smoking tobacco and cigarette papers. In this way you can satisfy his desire for smoking which seems to be greatest, and curb the desire for alcohol by cutting off the tobacco. I have found that I only required to do this once, and within three days they were willing to do anything for a sack of tobacco and papers.

In reference to ailments, the first three shipments were as choice a collection of sick animals as could be found—pulmonary infections with their various sequelae, were the principal source of trouble. With the limited space allowed (2 ft. 4 inches wide by 8 ft. long and a head-room at the most 8 ft. high, making a total airspace of 150 cu. ft. for each animal, with aisles 3 ft. wide and both rows of animals' heads projecting into it), it was no easy matter to treat them. An ugly animal made matters worse.

On leaving port I found it much to my advantage on Italian ships to get in touch at once with the commissary officer who had charge of the food, and ascertain from him the food rations allowed by the ship. In the meanwhile the foreman, under instructions, arranged the men in messes of not more than six and gave each man a berth supplied with a straw mattress, blankets and a pillow, for which they were held responsible. When this was finished, they lined up at the cook's galley, and the ship's commissary issued the mess gear to each man individually, and to two in each gang, selected by themselves, the large pans for their food, etc. These two men obtained the rations for the six in that mess, and in this way much confusion was avoided. Also, if the food was not what was desired, or what it should be, one could check back very easily. Wine I always issued myself with the assistance of the foreman, only on holidays and Sundays, and at night after feeding and watering. I found this little personal touch was very much appreciated.

In reference to the feeding and watering of the stock I found that, if the animals were fed a fair ration of good quality hay— about 6 to 8 lbs. in the morning and 10 lbs. at night—I did not get the same number of cases of azoturia which are so troublesome to handle aboard ship. A bran mash was given every third day and a generous portion of salt mixed in, and twice a week a handful of salt was given each animal—the same being placed on the iron deck immediately in front of each stall.

The day before arriving at Gibraltar, where we had to put in for inspection, as all ships are compelled to do, a count of all feed and hay was made and the animals got their first feed of oats in the ratio of bran four, oats one. This quantity of oats was increased each day for the next 3 days, when the bran was exhausted as per schedule, and the last two midday meals were usually oats straight. In this way the animals usually went off in fine fettle. For sick horses which would not eat oats or other fodder, I carried a few sacks of corn-on-the-cob; and as a great many of these horses were corn-fed before starting on their journey, I found it very helpful in restoring jaded appetites.

In reference to water, I was guided a great deal by the temperature of the holds, which was taken at midday, and in this way I could obtain a line of the requirements of the animals almost individually. In the winter months, or when the weather was cold, watering morning and night was sufficient, and they were not stinted in any way. If, however, the weather became warm, they were watered three times a day, and in the very hot weather four times a day—each horse, from an individaul round-bottomed bucket of galvanized iron suspended from the breast-board, which was also used for feeding the grain ration. It was the duty of the foreman and his assistants to take full charge of the feeding and watering. I always found the time to be on my rounds when this was being done, as in this way I was able to spot many an animal which was coming down with some ailment and be in a better position to combat it. It was the ventilation upon which I laid the most stress. On the S, S. Taormina I utilized the thermo-tank system of forced air wherever it was possible and 16 canvas ventilators or wind-sails. On the *S. S. Stampalia*, in addition to the thermo-tanks, 12 canvas ventilators, and on the *Caserta* I had to depend on the canvas ventilators only. It required constant vigilance and supervision to see that these were properly trimmed at each change of wind. In bad weather a man was stationed at each hold to watch the port-holes, which were open whenever possible. On these ships I was most ably supported in this work by the captains and their officers, who were untiring in their efforts to land as many animals as possible. They made things as easy for me as possible, and my association with these gentlemen will always be a source of pleasant recollection.

The cleaning out of the manure is a much-discussed question. Personally I do not favor the daily cleaning of the stalls. First: if it is rough weather you have the animals deprived of footing, and as the racks are wet and slimp, they will go down and in many cases injure themselves most severely. This could be avoided if a fair and reasonable amount of droppings were allowed to remain underfoot, which would give a good secure foothold whether the animal be shod or not. Second: to clean the stalls you have to take the animals out and crowd them into a space already as full as possible consistent with safety. Some of the men or some of the animals are usually hurt, either by kicks or getting down. The only objection to not cleaning is the decomposition of the manure and the urine, with the resultant ammoniacal vapors. This I counteracted as much as possible by daily spraying with a good strong disinfectant solution which I had put in a portable tank and forced out by air pressure in the form of a jet instead of a spray. In the form of a spray it would strike the legs of the animal already irritated by the splashing of the urine and produce nasty sores. This condition was obviated by the straight jet. The tank was placed in as competent hands as possible and the work was done at night, usually by one of the night watchmen.

In reference to the treatment of sick animals, as has been noted before, it was usually impossible to move them once they were placed in the holds. It was my custom to make as close and careful an inspection of the animals as possible when they came off the barge, and have any sick animals placed on deck or some other well ventilated portion of the ship where they could be under better observation and were convenient to get at. I always included any animal that lagged back upon the rope even if he showed no other symptom, as invariably these laggards were taken down with a serious trouble in a short time if not taken in hand at once.

Taking temperatures was out of the question, the principal dependence being placed upon the pulse, respiration and mucous membranes of the eye. Wherever a sick animal was placed, the diagnosis was marked on the headboard in black crayon and instructions to assistant and foreman were included from time to time. If animals were shifted in the cleaning of the stalls, great care had to be taken to see that the animals were returned to their proper stalls, for if changed great harm was apt to be done in that sick animals would be neglected. In such cases death is very often a result, and is another objection to daily cleaning.

As far as treatment is concerned, supportive measures in my opinion are always indicated. In the pneumonia cases, phylacogens were used with very excellent results. On one voyage a record was kept of each case and it showed that out of 150 odd cases of pneumonia, the loss was but 8, and post mortem showed well-developed cases of pleurisy with adhesions. It also showed extreme dilation of the heart which, in one instance, when put upon the scales, weighed 11 lbs. 14 oz. The walls of the ventricles were thickened out of all proportion and of a very inferior consistency. This condition was produced, in my opinion, in conjunction with other conditions present, by the injudicious use of strychnine, which seems to be the sovereign agent of those not competent to judge of its action. Purpura was quite prevalent, but of all the cases treated only one died, and that one lived less than 12 hours after being detected. The treatment consisted of ammonium chloride and potassium dichromate, in solution, internally and applications of tinct. iodine externally applied with friction. When the symptoms showed signs of subsiding dilute chloride of iron solution was administered. This treatment was never changed; the results obtained, as noted, being in my opinion satisfactory. On the last three voyages considerable annoyance and hard work was caused by infectious stomatitis. I had been aware that it was quite prevalent at the yards, and had been fortunate in having only a few isolated cases. The three voyages referred to saw it well established on board—so much so that I was enabled to detect some of these cases by the odor. These cases which at one time numbered over 350, treated on one trip, were first treated by a solution of potassium permanganate, alum and boric acid, but owing to the effect of the continued use of this mixture upon my hands and arms, I discontinued it for a solution of potassium chlorate and hot sea water. This I think gave me much better results upon a very severe case and required more than four washings of this. This was done by means of a force pump and an 8 ft. enema hose. The latter was passed into the mouth between the teeth and cheek as far back as the angle of the jaw and about 2 qts. of the solution slowly pumped from a pail by an assistant. Very little trouble was experienced if done quietly. Care was taken that the animals affected did not drink or feed from any other than their own pails, and to this end the sides of the stall were slatted to prevent them reaching to either side. The only instance in which this infection caused real damage was when it attacked an animal suffering from some serious depleting disease, such as pneumonia, and prevented his eating; the animal being weakened by lack of nourishment. As a direct and sole cause of mortality I never saw a case although a number were reported.

Abortion was quite common, a half dozen or more occurring every voyage, but in every case still-born; although we had a number that had almost reached maturity. To my mind, it is a crime against the shippers to ever put mares in advanced pregnancy aboard a horse transport, as invariably if there is heavy weather they will abort. It is running an unnecessary risk which could be easily avoided. Records have been shown me of deaths of mares after they had aborted.

As far as surgery goes, very little could be done—owing to surroundings—outside of opening abscesses from strangles and on the buttocks. In reference to abscesses on the buttocks, this is caused by continued chafing on the end boards and is apt to prove very serious if not remedied.

The animals, when unloaded in Italy, were taken in hand by soldiers at the land end of the gangway and loaded direct into box cars and taken inland to the various concentration and remount camps. It was here that I first saw the treatment that suggested the title of this paper. These box cars are about a third the length of our box cars which carry from 21-22 horses or 24-26 mules, according to size; but they packed 11 horses or 14-15 mules. To get them to enter, moral suasion plays no part. Anything that will administer a blow is used, be it a piece of 2x4, a halter shank with bale wire to reinforce it, or a 5-ft. length of Italian locust, which, when dried, I have never seen broken no matter how much one hammers with it. The horses are led singly up to the door, the shank thrown over his neck and every one who can reach him safely starts to beat him into the car. If the car is empty or half full the first blow is enough, but when there are 9 or 10 horses in, of course they block the door-way, and it is the work of the animal to force his way in by shoving aside those already in. If he is not strong enough he is almost beaten into a pulp until he, in agony, will plunge into the car. If there are others already weakened by the voyage, they are apt to go down, and once down, in the crowded condition of the cars, I have never seen an animal get up and be worth anything after a 30 or 40 mile railroad ride. I trust that our government will not make this error in transporting these humble, willing, and, in the majority of cases, efficient co-workers, but give them a chance to stretch their stiffened legs, together with a night's rest and pure air and water, before continuing their journey.

However, there are times when animals do not submit meekly to brutal beatings. I witnessed the death of a soldier and a broken leg of another by a horse of which I had warned a soldier, and my thanks was a blow from a locust stick across the horse's nose. The horse, a big black ridgling, which had given us considerable trouble until we found that we could do much more by kindness than by any other means, instantly reared and lashed out with his front feet, which were shod, and struck his tormentor full in the chest which you could see collapse. The man fell unconscious to be removed to the hospital where, I was informed, he died later in the day, the majority of his ribs being broken. When other soldiers attempted to catch him the same horse stampeded over 200 already landed and broke a man's leg with a kick for striking him with a stick while within reach of his hind legs. After a half-hour's futile work the animal was placed in a car by two horsemen from the ship in a few minutes.

The mules are loaded in the same way with this exception, that instead of being led singly, they are herded in gangs of six and the soldiers, usually about 100 to 150, form a half circle with the ends resting on the two sides of the car door. They gradually close in, and the beatings the stubborn animals received made me see red the first time I witnessed it. As in the black ridgling case, there were mules that asserted themselves, and when they did, things were lively. In one instance, I had a loop around the neck of a big brown mule of about 1200 lbs., which had been boss of his section all the way over and was in good physical trim. Sixteen soldiers tried to drag him into a car after he had burst things up several times. It was certainly a funny sight to see this mule, by a sudden plunge forward, catch the men off their balance and by a quick turn to one side every man was dragged off his feet. The officers in charge shouted to hold on and they obeyed orders and that mule, I think, took a malicious delight in picking the dirtiest and muddiest part of that corral where the overflow from the watering trough collected and dragging these men through it. Their uniforms were a sight. Of course the cattlemen offered their regrets which the soldiers returned in kind; and I was more than glad that neither understood the other. I made it a hard and fast rule that under no consideration was a soldier to touch an animal while he was yet upon the ship. I think in this way many weak animals, which would have been killed by the brutal handling of the soldiers, were landed. However, I always made it a point to call the attention of the officer in command to these animals, and after the first voyage they heeded my warnings.

A number of times I was called upon to assist in the unloading of other ships; and it was on these that I made the acquaintance of the ocean-going Horse Doctor and the ocean Cowboy, one in particular had as choice a collection of remedies as I have seen. I had to check up his drug list and found a gallon of tincture aconite, a pint tinct. nux vomica, a pint tinct. gentian, 5 gals. linseed oil, 2 gals. white liniment P. D. & Co., half-gallon aqua ammonia, 1 gal. turpentine. I noted a number of animals go off with a weak straddling gait and with the sheath much swollen, and in one instance with the penis extended fully and marked discharge and great swelling of the glans. On asking the cause I was given a very wise wink and the answer: "I know de treek", and nothing more. Later inquiries revealed the fact that nearly all of these animals died from cystitis and kindred urinary troubles; and one day when this veterinarian's assistant was badly in need of the price of a drink, I had revealed to me the secret of the "Treek". Nearly all of these animals were down; and as it would make a material difference in his bonus, he had given each horse a grain of strychnine sulphate hypodermically, and filled a two-ounce dose syringe with equal parts of white liniment, aqua ammonia and turpentine, and

had injected it into the urethra. What with the injection and the
agony caused by the ammonia and turpentine, the animal had
managed to get to his feet, and if he showed signs of weakening,
another grain of strychnine was given. This same man, by the way,
a Frenchman, has had mules whose hoofs have dropped off through
neglect, in my opinion. I had charge of loading them and remarked
at the time about the good condition of the animals; and when another veterinarian—this one a graduate—had the remainder of
the consignment, 1180 odd, while the Frenchman had but 442,
the losses were: for the graduate veterinarian, 5; for the Frenchman, 11, with the latter's stock all on the main and upper decks,
while the former was handling three decks down.

In another instance, while assisting in the unloading of 490
horses, 14 were unable to come up the brow. I was sent for to see
what should be done and found all of these animals suffering more
or less from aconite poisoning, all the symptoms being present.
Upon my asking what treatment had been given, I was told they had
been given exhaustion mixture, the contents of which I found were
equal parts of aconite, nitrous ether, belladonna and nux vomica,
the dose being one ounce, to be repeated in 15 minutes, and then a
grain of strychnine hypodermically. It is needless to say that they
received no more exhaustion mixture. The animals were placed
under my care for a week, when they were turned over to the government in fairly good shape.

Again, a mule was reported as having gone crazy and had been
destroyed as being too dangerous to keep on board, but fairly good
information indicated a case of spasmodic colic. At any rate the
veterinarian hit the animal with a hatchet, and as the animal
dropped, ordered the carcass thrown overboard. When it came to
the surface, lo! the animal supposed to be dead started to swim
after the ship.

When I was asked to make up a list of drugs for a ship, of
which the veterinarian in charge said, upon looking it over, he
thought it would do but that it lacked whiskey. When asked how
much, he replied: "5 gallons." When asked what kind, he replied: "O! I like Green River."

When crossing either way I was always given the best accommodations possible and always tried to be a gentleman. It was
hard to have to associate with some of these men who did not know
how to conduct themselves in any way except to drink excessive

quantities of wine. Those of us who desired to be judged by our actions suffered more or less by the comparison.

It was not only to Italy that these men were put in charge of animals. I have witnessed the unloading of several shipments in Bordeaux. On one occasion a consignment of very fine Canadian medium-draft horses was landed. I never saw such a sight—proper drainage had not been maintained, and as the animals were all housed on deck, but arranged in two tiers with a wooden floor, the urine seepage had removed the better part of the hair from the back and sides and great sores had resulted, so that it would be weeks before these animals would be in a condition to work. It cannot be said that this condition would redound to the credit of the veterinarian. I do know that if given healthy horses and good feed one can be reasonably sure of landing a consignment that will be a credit to veterinary science, if one will only use properly trained men. An assistant I had with me for four voyages went as foreman under a veterinarian for the British, but on sailing the veterinarian was removed for intoxication and another could not be obtained in time so my assistant was intrusted with the entire charge. By using stimulants and paying attention to ventilation, feed, watering, etc., he landed a complete cargo of 870 head, every one in good physical condition. He had no serious trouble as the animals were shipped in good condition and the voyage short.

In conclusion I would urge everyone present to use his influence with anyone and everyone connected with the transport of horses—whether for war purposes now or peace pursuits after the war—to have competent men in charge of their cargoes; to pay them a respectable sum as a salary and award them a fair bonus based upon results obtained. While it may cost a little more, it will be compensated for by the results obtained. It is only the just due of the animals over which they have been placed. These animals are called upon to do the most hazardous work and constitute one of the great supply trunks which the British term the "Silent Service". They go where the mechanical transport cannot go. They are called upon to assist the same mechanical transport when it has gone beyond its depth: i. e., the made road; and I call your attention to the fact that this War of Wars is not being fought on macadamized roads. Wherever there is an advance these animals are the sole source of supply for the immediate needs, for without their aid exhausted supplies could not be replenished in time to be of any service. When this war is won (and win we must and will) we will find that after we have had all our say about Liberty Motors and Standardized Army Trucks, we will have to take our hats off to the Liberty Army Horse and Mule.

—Lieut. J. E. Behney has been transferred from Kansas City, Mo., to Camp Hancock, Augusta, Ga.

—Dr. Frederick Low, formerly of Hankinson, N. D., is now with the Mobile Veterinary section at Camp Dodge, Ia.

—Major Olaf Schwarzkopf, formerly at St. Louis, Mo., is now stationed at Fort Snelling, Minn.

—Major Wm. Lusk is now with the American Expeditionary Forces in France.

—Lieut. H. K. Moore, formerly of Chicago, Ill., is stationed at Camp Logan, Houston, Texas.

—Lieut. C. W. Likely, formerly at Camp Funston, is with the American Expeditionary Forces.

—Lieut. W. H. Lynch of Portland, Me., is with the American Expeditionary Forces in France.

—Lieut. H. C. Nichols, formerly of Chicago, is stationed at Camp MacArthur, Waco, Texas.

—Dr. A. F. Malcom, formerly of Kansas City, Mo., is stationed at the Auxiliary Depot, Camp McClellan, Anniston, Ala.

—Dr. H. L. Shorten, formerly of Chicago, Ill., is now stationed at Camp Cody, Deming, N. M.

—Captain A. G. Fraser is stationed at Camp Logan as Camp Veterinarian.

—Lieuts. Jean Underwood, V. R. C., Spencer K. Nelson, V. R. C., and Guy M. Parrish, V. R. C., of the 88th Division, at Camp Dodge, Iowa, have made applications for membership to the A. V. M. A. This makes a total of eighteen applications for membership to the A. V. M. A. received from Camp Dodge, Iowa.

The veterinarians of that cantonment are a very progressive lot of young men. They have formed a Veterinary Medical Society which holds regular weekly meetings for the purpose of discussing scientific and professional subjects. They have further shown their interest in the welfare and advancement of their chosen profession by becoming members of its national association. May many more emulate their spirit of cooperation and enthusiasm and step forward and assist in keeping the A. V. M. A. a strong, well organized, efficient and progressive organization.

—1st Lieut. Ralph A. Moye, V. C., N. A., has been relieved from duty with the 88th Division and made Camp Veterinarian at Camp Sherman, Chillicothe, Ohio.

—1st Lieut. Lawrence A. Mosher, V. C., N. A., has received his promotion to Captain, V. C., N. A. Captain Mosher has been transferred from Camp Dodge, Iowa, to Camp Dix, Wrightstown, N. J., as Camp Veterinarian.

—Lieut. Clifford C. Whitney, formerly of College Station, Texas, is now stationed at Fort Leavenworth, Kansas.

—Dr. Bernard Johnson, formerly of Spokane, Wash., has been called to active duty in the Veterinary Reserve Corps and is now at Colville, Wash.

—Lieut. F. A. Drown, formerly of Kellogg, Iowa, is now stationed at Camp Greenleaf, Fort Ogelthorpe.

—Lieut. Edward Lapple, formerly at Camp Mills, L. I., is with the American Expeditionary Forces.

—Captain H. S. Eakins has been transferred from Camp Kearney, Calif., to Camp Funston, Kansas.

—Captain W. B. Maxson, formerly at Camp Lee, Va., is now with the American Expeditionary Forces in France.

—The summer meeting of the Missouri Valley Veterinary Association will be held at Omaha, Neb., July 15, 16, 17.

—Dr. M. F. Barnes has removed from Franklin to Philadelphia, Pennsylvania.

—Dr. H. V. Cardona has removed from New Orleans, La., to Mobile, Ala.

—The marriage of Miss E. Mildred St. John, Ithaca, N. Y., and Dr. Fred W. Cruickshanks, Fernsdale, Calif., occurred June 8, at the home of the bride. Dr. Cruickshanks reports for service in the Reserve Officers Medical Corps July 1.

—Dr. J. W. Joss has removed from Lincoln, Neb., to East St. Louis, Ill.

—Dr. O. C. Newgent has removed from Terre Haute, Ind., to Hume, Ill.

AMERICAN VETERINARY MEDICAL ASSOCIATION

ATTEND THE PHILADELPHIA MEETING

To the Members of the A. V. M. A.:

Undoubtedly you are already aware that the next meeting of the American Veterinary Medical Association will be held at Philadelphia from August 19th to August 23rd, inclusive.

If you have attended any of the previous association meetings I am sure that you are convinced of the great benefits resulting to the profession as a whole as well as to the individual veterinarian from such convocations of the members of the association. On the other hand, were you not so fortunate as to be able to attend on previous occasions, suffice it for me to refer you to anyone of those who did attend.

As we peruse the history of the veterinary profession in this country, we are not a bit surprised to find that the American Veterinary Medical Association has been the greatest factor in building up the profession to its present lofty state, and still is the pillar upon which further advancement is relied upon. But how did the association accomplish its glorious work? How was it in a position to know the needs, opinions, suggestions and advice of the individual members? The answer to these questions is, *by and through the annual meetings of the association.* This fact cannot be too greatly emphasized. The existence alone of the association could afford but limited aid to the profession were it not for its yearly gatherings, at which, in addition to the demonstrations of points of special interest to the practitioner, the voices of the individual members are heard, and suggestions and advice offered for the elevation of the profession and resulting betterment of the conditions of the individual members. Yes, the meetings have shaped the destinies of the veterinary profession in this country.

In these trying times, when history is being written before our very eyes, when hundreds of thousands of our boys are engaged in the blood struggle on the other side, the veterinary profession has not been found wanting. Thousands of our veterinarians are serving with the colors here, and "over there". They do everything in their power to make the world, in the words of our president, a decent place to live in. For this and other reasons it is even more imperative for each and everyone of us to attend the next meeting of the American Veterinary Medical Association.

Those that are across and many of those in the camps and other military establishments in this country will not be able to attend, owing to pressing duties devolved upon them. We must therefore fill their·places with those of us who can spare their time for this purpose. We must show those of our members who are in the military service that we shall not permit the decline of the interest in the association during their absence.

Therefore make it your duty to attend the next meeting of the A. V. M. A. at Philadelphia. Don't let trifling matters stay in the way of this great duty on your part.

The Committee on Arrangements promises the next meeting to be one of the most interesting we ever had.

I am certain that you will not regret the little inconvenience you may have to undergo to be present at this meeting.

L. Enos Day, Acting Secretary.

THE A. V. M. A. MEETING, AUGUST 19 TO 23, 1918, AT PHILADELPHIA

In this epochal year of 1918, Pennsylvania is to be accorded the coveted privilege of entertaining the 55th annual convention of the American Veterinary Medical Association.

In many respects this meeting will be the most important in the history of the association. In fact, the future welfare of the veterinary profession may be largely influenced by the spirit of cooperation and policies to be developed at the meeting.

War has wrought changes with us as with every other line of work concerned with the best interests of our communities and the nation at large. Our profession has assumed an importance, and is being accorded such recognition that we are now occupying a more prominent position, not only in army matters, but also in the important movements to conserve and increase the supply of food animals and those used in transportation by the armies and commercial industries.

If we are to meet these increased obligations successfully, it is essential that we keep abreast of the changes that are occurring and be prepared with fullest information on subjects that are intimately connected with our work.

There is no better way of keeping in touch with the progressive changes that are being brought about by the leaders of our profession, than a great international meeting of thinkers and work-ers. At a meeting of this kind there are many valuable thoughts expressed and policies promulgated which will never reach the great body of general practitioners through any other source than by being in attendance and coming in personal contact with fellow workers who labor in environments that differ in many respects.

At the Philadelphia meeting we will have with us a number of men who are intimately and actively concerned with matters that are of the utmost importance to the veterinary profession. There will also be in attendance, representatives from the great Allied Nations, who have seen war and experienced war, they will tell us of the requirements demanded of our profession by war conditions.

Although this meeting will be of serious importance it will not be all work. Extensive plans are being made for entertaining the members and guests, particularly the ladies, with instructive and interesting sight seeing trips in and about the city. Philadelphia and its environments are rich in historical association with the founding, growth and developments of the United States. The great war has made it the center of industrial activity in the production of munitions and ships. A ride along the Delaware River with its banks lined for miles with great ship yards in which many hundreds of vessels are being constructed, will be a rare and interesting sight. The close proximity of Philadelphia to Atlantic City and the Ocean, with excellent train service and beautiful roads, afford unusual opportunities for short outings.

Taken in all, this approaching meeting in August bids fair to mark an epoch in the history of the A. V. M. A. from which future association events will be reckoned.   W. S. GIMPER.

ASSOCIATION MEETINGS

MICHIGAN-OHIO VETERINARY ASSOCIATION

At a meeting of veterinarians from Monroe, Lenawee, Hillsdale, Jackson and Washtenaw Counties, Michigan, and Fulton County, Ohio, April 24th, the Michigan-Ohio Veterinary Association was organized. Dr. A. L. Tiffany of Monroe, Mich., was elected president; Dr. G. D. Gibson of Adrian, Mich., vice president; and Dr. A. J. Kline of Wauseon, Ohio, secretary and treasurer,

The meeting was largely given over to the subject of sterility in cows. Dr. R. I. Bernath presented an excellent paper on sterility. The paper was thoroughly discussed by Drs. Hallman, Kline and Dunphy. Dr. Hallman dwelt upon the uterine pathology and emphasized the importance of keeping in mind the fundamentals of treatment for sterility, i. e., drainage, disinfection and irrigation. Dr. Kline told of the necessity of educating the farmer along the lines of sterility treatment. Dr. Dunphy related some of his experiences in uterine irrigation and expressed a desire to see quince mucilage, containing one per cent of the iodide of silver, used after the uterus had been thoroughly cleansed.

Dr. Hallman of the Michigan Agriculture College demonstrated methods of diagnosing early pregnancy, and treatment for sterility, on subjects procured for the occasion.

A short evening session was given over to perfecting the organization and a discussion of prices. It was arranged to hold an outdoor meeting, which is to include the families of the veterinarians, early in August, at Wamplers Lake.

A. J. KLINE, Secretary.

LOUISIANA CONFERENCE

Louisiana's tick eradication forces of the U. S. Bureau of Animal Industry on a call issued by Dr. E. I. Smith, Inspector in Charge, assembled in conference at Shreveport, La., on May 18th. The City Hall, Shreveport's stately municipal structure, was donated for the purpose to the B. A. I. visitors, accompanied by a cordial welcome from the Honorable Mayor, John McW. Ford, and warmly responded to on behalf of the Bureau by the Inspector in Charge, Dr. E. I. Smith.

Nothing so inspires tick eradicators than a get-together meeting, as a conference is classed to be, and Dr. E. P. Flower, Executive Officer of the Louisiana State Live Stock Sanitary Board, enthused all present by his address on "Our State Livestock Possibilities". No one is better qualified to know what Louisiana holds forth as a livestock center, and the doctor stated the livestock cattle census on recent figures gave Louisiana a total of 1,250,000 head of beef and dairy cattle.

The state-wide tick eradication laws of Louisiana, Dr. Flower declared, were the best laws enacted for constructive legislation,

and all research by legal lights to test the drasticity of this measure
failed to find a weak link in the chain, and consequent action of
cattle owners by dipping will hasten the raise in standards and
importations of males that will undoubtedly put the State of Louisiana in the front rank as a cattle producer, with its splendid grasses
and climatic favors.

In the 14 parishes already in the free area the improvement
in the cattle is 75 per cent over the conditions when the same parishes were tick infested.

The conference was unexpectedly honored by the appearance
of Dr. W. B. Ellenberger of Washington, D. C., in the Tick Eradication Division of the Bureau, who regaled the assembly with
reminiscences of the older days when the doctor was working in
the field and tick eradication was in its infancy and had not attained its present broad scope; that was before the dipping vat
came into existence and ticks were eradicated by the laborious lu-
bricating method.

A distinctive point brought out by the doctor indicated that a
tick eradicator of necessity must dip the farmer's cattle whether
the farmer was in favor of it or not, while in demonstration work
all suggestions are optional with the farmer, showing conclusively
the harder task of eradication of ticks as compared to farm demonstration, that he realized long ago that the tick eradication was not
a sick man's job, but required vim and vigor, and plenty of back-
bone to succeed, so he came to listen to the discussions as he knew
the conference was of the right sort to give out valuable information along the line of handling tick eradication propaganda on a
state-wide basis.

Dr. H. L. Darby, Inspector in Charge in West Texas, in a
spirited address won the conference by his suggestions that tick
eradication is a war measure, a conservation of meat and milk, deserving the consideration that is accorded other foodstuffs and the
state food administrators and Council of Defense attention to be
brought to this fact; thereby materially increasing our meat and
milk supply, improving our cattle industries and aiding the early
completion of tick eradication, resulting in the saving of millions
of dollars. Dr. Darby is nothing if not original, always weaving
out something good and new that is food for thought.

A deviation from the regular grind of a business conference
was an address in French on tick eradication, delivered by Mr. J.

G. Richard, "A La Paroisse Evangeline", which was highly entertaining and instructive.

Doctors H. L. Darby of West Texas, Marvin Gregory of Arkansas, J. A. Barger of Mississippi, and W. B. Ellenberger of Washington, D. C., were visiting inspectors in charge, who clearly gave to the conference enlightenment on many intricate questions of importance in addresses generously applauded.

Louisiana is in the midst of a drive on the cattle fever tick and it is expected that over one million head of cattle will pass through the dipping vats twice each month for the balance of the 1918 season, and if the confidence displayed by the Bureau men in the field attending this conference is any criterion, it can be confidently stated that the day of the tick in Louisiana will in a short period be a thing of the past, and the State take its rank in the forecolumn of livestock centers. E. HORSTMAN.

PENNSYLVANIA DIVISION OF THE B. A. I. VETERINARY INSPECTORS' ASSOCIATION

At a meeting of the B. A. I. veterinarians of Philadelphia, held at the Veterinary Department of the University of Pennsylvania, June 5, 1918, there was organized "The Pennsylvania Division of the B. A. I. Veterinary Inspectors' Association". Addresses were made by Dr. W. Horace Hoskins of New York City, and Dr. Thomas Kean, travelling inspector for the B. A. I. All the veterinarians on the Philadelphia force joined the association. An effort is being made to have every veterinarian in Pennsylvania employed by the B. A. I. enrolled as a member. The object of the association is to have every member belong to the American Veterinary Medical Association and have that association, through its Legislative Committee, look after the interests of the veterinarians.

The following officers were elected:

President, C. S. Rockwell; secretary, M. J. Maloney.

NEBRASKA VETERINARY MEDICAL ASSOCIATION

The following resolutions were passed by the Nebraska Veterinary Medical Association, May 9, 1918:

Resolved, That the Nebraska Veterinary Medical Association in special session recommend:

1. That the University of Nebraska give only such instruc-

tion in veterinary medicine which is given so thoroughly that it
may be accredited towards a degree in veterinary science given by
any reputable veterinary college. That the veterinarians employed
in the University of Nebraska presenting such courses that tend to
lower the standard of the profession and not meeting the above
high standard, by creating empirics, be denied membership in the
State Association.

2.   That the resolution adopted by the M. V. V. A., Feb. 20,
1918 (a copy of which is hereto attached), relating to the activities of county agents be endorsed by this association and a copy of
same be sent to Secretary of Agriculture Houston. Also inform
Hon. Mr. Houston that no cooperation exists at this time between
the county agents and the licensed graduate veterinarians of this
State.

3.   That the Secretary of Agriculture direct that control and
educational work in veterinary science be conducted by the B. A.
I. and the State Live Stock Sanitary Boards and not by the State's
Relation Service and the extension departments.

4.   That a uniform high standard of entrance requirements
of at least a four-year high school course or equivalent for all veterinary colleges, State or private, be adopted. That State Board
of Examiners adopt such requirements for examination for licenses
beginning 1922 so that present students may not be excluded.

5.   That the Committee on Intelligence and Education of the
A. V. M. A. submit at the next regular meeting in Philadelphia the
above recommendations in regard to veterinary instruction in
agricultural colleges and the above entrance requirements in all
veterinary colleges.

The above to be considered in the interests of the livestock producers so that the most competent veterinary service available may
be secured.

<hr>

RESOLUTIONS PASSED BY THE M. V. V. A., FEB. 20, 1918

WHEREAS, Public necessity demands a high standard of qualifications in the learned professions, viz.: Law, the Ministry, Human
Medicine, Agriculture, Dentistry, Veterinary Medicine; and

WHEREAS, It is impossible as a general rule and practice for
any set of men to become proficient in more than one of these
learned professions; and

WHEREAS, The County Agent, unless he be at least a graduate

veterinarian, cannot efficiently and intelligently engage in the practice, teaching or demonstration of any branch of veterinary science; and

WHEREAS, The attempt on the part of County Agents who are not graduate veterinarians to so engage in the practice, teaching or demonstration of any branch of veterinary science is in violation of the principle of a high standard of qualifications in the learned professions; and

WHEREAS, The violation of this principle opens the way and leads to a lowering of the standard of veterinary science, incompetent veterinary service to livestock producers, and promotes empiricism and supplants those properly trained to deal with veterinary problems; and

WHEREAS, The livestock industry of America and the people of this Nation demand the most competent veterinary service available; and

WHEREAS, The lowering of the professional standard will in the end prove disastrous to the livestock industry; and

WHEREAS, The duties of the County Agent pertaining strictly to agriculture and horticulture require all his ability and energy without such agent engaging in veterinary activities; and

WHEREAS, The veterinarians, members of the Missouri Valley Veterinary Association, do heartily affirm the County Agent plan, provided County Agents will not violate the essential principles governing and regulating the learned professions by engaging in veterinary work; and

WHEREAS, The members of this association, realizing the immense responsibility to the nation in this time of national peril, do hereby pledge all their skill and energy and their lives to the service of our great country and do indorse a higher educational standard for the veterinary profession; be it

Resolved, That the Missouri Valley Veterinary Association, one of the largest bodies of practicing veterinarians in the world, hereby requests the Honorable David Houston, the United States Secretary of Agriculture, to issue a national order forbidding County Agents engaging in any veterinary activity whatsoever, either advisory or regulatory, and to refer all veterinary problems to competent graduate veterinarians; and be it

Resolved, That the secretary of this association make this resolution a part of the minutes of this meeting and that he send a copy to the Honorable David Houston.

COMMUNICATIONS

DIBOTHRIOCEPHALUS LATUS

Editor Journal of the American Veterinary Medical Association,
  Ithaca, N. Y.:

Dear Sir:

In an article by Hall and Wigdor which appears on page 355 of your June issue, there occurs the following statement: "The first record of which we are aware is one by Van Es and Schalk (1917) who report what they call *Dibothriocephalus latus* from a dog at Agricultural College, N. D. Their specific determination is apparently casual, being only incidental to work on anaphylaxis, and is presumably based on the fact that the worm was a bothriocephalid tapeworm and that *D. latus* is one of the commonest and best known of these worms from the dog."

May we not use a little of your space for a word or two of protest with regard to the manner in which attention is called to the occurrence of the parasite mentioned? While the finding of this tapeworm was of no primary importance to us, we object to having our published statement about it questioned without a stated reason. The terms "what they call"; "is apparently casual"; and "presumably based" certainly would indicate that Hall and Wigdor deem us capable to use in a scientific publication a specific name, merely because the tapeworm happened to belong to the bothriocephalids, and that "*D. latus* is one of the commonest and best known of these worms of the dog". We feel compelled to deny that we are guilty of such carelessness and lack of sense of responsibility.

Likewise we must deny that our publication contains anything which would in the least justify Hall and Wigdor to conclude that "their specific determination is apparently casual". In our publication we refer to the finding of the parasite as follows: "The autopsy disclosed the presence of two specimens of *Belascaris marginata* and one of *Dibothriocephalus latus*". (Page 184.) At one other place a similar statement was made. We believe that those sentences contain nothing "apparent" of a casual determination, nor anything else suggestive of the slip-shod manner of dealing with facts as Hall and Wigdor attribute to us.

It is true that we determined the *D. latus* as such but the very consciousness of the fact that we are not parasitologic specialists compelled us to caution, and hence we sought the counsel and assistance of Dr. B. H. Ransom of Washington, D. C., who was kind enough to confirm our determination. Only after those precautions did we undertake to name the parasite as we did.

Hoping, Mr. Editor, that this explanation in a measure clears away the result of the imputation of the carelessness on our part, and thanking you for your kind consideration, we beg to remain

Very truly yours,

L. VAN ES AND A. F. SCHALK,

STATEMENT CONCERNING PROPOSED AGREEMENT BE-
TWEEN THE KANSAS STATE AGRICULTURAL
COLLEGE AND THE KANSAS CITY
VETERINARY COLLEGE

For sufficient reasons, largely growing out of the war, the officers of the Kansas City Veterinary College have decided to abandon the field of education in veterinary medicine, and in order to conserve as much as possible the interests of the alumni, former students and students of the Kansas City Veterinary College, they have decided to transfer to the Kansas State Agricultural College all of the good will and the academic records of the Kansas City Veterinary College.

The Kansas State Agricultural College, in accepting the records of students of the Kansas City Veterinary College and the good will of that institution, engages: (1) To preserve the academic records of the Kansas City Veterinary College and to respond to all inquiries for information concerning the educational history and scholarship of graduates and former students of the veterinary college; (2) whenever it prints lists of its own alumni to print lists of the alumni of the Kansas City Veterinary College, accompanied by a suitable statement concerning the relations of the two institutions; (3) to receive as junior students all high school graduates who have taken the full freshman and sophomore work of the Kansas City Veterinary College from 1916 to 1918, and give evidence of sufficient training in the branches studied; (4) to accord sophomore standing to all high school graduates who as students of the Kansas City Veterinary College have taken within the period of 1916 to 1918, the full work required of a freshman student, and give evidence of sufficient training in the branches studied; (5) to receive on recommendation of the officers of the Kansas City Veterinary College students of that institution who are not high school graduates, and to allow them opportunity to make up deficiencies in the regular entrance requirements of the agricultural college; (6) to facilitate in all ways consistent with the standard requirements for graduation at the agricultural college, completion of the curriculum of that institution, and graduation with the degree of Doctor of Veterinary Medicine of any student of the Kansas City Veterinary College.

—Dr. E. M. Pickens has resigned from the N. Y. State Veterinary College at Cornell University to accept a position at the Experiment Station, College Park, Md.

—Dr. C. E. Mootz, formerly at Chicago, Ill., was recently transferred by the Bureau of Animal Industry to Wheeling, W. Va.

REVIEWS

MASTITIS OF THE COW

Sven Wall

Assistant in the Veterinary High School at Stockholm. Authorized translation with annotations by Walter J. Crocker, B.S., V.M.D., Professor of Veterinary Pathology, University of Pennsylvania.
pp. XI-166 with 29 illustrations.
J. B. Lippincott Company, Philadelphia and London. 1918.

The author of this book is known to students of comparative pathology, especially for his work in connection with infectious abortion. This volume on "Mastitis of the Cow" is based on the investigation of milk from diseased udders and subsequent autopsy of the udders. A large part of the material was of a tuberculous nature but there were about 50 cases of other infections. The bacterial content was determined from not less than 70 bacterial isolations and the histological changes were determined from a study of 30 different preparations. The clinical descriptions accompanying various forms of mastitis was determined by the author from his own veterinary practice and upon the cows in which he produced artificial infection, together with the data on uncommon forms of mastitis contributed by other veterinarians.

The contents of the book is divided into 18 chapters in which the following subjects are discussed: I, udder of the cow; II, mastitis in general; III, mastitis caused by external forces; IV, infectious mastitis in general; V, types of infection; VI, udder streptomycosis; VII, udder staphylomycosis; VIII, udder colibacillosis; IX, udder pyobacillosis; X, udder tuberculosis; XI, udder actinomycosis; XII, necrobacillosis; XIII, clinical diagnosis of mastitis; XIV, autopsy, post mortem technique; XV, importance of mastitis to milk control; XVI, importance of mastitis to meat inspection; XVII, post mortem report; XVIII, a few reports of contagious udder infections. The translator has placed in brackets a few annotations for the purpose of including valuable information on conditions prevailing in this country and in a few instances including new data on the subject.

The discussion of the various subjects is in most cases brief and to the point. In classifying mastitis the author refers to the parenchymatous tissue and the connective tissue or stroma. Bacterial invasion of the interstitial connective tissue is termed stroma infection or interstitial mastitis. Bacterial invasion of the tubulo-alveolar system or parenchymatous passages, and necessarily the milk which is contained in them, he calls *parenchyma infection* or *milk infection,* the presence of which is manifested by reaction on the part of the body to a bacterial irritation called *parenchymatous mastitis.* This may be primary or secondary, depending upon the manner of inception, acute or chronic, depending upon its duration, and, based on the character of its inflammatory exudate, it is classified as *catarrhal, sero-hemorrhagic, croupous, purulent,* or *croupo-purulent mastitis.* He also recognizes *interstitial mastitis* and *gangrenous mastitis,* which complete his classification.

In discussing the subject of milk invasion, the author states that in spite of the "before mentioned obstacles to infection, one or more bacteria may gain entrance but these may be taken up and destroyed by the ever present leucocytes which are more or less numerous. The leucocytes play a very important part inasmuch as they inhibit the invasion of the milk by the bacteria". The investigation of bacteria in milk in the normal, healthy udder of cows that have been made not only in this country but also in Europe indicate that milk as it leaves the udder is not as free from these organisms as the author's investigations indicate. The early work of Leopold Schultz and Gernhardt and later that of Bolley and Hall, Ward, Moore, Conn and others, indicate that milk in the normal udder contains a considerable number of bacteria. The fact should not be overlooked that Sven Wall has worked in a country farther north than any of the others and it is possible that the conditions there are different than in more southern latitudes.

It will be noted from the title of the chapters that in discussing the different types of infection, he has used the term *streptomycosis, staphylomycosis,* etc., to describe the lesions brought about by these organisms following the practice introduced by Ligniéres many years ago in connection with the *pasteurella* in which he used *pasteurelloses* to designate the disease produced by the septicemia hemorrhagica group of bacteria designated *pasteurella* by Trevasan. A good deal of space is given to the description of the invading organisms, methods for their cultivation and pathogenesis. Under colibacillosis he includes *Bacterium lactis aërogenes* with the colon bacillus. He has given a quite full description of *Bacillus pyogenes* and its presence in udder lesions.

In udder tuberculosis he has described two types (1) primary udder tuberculosis, including infection through the teat canal and infection through wounds, and (2) secondary or embolic tuberculosis. He estimates that about 10% of all cases of udder tuberculosis are primary and caused by infection through the teat canal but primary infection through wounds is very rare. Secondary or embolic udder tuberculosis is the most common and constitutes approximately 90% of all cases. In this connection he has given valuable information from his own experience.

The last chapters deal with the clinical diagnosis of mastitis and the technique of making the examination and a series of post mortem descriptions of udders affected with the different forms of mastitis as determined by their etiology such as streptomycosis, pyobacillosis, etc.

In dealing with the treatment of various udder troubles, he has not discussed the use of bacterins which are extensively used in this country and have been found to be beneficial in some cases but apparently useless in others. An authoritative opinion on this subject would have been helpful. The more recent practice of using formalin, which has been reported to be very beneficial when administered internally, is not discussed.

The volume contains the results of the author's investigations and the methods which he has employed. The illustrations are largely diagramatic but their reproduction is not of the best. Most of them, however, are helpful in illuminating the points at issue. The publishers have done their part in making this an attractive volume. It should be carefully read by veterinarians who have an extensive cattle practice.   V. A. M.

WOUNDS OF ANIMALS AND THEIR TREATMENT

HARRISON SMYTHE, M.R.C.V.S., Civil Veterinary Surgeon, Attached A. V. C.
Alex Eger, Chicago, Ill.

This book of 194 pages, including a fairly complete index, is of convenient size and contains a considerable amount of information. The author has kept abreast of the times and refers to special articles pertinent to his subject, which have appeared in recent veterinary literature.

The first five chapters are of an introductory and somewhat elementary character and deal with the pathology of wounds, infection, the general and surgical treatment and complications and sequelae. The author is not especially partial to antiseptics and doubts if the results gained by their use justify the great faith placed in them by a confiding public. He emphasizes drainage and summarizes as a routine treatment for ordinary wounds: (1) the provision of drainage; (2) maintenance of blood supply; (3) admission of air; (4) removal of pus and cleansing of the wound by the use of harmless fluids such as normal saline solution; (5) removal of necrotic and diseased tissues, when present. Other chapters deal with the wounds of the head and neck, trunk, open joint, wounds of the bursae, and tendon sheaths, limbs, feet, fistulae and sinuses, castration wounds, uterine and vaginal wounds and wounds involving bone tissue. The discussions are brief but interesting and practical. There is no claim of fresh and original theories nor the presentation of matter startlingly new, but he describes in a clear and concise way the methods which in his experience have given good results.

The final chapters on war wounds, use of vaccines and dietetics and hygiene could have been expanded with benefit to the reader. Because of its conciseness and up-to-dateness it should be of especial interest to veterinarians.   P. A. F.

NECROLOGY

THOMAS E. HUGHES

Dr. Thomas E. Hughes, a member of the American Veterinary Medical Association, died June 3.

—The officers of the Mississippi State Veterinary Medical Association for the present year are: President, Dr. W. R. Edwards, Vicksburg; vice president, Dr. E. S. Norton, Greenville; secretary-treasurer, Dr. J. A. Beavers, Canton.

—Veterinary Inspector F. Kickbusch has been transferred from Grand Rapids, Wis., to Milwaukee.

—The Wisconsin Veterinary Medical Association will meet at Monroe, July 16, 17, 18.

MISCELLANEOUS

—HIGHER STANDARDS. In the interest of higher education the War Department has recommended, and this recommendation has received the concurrence of the Civil Service Commission, the Secretary of Agriculture and the Committee on Intelligence and Education of the American Veterinary Medical Association, that Regulation I of the Regulations Governing Entrance to the Veterinary Inspector Examination (Circular A-16) of the Bureau of Animal Industry be amended. In accordance therewith it has been ordered that Regulation I of the above circular be amended to read as follows, to become effective at the beginning of the 1918-19 session of veterinary colleges:

REGULATION I—MATRICULATION. The matriculation requirement which shall be adopted by each accredited veterinary college shall be at least two years of high school education of at least seven credits (units) or their equivalent as certified by the commissioner on education or a similar official of the State where the student resides.

—Dr. H. W. Witmer, with the State Department of Florida in cholera work, has been transferred from Fort Pierce to Bradentown, Fla.

—Dr. E. A. Cahill has resigned as Resident State Secretary of the A. V. M. A. for Massachusetts and has accepted the position of Manager of the Biological Farm of the Pitman-Moore Co. of Indianapolis, Ind.

—Dr. T. J. Eagle is representing the Government in the States of Kansas and Missouri where the Department of Agriculture is endeavoring to formulate plans whereby there may be cooperation in the eradication of tuberculosis.

—Dr. B. E. Cheney has removed from Corpus Christi, Texas, to Plaquemine, La.

—Dr. J. H. Knox has removed from Great Falls, Montana, to Warner, Alberta, Canada.

—The Municipal Civil Service Commission will receive applications for examination for veterinarian at the Municipal Building, Manhattan, Room 1400, until July 1, 4 p. m.

—The next meeting of the Maine Veterinary Medical Association will be held at Portland, July 10.

—Dr. H. L. Darby has removed from Fort Worth, Texas, to Cleveland, Ohio.

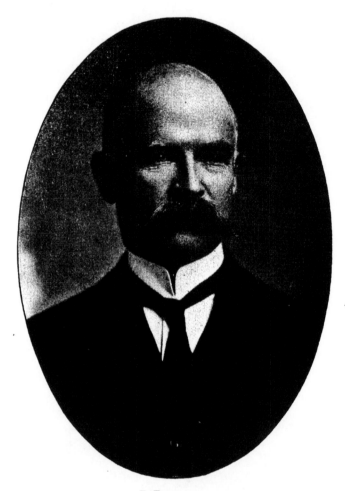

F. TORRANCE
President of the American Veterinary Medical Association 1917-1918

JOURNAL
OF THE
American Veterinary Medical Association
Formerly American Veterinary Review
(Original Official Organ U. S. Vet. Med. Ass'n)

PIERRE A. FISH, Editor   ITHACA, N. Y.

Executive Board

GEORGE HILTON, 1st District; W. HORACE HOSKINS, 2d District; J. R. MOHLER, 3d District; C. H. STANGE, 4th District; R. A. ARCHIBALD, 5th District; A. T. KINSLEY, Member at large.

Sub-Committee on Journal

J. R. MOHLER   R. A. ARCHIBALD

The American Veterinary Medical Association is not responsible for views or statements published in the JOURNAL, outside of its own authorized actions.

Reprints should be ordered in advance. A circular of prices will be sent upon application.

VOL. LIII., N. S. VOL. VI.   AUGUST, 1918.   No. 5.

Communications relating to membership and matters pertaining to the American Veterinary Medical Association should be addressed to Acting Secretary L. Enos Day, 1827 S. Wabash Ave., Chicago, Ill. Matters pertaining to the Journal should te sent to Ithaca, N. Y.

A MATTER OF DUTY

The President of the United States has recommended that, even in time of war, educational facilities should be maintained; that scientific and professional organizations should continue and perhaps increase their activities. The basis of this is doubtless the view that actual assistance is rendered the government, either directly in connection with the war or in the discussion and mastery of problems that will inure to the benefit of our country and thus indirectly assist in the war.

One of the important features of war is elasticity. Many are called from their usual activities for combatant purposes. From producers they are converted into consumers, with the result that more supplies are demanded with a diminished number left to produce them. This is the test of elasticity. Our productive power must be stretched to greater and greater limits as the war goes on. All of the fighting is not done at the front. We can all fight in one branch or another of patriotic service and to that every real American has dedicated himself.

Seventeen hundred veterinarians have been commissioned as officers and more will be commissioned as their services are needed.

Those remaining in practice have the opportunity of stretching their capacity to care for the practices of their colleagues who have gone.

There are veterinary problems concerned with the war and the welfare of our country which can be handled satisfactorily in an association meeting—which serves as a clearing house for ideas. Particularly is this true of a national meeting where representatives from all parts of the country are gathered together. This year, more than ever, and because of war conditions, especial effort should be made to attend the meeting of the American Veterinary Medical Association at Philadelphia. There will be an earnest effort to deal with problems that will benefit our country and help it to win the war. Philadelphia is the "cradle of liberty". Its historic associations of one hundred and forty-two years ago have a peculiarly intimate relation with the principles involved in the present struggle, and make it a fitting environment for the annual meeting.

The American Veterinary Medical Association is clearly included in the President's recommendation. Its meetings are educational and its purpose is helpful and progressive. It is represented at the front, and three thousand miles behind the front it puts forth its loyal effort for the welfare and success of the great work in which our country is engaged.

The association expects every member to do his duty.

P. A. F.

VETERINARY RELIEF

If we visualize the struggle abroad as we should we shall become more and more determined and self-sacrificing for an allied victory. While our brothers and sons are giving their lives, we shall give our luxuries, our necessities, our money, our food, our comfort, our all, if need be, in order that those who have given more shall not have died in vain. We shall learn new lessons in the lavishness of our giving for the cause of humanity and civilization, and new lessons in self sacrifice in order that we may have the wherewithal to give.

Impossible things have happened and unbelievable crimes have been committed in the effort to torture civilization. The inhuman is differentiated from the human in that the former inflicts suffering while the latter alleviates it. The desire to extend relief is natural but the appeal strikes a little deeper, when members of our own professional brotherhood are affected.

We have known that the invasion of Belgium and northern France has separated and pauperized the families of veterinarians in common with others. We know that Americans have been and are assisting in the reconstruction of devastated towns and in the rehabilitation of the people. Aside from this general relief there should be special relief to the unfortunate but unconquered veterinarians. Special equipment is needed by them in the way of instruments, medicines and sundries essential for practice after their homes have been recovered, and special assistance may be needed even now to keep them alive until the invader can be driven back.

The first to appreciate the situation and to take active steps in assuaging the pitiable condition of our Belgian and French confrères was Alexander Liautard. At first there was established the Franco-Belgian fund. After the cooperation of the British in this work of mercy the title was lengthened to the Anglo-Franco-Belgian fund. Last year our American veterinarians quickly raised a fund of $3000 at the annual meeting of the American Veterinary Medical Association, and the fund has now grown until it amounts to about $4600. The title of the fund will not bear much further lengthening. In our tribute in the May issue relative to the death of Dr. Liautard, we stated that these funds stand as "a memorial to his great heart". As Dr. Liautard was, in reality, the originator of the fund in America, as well as in Europe, the thought was in our mind that it would be eminently proper to link his name with this great humanitarian work under the name of the Liautard Memorial or the Liautard Fund. To us it seems there is no better way to perpetuate the memory of this great and good man than to associate it with such a worthy cause. There need be no lapse in such a memorial. When peace arrives and we have done our duty toward our war stricken brothers, there may be worthy but unfortunate members of our profession at home to whom it might be applied.

Dr. Liautard's life was a life of service for his fellow man. Such a memorial would perpetuate his service and although gone from our midst his spirit would remain a living force in the ranks of our profession.

The suggestion of the use of Dr. Liautard's name in connection with the fund has been made independently of our own. At a meeting of the executive committee, of the European fund, held at Paris, May 8, Monsieur Rossignol spoke of the growing length of the title and suggested that it be abbreviated by the use of Dr. Liautard's name.

Efforts toward increasing the fund should not be relinquished. As the war goes on more and probably greater demands will be made upon it. Since our last annual meeting the northern portion of Italy has been invaded and doubtless a number of Italian veterinarians find themselves in the same situation as do the veterinarians of Belgium and northern France. As in France there may be some veterinarians in the uninvaded portion of Italy who may be in a position to assist those less fortunate than themselves and the scope of the fund thereby increased.

As the sending of only a portion of the American Army to the shores of France has brought cheer and renewed vigor to the allies, so might we expect that a portion of our fund placed at the disposal of the administrative officers of the European fund will bring renewed confidence and appreciation of our purpose to bear a share of the burden of rehabilitation and demonstrate that American veterinarians are second to none in responding to humanitarian appeals for aid to members of their profession.

P. A. F.

GAS MASKS FOR HORSES

Poisonous gas, one of the horrors of the war, introduced by the Central Powers, has taken its toll from horses as well as men. A factory in this country is now finishing 5,000 masks a day especially designed for the American horses and mules on the battle front and it is expected that soon all the transport and artillery animals will be equipped with this life-saving device. Although much of the hauling of supplies and ordnance is effected by motors, it has been found that the horse cannot be dispensed with and that the motors do not supplant but supplement his work. The dogs used in the service of the Belgian Army are also supplied with masks. It is a matter of profound satisfaction that these useful friends of man can be protected from one of the atrocities of the war.

RECIPROCITY AND EQUALITY IN VETERINARY INSTRUCTION*

H. E. BEMIS, Ames, Iowa

Since having opportunity to make a few first hand observations during the last few years in connection with the classification of students in veterinary medicine and the examination of graduates of various veterinary colleges for the Veterinary Reserve Corps, it has seemed to me there were at least three great needs in our educational system which are necessary to uniformity of product. The first as we are all agreed is uniformly high entrance requirements which should be not lower than graduation from a four-year high school which requires that at least a large proportion of time be devoted to the languages and sciences to the exclusion of agriculture taught from a text book by some lady who probably was raised in the town or city. We all recognize the value of agriculture in connection with veterinary medicine but not as a foundation for veterinary medicine when other subjects more important must be sacrificed.

To my mind, the value of a high school education is not wholly in the accumulation of so many facts, but in part is due to the test which is put upon a young man to finish his high school education. Many who take a short cut to college often do not do so from necessity but from lack of application and vision necessary to complete the course. Such a person can never have the vision of a professional man even though he may graduate from a veterinary college.

The second important step is to have sufficient uniformity in methods of teaching, in length of time devoted to each subject, and in sequence of subjects within the course so that students who voluntarily or of necessity change from one school to another, might be able to continue their course without loss of time or instruction. Veterinary faculties should agree upon what shall constitute a course in veterinary medicine which is worthy of the degree of D.V.M. and should agree approximately upon the length of time to be devoted to each subject and the sequence of subjects within the course. Time should be allowed for electives so that students, or

---

*Presented at the 54th Annual Meeting of the A. V. M. A., Section on College Faculties and Examining Boards, Kansas City, Mo., August, 1917.

colleges, who wish to emphasize certain branches may be free to do so. This would give individuality to colleges but would still provide the essentials in all and make reciprocity possible.

The third refers to greater uniformity of teaching talent and of methods of teaching within each college. Dean White of Ohio has made the statement, or at least quotes it, that there are scarcely enough good teachers in the country to man one veterinary college and we realize the force of the statement. A teacher should have teaching ability plus a broad general foundation acquired either by college training or natural inclination to study the foundation subjects. The final essential is a thorough *veterinary* education. The dean of a veterinary college should make an effort to develop all departments as equally as possible and to see that the teaching methods in each are as near alike as the nature of the work will permit. Examining students from various schools show that some schools are uniformly strong in some branches and weak in others. I believe there is too great a tendency to slight the foundation subjects and emphasize the more practical or more interesting subjects. A man nowadays should not be called a veterinarian who cannot analyze his cases from the foundation up if necessary. For instance, how can men practice successfully who, as shown by recent reserve corps examinations, never heard of the pododerm, who state that the superficial and deep flexor tendons are lateral ligaments of the shoulder joint, that the biceps brachii is the "motor engine" for the shoulder joint, and are unable to say anything more about it; who know nothing about the bicipital bursa and its diseases and cannot name the divisions of the intestinal tract? On the other hand, what are we to think of the veterinarian who may have a working knowledge of anatomy but knows nothing of the lymph system or the functions of the liver, except that it secretes bile, who never heard of malignant edema and always advises strychnine as a stimulant in cases of pneumonia? These statements have been taken from answers given in examinations and indicate either lack of capacity on the part of the student or lack of adequate, systematic teaching of both foundation and advanced subjects on the part of the faculty.

To summarize, the three needs are: 1, thorough preparation; 2, uniformity or standardization of courses; 3, better balance of teaching ability, and teaching methods within each college.

EDUCATION OF A VETERINARIAN*

E. L. QUITMAN, Chicago, Ill.

My position as a member of the Board of Examiners of the Veterinary Officers' Reserve Corps taught me much, and has made me ponder much, and has caused me to wonder how some veterinarians could learn so little in three years at college, and how others could "learn so little and forget so much" within a year or two after graduation.

I have examined men from nearly all colleges and find the same average condition prevails among the various graduates. This caused me to attempt an analysis of the cause of the deficiences, and brought to my mind the question—is it the fault of the veterinary college, or of the individual? Aye, there's the rub—*yes* and *no*—it is.

The result of my analysis of the deficients are as follows:

Poor or improper teaching methods........ 50%
Deficient education of student............ 25%
Deficient intellect (though educated)...... 25%
Total...............................100%

So you see the fault lies half with the college and half with the student body.

THE REMEDY: First, closer lines on the entrance examination, a few less dollars each session spells a longer life to the private school; attention paid to the fitness of an intending student regardless of education.

Second, the teacher should be taught how to teach—I found in many cases that the graduates of a certain college were deficient in some certain branch or branches, while the graduates of another college were poor in other branches; this condition in the 50% of the cases put the deficiencies clearly up to the college—the teachers of certain subjects either did not command the respect of his students or he did not know how to sow his seed; how to drive his points home; how to make his subject impressive or how to make the more important parts of his subject remembered.

The really good teacher can make the least important subject appear as important and impressive as any subject in the curricu-

---

*Presented at the 54th Annual Meeting of the A. V. M. A., Section on College Faculties and Examining Boards, Kansas City, Mo., August, 1917.

lum and make his students remember the salient features—if he has the proper soil.

I would suggest that just at the opening of college sessions a meeting of the *entire* faculty be called and some member of the faculty or directorate, preferably the dean, if he is properly qualified for this function, deliver a lecture to the faculty wherein he will call a spade a spade, and call the attention of the individual members of the faculty to their short comings, then tell how certain subjects should be taught; how to make them impressive; how to lessen cheating in quizzes and examinations and finally inviting a free discussion of the subject.

I believe that frequent quizzes are of the greatest help in forcing neglectful students to keep up in their work and I suggest, in order to prevent students being helped or prompted by neighboring students, that the teacher leave his rostrum and walk down among the students, always getting as close as possible to the one being quizzed.

Those who have not tried this method can have no idea how much it helps the student and how much it will correspondingly add to the reputation of the teacher as a teacher.

And of almost greater necessity is the fact that freshmen should be taught how to study; they should be taught that memorization alone is not sufficient, but that correct study means a full comprehension of the subject. No words should be used that are not explained or understood by the student. I frequently ask students to tell me the meaning of certain terms they may be using in answering questions in my quizzes, and at the beginning of a session I find that commonly they do not know the meaning, then a nicely put "roast" and an explanation as to the futileness of Poll-parroting follows, and in the future this rarely occurs.

The writer also wishes to emphasize the great necessity of *more practical* instruction and that the teachers at all times call the student's attention to the *practical* importance of the subject under discussion, remembering that the student is not in a position to always see this for himself.

More clinics should be given, and I am a firm advocate that a veterinary college should and is justified in advertising free clinic days for all animals, or better, a certain day for free horse clinics; a certain day for free dog clinics and a certain day for free cattle and other farm animals' clinic.

This method, of course, always brings out a storm of protest from the local veterinarians, as some unworthy people take advantage of these free clinics, which of course, should be for the benefit of the poor and care should be used to prevent the unworthy . or able-to-pay people from taking such advantage.

With this discrimination always in mind, I would say that inasmuch as said free clinics would be ''for the greatest good, for the greatest number'' that no attention should be paid to such protests.

I would suggest that teachers frequently impress students, especially those of the graduating class, as to the necessity of reading and studying after their graduation, so as to keep up with the times, to impress them with the fact that a *month's* neglect in reading veterinary and medical journals and new or standard publications, may put them years behind.

Encourage them to form community associations with frequent meetings; for 'tis competition that spurs to best efforts.

The most potent and frequent excuse of the veterinarian for being ''behind the times'' and for ''forgetting'', is ''isolation'', alone in a country practice—and I know of no better remedy to remove this condition than community associations with frequent meetings.

———◆———

THE VETERINARY CURRICULUM AND ARMY VETERINARY SERVICE*

JOHN P. TURNER, Washington, D. C.

A year ago, the consideration of this subject would have been considered by this body as rather superfluous, owing to the well-known attitude of many veterinary schools relative to their graduates entering the army veterinary service.

As far as the writer knows, only one school has given this matter any consideration whatever, and that was given in a short course of lectures, and was made possible by the proximity of a cavalry post, where army veterinarians were always stationed.

Without rank, promotion or organization of any kind, the army did not appeal very strongly to young veterinary graduates. Now that the results of our 25-year campaign for recognition in the mili-

*Presented at the 54th Annual Meeting of the A. V. M. A., Section on College Faculties and Examining Boards, Kansas City, Mo., August, 1917.

tary service, a fight started by the brilliant Huidekoper, has brought forth good results, it is high time that the profession and more especially the schools, should prepare their young men to meet the high requirements of this service.

The question is frequently suggested that there is no difference in the practice of veterinary medicine and surgery in the army and in civil life. The cause, symptoms, diagnosis, prognosis and pathology of disease is exactly the same for the same disease whether it affects the lowly mule of the poor negro cotton worker or the flashy charger of the General. The treatment and handling of the disease in either case by the civilian practitioner and the military veterinarian call for far different methods.

In the former case, severe criticism would be meted out to the civilian practitioner who fails to roll up his sleeves and get into his jumpers and hustle. For some reason or another, probably military, the same procedure would be somewhat criticized in military practice, where in many cases it seems to be the rule to make the other fellow do the work.

The writer remembers very distinctly a severe reprimand given by a very strict old colonel of cavalry, who entered the post veterinary hospital and found the regimental veterinarian drenching a horse, instead of ordering a somewhat stupid farrier to perform this work.

Then again, there is quite a large amount of work such as the handling of contagious disease, which is handled somewhat differently in the army than in civil practice.

In civil practice, these horses belong to an owner or firm who may or may not follow your advice as to the handling, treatment and isolation of horses with infectious disease, and disinfect their barns according to their own primitive ideas and methods, in spite of the efforts of the attending veterinarian.

The only satisfaction received by the attending civilian veterinarian is in receiving more fees for another outbreak in the near future, due to faulty methods of handling and disinfecting. This condition does not apply to the army man, where absolute efficiency is expected and required. It is expected of an army veterinarian that he can teach hippology and be a horse master. Where does, or where can, the veterinary student get instruction in the colleges to prepare him for this work?

The writer found shortly after his entrance into the service that he must prepare for work far different from that expected of the civilian veterinarian, and along many lines that were new and unfamiliar to him.

As early as 1884, the late Dr. Rush Shipper Huidekoper realized the necessity of a trained army veterinary service, and began his effort in its behalf and never ceased as long as this brilliant man and prodigious worker lived. Having been trained in the great Alfort school of France, it was only natural that he should look on the military aspect of veterinary training. Horsemanship, zoology, zootechnics, especially as related to the horse as a military animal, all appealed to this wonderful man, and in turn he did his utmost to impart his knowledge to those fortunate students of the classes of 87-88-89-90 at the Veterinary Department of the University of Penna.

It is doubtful if many of them realized the ideals of this man or the reasons that caused him to devote so much time and drill us in the subject of zootechnics.

Those of us who for shorter or longer periods entered military life, realized at once the importance of this great teacher's work. Taking us back into the dawn of animal life, he gradually brought the development of the horse into his present usefulness. Then he lectured on horse breeding, equitation (both theoretical and practical in the ring); the importance of physiology, and hygiene in veterinary practice were continually rung into our ears, and later the control of contagious and infectious disease among animals. Quarantine—shipping by rail and sea—all of these were comprehensively covered by this teacher. Those of us who have wrought with what he taught many years ago hold this great man in the highest veneration, and realize that his untimely death was a great blow to the development of the military side of our profession.

If our colleges are to meet the requirements of the army, what must they do?

First: the matriculation examination must be so high that only men of broad education and brains big enough to absorb knowledge should be entered. Army officers, either from the military academy or in the staff department, are educated men and there is no place officially or socially in the service for the uneducated or narrowly educated veterinarian.

Second: after the first two years of study in the veterinary colleges, the specialization work should commence. The sooner our profession realizes and acknowledges that this is the day of specialties, the sooner we can properly train the young man for his life's work. The man who is preparing to enter food inspection work in the Bureau of Animal Industry or dairy farm inspection work for municipalities needs all the instruction he can get in pathology, hygiene and animal husbandry.

The student who is specializing for bacteriologic work should have his special work mapped out for him.

Likewise the general practitioner and surgeon.

The student preparing for army service should primarily be a horseman and horse master, and in the line of such work, he should receive lessons in equitation in either the veterinary or riding school. Then should begin his special training. Hygiene and then some more hygiene as laid down by the illustrious English teacher, Gen. Fred Smith, himself a distinguished army veterinarian.

Feeding, watering, ventilation and construction of stables and veterinary hospitals should be given special consideration.

The examination of feeds for quality and molds; the study of water supply and its origin.

Students should be instructed in the general rules of construction work and the proper shapes and locations for stables. Ventilation should be thoroughly given and special training as to ventilation on shipboard. The feeding, watering and care of animals on board ship should receive consideration.

Instruction in horse shoeing, now given in many schools by lectures only, should be given by practical instruction at the forge with the actual making of shoes and shoeing of horses, such training as was given in one of our schools 30 years ago.

The recognition and control of contagious diseases among horses, mules and food animals should be thoroughly taught by both lectures and practical field work. The instruction in the control of contagious diseases should be very broad and comprehensive, and should begin with the transportation of animals from the farm to the markets.

The control and disinfection of horse markets, railroad cars and dealers' stables should be given close and thorough study and attention.

Veterinarians should be instructed in the proper classification of sick animals for isolation and treatment; such work could be given in the form of military problems and taught to students as other military problems are taught to military students.

Some may object and say that these subjects are more properly the work of post graduate or army service schools, and very probably they are, but in the absence of such institutions, and in the present great need for veterinarians with some military knowledge, the schools must do their best to give the students the best they have with the limited facilities on hand for such instruction.

Army veterinarians act as instructors of hippology to the young cavalry and artillery officers. Such a position requires that a man be broadly educated and at home in the lecture room.

The word hippology is very broad in its meaning, and doubtless every veterinarian has his special ideas as to the subjects that should be taught.

The writer suggests a course somewhat as follows:

(1) The origin of the horse and mule.

(2) Genus, species, families of the Equidae.

(3) Gross anatomy of the horse. This should be given along broad lines, such as showing the actions of different groups of muscles. The bones, especially of the leg and foot. The special anatomy of the horny box of the foot. The anatomy of the mouth, in order that the physiology of bitting may be understood. The anatomy of the shoulder in its relation to draft and the anatomy of the withers and loins, in order that the physiology of saddling may be understood.

(4) The mechanical principles involved in bitting a horse and the measurement of horses' mouths.

(5) The construction and fitting of military saddles and packs, showing the relation of saddle pressure to the muscles, and the relation of the bearing points of the saddle to the ribs.

(6) Watering, feeding, ventilating, drainage, lighting and general construction of military stables.

(7) Judging feeds.

(8) A short course on digestive troubles of the horse, showing the relation of the anatomy of the equidae as a predisposing cause of colics.

(9) Contagious diseases. How recognized, and the general rules of sanitation and quarantine.

(10) The treatment of wounds, sore backs, and shoulder, and the prevention of the latter by properly fitting saddles and collars.

(11) Instruction in plain horse shoeing to both officers and enlisted men.

(12) Writing proper descriptive lists of horses. Text books recommended: Smith's Veterinary Hygiene (Gen. Fred Smith). Gen. Fred Smith's "A Manual of Saddles and Sore Backs". Henry's Feeds and Feeding. Fitzwygram's "Horses and Stables". Smith's (Gen. Fred Smith) Veterinary Physiology.

DISCUSSION

DR. QUITMAN: When I was examining these fellows who were anywhere from a few months to fifteen years beyond their graduation, I thought I could see them from the view point of the State board examiners, and I have said and heard said "how did so and so ever come out of that school"? I don't blame some of these State board examiners for some of the ideas they have on the subject.

I have to say that in my paper—Dr. Bemis' paper was very much along the same line—it seems we advocated a well-rounded faculty resulting in a well-rounded graduate. I want to say this in view of some of the things that were said in Dr. Turner's paper. I do not believe, however, it lies within the effort of any veterinary college to turn every man out a specialist in every different branch. Dr. Turner evidently sees the veterinarian only through the army eye, while Dr. Bailey, in his paper, sees the veterinarian only through the eyes of a milk hygienist. It certainly would mean about a seventeen-year course to follow out the ideas of these two gentlemen, if every specialist had the same idea. In human medicine they do not turn out specialists. If a man wants to specialize in human medicine he has to continue his studies after he graduates. If he takes an engineering course he cannot always specialize from the general course in engineering, but after having completed that general course he becomes an electrical engineer or a civil engineer, as the case may be. I think it is asking too much of a veterinary college whether it be a State university or a private school, to turn out men who are specialists in every different branch.

DR. HOSKINS: I was impressed, in listening to Dr. Bemis' and Dr. Quitman's papers, with their several points; one was in regard to what the high school represents in the entrance examination. I have had considerable experience upon State boards, and for the last six months I have had experience in dealing with a body of students in a State college that holds the highest entrance requirement of our country. You know in New York State we have nothing to say about the requirements of men entering veterinary schools there. The Board of Regents establish the requirements for us. They require that they shall be graduates of four years of high school work and shall have seventy-two counts; and I am not yet convinced that high school requirements will solve the difficulty that we have been contending about for a good many years. In all large cities like the City of New York, the high school there does give a very wide latitude of instruction; but I have been disappointed considerably by the fact that many of these men that come to us with high school entrance requirements are still very lacking in the proper knowledge of the fundamentals. I have marked a good many papers in my time, as a member of the State board, of men who came to the college without the need of any entrance examination, but with the qualifications of high school men. I have been quite disappointed in a reasonable per cent of those men that they did not write either an intelligent paper nor were they able to write correctly or to express themselves in their papers grammatically. In large cities the whole trend of high schools is to fit men for commercial pursuits. I glory in the address of the president which we listened to this morning, because I always admire the man who preaches the gospel of discontent, since he is sure to get somewhere; while the man who preaches to those who listen to him that they should be contented with their lot does not get very far and in fact has commenced to retrograde.

When men come to us in our veterinary schools in great states like that of New York, or a great city like New York City, they come to us lacking, to my mind, a very essential thing to make a well rounded veterinarian. They come to us from back of counters or from desks in counting houses; they come to us from the great commercial industries of the cities, from the stores and other places, without a particle of knowledge of animal industry, with no knowledge of farm life, with no particular love for animals, but too many of them come to us with purely a commercial thought in mind. It is one of the difficult problems to eliminate that from these men's minds, and I have decided that this year, in opening the four years' course at the New York City Veterinary College, from the 5th day of September to the 26th day, we will devote that entire period with the four classes, teaching them and getting into their minds the thought that the field of veterinary medicine is not a commercial one, but is one of service—of service to humanity, of service that will bring them a rich reward in a feeling when they have closed their career that they have been helpful to mankind, that they have done something to lift the burdens off the shoulders of the great masses of people, and done something for what our president has spoken of, a world-wide democracy based upon a world-wide christianity. And so I feel today that we are not going to solve all of the problems by demanding just a high school entrance to our veterinary schools, nor are we going to make the well rounded veterinarian that Doctor Quitman has so practically pointed out.

Another point that we might take notice of from our president's address is that we must realize the importance of maintaining our courses in keeping with the courses of engineering and with the course of human medicine. We cannot hope, understand, that the future of any of our men can have the possibilities of engineering that oftentimes brings great fortunes over night, nor the possibilities of human medicine in the great cities where men command as much as $500.00 to wait upon the birth of a child on Fifth Avenue, or perhaps on Walnut Street of Philadelphia. Our men are going into a field that only promises perhaps with care and frugality and thrift a competence in old age—not riches or affluence; and we, who are engaged in the teaching of veterinary medicine, we who are trying to lift up veterinary medicine and build it up as we should must take into consideration, in dealing with student bodies, this phase of it.

While I am desirous of moving just as fast as we possibly can I am not unmindful that there are barriers to veterinary education, that locality and geography have to be considered. There are advantages enjoyed by the State schools in the agricultural districts over those in the large cities, and so it is a great subject that we ought to approach and deal with in the most thoughtful manner, lifting up every department of veterinary medicine and learning that it is possible to do; being careful not to destroy anything that has served us well in the past though perhaps not as fully as we would like, in the field of veterinary medicine in North America.

DR. S. STEWART: In some of the states, as you have heard to-day, a graduate of the veterinary college is granted a license to practice upon presentation of his graduation certificate or diploma, which is recognized by the State board. However, in the State of Minnesota they do not recognize anybody's diploma other than to the extent that it makes the holder eligible to enter the examination for a license to practice. The peculiar state of affairs as developed in Minnesota, in that particular, differs from any other State board of which I have knowledge, in that they believe it their duty to examine the candidate's basic educational qualifications as well as his scientific qualifications. The fact appears to be that about eighty per cent of the men who have appeared before that State board in the last two years have failed to pass, largely because of their failure to meet the basic educational requirements as set forth by that board.

If the proposals in part as set forth in the secretary's report as coming out from the Detroit meeting, that State boards should permit reports of their examinations to be made from which might be collated data to be sent to the various colleges so that they might be informed as to what the State boards demand from graduates of these colleges could have been carried out we would have reached a little farther along the road of progress. However, when I come to the examination of the Minnesota State board, the best they will do is to give the names of the men and the subject in which they failed. I sought through different channels to get a set of questions submitted to these men so as to ascertain upon what probable basis they failed and was told by the secretary of the board that it was contrary to the rulings of that board to send out any of the questions used by that board. Thus it is a closed corporation so far as general information is concerned.

My feeling is that colleges have stepped along pretty rapidly, but they have not realized nor felt the force of their own defects, and that the State examination boards have the opportunity, when they shall all correlate their efforts as a body in veterinary education to lead the veterinary colleges to a better comprehension of their short comings and in a measure make a potent source of information to those colleges that must necessarily make for better things for their graduates who are asking to be granted licenses in the respective states.

If the State of Texas holds an examination that you would say was primitive and the State of Massachusetts holds an examination that you would call super-technical, you will see the great difficulties that the colleges labor under when they feel that they must in some way prepare students to meet the varied demands of these State examination boards.

State boards have been guilty in some instances of some peculiar, eccentric catch question and they have been guilty of asking or propounding questions on theories that have long ago been exploded. They are not aware of that fact and are not up to where they ought to be. They ought not to complain of the veterinary colleges as failing to prepare students to answer questions of that sort in this day of advanced veterinary progress. One professor in a State college remarked to me one day that he considered it his business to give the graduating class under his care a series of instructions as to how to answer catch questions propounded by State examining boards, including in that a vocabulary which some State boards now use but which is antiquated and which the student did not get in the regular course.

All that sort of thing can be eliminated if the State examining boards will get together actually and discuss the features of the examination which it is possible for them to give under the laws of the State under which they are operating. If they will prepare and edit a series of questions as samples or guides for boards from which State boards may prepare their examinations, it would be of great service. Some of these State boards have very little experience— the State board of Texas has had possibly two years' experience and it is made up of men who never did any teaching, and who have no ideas concerning the work of instruction. They may never have prepared a set of questions and may not know the difficulty of making questions perfectly plain; may know nothing of how to equalize the value of various questions in the various departments, which is a very serious trouble indeed. I believe if it were the province of this body to prepare such sets of questions and offer them as suggestions of what kind of questions would be proper questions and such as would be fair to the student preparing to apply for a license, and which would be just as fair really in the State of Texas as in the State of Pennsylvania, it would be of very great advantage. We find at times such peculiar questions propounded by these State examining boards as to describe the hearts, lungs and liver of a horse, for one of ten questions in anatomy, the others of the ten being about equally as broad. You can readily see how a man might spend a great deal of time trying to write out an answer to a question of that kind.

Just one more matter, and that is, whether State examining boards might not develop the student's knowledge by a practical examination as, for instance, if they should require him to pick up a horse's foot and examine the bottom of it and show that he knows how to go about his business; so that they could ascertain whether he could really, put a bridle on a horse or whether he knows about harness and how a double-team harness was put on for instance, so that he would show the examiner by his methods that he knew what auscultation and percussion really means and what might be learned by them. In that way the examiner gets a definite notion of whether the student knows anything about the theory practically applied. Here is a great field which has been left uncovered. There is good ground for complaint because of our failure to publish our proceedings promptly and distribute them to the various State board members and various college faculty members. Some of these proceedings relating to State examining boards might be in a measure resurrected yet and properly edited and serve a very good purpose. They ought to be printed in convenient form and in a sufficient number of copies to supply the new incoming boards of examiners, because there are fifteen or twenty every year entering upon their duties without any personal understanding of the obligations they assume. When we do that the State examining boards will begin to comply with their duty and then the veterinary college will begin to do things it has not yet done to prepare men to be practical veterinarians.

DR. DONALDSON: Dr. Stewart had something to say about the Minnesota State Board, and its refusal to grant him copies of the questions. I wish to say that at the meeting of the Minnesota Veterinary Association Dr. Kinsley was present at one time and I myself instructed the secretary at that time that he could hand to Dr. Kinsley, or any other representative of any college there, a copy of those papers to see whether there was a catch question or an unfair question in the whole thing. Dr. Kinsley, I think, had an opportunity to look at some of the papers and admitted that there was not a question in those papers that a young man coming out of a college ought not to be able to answer. We claim that we never allow catch questions in the Minnesota board examinations. We follow closely the rules of the civil service examination. We examine by number only. No member of the examiners, until the papers are all in and gone over, has any way of knowing whose papers he is examining. Those numbers are not opened until after that time. We have no reason one way or another to hide our questions; but we certainly did not want to hand out a whole batch of questions extending over a number of years. That would certainly be a foolish thing to do. Then the prospective candidates could go to work and post up along that very line with very little knowledge of anything else behind it.

In regard to the Minnesota examination board's putting up an examination in preliminary education, I assure you some of the answers we get and some of the papers show that it is very necessary. I do not want to be very specific in this, but it is plainly evident that something is needed along that line. Not very long ago I had the 1917 prospectuses that were sent out to me from the different colleges, which tell what their entrance requirements are. One thing I want to say is, that judging from what we get in Minnesota, some of those colleges are not coming up to what they say in their catalogues. They could not be, or we would not get men like that coming out of those colleges. I am not here to criticize or tell what ought to be done. That has been spoken of enough already. There are institutions that are not examining their men properly before they go in. I am not advocating a high school education. As far as I am concerned I do not think it is necessary. Dr. Hoskins covered that beautifully. I think, however, there ought to be a line drawn as to where a man ought to have education enough any way to understand the language that is being used in the college; and I think he ought to have enough education so as not to come up to the Minnesota State board and spell such words as stomach "s-t-u-m-i-k".

I haven't a full copy of a set of questions in my pocket, but I have a few of them that I am willing to hand over to Dr. Stewart or any other college man, and let them look them over; and if there is an unfair question or a catch question or anything of that kind I would like to find it and we will have such things eliminated.

Dr. S. Stewart: I am very glad indeed I said some of the things I did, because it brought the remarks we have heard from Dr. Donaldson. It also brings to mind several other little things. Personally I did not wish to intimate that the State of Minnesota asked catch questions, and I did not have that State in mind when I made the statement. It was an eastern State. I have no way of knowing whether Minnesota has catch questions or not, because I never saw their questions; but what I most desired was a set of questions on the basic subjects and to get an inkling of what examination they give, not in criticism of the board, but for enlightenment to myself and our faculty. That is why I wanted them.

In relation to this matter, I met a man on the street in Minneapolis in July who was a graduate holding a degree of veterinary medicine from the Kansas City Veterinary College, two years ago last spring. I met him and inquired how he happened to be in Minneapolis. He said, "I have just been here to take the State examination again", and I said to him, "How many times have you taken that State examination"? He said "This is the fourth time"

I got a record that he took the examination and failed and he told me that he failed every time on the basic examination, but that he hoped this fourth time he would get by. I looked up his record and found he entered the Kansas City Veterinary College with a high school diploma credit and never was examined here. Looking up that same record I found another man who said he had never had any high school training at all but who took the examination and passed with a good grade on every subject with the State of Minnesota board, where the other man had failed.

DR. DONALDSON: Was he a graduate of a Minnesota high school?

DR. S. STEWART: No. That brings out the point that Dr. Hoskins made that a high school course—particularly two years, or even three years in the high school—is not all the basic education that a man needs to prepare him to pass a first grade civil service examination or the examination given by some of the veterinary colleges.

A man who can pass an entrance examination such as the Minnesota State board possibly gives today, but who has taken a course of veterinary medicine and has undertaken to jot down by rapid notation what the instructors say is very likely at the end of the course to be a poor speller. They do not write any word hardly in full. They do not have time, but must abbreviate and find short ways to spell the words, right or wrong; and that is possibly some explanation of the condition we find. I am not offering that as an excuse for it, but as an explanation. In my own practice I tell the student never to take a note. Listen and digest what is being said and then go to the text book and read and he will read it more intelligently and don't spend time writing out what I am saying because they are not good enough short-hand reporters to take it down rapidly, and I think the results are less satisfactory. All men do not view that work as I do. However, it is my experience that men do take short cuts in their spelling and the tendency of rapid note taking is to make them defective spellers, even if before they were reasonably good.

There is another point of course that in taking an entrance examination a man may pass 50 on spelling and 90 on arithmetic and the average gets him over, and he never does become a good speller; or he may spell 90 or 95 but his writing is almost illegible, and he never does become a good writer during the course of the instruction. We have many difficulties, as Dr. Hoskins has said.

DR. S. L. STEWART: I was very much interested in Dr. Hoskins' talk about the qualifications of men who make application to a college for entrance. We have had high school men who were the very poorest students you could attempt to teach; and I have in mind one in particular. Not so very long ago this man could not pass the final examinations in one year. On the other hand in the same class was a fellow that really had trouble to pass the entrance examination to get into the school. The fellow that had the trouble in passing the entrance examination came out at the end of the year with good grades, while the other fellow who came in without any examination because he was a high school graduate did not pass. Of course, you understand, these are exceptions; but they are the facts.

I hope to see the day when all the States in this country will have the same rules for their examining boards or give practically the same examinations that Minnesota does, because in doing that it is going to make the colleges compete on their entrance requirements. I have said, and I still maintain, that I do not see any possible chance of the State examining boards ever getting anywhere near each other or giving examinations which are any where near equal unless some reciprocity be brought about. Wherever the B. A. I. examination could be substituted for the State board examinations, it would be a good thing. That would give the man in Missouri and Connecticut and Minnesota a chance to practice without taking an examination. As it is now if a man moves from one State to another it is up to him to take the State board examination in the State to which he goes, and you gentlemen know that when a man is out of school fifteen or twenty years, even though he is a good practitioner and even though his grades may have been in the nineties, when in school, it will hustle that man to take the State board examination in any State, although he may be one of the best veterinarians. I would not want to go to Minnesota to take an examination, because I have been too long away from these studies; and that is why a good many fellows would like to see reciprocity and an effort toward uniformity and standardization if there is any way of bringing it about.

Again bringing up the subject of passing examinations, if you will go to the records of the students in the public schools and in the high schools you will find very few good spellers. They are exceedingly poor in spelling and in clear handwriting. I don't know how a veterinary college is going to turn out men who are good spellers and good copywriters unless they have attained these accomplishments in the public and high schools. It is a surprise to see the words that a high school graduate will mis-spell, and it is surprising to know that few people can really write a clear copy hand and make a correct copy. I think those things ought to be corrected in our public schools and in our high schools. I cannot see, for myself, why State boards require men to pass a certain high basic educational examination when these things never were taught them.

Dr. Donaldson: Dr. Stewart said something about a young man from the Kansas City Veterinary College being up for examination the fourth time. I think the fact is that every student who fell down in the preliminary examination also fell down on the other requirements. Nobody has been flunked in Minnesota for failure on basic education alone. The scoring is very easy on copying and on spelling. I still stick to it that I think some of them must have slid through awfully easy. I had at one time a young man in the examination whose first excuse was that he could not take a written examination because he had forgotten his glasses and could not see to write. It was agreed that we would give him an oral examination and ask him the same questions. Well, we asked him the same questions as were on the paper. I strung him along until I asked him if there was any particular difference between the liver of a horse and that of an ox, and he said the gall bladder of a horse was a good deal larger than it was in an ox. In talking the matter over with Dr. Hay I said, "I cannot, for the life of me, see how that man escaped from college". Hay said, "I'll go you one stronger. I don't know how he managed to break in". I said, "I will try to find out", and I went and asked the gentleman just what kind of entrance examination he took. "Oh," he said, "I didn't even take that." "He said, "Why, I had a high school certificate". That is all there was of it—just what Dr. Hoskins said in his remarks.

I don't believe for a moment that any college can make a veterinarian out of every student. The man must have it in him to go after it himself, to make him a winner. If you are any judge of humanity at all you can see whether the possibility is there.

DR. W. E. STONE: I heartily agree with the gentleman who has just spoken. I remember distinctly one student with quite a little preliminary education and there were many boys in my class with no education, but were just as good students as he was and mastered the subject as well as he did and I believe much more easily. I remember last winter having a young man in my class who came into the college by examination but did not have the finances sufficient to buy himself any textbooks, and who had to work during the time that he possibly could spare from his classes, and who never took a note in one of my classes; and let me ask that man a question and it would come back to me just exactly as I put it out to him. That man occupied a back seat in the class room, and he would sit there with his head down and did not seem to be paying very much attention to what I was saying in my lectures; but when it came to quizz time he was there with the goods. That man, I learned, on inquiring into his early life, had been raised in an agricultural district and had a natural love for animals and was there in the school to make good; and I want to say to you gentlemen that he did make good in his work.

In drawing the line on entrance requirements in our veterinary schools it is certainly a very difficult problem to eliminate the unpromising material. If we were to take only high school graduates, we would take away the opportunity of many boys who have not been able to afford to go into the high schools, and yet many of whom will become our best practitioners. It would be placing it in the hands of the more fortunate boys financially and otherwise. I have no remedy to offer to you gentlemen for this problem, but I believe it is the great problem that confronts the veterinary schools today.

Another thing to which I wish to refer is honesty in examinations in veterinary colleges. This is true not only in veterinary schools, but in other colleges as well. I remember when I was in veterinary college we used to call it rutting. I have been a student of a couple of the largest veterinary colleges in the country. I found in these two schools, and I might say in the school with which I am connected, a great amount of "ponying" which takes place in examinations where the students depend upon help other than what they have within themselves. In other words, the men in the faculties of our colleges are too lenient with those students and do not hold them to the line sufficiently. I think the schools are derelict in this line. I believe if the faculty would come right down and refuse to grade a paper where they have a suspicion of its not being original it would tend to help eliminate "ponying" out of our schools.

Again, I do not believe that the majority of our veterinary faculties grade in the subjects of spelling and writing when they are correcting examination papers. Dr. S. Stewart has referred to the fact that the rapid taking of notes had a tendency to overcome good spelling and writing. I heartily agree with him, because I know that oftentimes in writing examinations I would abbreviate my word or write it regardless of the correct way of spelling, just so that the instructor could make out what I meant. If I had been corrected and a demerit put after such a word, the next time I would not have done that. That may be due to the fact that our examinations are hurried, that we give too long examinations, that the time required to take them is not sufficient. If that be the fact, then it is up to the veterinary faculty to give examinations more in accord with the time available and give the student ample time to write out in full the answers he writes without using a single abbreviation in the spelling of a word.

There are a number of things I would like to speak of and another thing is reciprocity. I would hail the day with much delight when we could have a government board examination. All veterinarians would be glad of one universal board before which all veterinary students could go and take an examination and do away with the State boards entirely; or else have uniform State questions so that if a man is registered in the State of Missouri he could pass into the State of Minnesota and practice. If I am capable of practicing in the State of Missouri surely I am capable to practice in the State of Minnesota and I believe reciprocity is one of the great things. If it could be put into practice throughout this country it would be welcomed by all veterinarians and veterinary schools.

DR. HOSKINS: I feel I would be forgetful of what I believe personally today if I did not refer to Dr. Turner's paper and what he said as emanating from our lamented Rush Shippen Huidekoper concerning some of the essentials of a thorough veterinary education. He had conceived the idea back in the early eighties that men who were going to enter the veterinary profession should have certain preliminary training or education and even then he hoped to live to see the day when there would be established a veterinary school at the University of Pennsylvania where the first year of every entering student would be devoted entirely to determining his aptitude for the profession. He considered, in the way of aptitude, that that student ought to know a great deal about animal life; he ought to know all about taking care of horses; and his thought was that he would put him into the stable and he would teach him how to use a fork for cleaning out the stall and teach him how to use the brush and curry comb and he would compel him to take a set of harness apart and put it together again and be prepared before going on with the more theoretical studies to know how to harness every kind of a horse and for every purpose and how to saddle a horse and how to ride one. After the expiration of that year, if he had shown that aptitude that he deemed necessary to fit him for the profession, he might then go into the other three years in order to obtain the technical education. We may still hope, or I sincerely do, that some such plan may yet emanate from some of our schools. For I consider it of far greater importance in qualifying a man to go out and perform the service he will be called upon for the people and for the State than a mere high school education.

I cannot help but take advantage of what has been said by Dr. Stewart and Dr. Stone on the subject of reciprocity. I have no doubt that neither of these men are aware of the fact that we have wrestled with that problem for twenty-four long years; but I am glad to see that we are getting nearer to the only possible solution of it under our form of government. We are getting to the time when we are going to ask and demand, as far as possible, of our federal government that she should raise continuously the standard for those who are going into federal service; and I am hopeful that she will establish very soon some standard of requirements for the veterinarians who are acting under the B. A. I., for the men who are going into the army, and into veterinary service, or any other position under our government. I am also hopeful—and I do not believe that it is a dream any longer—that when we are asked to give a certificate it will be a certificate based upon an examination and that examination planned by a committee of this association and when they give that certificate it will represent the standard of veterinary medicine in the United States and will tell every nation of the earth what our standard is. Then we may well go into the State legislatures and ask them to modify their laws and accept this certificate in lieu of an examination. Then we will see men rushing first to get this examination, and then we will see the schools preparing themselves to fit men to pass this examination. Then the man who has been ten or fifteen years out of school will have no fear that if ill health or some other misfortune comes ten or fifteen years after he has been in practice in a certain state and makes it desirable for him to go to another, that he may not be able to take some State examination, but will find that State has passed an amendment to its laws recognizing that the certificate he obtained when he was best able to obtain it entitles him to go into the State he desires without any of the barriers that exist today, and there practice and enjoy whatever features that State may offer to him, or which he seeks to enjoy.

PALPEBRAL MALLEINIZATION*

PROF. DOUVILLE, Veterinaire Aide-Major, mobilized with the armies

It will soon be two years since hostilities caused the mobilization of the equine effectives of France, and, as had been foreseen, their sanitary condition, although perfect at the beginning, was soon disturbed by the two diseases incident to all wars, glanders and mange.

Although the latter affection did not tend to spread until after the winter of 1914-15, glanders broke out in certain corps in October, 1914, transmitted to them perhaps by German horses which were abandoned, or captured in battle; or perhaps it resulted from the dissemination of latent infection in some of the requisitioned animals. The great problem of applying mallein to the contaminated effectives was considered and, to be frank, it was seen from the beginning that it could not be solved: insurmountable difficulties were encountered because of the conditions which must prevail for the proper execution of the subcutaneous mallein test.

The intradermal mallein test was to save the situation. The different duties which have been confided to us since the beginning of the war have permitted us to assist from the beginning with experiments on a very large scale to test it parallel with the subcutaneous method and, at the same time, to verify every positive result by autopsy.

Now that it has been tested for 15 months and has displaced the previously recognized test we have acceded to the request of

*Translation from Recueil de Medecine Veterinaire, V. 92, p. 257, May 15, 1916. By. M. Dorset.

the Editor of the *Recueil de Medecine Veterinaire* to describe it to his readers. We make absolutely no claim for original work: the technique, the judgment of the results, the classification of the sub-jects and the measures to be taken, are set forth in the Ministerial Circular of December 23, 1914, which only codifies the publica-tions of MM. Drouin and Naudinat.

We review these, adding thereto a typical case, some details, certain personal observations, some exact experimental data which may guide or instruct colleagues who have little familiarity with this method, and which, finally, may convince the skeptics if they still exist.

The method of intradermal malleinization is merely a combina-tion of the procedures employed by Prof. Lanfranchi[1] for glanders and by Prof. Moussu for tuberculosis.

Early in 1914, the former published the excellent results which he obtained in the diagnosis of glanders by the subcutaneous injection of the classical dose of diluted mallein at the border of the lower eye-lid.

Similarly, on the same date, M. Moussu, whose name will re-main associated with the intradermal tuberculin test, recommended the injection of 0.1 cubic centimeter of diluted tuberculin, not into the sub-caudal fold but into the dermis of the lower lid. The results were distinct and much more striking than at the old point of election.

The extreme rarity of glanders in France at that time did not give to experimenters the opportunity to apply either one or the other of these methods.

Nevertheless the French veterinary missions in Greece (Mili-tary Mission: Veterinary Major Laumarque; Civil Mission: MM. Drouin and Naudinat) found a field for experimentation in the Grecian cavalry infected with glanders as a result of the Balkan war. The results of their experiments, which confirm those ob-tained by Professors Lanfranchi and Moussu, were published by MM. Drouin and Naudinat.[2]

The mobilization having placed us by the side of M. Lau-marque, we are, in truth, compelled to say that he was the intro-

---

1—Lanfranchi—A new method for the diagnosis of glanders—Intrapalpe-bral Reaction to Mallein (Il Moderno Zooiatro, January 31, 1914), Review in Recueil d'Alfort.

2.—Bulletin de la Societe Centrale de Medicine Veterinaire, Decembre, 30, 1914; Revue Generale de Medicine Veterinaire, Aout, 1914.

ducer of the intradermal test in France and in the Army. From
October, 1914, he demonstrated the technique and the results upon
the glandered horses of *C. A.*, of which principal Veterinarian
Schelemeur had the veterinary control. With remarkable diligence
M. Schelemeur applied the process to all his effectives and the epidemic was checked when the Ministerial Circular of December 23,
1914, appeared.

At the same time we applied the test systematically to the
horses evacuated from the front to the depots for sick horses and
an assignment to apply the palpebral mallein test in the latter,
permitted us to apply it on a large scale and, accordingly, to judge
of its value.

The staff of a quarantine hospital for suspected animals
(groups C and B) permitted us to test it and to compare it with
subcutaneous malleinization. We have taken care to autopsy all
of the slaughtered subjects in order to determine in each case the
nature and the extent of the lesions, and we do not hesitate to pro-
claim that our faith in the palpebral malleinization has only increased with added experience.

In July, 1915, we had the honor to be sent on a mission by the
G. Q. G. to Brigadier General Moore, Director of the Veterinary
Services of the British Army, for the purpose of having a conference with him and his veterinary officers and of making a practical
demonstration of the palpebral method. The results were conclusive and upon our departure the Brigadier-General gave us the
assurance that the procedure would be immediately applied in his
services. This spirit of initiative and prompt decision are an
honor to such a chief and it is one of the happy consequences of the
autonomy of the British Veterinary Service.

TECHNIQUE.—1st. The necessary material comprises: a one
cubic centimeter syringe with a set screw, graduated in tenths,
and provided with fine and short needles (length: 10 to 15 millimeters); 2nd, mallein diluted to $\frac{1}{4}$ (crude mallein=1; 0.5% solution of phenol=3), as prescribed by MM. Drouin and Naudinat, is
employed generally in the Army. The Pasteur Institute delivers
it in tubes labeled specially ''mallein $\frac{1}{4}$ for intradermal reaction''.
In default of this we have used mallein diluted to 1/10; the results are practically the same provided the dose is doubled so as
to be 1/5 of a cubic centimeter.

The application of the twitch to the upper lip or to the ear is indispensable in order to operate quickly and conveniently; a staff of three assistants enables the somewhat experienced operator to apply the mallein to at least 100 horses an hour.

Either eye may be used for the injection. It is as easy on the right as on the left. Nevertheless it is contraindicated to operate upon lachrymating eyes or those affected with keratitis, acute conjunctivitis, or epiphora. On the contrary, old lesions (leucoma, cataract, dislocations of the crystalline lens) interfere in no way with the result. When operating upon a great number of horses it is prudent to note the side selected and, if there is occasion, the animals in which the opposite lid is selected and the reasons therefor. One thus avoids embarrassment the next day and faulty interpretations which may result therefrom.

The injection is made into the dermis of the lower lid about one centimeter from the free edge. Disinfection of the point of injection is not absolutely necessary; we practiced it at the beginning and little by little we dispensed with it without ever observing local infections. In the case of certain dirty or greasy lids, wiping with a cotton tampon wet with alcohol or ether is advantageous.

The dose to be injected is 1/10 of a cubic centimeter. The syringe, filled, with needle attached and with set screw regulated to 0.1 cubic centimeter, is held in the right hand between the thumb and middle finger, while the index finger rests upon the milled head of the stem of the piston. The left thumb and index finger make a horizontal fold on the lower lid into which the needle is introduced for a distance of three millimeters, and as near as possible to the surface of the skin; "the injection should be made into the dermis." This requirement, which has disturbed numerous beginning operators and has caused the technique to be regarded as delicate, is by no means a *sine qua non*. MM. Drouin and Naudinat have obtained the same results by injection into the deep layers of the skin.

When the injection is well made it produces a small lenticular swelling; it seems to us that this is easier to obtain and to verify when instead of making a fold in the skin, the index finger is passed into the lower conjunctival cul-de-sac in such a way as to stretch the lid, the thumb immobilizing it and rendering it more easily perforated. However that may be, the technique remains extremely simple and available to every practitioner.

PHENOMENA FOLLOWING THE INJECTION: In the majority of horses, in the first hours following the injection, a circumscribed edema appears on the lower lid; it is of an irritative nature, non-toxic, only slightly painful and of quite short duration. When the mallein is applied in the morning it disappears during the night or it is found in the process of distinct retrogression the next day. No significance should be attached to it. It suffices to know of its existence or the possibility of it. In healthy animals the eye preserves its normal appearance. In glandered animals the reaction becomes defined about the 10th or 12th hours, attaining its maximum from the 24th to the 36th hour. It lasts two or three days on the average, subsides, and disappears without leaving any trace, except for a certain amount of local thickening of the connective tissue.

The typical reaction is distinctly striking.

A voluminous edema involves not alone the lower lid but also the tissues surrounding the eye, almost closing it and reducing the size of the palpebral opening. This edema is always hot, sometimes burning and extremely sensitive: the patient flinches at the slightest attempt to touch it.

The conjunctiva is markedly congested and from the internal angle of the eye there flows a muco-pus more or less abundant, which becomes transformed into a sulphur-colored exudate, at the border of the eyelashes.

There are occasions where the reaction seems to localize itself in the lower lid. The conjunctivitis and the exudate are as distinct as in the complete reaction, but the edema, although quite voluminous, is circumscribed in the angular space above the zygoma; of characteristic importance, and to which we attach great value, is the fact that this region exhibits to the touch the same characters as in the complete reaction (heat and marked hyperesthesia). The edema is as persistent as in the typical reaction; often it extends below the zygoma and is accompanied by fine sinuous lymphatic lines converging toward the sub-lingual glands. Palpation of the surface of the masseter is painful and the gland is sensitive.

Such a reaction, although exclusively of the lower lid, should cause the horse to be regarded as affected with glanders and we believe that it should be classed in the group of positive reactions. Its establishment is easy by comparison with the opposite eye; by taking care to administer the mallein in the morning and to make the judgment of the test the afternoon of the next day, it cannot be missed.

In the bulletin of the Central Society of Veterinary Medicine (30th December, 1915) M. Fayet reported delayed reactions which appeared only toward the 3d, 4th and 5th days following the injection; he considered them as very rare and we freely agree with his opinion; among 12,000 mallein tests which we have applied ourselves, including 104 horses (affected with clinical or latent glanders) we have not been able to record a single one.

DOUBTFUL REACTIONS. By considering the edema of the lower lid, having the characters which we have described, as a positive reaction, the number of doubtful reactions and the size of group B of the Ministerial Instructions are considerably reduced[3]. Does that mean that they do not occur? No, but they are very rare.

Between the reaction previously described and the swelling without diagnostic value, which persists at times in some healthy animals, one may observe some intermediate grades with regard to which the operator must exercise his common sense and his clinical knowledge.

Conjunctivitis is generally absent or is very slight. The palpebral edema affects only the lower lid, it is diffuse, or at times is circumscribed about the point of injection in the form of a crescent with a tendency to extend over the zygoma.

In doubtful cases we test the other eye after 5 or 6 days, making the intradermal injection into both lids, the upper and lower.

We have stated that during the period of incubation of glanders the infected subject may present atypical reactions although it will react clearly some days later, its body having had time to become sensitized to the reacting toxin.

In addition, the examination and control of a lot of horses classed in group B, evacuated from the front, has shown us that as a result of the edema of the lower lid the connective tissue becomes thickened, the skin adherent, to a certain degree, to the zygoma and

---

3—TRANSLATOR'S NOTE. The author here refers to French Ministerial Instructions, dated December 23, 1914, in which the horses subjected to test are placed in three groups, as follows:

"*Group A.*—Subjects which either do not present any edema, or else only an insignificant reaction.

Group B.—Subjects in which the reaction affects only the lower lid and may be considered as doubtful.

Group C.—Subjects which present a typical reaction (edema of both lids, and a purulent conjunctivitis)."

for some time the region is unsuitable for good reactions. If one attempts a second test, the edema remains diffuse, the conjunctivitis is slight, and one is justified in having doubts as to their significance. These doubts have always been relieved by testing the upper lid simultaneously. In infected cases this becomes swollen, the supra-orbital fossa fills up, and there is a ptosis of the lid. We believe that it is advantageous to utilize this additional source of information for doubtful or suspected cases; personally it has given very much more satisfaction than the hypodermic control.

* * * * * * * *

VALUE AND ADVANTAGES. With the object of determining the relative value of the two methods, we have submitted all of our horses successively to palpebral malleinization and to the subcutaneous test; each positive reaction has been checked by autopsy.

The first conclusion which forces itself upon one is that the glandered horse or the horse in the incubative stages of glanders, reacts marvelously to infinitely small doses of mallein. The toxin indicates the presence of lesions without relation to their location, their extent or their age. In horses with latent glanders the intensity of the reaction has not seemed to us to be always "in inverse ratio to their extent or their chronic character".

We have produced superb palpebral reactions as well in horses with two or three recent nodules as in animals whose pulmonary substance was filled with glanders nodules of the size of a hazel nut and whose tracheo-bronchial glands revealed numerous miliary abscesses. All of our clinical cases of glanders (40) have reacted to the intrapalpebral test, although five of them gave atypical subcutaneous reactions, insufficient in themselves to establish the diagnosis if that had not already been established by the clinical examination. It is possible that in rare cases of undoubted glanders the intradermal test has sometimes failed: the organism, saturated with toxin by the natural disease, remains insensitive to the introduction of a small supplementary dose of mallein. In such a case, where the palpebral method remains negative, one cannot expect anything from the classical procedure, but the clinical diagnosis is almost always forced upon the experienced practitioner. In the case of latent glanders, positive palpebral reactions have not always been confirmed by subcutaneous test, although we have taken all precautions to avoid chances of error.

In 120 eye reactions we have had 104 confirmations by the subcutaneous test.

In subjects with fever which have responded poorly to the classical procedure (old method), we have had no exceptions to the intradermal test.

Notwithstanding the increasing importance, which for ten years has been attached to the local reaction in the subcutaneous test, doubts have arisen in the minds of numerous observers when the tri-fold reaction was incomplete. We know, nevertheless, how uncertain the general organic reaction is, and what limited significance should be attributed to a rise in temperature. The intradermal method has considerably simplified the problem if it has not entirely solved it. Its superiority lies in basing the diagnosis exclusively upon the local reaction and in having this develop in striking form in a region where its presence can hardly be mistaken. With it, doubtful reactions are much less frequent.

All of our colleagues who have made numerous subcutaneous mallein tests have been able to establish that in certain horses mallein may cause a more or less considerable rise in temperature, attaining at times 40° C., oscillating for the most part about 39.5° C. for some hours. Notwithstanding the absence of local and general reactions, this rise of temperature is liable to influence some observers. All subjects with fever of this kind that we have tested by the intrapalpebral method have always given clearly negative reactions, and after some weeks of observation with repeated tests, we have not hesitated to sign their discharge. It is well to remember that this hyperthermia is generally provoked by affections quite distinct from glanders. Melanosis (Comeny, Nocard, Mauri) chronic broncho-pneumonia (Trasbot) pulmonary emphysema (Schindelka) strangles particularly (Cagny) are among the number. We consider that, from all points of view the intradermal mallein test constitutes a distinct improvement over the classical procedure. Its diagnostic value, although based exclusively upon the local reaction, is certainly equal to that of the test formerly used; personally, we have found it superior and when employed exclusively, with system and at the right time, it has always enabled us rapidly to eliminate infected animals.

From a practical point of view, its advantages are even more numerous and frequent. They are those which M. Moussu has pointed out for the palpebral tuberculinization: no necessity for taking temperatures; no chances of error through abortive temperature reactions or through erroneous reading of the thermometer; no obligation to work at fixed hours; the veterinarian chooses the hour for injection and for the interpretation of the test; the possibility of immediate application to febrile animals; the possibility of making a great number of successive tests (several hundred a day) with economy of personnel, the possibility of application to all horses under all conditions of surroundings, of quarters (stable or bivouac) and of exterior temperature; the possibility of repeating the tests periodically; almost complete elimination of injuries to assistants from kicks, always to be feared with the classical method; economy of thermometers, of mallein and of time. .

These multiple advantages have quickly appealed to our British allies. Our distinguished colleague, Prof. Hobday, commanding officer of a veterinary hospital, wrote us recently: "Since your conference thousands of horses have been tested by this method; as to the results and our opinion, I believe I am justified in saying that we all think that it is the most excellent and the most accurate.

"We employ it now as the regular method of testing and I am certain that the Brigadier-General Director of the Veterinary Service will send you a reply confirming all that I have written you." General Moore had in truth the kindness to advise us that "according to the reports of all his officers they had no objection to make".

Is not all of that sufficient to permit the statement that at the present time the intradermal malleinization is "the most simple, the most expeditious, the surest, and the most practical" in order to check glanders under all conditions?

TOLERANCE TO MALLEIN—ASSOCIATION OF THE TWO METHODS: —Our numerous mallein tests combined and reversed have permitted us to study under all conditions the question of tolerance to mallein.

Here are the different problems which we have considered and the solutions obtained:

1. Is there a tolerance to the palpebral mallein test? The horse infected by glanders reacts to the palpebral test as many times as one applies it, whatever be the period which elapses between the successive tests. Let us remember, however, that if one uses a lid which has been recently tested the second reaction may be diffuse and doubtful on account of the thickening of the connective tissue.

The intradermal reaction applied to the upper lids or to the shaved surface of the neck or shoulders has always confirmed the reactions on the lower lid. They take place within the same time and are easily interpreted.

We have established many times that the weak dose of mallein used in the intradermal test is sufficient to produce an appreciable and lasting rise of temperature in horses with virulent lesions.

*   *   *   *   *   *   *   *

2. Does tolerance exist in the case of the subcutaneous test? Although it is prescribed and is the custom to allow an interval of three to four weeks between two mallein tests intended to check each other, we have reduced this time little by little to a ten-day and sometimes to an eight-day period. Our conclusions confirm those already expressed by Nocard, Drouin and Galtier: *there is no tolerance to mallein.* Two injections made several days apart give identical results. Before determining upon this reduction in the time between tests, and, we must admit, a little influenced by what we knew about tuberculin, we applied to glanders the method of the double dose recommended by Vallée for tuberculosis. Animals which we knew to be affected with latent glanders as a result of one palpebral and one original subcutaneous test, have reacted in the same time and in the same way with a double dose of mallein ; the reaction was in no case earlier.

Tolerance to mallein does not exist. It therefore follows:

1. That a palpebral mallein test may be followed without delay by a subcutaneous injection.

2. That after a subcutaneous test, even though positive, the subject remains sensitive to the intradermal.

The facts which we record herewith are absolutely genuine and are in conformity with these conclusions. Among contaminated effectives in the case of doubtful or suspected subjects when one desires to repeat the palpebral tests or to associate the two tests with the object of control, it is indispensable to allow a lapse of time of at least 12 to 15 days between them. This delay corresponds to the period of incubation and to the sensitization of the subject to mallein. It is extremely probable that the supposed failures of the palpebral test, revealed by a subcutaneous test some days later, are due to failure to observe this delay.

*   *   *   *   *   *   *   *

[The article by M. Douville has been translated in full, there being omitted merely a chart and table, together with the records of several illustrative cases.]

A PRELIMINARY REPORT ON THE INTRAPAL-
PEBRAL MALLEIN TEST*

L. PRICE, D.V.M.
Department of Health, New York City

In recent veterinary literature the intradermal palpebral or intrapalpebral mallein test has occasionally been mentioned as useful
in the diagnosis of glanders.

This method seems to have been first reported in 1914 by Lanfranchi in Italy.* The French Commission in Greece under Drouin
carried on extensive experiments with this method.** Finally in
France after the preparation of intradermal mallein was modified,
the method was considered as second only to the subcutaneous test.

Captain Goodall in Africa found the intrapalpebral test a valuable method for the diagnosis of glanders under severe campaign
difficulties.*** Some cases of glanders gave no reactions and some
doubtful reactions to the subcutaneous test. These cases gave positive reactions to the intrapalpebral method. M'Fadyean reports
on the value of the palpebral method on two million cases, after it
was adopted by the British Army. He considers this method at the
present time, superior to any other.* Captain Holmes found this
method to be very valuable in his experiments.*

In a preliminary note upon the intradermal palpebral test, the
Veterinary Journal for August, 1915, states that this method never
failed in 5-6000 tests. In almost every instance the palpebral and
subcutaneous methods agreed. However, in a few cases of glanders,
the palpebral method gave positive reactions while the subcutaneous
test was indecisive.

Having had an opportunity to observe the veterinarians of the
French Army apply this test to horses purchased in this country
and having had an exceptional opportunity to give this method a
trial on horses presented to be slaughtered for food purposes, I note
my observations and findings.

This method has been applied to over 500 healthy and 27 glandered horses. The complement fixation, agglutination and ophthal-

---

*Vet. Journal, 1915-1917.
**Amer. Vet. Rev., 1914.
***Jour. Comp. Path. & Ther., 1916.

---

*Prepared for the New York State Veterinary Medical Society meeting at
Ithaca, N. Y., July, 1918.

mic mallein test were also applied as a routine procedure. The subcutaneous method was applied in a number of instances. Careful and detailed post mortem examinations were performed on the non-reacting as well as the reacting animals. Laboratory diagnosis was frequently made of typical as well as questionable material. Only that data is considered where there remains no question as to the facts of the case.

There were some doubtful reactions to the palpebral test among the healthy horses. In most of these cases the other tests were either negative or suspicious. On post mortem examination if there were any lesions, they were found not to be glanders.

Of 24 cases of glanders considered with the one exception noted later in the paper, 23 gave positive intrapalpebral local reactions. One case noted in the paragraph on temperatures gave a typical thermic reaction but not a satisfactory local reaction.

MALLEIN. The mallein employed was the same as that prepared for the veterinarians of the French Army, according to their directions. One volume of ophthalmic mallein diluted to three volumes of a 0.5 per cent carbolic acid solution. The dosage used was 2 minims or 1/10 c.c.

TECHNIC. A metal hypodermic syringe with a glass barrel of 1 c.c. capacity, fitted with a stop on the piston rod and graduated in tenths of a c.c. was found most convenient in performing the test. A fine bore needle of steel, 5/8 of an inch in length and strengthened by being soldered in deeply at the cup, was found to be the most desirable.

The test may be applied to either eye. The lower eyelid was the usual site of injection, though some have applied the test to the upper eyelid.

In most cases the holding of the horse's head by an assistant is sufficient means of restraint; however, in restless animals a twitch may be applied.

A fold of thin skin of the lower lid of the eye is grasped by the fore finger and the thumb, as near to the margin as possible. The needle is inserted into the dermis, parallel to the margin of the eyelid and midway between the inner and outer canthus. The syringe is inserted into the head of the needle and 1/10 c.c. of mallein injected.

A little practice soon develops the necessary skill in the technic of the operation. The possibility of injecting the mallein under the skin, while likely to obscure and delay the reaction, does not materially interfere with the test. In such instances the temperatures assist in the interpretation, and limit the danger of error. With ordinary precautions of cleanliness and antisepsis no danger of injury or infection is likely to occur.

The intrapalpebral mallein test produces a thermal and a local reaction, and occasionally a general reaction.

LOCAL REACTION. The positive local reaction is obviously the most striking and important. In glandered animals it commences a few hours after injection. Sometimes an inflammation is observed as early as the second or third hour. The height of the local inflammation is reached at different times in the course of the reaction. At times it is most marked at the eighth to the tenth hour after injection, at other times it may be most marked as late as the forty-eighth to the fifty-sixth hour. The reaction has been observed to last seven days after injection, but usually evidence of the reaction may be noticed up to the fourth or fifth day.

A positive reaction comprises a hot painful diffuse swelling of the lower lid and may involve a considerable area about the eye. The conjunctival mucous membrane is usually congested and a purulent conjunctivitis occurs as a rule, with a dirty purulent or muco-purulent discharge from the inner canthus. The free edge of the eyelid is swollen and tends to protrude upward at the inner canthus. The inflammation often extends to the upper lids, sometimes it extends as far as the zygomatic ridge appearing to involve the whole side of that portion of the face. The eye seems to be sunk deep in the orbit due to the swelling which tends to make its fellow appear much smaller. Occasionally, corded lymphatics may be noted radiating from the local swelling. The untested eye at times may show some discharge at the height of the reaction. The corresponding submaxillary lymph gland is usually swollen and painful on palpation.

The local reaction in cases of glanders may vary in extent, intensity and degree. The inflammation may be so severe and extensive as to involve the side of the face completely closing the eye and producing a copious purulent discharge. On the other hand the inflammation may be but slight and affect just the area about the point of injection, and in some cases the discharge may be barely noticeable or entirely absent,

In animals not infected with glanders an inflammatory edema appears at the point of injection, which reaches its height at the eighth to the tenth hour and then subsides. This edema seldom persists for more than 24 to 36 hours. This swelling is not painful or diffuse and takes on a crescentric shape. Frequently a slight mucous or serous discharge, different in character from a reactor's dis-

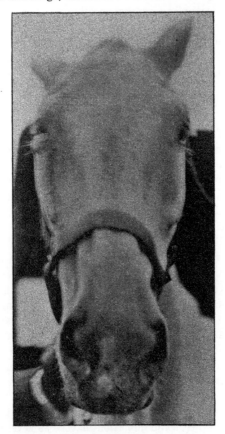

FIG. 1. Positive reaction at 20th hour.

charge is also present. The conjunctival mucous membrane is not injected or congested.

This non-specific swelling is easily recognized if present at the time of reading the test. In the majority of cases there is practically no obvious change at the point of injection.

TEMPERATURE. In positive cases the temperature has been observed to rise as high as 105.7° F. and usually takes on a definite curve. The temperature may rise as early as the sixth hour after injection and, as a rule, follows the appearance of the local reaction. The height of curve seems to be reached from the 12th to the 18th hour. A fever temperature is frequently observed as late as the

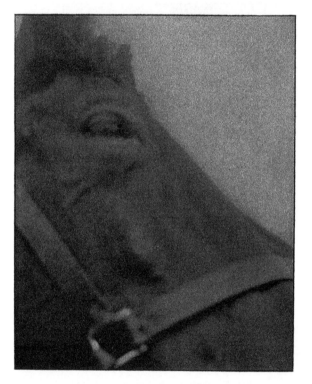

FIG. 2. Positive reaction at 20th hour. Note corded lymphatics.

24th to 36th hour and sometimes even later. In some cases where the local reactions were marked and continued, the high temperature lasted as long as the third day. The temperature curve has occasionally been observed to make a sharp drop after it has remained high for a period. A rise would follow for a short time, then there would be a gradual drop to normal. In some positive cases a very slight rise in temperature was noticed, but in these cases the readings were not taken frequently enough or at the most desirable times.*

In one case of glanders a typical temperature curve was observed while the local reaction would have been over-looked. In this case at the 14th hour when the temperature was over 105° F., the swelling and discharge were marked. In fact a slight purulent

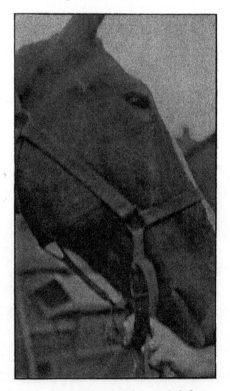

FIG. 3. Positive reaction on 3rd day.

discharge was also present from the untested eye. The local reaction of the retest was not entirely satisfactory while a subcutaneous test gave a typical positive reaction.

Non-glandered horses usually show no rise in temperature after injection with intradermal mallein. There has been a slight tem-

*NOTE.—It was impossible to obtain the temperature of all cases for the full period of the test. Accordingly my observations are based on those temperature readings which I was able to make as complete as possible.

perature rise in a few instances of doubtful local reactions which showed no lesions of glanders on post mortem examination. Retests on these animals gave negative local and thermal reaction. The possibility of these horses having been tested before is likely and the temperature rises being the result of sensitization.

Most of the writers on this method of malleinization have given the temperature readings secondary or no consideration in the in-

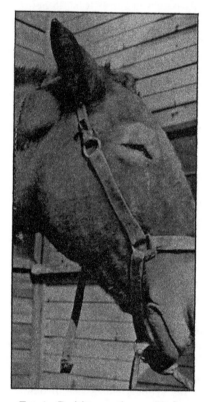

FIG. 4. Positive reaction on 4th day.

terpretation of the result. Undoubtedly the greater majority of cases of glanders may be recognized by the local reaction alone. However, careful and repeated temperature readings will unques-tionably decide doubtful reactions and, perhaps, occasionally point to the necessity of repeating the tests on certain animals.

GENERAL REACTION. The general reaction is not very marked

and, as a rule, not observed at all. Dullness and loss of appetite have been noticed and seem to depend upon the intensity of the local and thermal reactions. Lack of condition and loss of weight as result of the test have occurred in a few instances.

INTERPRETATION. The reaction is as a rule definite and characteristic. The diagnosis may be made upon observing the local reaction 24 to 36 hours after the injection of mallein. Doubtful reactors must be carefully observed for at least 48 hours. Taking a few temperatures between the 12th and 36th hours will often eliminate any indecision and occasionally help detect a case of glanders. Repeating the test to the other eye may settle any questionable reactions. To detect glanders it has often been necessary to apply more than one test or one method. To effectively control or eradicate this disease, matters of convenience and facility must at times be sacrificed.

EFFECT ON OTHER TESTS. The intrapalpebral mallein test has a transient effect on the serological tests after 24 to 36 hours. When applied shortly after the ophthalmic test it frequently brings out a reaction more prominently. Sensitization must be considered when repeated tests are applied. Otherwise the intrapalpebral method applied subsequently or in conjunction with the other mallein tests cannot be said to have any action of interference.

COMPARISON WITH OTHER TESTS. The intrapalpebral method being a clinical test, cannot be very well compared with the serological methods for diagnosing glanders. However, it may be said that the many inconveniences and occasional indecisive and unsatisfactory results of the latter tests have caused the veterinarian in the field to depend more upon clinical methods.

The single application of the ophthalmic test has proved rather unsatisfactory. In order to condemn a horse for glanders on the result of this test a distinct purulent conjunctivitis should be present. A copious discharge of pus, deep reddening of the mucous membrane, a swelling of the eyelids, and a rise in temperature if taken at the proper time, are the usual symptoms of a decisive reaction. The *suspicious* reaction with either a congestion, sero mucous discharge or perhaps purulent flakes occur too frequently. In performing the ophthalmic test, repeated examinations over a longer period of time as well as the taking of a few temperatures would undoubtedly uncover more cases of glanders and lessen the convenience attributed to this method of testing.

Mallein from different sources was used on 27 cases of glanders. Nineteen gave positive reactions to the ophthalmic test, seven of these had to be retested to obtain a positive result. The remaining eight cases were suspicious, four remained suspicious when retested. (All reacted to the palpebral method.) Among the many healthy horses tested too large a percentage gave suspicious reactions. A false positive occurred very rarely.

The accuracy of the palpebral and subcutaneous methods for the diagnosis of glanders compare very favorably when performed carefully by experienced operators. There is a disadvantage and a danger in the use of the subcutaneous method by the inexperienced in testing healthy horses. The false positives and atypical reactions are too numerous and confusing and are likely to be misinterpreted.

CONCLUSIONS. The intradermo-palpebral test is comparatively a simple, accurate, convenient, and reliable method for detecting glanders in horses. It is the most suitable method of testing with mallein in war times or when large numbers of animals must be speedily tested. If the local reaction alone is considered a large number of horses may be examined in a short period of time.

ADVANTAGES OF THE PALPEBRAL METHOD. 1. Simple in application.

2. Convenient in arrangement of time, especially if local reaction alone is considered.

3. Positive reactions are definite and doubtful or indecisive reaction not very frequent.

4. Reaction continues as a rule for forty-eight to seventy-two hours.

5. The reaction cannot be removed or modified.

6. May bring out a latent ophthalmic test.

7. Does not interfere with subsequent or other clinical tests.

8. The local condition of the conjunctival mucous membranes or a high temperature do not necessarily interfere with this method of testing.

9. Less mallein is used than in any other mallein test.

DISADVANTAGES. 1. Affects the serological tests.

2. Requires the use of a hypodermic syringe and needle.

3. The question of skill and care in the performance of this test may also be noted. However, the other methods also require this consideration if successful results are desired.

Interpretation of the reaction of various methods have much to do with the value of the tests. Not giving thorough unbiased and careful trials have caused unfair condemnation of many different methods.

In conclusion I wish to say, if the opportunity continues, more detailed work will be done with the intrapalpebral method. An effort will be made to make a more complete comparison of the methods more commonly used before estimating its value. It is hoped that this method will be tried by others to establish its real worth.

VETERINARY DISEASES IN SOUTHERN RHODESIA*

Ll. E. W. Bevan, M.R.C.V.S., Salisbury

The *routine work* of the laboratory has considerably increased during the past year, and in the absence of the laboratory assistant on war leave most of the technical work has fallen upon the bacteriologist himself, the lay members of the staff having rendered any assistance within their power. The work has included the examination of over two thousand five hundred smears and specimens from the "field" and almost as many from animals under experiment at the laboratory. Of the former, one hundred and twenty smears have revealed the parasites of African coast fever, one hundred and twenty-five the parasites of other diseases, and thirty-three specimens of serum have indicated the presence of contagious abortion in cattle. It may be pointed out that each specimen has to be examined with the greatest care and that it is not those preparations in which the causal organisms of diseases are readily found which occasion the greatest labor and anxiety, but those in which after prolonged search no parasites can be detected, because failure to find them if present, may lead to a faulty diagnosis misleading to the veterinary officials responsible for the administrative side of the work. Moreover, smears are frequently forwarded carelessly taken and without the necessary clinical details upon which to base a microscopic examination. The importance of careful and accurate laboratory diagnosis in assisting the administrative side of the veterinary department has been emphasized during the past year on many occasions.

*Report of the Government Veterinary Bacteriologist, Southern Rhodesia, for the year 1916.

EXPERIMENTAL RESEARCH WORK has been considerably handicapped by the demands of the routine and technical work, and it has been impossible to devote to it the undivided and concentrated attention it deserves. Thus much of the research which has been attempted has had to be abandoned. Nevertheless, it is felt that in spite of these difficulties considerable progress has been made in the solution of some of the chief problems which handicap the pastoral industry of the country. For reasons of economy full details of the experiments carried out cannot be published, and only the results attained can be referred to in this report.

HORSE-SICKNESS. In the report from this division for 1915 it was stated that in the absence of suitable animals for experiments in connection with this disease, the Commandant General had placed at our disposal, on generous terms, horses recently imported as remounts for the police. At that time eighteen horses had been thus supplied. The system was continued during the present year and the results obtained were considered so satisfactory that it was decided to apply the process to horses already on the strength. Batches of six or eight animals were at first sent to the laboratory for inoculation, but later large numbers were stabled at the Police Headquarters Depot, Salisbury, and were treated there under a Farrier Sergeant Major and staff. In this way one hundred and fifty-six police horses were inoculated, with a loss of twenty animals. As these have been collected from all parts of the country and have been inoculated without regard for their age or condition it is felt that the death rate of 12.82 per cent is not excessive. The average age of those animals which have died, as shown by the police records, is eight years and nine months, but as aged horses when purchased are recorded as eight years old, the average is probably somewhat greater. The immunity of these horses when distributed and exposed to natural infection remains to be seen. Experiments have been conducted to determine the degree of immunity conveyed by this method. Three horses were taken, two previously inoculated and one as a control not previously treated; into each of them was introduced a quantity of virus taken from an animal which had died as the result of inoculation by Theiler's method. The control horse died on the sixth day while the two vaccinated animals remained unaffected. Again, police horse No. 092, inoculated in October, 1915, was brought in from Makwiro District during September and was given a quantity of the same deadly virus; no reaction followed.

Mules inoculated by Theiler's method have proved resistant to horse-sickness in most districts of Southern Rhodesia, and it is hoped that since vaccinated horses resist the virus used in protecting the mules, that they will enjoy a similar degree of immunity. Nevertheless, it is known that one virus differs from another and that the immunity against one may not necessarily hold good against infection from another, and thus it is anticipated that when inoculated police horses are distributed throughout the country many of them may become infected with a strain of virus peculiar to the district to which they are sent. This has been known to happen but past experience has shown that if this reinfection is detected and the animal is put by during the reaction its chance of recovery is considerably greater than that of an animal not previously treated. Thus the market value of an inoculated horse is increased and its usefulness for police purposes is considerably enhanced. During the year 1912-1913, of two hundred and seven police horses forty-five died of horse-sickness and in 1914-1915, of one hundred and ninety-three animals, forty-one died of the disease; as the present season bids fair to be exceptionally severe owing to the early and continuous rains, it is satisfactory to know that as many as one hundred and thirty horses are thus to a large extent protected against infection. It should be recognized that the inoculation of police horses in the first place was only undertaken with the object of carrying on certain experiments, and that the application of the process on a large scale was decided upon because of the excessive annual losses of police horses, which justified the operation so long as the inoculation death rate could be kept below a certain figure. The method, however, is by no means perfected, and much experimental work is still required to place the process upon a strictly scientific basis. Until the causal organism of horse-sickness has been identified and the many problems associated with it solved by careful research, any method of immunizing against it must rest upon a more or less empiric basis.

THE PLASMOSES OF CATTLE. The more general application of the principle of "short-interval dipping" has to a large extent reduced the losses due to these diseases, and at the present time there are farms to which cattle imported for the improvement of local herds can be introduced with safety without inoculation, and upon which the improved progeny grow up free from the tick-borne diseases. Although the advantages thus derived are great, it must be remembered that the dipped areas in the country are far exceeded by those where the principle is not carried out and ticks and the diseases transmitted by them are prevalent. Thus in practice there would appear to be three stages in the development of a herd: the first or pioneer stage, when imported animals cannot be used for the improvement of the nucleus of native cattle unless inoculated, and when a heavy mortality of young stock must be expected from redwater and allied diseases; a second stage when by systematic dipping the veld becomes tick-free and imported stock can be introduced with impunity and the young progeny grow up and thrive free from disease; and lastly the stage when the animals bred upon such areas, being susceptible to tick-borne diseases, cannot be exposed to tick-infested veld, so that the market for them becomes restricted. Therefore, in spite of the progress and advantages of systematic dipping there are certain disadvantages associated with it until the system becomes universally practiced. In the meantime there remains the necessity for a satisfactory method of inoculation for the protection of imported bulls exposed on infected veld, and of young stock born upon tick-free farms, in order that they may be disposed of with safety beyond the limit of such areas. During the past ten years efforts have been made to discover a satisfactory means of conveying immunity, but experiments have unfortunately been handicapped by the extreme cost of experimental animals which have of necessity to be imported from countries free from these diseases; but from time to time consignments of cattle have been imported by progressive breeders anxious to improve the class of cattle in this country and the veterinary department has been called upon to inoculate them to the best of its ability. Thus in 1911 ninety-four bulls were imported and were inoculated with a loss of 5 per cent only, but many of these were inoculated with a virus supplied from the south and did not prove immune when exposed to natural conditions. Others, inoculated with a local strain of virus, suffered more severely at the time of treatment, but subsequently proved immune. The utility of such animals is somewhat impaired during their first year in the country, but a record of many of them is available and shows that some of them have taken honors in the show ring, notably the bulls "Baronet" and "Aerial Knight", and a considerable number have been responsible for as many as two to three hundred progeny, of improved type and bearing the impression of the sire. Again, in 1912, about

sixty-eight animals were imported from overseas, twenty-five home-
bred animals died, but it should be pointed out that their owners
had been previously warned that such stock was unsuitable for inoculation on account of age, soft condition, pregnancy, or in-breed-
ing, and the inoculation was undertaken under protest.   Nevertheless, in spite of the heavy mortality the survivors have proved a
profitable investment, more than paying for the losses, the progeny
of some of the inoculated females having been sold for three figures.
In 1913 ninety-four cattle from Great Britain were inoculated with
a loss of twenty-seven; this mortality which took place during the
absence of the bacteriologist was probably due to some unaccounta-
ble exaltation in the strength of the virus used, and it was thought
wise to suspend further inoculations until the process could be
placed upon a safer basis.   Since then no privately owned imported
stock has been accepted for inoculation until October last, when
eleven animals were received for treatment at the laboratory, the
inoculation of which is not yet completed.   During the interval,
however, two small consignments of young cattle from England
have been imported for experimental purposes and different strains
of virus have been tested with the result that it is now hoped that,
given suitable animals and proper accommodation, the principle can
again be applied upon a large scale.   It has been abundantly proved
that to obtain the best results, animals submitted for treatment
shoud not be too fat or pampered, or too highly bred, and should
not exceed fifteen months of age.   The mortality among such animals
should be insignificant and recovery from the slight set-back caused
by the operation should be rapid.   Now that Rhodesia has, with her
limited supply of high-grade animals, entered the meat markets of
the world, no time should be lost in bringing up the bulk of her
stock to the same standard of excellence as that exhibited by the
sample consignments.

   TRYPANOSOMIASIS.   In January it was reported to the veterinary department that a large number of pigs were dying from some
unknown disease at two farms on the northern border of the Umfuli
River.   In one herd of one hundred and fifty as many as twenty pigs
had died, and a large number at the time were showing symptoms of
the disease, and in the second herd of about fifty pigs five had died
and many others were severely sick.   Examination of smears submitted from sick animals revealed large numbers of trypanosomes
of pecorum group, but differing slightly morphologically from the

trypanosome commonly met with in cattle in the Hartley District, notably in the fact that the body appeared more flexible and the undulating membrane more highly festooned, so that in fair specimens it was afterwards possible to distinguish the two by microscopic examination. One particular feature of interest in connection with the outbreak was that although the Hartley District has been known since the early days to be an area infested by' *Glossina morsitans*, no tsetse fly had ever been encountered in the particular position where this outbreak was occurring and there was every reason to fear that the disease might be transmitted by biting flies other than the tsetse, or by some other means. Such a possibility was alarming, since the experience and research of the past ten years has led to the conclusion that as far as the trypanosomiasis of animals in Southern Rhodesia is concerned, it is seldom if ever transmitted from sick to healthy in the absence of the tsetse fly. That certain forms of trypanosomiasis can be so spread is admitted, and examples have been met with in neighboring territories; but it would appear that in such instances certain conditions are necessary, which may almost be laid down as axiomatic, namely, an original source of infection, generally an animal infected by the tsetse fly; an abundance of trypanosomes in the peripheral blood of the animal; very close contact between sick and susceptible animals; a vast number of transmitting agents, and finally certain climatic conditions of warmth and humidity. These essential conditions are seldom if ever met with in Southern Rhodesia. In order to study this disease of pigs one or two infected animals were sent to the Laboratory. With the virus thus supplied experiments were undertaken to ascertain the nature of the parasite and its infectivity to domestic stock, its transmissibility other than by the bite of the tsetse fly, and to obtain as quickly as possible a means of treating and preventing the disease caused by it. It was found that this disease could easily be transmitted from pig to pig by artificial inoculation of small quantities of blood, giving rise to a disease rapidly fatal, killing untreated animals in less than thirty days. Small laboratory animals did not become infected even by repeated doses of virus from a natural case, and sheep and cattle exhibited a marked degree of resistance. Transmission experiments undertaken proved negative and a natural experiment showed that infection from sick to healthy was not readily effected by biting flies. At the laboratory sick and healthy were closely styed together and were continually pestered by swarms of stomoxys which were noticed to pass from one to the other. Nevertheless no infection of the healthy took place except by means of the syringe. Thus the manner in which so gross an infection can have been brought about under natural condition's remains to be shown. The problem of greatest importance to be solved was to find a means of protection and treatment. For several years the trypanosomiasis of Hartley cattle had been found to yield to massive doses of antimony and arsenic. But the former drug had to be carefully injected into the vein, because if it made its way under the skin it gave rise to severe abscesses and sloughs; it could not therefore be applied in the same way to pigs, and further, its beneficial effect upon bovine animals was largely due to their peculiar tolerance to antimony. It was necessary therefore to discover a form of the drug which could be administered to pigs without harmful effects and this was finally met with in a combination of emetic and arrhenal which was applied with most favorable results; but it has to be admitted that in the great majority of cases a complete cure was not effected but merely, as in cattle, a state of tolerance established, enabling treated animals to live in apparent health until adverse conditions reduced their resistance and once again the trypanosome reasserted itself and produced its harmful effects. Thus in one herd the results were most favorable and the disease was arrested so that the great majority of animals could be fattened off and disposed of, but in the second herd, where the owner failed to supply an adequate diet, the good results of the treatment were but temporary and most of the animals died. During the year a few experiments have been conducted in connection with other forms of trypanosomiasis; the appearance of *T. bruci* var *rhodesiense* in donkeys working at the junction of the Umfuli and Umnyati Rivers indicates that the distribution of this form of infection is greater than was supposed, and in view of the possible transmission of the parasite to man by *G. morsitans* and the invariably fatal disease set up, experiments were conducted with remedies for which success has been claimed by workers in European laboratories. The most important of these was that recommended by Daniels and Newnham in the Lancet, January 8th, 1916, page 102, who claim to have permanently cured a case of human infection with *T. rhodesiense* by subcutaneous injections of 30 minims of Martindale's solution (injectio antimoni oxidi) given subcutaneously twice a day. This drug, when applied to pigs infected with the small trypanosome of pecorum group, in the dose recommended, produced no appreciable effect. Martindale's solution is supposed to contain one hundredth of a grain of antimonious oxide in 1 c.c. of glycerine and water equal parts. Nevertheless infected pigs and sheep received quantities containing as much as 0.5 gm of antimonious oxide without harmful effect, but without beneficial results or apparent influence upon the course of the disease. An ox naturally infected received up to 2 gm of the salt in suspension but the parasites did not disappear from its blood and the animal died from trypanosomiasis six days after the last injection. The results with this agent were very disappointing, as difficulty was being experienced by the military authorities in passing animals through the fly-belts of Northern Rhodesia on their way to the northern frontier of operation, mules becoming infected and useless for transport work and fly-struck cattle proving unsuitable for human consumption. The use of tartar emetic, although beneficial, had its disadvantages owing to the difficulty in application and dangers of local injury, and it was hoped that if the tri-oxide of antimony was equally effective and could be applied subcutaneously in the form of a cream, it might take its place with advantage. Unfortunately experiments showed that the results obtained were by no means as good as those following the use of emetic, and the treatment could not be applied in practice.

DIPPING OF SHEEP. Reference may be made to an experiment carried out at the request of the Chief Veterinary Surgeon to ascertain the effects of ''short-interval dipping'' upon sheep and lambs. A small flock made up of thirty-nine sheep and lambs of mixed breeds, the majority being half-bred Persians, but six of long-wooled varieties, were purchased for the purpose. All these animals were in a most emaciated condition and suffering from fluke, wireworm, tape-worm and the nodular-worm of the intestines. It was with difficulty that they were driven from the farm from which they were purchased, to the laboratory. On the 5th of February dipping was commenced in Cooper's dip, one in three hundred strength, in which they were immersed three times in ten days; the strength of the dip then being increased to one in two hundred and fifty. Dipping was carried on regularly twice a week in this strength until the 16th of April, making nineteen dippings in all. During this period ten animals died, namely, four sheep (one wooled) and six lambs, these being the weakest of the flock. The rest of the flock improved markedly in health. The experiment was then discontinued but the result is still apparent in that the survivors are still alive and in the best of condition, and the ewes have given birth to lambs which have thrived and grown out in spite of the fact that most of them have been born during the dry season. The experiment was originally intended to determine to what extent small stock could be dipped with safety in areas which have to be freed from African coast fever. It is probable that such drastic measures could not be applied in a damp atmosphere, or to woolled varieties because of the damage to the fleece, but in practice this would not be necessary. The experiment, however, has gone further in affording support to the observation of officers in the field that dipping exerts a beneficial action upon sheep infected with worms. The results have been so remarkable that when opportunity arises further experiments of a more exact nature will be carried out.

CONTAGIOUS ABORTION. This disease has been detected by means of the agglutination test in several new centers during the year, and owing to the local peculiarities presented by it has caused some uncertainty as to the best means of dealing with it. The application of the pipette method of collecting blood has proved of great value in allowing specimens to be taken by laymen, which in the great majority of cases have arrived at the laboratory in a suitable condition for the test. In addition to quarantine, isolation, and the removal of the bull from the herd, vaccination has been practiced in several instances. The results reported by officers in charge of the outbreaks have on the whole been favorable, but whether these can be attributed to the vaccination or to the other measures adopted cannot be definitely stated. As the result of an investigation into the outbreak of this disease in the Marandellas District, D.V.S. Johnston reports upon the use of vaccine as follows: " * * * it will be noticed that on those farms where the cattle were treated with vaccine there have been no cases of abortion, whereas, on Mr. Bradshaw's farm, where only antiseptics were used, the abortion broke out again after a lapse of several months" * * * " * * * on Nua farm the cows aborted after being treated with corrosive sublimate solution, but after the vaccine treatment there have been no cases—unless the calf which was born and was never found, was a case." At a recent meeting of the Umvukwe Ranches Association the vaccine treatment was favorably referred to. As the result of experiments conducted by the Board of Agriculture in England, the protective inoculation of cattle against contagious abortion has proved successful when the vaccine has consisted of "massive" doses of living organisms, but equally good results have not been obtained when vaccines have been killed by heat. On the other hand, a certain firm of repute continues to issue a dead vaccine and claims good results from it. Although agglutinins are not identical with immunity they do to a great extent run parallel with it, and may be accepted as an index of the production of immune bodies in an organism. Experiments were conducted to test the relative value of (a) living vaccine, (b) carbolised vaccine and (c) vaccine killed by heat, from which it was found that a vaccine of *B. abortus* killed by extreme heat gave rise to a reaction almost as great as that produced by a living vaccine, but of a somewhat shorter duration. It would be unsafe to issue a living vaccine in this country where transport facilities are often primitive and where it is often impossible to determine whether an animal is pregnant or not; but since a small dose of vaccine killed by heat does cause a marked reaction it is probable that frequent injections of massive doses would prove efficacious. Unfortunately the number of veterinary officers to perform the operation in the "field" is limited and the maximum capacity for cultivation of the organism in this laboratory is at present about one hundred and fifty massive doses per mensem.

VARIOUS. A number of experiments have been conducted with material suspected to be poisonous, some supplied by the agricultural chemist for test upon laboratory animals and others sent in from the field. An outbreak of disease at Rusimbas Kraal, Chibi District, was at first suspected to be due to African coast fever, but when this diagnosis could not be supported by the microscopic examination of preparations, certain poisonous plants were suspected. One of these, a kaffir onion known as "Chitupatupa", used by natives for poisoning pools when catching fish, was incriminated, but large quantities did not set up any poisonous symptoms in test cattle. Similarly the root of a bush known as "mutsuri", used by the natives for the same purpose, proved harmless in comparatively large doses. An interesting case of tuberculosis was detected in a nine-year-old cow in a herd in the Umtali District; the mother of the animal died of the disease in 1913 and the grand-dam in 1911, both of them presenting lesions which in all probability were those of tuberculosis. The herd was tested with tuberculin and several animals were found to be tuberculous.

ACCOMMODATION. The inadequacy of the existing accommodation was pointed out in the annual reports of this division for the years 1913, 1914 and 1915, but has not yet been improved.

EXPENDITURE. Details of expenditure are given and show that exclusive of salaries, the work of the laboratory has been maintained at a cost of a little over $1500, and has been undertaken by the bacteriologist with the assistance of a lady clerk and a stockman.

----◆----

TWO NEW FLUKES FROM THE DOG*

MAURICE C. HALL, PH.D., D.V.M. AND MEYER WIGDOR, M.A.
Research Laboratory, Parke, Davis & Co., Detroit, Mich.

So far as we are aware, the only fluke reported from the dog in the United States is *Paragonimus kellicotti.* This fluke occurs in the lungs of dogs, cats and swine. Ward and Hirsch (1915) note that the worm was discovered in the lung of a dog from Ohio by Kellicott. They also note, regarding lung fluke: "Null stated casually that it occurs in dogs and cats from the Oriental quarters of San Francisco, but gave no further data regarding the parasites."

In a series of 300 dogs examined post mortem here at Detroit, we have found intestinal flukes in 7 animals (Nos. 122, 133, 134, 195, 229, 237 and 281). The flukes of these dogs belong to 2 different species. The 2 species of flukes appear to be undescribed, and we have accordingly created new species for them.

An examination of our flukes shows that they belong in the genus *Hemistomum,* but an examination of the status of this generic name, which is the one in common use, indicates that the name is not in good standing, and while we are reluctant to tamper with nomenclature, a proceeding which always invites criticism from some school of zoologists, we are even more reluctant to refer new species to genera which are without standing. According to Stiles and Hassall (1908), *Hemistomum* Diesing, 1850, has as its type species, by inclusion and by the first species rule, *H. alatum* (Goeze, 1782) Diesing, 1850. But Railliet (1896) has renamed *Hemistomum* Diesing, 1850 (not Swainson), proposing the name *Conchosomum* Railliet, 1896, with *C. alatum* as type species. However, a

----

*Read before the Zoology Section of the Michigan Academy of Science, March 29, 1918.

further examination of the extremely useful bulletin by Stiles and Hassall (1908) shows that the genus *Alaria* Schrank, 1788, has as its type, and only, species *A. vulpis,* which is a renaming of *Planaria alata* Goeze, 1782, the fluke which has been called *Hemistomum alatum* since the publication of that name by Diesing, 1850. In default of any earlier nomenclature affecting the status of the generic name *Alaria* Schrank, 1788, or the specific name *alata* of Goeze, 1782, it appears that the fluke from dogs and other carnivores in Europe should be known by the name *Alaria alata* (Goeze, 1782) Hall and Wigdor, 1918. This fluke has been assigned to the family Holostomidae E. Blanchard, 1847, and to the subfamily Hemistominae Brandes, 1890 (name used by Brandes on Plate 40 and overlooked by Stiles and Hassall, who credit this name to Braun, 1893), and the tribe Hemistomeae Brandes, 1890. Since the name of the genus on which the subfamily and tribe names are formed must be changed from *Hemistomum* to *Alaria,* the subfamily and tribe names must be changed to Alariinae and Alarieae.

These flukes belong to the Holostomata, or metastatic trematodes, those which develop without intermediate generations arising by asexual methods. Two larval forms develop and pass through an intermediate host.

The family diagnosis is as follows:

Family HOLOSTOMIDAE E. Blanchard, 1847.

Family diagnosis.—Holostomata: Oral sucker terminal or subterminal; ventral sucker usually but slightly developed. Behind the ventral sucker is a peculiar attaching apparatus, varying in shape in different species. The body is commonly divided by a cleft into an anterior and a posterior region. The sex organs are principally in the posterior region and have their common openings at the posterior end in a depression, opening dorsally, called the bursa copulatrix. The oral and ventral suckers, the attaching apparatus, and part or all of the highly developed vitellaria are in the anterior portion. The simple intestinal ceca are without diverticula and extend the entire length of the body. The uterus is but slightly contorted and contains only a small number of relatively large eggs, which develop in water. The adult worms occur in the intestine of mammals, birds and reptiles, rarely in fish and amphibia; the intermediate hosts are mammals, birds, amphibia, fish and mollusks.

Type genus.—*Holostomum* Nitzsch, 1819.

Subfamily ALARIINAE Hall and Wigdor, 1918.

Subfamily diagnosis.—*Holostomidae*: Forms with flattened anterior body portion, of which the lamellar lateral edges are strongly bent ventrally, forming a sort of sac with a long ventral aperture between these lamellar edges. The ventral sucker is often covered by the attaching apparatus and is usually not larger than the oral sucker or the pharynx. (The ventral sucker is lacking in at least one species). The attaching apparatus is in the form of a compact mass, often covering the greater part of the anterior body. The apertures of some glands are at the sides of the oral sucker. The genital cone and bursa copulatrix are notably developed only in exceptional cases. The opening of the bursa is constantly dorsal. Parasitic in birds and mammals.

Type genus.—*Alaria* Schranck, 1788.

Tribe ALARIEAE Hall and Wigdor, 1918.

Tribe diagnosis.—*Alariinae*: With the characters of the subfamily.

Type genus.—*Alaria* Schranck, 1788.

Genus *Alaria* Schranck, 1788.

Generic diagnosis.—*Alarieae*: Posterior portion of the body approximately cylindrical; anterior portion flattened and with its lateral borders curving toward the ventral surface. The ventral sucker is usually larger than the oral sucker. The attaching apparatus is a compact structure which often covers the greater portion of the ventral surface of the anterior part of the body, and may entirely or partly cover the ventral sucker.

Type species.—*Alaria vulpis* Schranck, 1788 (=*Planaria alata* Goeze, 1782, renamed, =*Alaria alata* (Goeze, 1782).

The fluke which we found in 4 dogs (1.33 per cent) of the series of 300 dogs is the larger of our two species and is most closely related to *Alaria alata*, the intestinal fluke from dogs and other carnivores in Europe. We propose for this species the name *Alaria americana*. The smaller of our two flukes, which we found in 3 of our 300 dogs (1.0 per cent), we propose to call *Alaria michiganensis*. The three species may be differentiated as follows:

KEY TO SPECIES OF ALARIA FROM THE DOG

1. No projecting structures at each side of the oral sucker; right testis bilobed, left testis irregular in outline but integral..*Alaria michiganensis*.
   Projecting structures at each side of oral sucker; both testes bilobed........2

2. Attaching apparatus covers the posterior portion of the ventral sucker;
   the field of the vitellaria extends to the ventral sucker; the ventral
   sucker slightly larger than the oral sucker.............*Alaria americana*
   Attaching apparatus distinctly posterior to, and not touching or covering,
   the ventral sucker; the field of the vitellaria in the median line all
   posterior to the anterior end of the attaching apparatus and to the
   oral sucker; the oral sucker larger than the ventral sucker....*Alaria alata.*

Part of the above key is based on Brandes' (1890) figures
and depends for its accuracy on the accuracy of those figures and
of our interpretation of them.

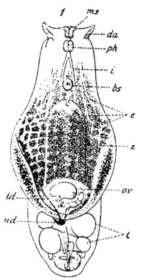

FIGURE 1. *Alaria alata.* Ventral view. *ms,* oral sucker; *da,* site of gland aperture; *ph,* pharynx; *i,* intestine; *bs,* ventral sucker; *e,* excretory system;
z, vitellaria; *ov,* ovary; *td,* transverse vitelline duct; *ud,* unpaired
vitelline duct; *t,* testes. Magnified. After Brandes (1890).

More extended descriptions of these species are as follows:
Species *Alaria alata* (Goeze, 1782) Hall and Wigdor, 1918.
Specific diagnosis.—Alaria: Flukes 3 to 6 mm. long (Fig. 1).
The posterior body much shorter than the anterior. The oral
sucker and pharynx quite distinct and each of them larger than
the ventral sucker. Some distance posterior of the ventral sucker
is the attaching apparatus, a high structure, notched anteriorly,
according to Brandes' figures, and with prominent lateral margins. The greater part of the vitellaria are contained in the attaching apparatus. In the median line there is a row of apparent

cavities, which are actually interruptions in the vitellaria and
which are bounded by the dorso-ventral anastomoses of the excretory system. (The cut for Fig. 1 has been tooled in a way that has
effaced the representation of these somewhat.) On each side of
the oral sucker is a crescentic projection and in these are located
the apertures of glands. There is a large bilobed testis on each
side of the posterior body. The ovary gives the appearance of being in the anterior body portion, owing to the fact that the lateral
lamellae of the flattened anterior portion unite on the ventral surface far back over the cylindrical posterior portion of the body,

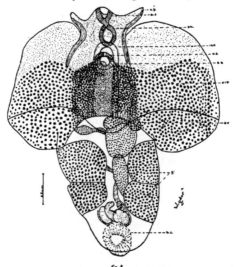

Fig. 2. *Alaria americana.* Ventral view. *a. p.,* anterior projection; *o. s.,* oral
    sucker; *ph.,* pharynx; *int.,* intestine; *v. s.,* ventral sucker; *a. a.,* attaching
    apparatus; *vit.,* vitellaria; *ov.,* ovary; *t.,* testes; *b. c.,* bursa copulatrix.

with the entire ovary anterior of the line of union, according to
the figure given by Brandes. The uterus and vas deferens open in
the middle of a small genital cone. The bursa copulatrix opens
dorsally, as in other species of this genus, and is relatively insignificant.

Hosts.—*Canis familiaris, Canis vulpes, Canis lupus, Canis
lagopus, Thoas cancrivorus,* and *Megalotis cerdo.*

Location.—Intestines and, occasionally, stomach.

Locality.—Europe. (Natterer is said to have collected it from
Thoas cancrivorus, which suggests that the fluke was collected in
South America).

Species *Alaria americana* Hall and Wigdor, 1918.

SPECIFIC DIAGNOSIS.—*Alaria*: Mounted specimens less than 3 mm. long (Figs. 2 and 5); live specimens appear to be between 4 and .5 mm. long. The posterior portion of the body appears to be shorter than the anterior, but owing to the contractility of the animal, the two parts may appear to be of practically the same length in some specimens. A transverse wrinkling of the cuticle of the equatorial region of the posterior body seems to be common. The oral sucker and pharynx are quite distinct, but their transverse diameters are less than that of the ventral sucker, contrary to the condition in *Alaria alata*. The ventral sucker is relatively

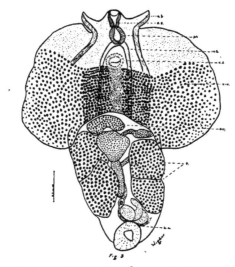

FIG. 3. *Alaria americana.* Dorsal view. Lettering as in Fig. 2.

well forward, less than its own diameter from the angle formed by the intestinal ceca, whereas the sucker in *A. alata* appears to be placed a distance distinctly greater than its own diameter behind this angle. The attaching apparatus is similar to that in *A. alata*, but the anterior end is smoothly rounded and does not show the notch which is figured for *A. alata* by Brandes (1890). In the median line of the vitellaria in the attaching apparatus, there are a series of apparent cavities, not presenting sharply defined, occasionally rectangular outlines as in *A. alata*, and usually 3 to 5 in number and not 9 in number as figured for *A. alata* by Brandes.

In the median line the vitellaria in flattened specimens extend
forward to the same transverse plane as the ventral sucker, the attaching apparatus extending slightly forward of the vitellaria
and partly covering the ventral sucker. In *A. alata*, the ventral
sucker is well forward of the anterior end of the attaching apparatus of the vitellaria in the median line. Specimens which have
curled up, apparently in response to some irritant stimulus, show
the attaching apparatus shoved forward till its anterior end is in
the vicinity of the oral sucker, the lateral lamellae of the anterior
body being folded over toward the mid-ventral line, and the posterior body being bent back in a way that tends to bring its dorsal

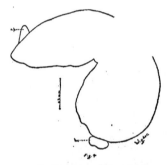

Fig. 4. *Alaria americana.* Outline view from side. *a. p.*, anterior projection;
b. c., bursa copulatrix.

portion in contact with the dorsal portion of the anterior body.
On each side of the oral sucker are crescentic projections as in *A.
alata*, presumably bearing the ducts of glands as the similar structures in *A. alata* are said to do. There is a large bilobed testis on
each side of the posterior body. The ovary appears to lie partly
anterior to and partly posterior to the line of union of the lateral
lamellar margins of the anterior body. The bursa copulatrix is
less than twice the diameter of the ventral sucker, whereas in *A.
alata* it is about three times the diameter of the ventral sucker,
according to Brandes' figures. The eggs in the uterus are 90 μ to
120 μ by 80 μ to 86 μ in diameter. Eggs from the feces measured
106 μ to 134 μ by 64 μ to 80 μ (Fig. 5). Other details of the reproductive system and other systems were not determined, as this
study was only incidental to other investigations which would not
permit of taking time for the work of making and mounting sections.

Host.—*Canis familiaris.*

Location.—Small intestine.

Locality.—Detroit, Michigan.

The largest number of *A. americana* found in one animal was 91 (in dog No. 281).

Species *Alaria michiganensis* Hall and Wigdor, 1918.

Specific diagnosis.—*Alaria*: Flukes 1.8 to 1.91 mm. long when mounted (Figs. 6 and 7). Posterior portion of body longer or shorter than the anterior portion, according to the state of contraction. The anterior portion of the body appears to be covered with minute, posteriorly-directed spines. Well developed oral sucker and pharynx. Oral and ventral suckers of approximately the same size, sometimes one and sometimes the other the larger. The attaching apparatus is usually immediately posterior of the ventral sucker in flattened specimens and has no notch anteriorly.

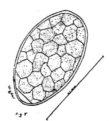

Fig. 5. *Alaria americana.* Egg from feces.

Occasionally it is considerably posterior of the ventral sucker and in a number of mounted specimens we are unable to detect an attaching apparatus. In the median line the vitellaria extend anterior of the ventral sucker to a point between the ventral sucker and the posterior end of the pharynx. There are no such apparent cavities in the median field of the vitellaria as there are in *A. alata* and *A. americana*. There are no crescentic projections on the sides of the oral sucker. The right testis is bilobed and lies transversely across the posterior body, extending across the median line in such a way that one lobe lies on the right side and one lobe lies on the left side of the worm posterior to the left testis. What appears to be the cirrus can be distinguished on the left side, connecting with the bursa copulatrix. The ovary lies somewhat to the left, instead of median, and is entirely posterior of the line of union of the lateral lamellar margins of the anterior part of the body. The transverse vitelline duct crosses to the right side near the union of the anterior and posterior body and the main vitelline duct extends along the right side of the posterior portion of the body and apparently crosses ventrad of the right testis to the left side, forming a dilation in the median line. The bursa copulatrix is more than twice the diameter of the suckers. The eggs in the uterus are 80 μ to 104 μ by 76 μ to 80 μ in diameter.

HOST.—*Canis familiaris.*

LOCATION.—Small intestine.

LOCALITY.—Detroit, Mich.

The largest number of *A. michiganensis* found in one animal was 80 (in dog No. 195).

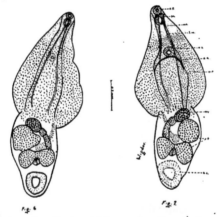

FIG. 6. *Alaria michiganensis.* Dorsal view.
FIG. 7. *Alaria michiganensis.* Ventral view. Lettering as in Fig. 2.

The resemblance between *Alaria alata*, the form described from Europe, and the species we have designated as *A. americana* is very considerable and the possibility of their being the same species should be given consideration. We find certain differences on comparison: Although the measurements overlap, *A. alata* appears to be larger as regards average size and maximum size. In *A. americana* the vitellaria in the median line and the anterior border of the attaching apparatus both lie in the transverse field determined by the antero-posterior diameter of the ventral sucker, whereas in *A. alata* the ventral sucker lies anterior of the forward end of the attaching apparatus, which in turn seems to extend well forward of the anterior limits of the vitellaria in the median line. This difference, the absence of a notch in the anterior margin of

the attaching apparatus, and a few other differences in relative
sizes of suckers, etc., make it unwise to claim the identity of the
European and American form. In this matter we follow the advice of Dr. Ch. Wardell Stiles, who considers it better to take a
chance on making a new species for an old one, where there is a
doubt, and assuming that an error will be pointed out and the new
name assigned its proper status as a synonym, than to record such
a doubtful finding under the name of an old species with which it
may easily be long confused and from which it will be very difficult to separate it if there is an error.

The measurements of mounted specimens of the two American
species of flukes are given in the following table, nothing of the
sort, except the body length of 3 to 6 mm., being known to us for
A. alata:

Structure	A. americana					A. michiganensis				
Entire body	1.16	mm. to 2.32	mm.	long		1.89	mm. to 1.91	mm.	long
Anterior body	0.69	mm. to 1.07	mm.	long		0.80	mm. to 1.17	mm.	long
	0.71	mm. to 1.95	mm.	wide		0.85	mm. to 0.94	mm.	wide
Posterior body	0.48	mm. to 1.25	mm.	long		0.72	mm. to 1.11	mm.	long
	0.65	mm. to 0.95	mm.	wide		0.85	mm. to 0.92	mm.	wide
Oral sucker	0.090	mm. to 0.137	mm.	diam.		0.086	mm. to 0.157	mm.	diam.
Pharynx	0.120	mm. to 0.196	mm.	long		0.142	mm. to 0.152	mm.	long
	0.080	mm. to 0.137	mm.	wide		0.118	mm. to 0.127	mm.	wide
Ventral sucker	0.070	mm. to 0.176	mm.	diam.		0.090	mm. to 0.176	mm.	diam
Bursa copulatrix	0.114	mm. to 0.245	mm.	diam.		0.088	mm. to 0.235	mm.	diam.

The flukes reported from the dog outside of North America
include the following: *Opisthorchis felineus*, *Opisthorchis caninus*,
Clonorchis endemicus, *Metorchis albidus* (?), *Pseudamphistomum
truncatum*, *Ascocotyle minuta*, *Ascocotyle italica*, *Loossia romanica*,
Heterophyes heterophyes, *Heterophyes aequalis*, *Heterophyes dis-
par*, *Isthmiophora melis* (?), *Echinochasmus perfoliatus*, *Dicro-
coelium dendriticum*, *Schistosomum japonicum*, *Yokagawa yokagawa* and *Hemistomum alatum*.

In passing it is of interest to note that Stiles and Hassall
(1894) report the presence of *Hemistomum alatum* in the collection of the U. S. Bureau of Animal Industry at Washington, D. C.,
but the material is European, not American. The specimens are
from Rudolphi's collection and probably have an historical interest
far greater than their scientific value for study after preservation
for a century; no effort was made to examine this material for
comparison.

BIBLIOGRAPHY

BRANDES, GUSTAV. 1890. Die Familie der Holostomiden. *Zool. Jahrb., Abt. f. Syst.*, v. 5 (4), 24, Dec., pp. 549-604, pls. 39-41.

RAILLIET, ALCIDE. 1896. Quelques rectifications à la nomenclature des parasites. *Rec. de Méd. Vét.*, v. 73, 8 s., v. 3 (5), 15 mars, pp. 157-161.

STILES, CH. WARDELL, and ALBERT HASSALL. 1894. A preliminary catalogue of the parasites contained in the collections of the United States Bureau of Animal Industry, United States Army Medical Museum, Biological Department of the University of Pennsylvania (Coll. Leidy) and in Coll. Stiles and Coll. Hassall. *Vet. Mag.*, Phila., v. 1, (4), Apr., pp. 245-253; (5), May, pp. 331-354.
———— 1908. Index-catalogue of medical and veterinary zoology. Subjects: Trematoda and trematode diseases. *Hyg. Lab. Bull.* (37), 401 pp.

WARD, HENRY B., and HIRSCH, EDWIN F. 1915. The species of *Paragonimus* and their differentiation. *Ann. Trop. Med. & Parasitol.*, v. 9 (1), Mar., pp. 109-162, pls. 7-11.

A NEW CENTER FOR VETERINARY RESEARCH

R. W. SHUFELDT, M.D.
Major, Med. Corps, U. S. Army; Membr. Anthropological Society of Florence; Corr. Membr. Zoöl. Soc. Lond., etc., Army Medical Museum, Washington, D. C.

It will be of interest to veterinarians to learn that very recently steps have been taken at the Army Medical Museum, of the Surgeon General's Office at Washington, to improve the status and further the interests of veterinary science in that institution. As in the case of so many activities, the present war is largely responsible for giving greater prominence to this important department of science. Our armies are using a great number of horses and mules, not only in the cavalry service, but as draught animals and for other purposes. It also becomes a matter of great importance that the veterinary department of the Government should bestow the strictest attention to the meats that are issued to our men and officers in France as well as in this country—a precautionary measure that is too obvious to require any debate in this place. Finally, we have come to use the dog in many capacities at the front, and dogs require that just as much care is bestowed upon them as do men, in that they may be kept fit for service and ready for duty at all times.

With these activities and necessities before the Government, it will be a surprise to no one to learn that, with the means so conveniently at hand, the required action was promptly taken to meet

what was so obviously demanded in the premises, in that efficiency
and the requirements of hygiene might be realized to the fullest
extent. To deal with the problems of practice and therapeutics, in
so far as they apply to the care of any one of our domestic animals,
it is clear that such an institution as an army medical museum can
undertake but certain steps in the matters of teaching and the exhibition of material, in that officers and men of the veterinary service may profit by what is placed within their reach.

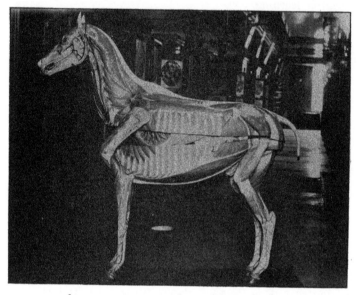

Fig. 1. Life-size manikin or model of a horse, manufactured by Auzoux
of Paris; muscles, organs, etc., all detachable. Circulatory system, etc., perfect.

This applies, however, with equal truth in the case of our own
species, be they civil or military subjects. By this is meant that a
medical museum fully serves its end when it has properly placed
on exhibition all the material that it can accumulate, and all that
its space will accommodate, which brings before the student and the
practitioner the morphology and physiology of the forms they
strive to maintain in as thoroughly healthy a condition as possible,
and render of the greatest service to their kind; these elements of
structure and function are likewise fully illustrated with respect
to their pathological condition. When these ends are met to the
fullest extent, there is but little left for a medical museum to do,

beyond thoroughly keeping abreast of the profession's advance, and offering all possible facilities for educational extension, through employing, for teaching purposes, all the material the institution contains.

This last statement is as true of veterinary science and its demonstrational material as it is of the corresponding collections as they relate to our own or any other species, when we come to apply it to the teaching of the professional branches of that department of learning.

We may now pass to a brief consideration of such specimens

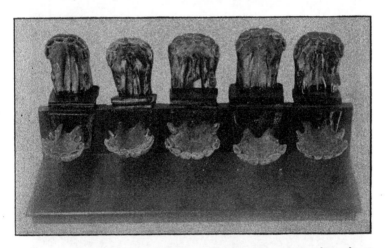

FIG. 2. A very ingenious contrivance to show the age of a horse by the teeth. Anterior parts of the actual maxillæ (upper and lower jaws) of five horses, so hinged that they can be shut together. Anterior teeth all perfect, the characters showing the ages of this animal at 11, 12, 16, 18 and 20 years. (Nos. 749-753.) Dr. Brailey, Vet. Surg., U. S. A., contributor.

as are to be found in the Army Medical Museum, and the facilities it offers for study and research work. In the first place, there are to be found in the library of this institution several hundred standard works, devoted to the various branches of veterinary science, while the reading room receives many of the leading journals on such subjects. These works are regularly loaned to veterinarians under the same rules and restrictions as are medical works to physicians and surgeons on our own species. Later on, when the proposed new Army Medical Museum becomes an accomplished fact, there will be dissecting rooms for veterinary students and practitioners, as well as facilities for microscopical and pathological research and case examinations; but it is a little too early to look for such advantages as these. When we turn to the collections, however, it will at once be appreciated that the museum has taken a long step in the direction of laying the foundation upon which to build up this part of the requirement for investigations in veterinary science.

One of the most expensive as well as one of the most useful specimens in the museum is that of a model of a horse, here shown

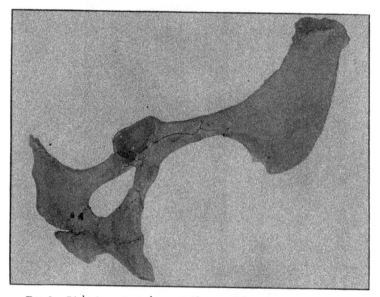

FIG. 3. Right innominate bone of a horse exhibiting a case of comminuted fracture, involving the acetabulum. Result of a fall. Animal was at once killed. (No. 9663.)

in Fig. 1. This is an Auzoux of Paris, and was purchased a long time ago. It occupies an entire special glass case all to itself, and is of the size of life. Nearly all of its anatomical parts are detachable, thus affording students and demonstrators opportunity to handle them separately. This does not apply to the superficial muscles and other parts exclusively, for the model is so constructed that it opens up entirely along the horizontal plane shown in the cut. When thus opened, all of the internal organs and viscera may be taken out, piece by piece, allowing the form and relations of each organ to be studied separately. A model of this sort is of some value when studied through the four sides of its big glass case; but it would be of far greater value were it used in a room where veterinary lectures on equine anatomy were being delivered regularly, and the class of students had the opportunity to take it apart. Such a lecture-hall will doubtless form a part of the proposed new

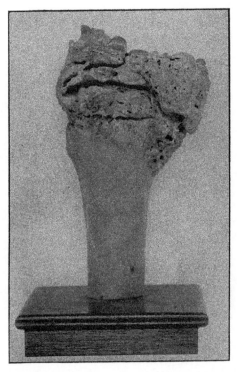

FIG. 4. Right carpal bones and proximal end of metatarsus, showing large exostotic growths. From a mare, age 15 years, which fell, injuring the joint. Synovitis ensued. (No. 10657.) Contributor C. B. Robinson, V.S., Washington, D. C.

building, and it should be a modern room with respect to acoustics, lighting, and size. It goes without the saying that such an auditorium or lecture-hall could be used for all lectures pertaining to the various activities that the institution exploits; in fact, no museum worthy of the name would in any way be complete without it.

We further find in the collections of the museum now being

considered many fine Auzoux models of separate organs of many different species of animals other than those of the horse. Not a few of these are several times their normal size and very perfect in their way. The increase of size is often of advantage; for, in the case of large audiences, those far from the lecturer's desk may be able to see the model and its smaller parts. Such a series of models should be sufficiently extensive to make necessary comparisons. For example, the stomach of a horse, a cow, a pig, and several carnivores, should all be thus compared and intercompared. Anatomy attains its full teaching value only when every structure is contrasted with the same structure of all animals in any way related to the one being described. Without this, philosophy gives way before the incomprehensive single-species method, which is now gradually being abandoned in centers of such instruction at all worthy of the name.

The teeth of horses have always held an important place in the study of the animal, particularly as they materially assist in determining the age of the species, which is an important factor in the marketing of horses, or the buying of a large number of them by the government for use in the Army. In Fig. 2 is given a device that fills a useful purpose in this matter, and one that is a good demonstration model for class work.

There are many specimens in the cases of a teratological nature, and these refer not only to the horse but to the majority of our domestic animals; they are wonderfully varied in character, and of great interest, especially those of the skull and the feet (polydactylism). Osteologically they are of value when compared with similar departures from the normal, as we find them to occur in our own species and among the lower types of mankind.

—Dr. Richard Ebbitt has removed from Grand Island to Papillion, Nebraska.

—Dr. G. H. Grapp has removed from Port Deposit to Baltimore, Md.

—Dr. T. E. Wilke has removed from West Plains, Mo., to Chicago, Ill.

—Dr. A. J. Dinse has been transferred from Warrenton to Hamilton, Ga.

SOME BLOOD-SUCKING FLIES OF SASKATCHEWAN

A. E. CAMERON, M.A., D.Sc.
Technical Assistant, Entomological Branch, Department of Agriculture

INTRODUCTION. Last summer (1917) the author in cooperation with Dr. S. Hadwen of the Health of Animals Branch, Department of Agriculture, made a preliminary survey of the blood-sucking flies affecting stock and man in the vicinity of Saskatoon. Because of other important investigations occupying their attention, including the study of bot-flies, and so-called "swamp fever" which causes serious losses among horses, the time allotted to the survey was necessarily limited. It is therefore proposed to discuss tentatively only a few of the more frequently occurring forms that were encountered within a radius of 50 miles of the city of Saskatoon, Sask. Inasmuch as the environmental conditions existing in this area are fairly representative of those throughout the southern half of the province, the remarks that follow will be found to be more or less applicable to the whole of this region, where wooded bluffs are relatively few and far between. In the northern territory, as yet unexplored by the author, it is not unlikely that in the more sheltered wooded districts, more favorable environmental conditions will prove such as ·to have an important bearing on the constitution of the fauna of blood-sucking flies, with a probable consequent greater fertility in species numbers. It could not but be remarked that the area studied yielded a surprising paucity of form especially of horse-flies, although in actual numbers their dominance could not be denied.

Attention was principally paid to the three families known as the Culicidae or Mosquitoes, the Simuliidae or Black-flies and the Tabanidae or Horse-flies, all of which have aquatic larvae.

MOSQUITOES.* Until Knab published his paper "Observations on the Mosquitoes of Saskatchewan", Smithsonian Miscellaneous Collections, Vol. 50, Pt. 4, 1903, pp. 540-547, very little was known about the prairie species or their habits. There still remains much to ·be learned. The great majority of the species of the prairie region of the northwest belong to the genus *Aedes*. These typically northern forms develop in the melting snow-water of early spring.

To some, the great abundance of the prairie mosquitoes has pre-

*The author desires to express his thanks to Dr. H. G. Dyar of the Smithsonian Institution, Washington, D. C., for kindly identifying the species of mosquitoes.

sented a puzzling question because of the comparative scarcity of water—essential to mosquito breeding—on the prairies during the summer months. There is only a single annual brood of prairie mosquitoes, and the adults are apparently long lived. The eggs are laid in the late summer on the ground where they remain until the following spring, when they readily hatch into "wrigglers" in the water produced from the melting snow. Many sloughs persist well into the summer, but frequent investigation during July and August failed to reveal the presence of larvae in these stagnant waters, the first and only generation having departed earlier. Knab, however, found the larvae in large numbers in alkali swamps and ditches in May and June (1907). In one or two instances *Aedes canadensis* Theob. and *Aedes sansoni* D. and K., were particularly prevalent in the immediate vicinity of these sloughs during July. Peculiar to swampy creeks and ravines opening into the Saskatchewan River one finds *Aedes mimesis* Dyar, *Aedes vexans* Meig., and *Aedes aesti-vali* Dyar, all of which are more or less persistent in their attacks on man. *A. canadensis* and *A. sansoni* were occasionally encountered in large swarms when disturbed from their shaded resting places among the grasses in these ravines.

The most widely distributed species on the prairies are *Aedes spenceri* Theob., *Aedes fletcheri* Coq. and *Aedes curriei* Coq. The first two are very prevalent around Saskatoon, and it is principally due to their vicious habits that the existence of the prairie inhabitants is rendered almost intolerable at times. They are rarely to be encountered in the towns, although they enter the porches of houses on the outskirts and attack the occupants. Their attacks on stock are equally troublesome, and the provision of protective fly-nets on horses is a wise precaution now generally adopted.

From the nature of the life-history facts here outlined, it will be readily imagined how difficult is the problem of mosquito control on the prairies. None of the species appear to undertake long migratory flights so that the problem is more or less a local one, but a local one of immense size. Undoubtedly, much could be accomplished in the vicinity of townships by oiling the temporary pools of the early spring wherever larvae are found. The judicious application of kerosene, crude oils of paraffin or asphaltum base will provide a surface film which will readily kill the larvae by suffocation as well as by their toxic properties. An alternative method, which has been employed in anti-mosquito work with great effect, is the application of a preparation known as "larvacide" manufactured according to the following formula:*

              Resin.....................150 to 200 pounds
              Soda (caustic)....................30 pounds
              Carbolic acid....................150 gallons

The product readily emulsifies in water, but unfortunately brackish or alkali waters render it inert. Combined with its marked toxicity, it has the advantage of cheapness, a fact which makes it preferable to the more expensive kerosene oil.

Sloughs near towns should be readily filled up with refuse wherever possible, the work to be accomplished during the summer and fall in preparation for the thawing of the following spring.

BLACK-FLIES. The virulence of the bite which the species of this family are capable of inflicting is in inverse ratio to their size. In different parts of the continent they are known variously as "buffalo-gnats", "turkey-gnats" and "sand-flies", but the designation of black-flies is by far the most suitable in that it is not so narrow in its content as the others, each of which emphasises one particular habit of a single or limited number of species.

In the early stages of their life-histories black-flies are aquatic and their gregarious, greenish-gray larvae may be found attached to stones in the rapids of streams and rivers. They maintain their position in spite of the current by means of a suctorial disk at the posterior end of their body, and by means of the peculiarly adapted head-fans they contrive to sweep minute vegetable organisms such as diatoms and desmids into their mouths. Should they, by any chance, become dislodged from the security of their position, they have the power of secreting a silk-thread. By fixing it to a stationary object, the chances of their being washed downstream before they encounter another suitable anchorage are considerably decreased.

Before pupating the larva spins a closely-woven, slipper-shaped cocoon, open anteriorly. It is securely fixed to the stones, and the thread-like breathing filaments are exposed.

The velvety black-flies lay their eggs on the exposed surfaces of stones or weeds, and some penetrate beneath the surface to deposit their eggs on the water-washed surface of stones. The whole life-history occupies a period of about six weeks.

---

*Le Prince, J. A., and Orensteen, A. J., Mosquito Control in Panama, New York, 1916, p. 174.

We were able to witness how intense is the annoyance and injury inflicted on cattle by the persistent and tenacious attacks by myriads of these black-flies. At the beginning of July, the species most abundant was *Simulium similis* Mall. On the evening of July 4 some cows staked out on the prairie in close proximity to the Saskatchewan River and not more than two miles from Saskatoon, were observed to be straining on their tethers and lowing pitiably. A closer view revealed the presence of dense swarms of this species, which extended all round the animals for at least eight to ten yards. The animals were very restless, and a close examination revealed the fact that on their forequarters, abdomen, and udders, the flies were congregated in dense masses and were distended with blood. On these regions the skin was broken, and blood oozed from innumerable punctures. The flies were also entering the nostrils, ears and eyes.

The damage caused by black-flies results from their painful bites and the loss of blood which ensues. They have frequently been guilty of inflicting extensive losses among livestock, but so far have not been incriminated as vectors of disease-causing organisms. At Duck Lake in Saskatchewan it was stated on good authority that in 1913 about 100 head of cattle died from the attacks of black-flies. The first swarms are generally in evidence about the beginning of June, and the infestations may recur at intervals as late as September and October. One witness testified to the pungent, mustard-like taste of the flies.

The Saskatchewan River, the only apparently suitable water for the breeding of black-flies, is six miles distant from Duck Lake and there is little doubt but that the flies either voluntarily or compulsorily undertake migratory flights which carry them long distances from their places of breeding. Probably they are assisted in this by mild, favoring breezes.

At the present time the only measure of control that commends itself is either to burn "smudges"—which many farmers do—and thus ward off the flies from the animals by the resulting dense smoke, around which they congregate for protection, or to dress their coats with some disagreeable preparation of oil or grease. Fish oil alone or in combination with other strong-smelling substances is one of the best repellants. A mixture* consisting of three parts of fish oil

---

*Washburn, F. L., Diptera of Minnesota, Bulletin N. 93, Agr. Exper. Sta., Univ. Minn., 1905, pp. 75-76.

and 1 part kerosene spread over sores gives excellent results. In smearing animals with the various strong-smelling oils care should be taken not to use machine oil or other powerful oils, the repeated application of which tends to remove the hair. The dressing should be renewed once a day in the fly season.

The most satisfactory means of control would be to kill the larvae in the streams, but in large rivers the practicability of making any extensive application of toxic substances is out of the question. Further, the danger to stock and human beings, who may use the treated water, must be duly emphasized. In some experiments recently carried out with Phinotas oil** in streams, it was found that a film of oil may be found upon stones 48 hours after application, and the black-fly larvae may be killed one-eighth of a mile below the point of application.

A small stream which drains a swampy area and debouches into the Saskatchewan River, about 3 miles south of Saskatoon, was found to contain the larvae of three different kinds of black-fly and, in this particular instance, treatment with Phinotas oil would have supplied the necessary remedy.

HORSE-FLIES. The flies belonging to this family are also variously known as breeze-flies, clegs and deer-flies. The name, however, by which the larger horse-flies of the prairies are most generally known is "bull-dogs", which conveys some idea of their pertinacious biting habits. The adults frequent marshy places and are commonly encountered in the vicinity of sloughs in large numbers. Here they lay their eggs on the leaves of aquatic plants, and the larvae inhabit the muddy bottoms and margins of these ponds. The larvae are carnivorous, preying upon slugs, worms and the larvae of other insects, whilst in captivity they do not hesitate to devour their own kind.

The most prevalently occurring species in the environment of Saskatoon is *Tabanus septentrionalis* Loew., which is extremely variable in its coloration and size. It was our experience that this species displayed a marked tendency to seek shade. When an automobile was stationed near a slough with the cover up, they swarmed around it in large numbers, circling it in rapid flight and finally entering and resting on the roof or on the mud-guards and sides

---

**Phinotas oil is a preparation made by the Phinotas Chemical Company of New York and is a powerful larvacide. The great objection to its use is that fish also succumb to its poisonous properties. It costs about 40 cents per gallon (Smith, J. B., Mosquitoes of New Jersey, Trenton, N. J., 1904, pp. 128, 129).

outside. By the same token, they were often found at rest on the outside walls of dwelling-houses and inside on the windows, associated with *Tabanus illotus* O. S., and *Tabanus hirtulus* Bigot. In lesser numbers *Tabanus phaenops* O. S., *Tabanus rhombicus* O. S., *Tabanus cantonis* Marten, and *Tabanus epistatus* also occurred.

None of these species were found to be aggressive in their attitude to human beings, but they were persistent in their attacks on horses and cattle grazing on the prairies. The provision of fly-nets for horses at work is ample protection against these flies.

Of the genus *Chrysops*, all of which have pictured wings, *Chrysops moerens* Walk. and *Chrysops fulvaster* O. S. were the only two species found during the summer. Around the sloughs near Dundurn the former was very common. In the grass at the margins of these sloughs, they were readily disturbed as one walked along and they were not slow to attack human beings. The latter was only encountered in low, swampy ground and was taken in large numbers. It does not hesitate to attack those who intrude in its preserves.

The delicate, grayish-black breeze-fly *Haematopota americana* O. S., with grayish pictured wings, is occasionally found around horses and readily settles on people in the vicinity. In its flight it makes very little noise and it is very quiet and unobtrusive as it settles to bite.

For those horse flies which attack the ears of horses nets will be found useful as a protection. In case where the eyes are also attacked, the ears and skin about the eyes may be smeared with the following repellant solution as recommended in Bull. No. 93, Agr. Exper. Station, Univ. Minn., 1905: Pine tar one gallon; kerosene or fish oil, or crude carbolic acid one quart; powdered sulphur two pounds. This mixture, also, applied to wounds made by barbed wire or otherwise, will ward off those flies which might be disposed to lay their eggs therein.

In Russia, Portchinsky* has taken advantage of the habits of

---

*Portchinsky, L. Tabanidae and the Simplest Methods of Destroying Them. Memoirs of the Bureau of Entomology of the Scientific Committee of the Central Board of Land Administration and Agriculture, Petrograd, Vol. II, No. 8, 1915. Abstract in Rev. App. Entom., Ser. B., Vol. III, 1915, pp. 195-196, 1916.

Dr. L. O. Howard, Bureau of Entomology, Washington, D. C., was the first to attract attention to Portchinsky's discovery in "A Remedy for Gadflies: Portchinsky's Recent Discovery in Russia, with Some American Observations". This was published in Bulletin No. 20, Division of Entomology, United States Department of Agriculture, 1899. The Russian author had previously published an account of his findings this same year.

horse-flies of concentrating in damp places and near pools at which they drink. He found that during the heat of the day the flies rapidly skim the surface of the water in order to drink, only the underside of their bodies touching the water. Very good results were obtained by pouring kerosene on the surface of these pools of stagnant water, and it was found that these "pools of death", as he called them, soon became covered with the dead bodies of horse-flies which frequented them. Contact with the kerosene, which adhered to their bodies, rapidly poisoned or suffocated the flies. The author advocates the use of "pools of death" in pastures where cattle graze, but they should always be securely fenced off.

In Canada, Mr. Norman Criddle of the Entomological Branch, Manitoba, made independent observations and experiments in 1914 and 1916 in Manitoba similar to those of Portchinsky in Russia. In 1914 he noticed the habits which horse-flies display of making rapid, skimming flights along the surface of exposed water. Like the Russian author, too, he found that the great majority of the flies that thus behaved were males, only a small percentage of females coming to drink at open water. In experiments covering a period of 5 days in a pool but one square metre in surface area, Portchinsky counted in all 1967 horse-flies, of which only 14 per cent were females.

My thanks are due to Professor J. S. Hine, Ohio State University, who kindly confirmed the identification of some of the specimens of horse-flies and also named others about which there was some uncertainty.

—Veterinary Inspector D. B. Pellette has been transferred from Oxford, Ala., to Colfax, La.

—MAKING THE CATTLE TICK HOOVERIZE. While civilians are depriving themselves of meat, so that our soldiers and our allies may have sufficient meat rations, the cattle tick is also compelled to give up his continuous meal of cow blood in counties doing Tick Eradication work.

During the past month 698 vats were used and 275,000 cattle dipped for ticks in South Texas. Every tick gotten rid of by the dipping means that much blood saved for beef production.

—The marriage of Miss Lois Mary Smith of Columbus, Ohio, to Dr. J. P. Scott of Manhattan, Kansas, is announced. Dr. Scott is on the staff of the Veterinary College at Manhattan.

ORGANIZING AND CONDUCTING STATE-WIDE TICK ERADICATION IN LOUISIANA

ERNEST I. SMITH, D.V.M.
Inspector in Charge, B. A. I.
Baton Rouge, Louisiana

On July 25, 1917, Hon. Ruffin G. Pleasant, the distinguished Governor of the State of Louisiana, signed and approved one of the greatest constructive measures ever passed by any legislative body. It is known as Act No. 25, Senate Bill No. 10, by Senator Norris C. Williamson, under the caption as follows:

AN ACT

To provide for the eradication of the Texas fever carrying tick, commonly known as the cattle tick, (Margaropus annulatus); to provide for the expenses of conducting and carrying out said work in the State of Louisiana; to provide process to compel compliance by Police Juries and the members thereof with the provisions of this Act; and prescribing the manner in which Live Stock Sanitary Inspectors shall be appointed and compensated; defining their duties and fixing the authority of the Louisiana State Live Stock Sanitary Board relative to cattle fever tick eradication in the State of Louisiana, and to provide penalties for the violation of this Act; and to repeal Act 127 of the General Assembly of Louisiana for the year of 1916; and all laws or parts of laws in conflict with this Act.

During the time the bill was on trial before the agricultural committees of the Senate and the House, planters, cattlemen and others in the State hastily sent to their various law-makers a flood of telegrams urging them to make a favorable report, which proved beyond a reasonable doubt that the majority were desirous that such an indictment be drawn against the tick sufficient to insure that no competent jury could ever succeed in returning a verdict of acquittal. The language in the Act had been carefully phrased to affect every parish in the State, in the event those already released should become reinfested. However, it directly affected forty-two new parishes which, heretofore, had never taken any official action along the lines of tick eradication.

The proper legislation was finally enacted, and it specifically stated that all parishes must be equipped with sufficient number of

vats and chemicals to commence systematic tick eradication by April
1, 1918. The gigantic wheels of progress began to revolve, and in
order to smoothly pave the highway of success in advance, it became
immediately imperative for Dr. E. P. Flower, Secretary and Executive Officer of the Louisiana Live Stock Sanitary Board and the
Bureau forces to make a survey of every one of the forty-two new
parishes, meet their governing bodies on scheduled dates and explain to them the fundamental principles of the law. Notably, their
part in the undertaking; what the State would do, and what would
be the attitude of the United States Bureau of Animal Industry.
This procedure was a campaign within itself which forced many fat
mileage books to swiftly fall away into two thin pasteboard covers.

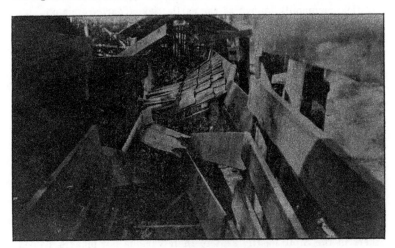

FIG. 1. A miscreant dynamites a dipping vat
Photographed by C. F. Lipp

In the meantime, executive bodies summoned our assistance, and in
a number of instances, special sessions were called for the purpose
of conserving time. We were extended a cordial reception by each
local executive board and, as a result of the conference, they immediately made arrangements for a liberal appropriation to build vats,
purchase chemicals and provide for local inspectors to work under
the direction of the federal supervising inspector.

In the early winter, many of the parishes began to call for a
leader to aid them in locating the vats and explain the details of
construction. Then an efficient Bureau organization had to be as-

sembled and systematized to meet the requirements in order that every parish might have close individual supervision including fifteen other parishes which had carried on the work in 1917 under a local ordinance with not the highest degree of efficiency.

In November, 1917, vat building made a small but healthy start and so continued until it reached the climax, when during the month of April, 1918, alone, the various parishes over the State, both by cooperative labor and the contract system constructed, complete, ready for instant operation, eight hundred and twenty-seven dipping vats. Adding this number to those which had been previously constructed and to those which have been built since May 1st, makes the splendid total of about five thousand for the entire State.

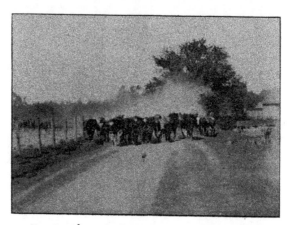

FIG. 2. Along the dusty road to the dipping vat

In consequence of this great number of vats, chemicals have been purchased by all the parishes equivalent to about one hundred and fifty tons of white arsenic.

The machinery has now speeded up to the point where the Bureau has sixty-five employees in Louisiana consecrated to the service of tick eradication, and the State and parish furnish between six and seven hundred more. The State-wide law did not become effective until April 1st, 1918, but notwithstanding that fact, our records show 250,000 dippings under supervision during the month of March and in April the figures leaped to 1,700,000 with the machinery running smoothly and capable of trebling the load. As horses and mules harbor the tick, they were not overlooked and many of them took their regular swim through the vats with the usual joy of satisfaction.

In one parish a few miscreants from the piney woods resorted to dynamite to help the cause along, but their un-American, cowardly tactics precipitated a reaction which resulted in the Chief Executive of the State informing the local officials to prosecute to the

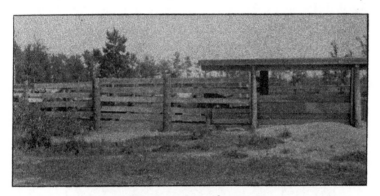

FIG. 3. Ready to plunge in

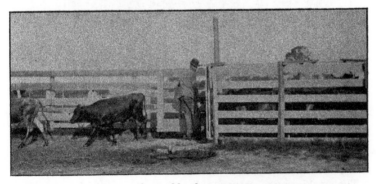

FIG. 4. Thoroughly cleansed to the skin

limit any individuals who exhibited an ugly face toward tick eradication by cooperating with dynamite. Act No. 68 passed by the 65th Congress played an important part, in that it forbade any individual from having in his possession explosives, except he be licensed accordingly by the federal government.

The busy season has arrived and soon after sunrise if one were in the proper place, large herds of cattle could be observed hurrying along the dusty road to their semi-monthly bath, and when they arrive there is little left to do but head them toward the chute leading to the dip where they will plunge in safely, one after another with accurate precision and finally come out of the dripping pen at the other end of the vat thoroughly cleansed to the skin and the tick

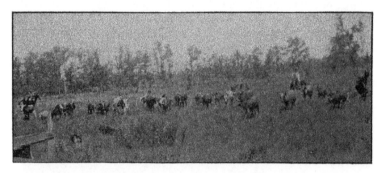

FIG. 5. Free rangers from the piney woods

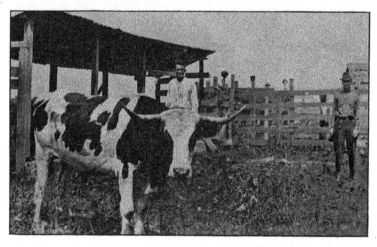

FIG. 6. With horns too broad to dip

administered a powerful toxic dose, sufficient to kill it within the next forty-eight hours.

The vast areas of cutover pine lands in Louisiana furnish excellent grazing for thousands of cattle and to the student and lover of nature it is interesting to hear the first faint tinkle of bells somewhere in the dense woodland. Finally, the medley becomes louder, sounding like a thousand bells of all dimensions attached to so many wild beasts of the jungle. Suddenly the free rangers break out into the open and, with the horseback riders in the rear, leisurely wend their way to the vat pens for the ultimate purpose of breaking the long, uninterrupted game of extortion played by the tick in its annual toll of death.

In a State-wide campaign of cattle dipping it would, indeed, be very exceptional if we were unable to find a steer with natural instruments of defense too broad to permit him to pass through the vat without his horns becoming locked between the walls. He is a

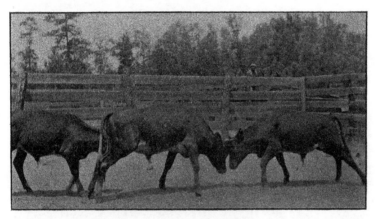

Fig. 7. Two native gladiators

descendant of the early bovine settlers of Texas when the cattlemen bred largely to horns and head. Nevertheless his generous equipment of horns does not permit him to escape the treatment; he is placed in the dripping pen, given a good shower bath and, as a result, he apparently craves to be normal so he could follow the regular procession through the vat.

In the common cause to eliminate the dreaded cattle tick the regular herding of cattle for each dip day has its perplexities and amusements. The man who rides all day through thick bushes, shrubs, and sharp briars, in and out of the almost impenetrable jungles and finally lands his cattle at the vat by nightfall, deserves much credit and consideration. It is an undertaking that will, temporarily, ruffle the most gentle disposition. However, after dipping and the day's work is completed, the humorous side may present it-self, as it is not an infrequent sight to see two native gladiators from the piney woods, with their referee, striving to decide who shall be master of the open range for the next two weeks.

Tick eradication this year in Louisiana is, undoubtedly, the most gigantic undertaking ever inaugurated by the Bureau in any one state. Previously, the opportunity to do any preliminary work had not presented itself and, as mentioned above, forty-two new parishes had never spent a single dollar from their treasury to build vats for the purpose of educating the people to the advantages of dipping. After all, the people throughout the entire state had ab-sorbed considerable knowledge about the tick, either from the press, or listening to others discuss the situation. In this connection it may appear that Louisiana has exploded the theory that years of preliminary effort is necessary before systematic work can com-mence, but the fact must be remembered, and ever kept vividly be-fore the eye, that the Pelican State has a distinguished leader in veterinary science who has never lost an opportunity to show the great commonwealth how they could better their sanitary condi-tions. Dr. W. H. Dalrymple has contributed his full share toward preparing the way for state-wide tick eradication and to him the people owe much, much more than they can ever repay.

The only practical solution of tick eradication is a State-wide act, and after its passage, it is amusing to note how quickly some of the most backward parishes will meekly fall in line and be the strongest cooperators. If the existence of the tick is left to local option, scattering territory can only be cleaned up, which leaves annoying border lines to contend with, and a mass of obstinate peo-ple no stronger for the work than in the beginning. When the tick is a menace to all the country, no class of ignorant and prejudiced citi-zens should be delegated the power at the ballot box to decide the destiny of the cattle industry.

—Dr. V. W. Knowles, formerly of Little Rock, Ark., has taken up veterinary practice at Livingston, Mont.

—Veterinary Inspector H. T. Juen has been transferred from Chicago, Ill., to El Paso, Texas.

—Dr. V. H. Knutzen has removed from Cleveland, Miss., to Chi-cot, Ark.

DIPLOMACY IN THE FIELD*

EDWARD HORSTMAN, Veterinary Inspector

Diplomacy in the field, or diplomacy in any branch of industrial life, is characterized by special tact in the management of affairs. We cannot all hope to excel in this quality, because we may not be sufficiently skilled in the art of handling men and affairs, but an inspector in the field has a wonderful range for using good judg-ment or tact if he will stop to study the man he is attempting to persuade to dip his cattle.

There are two sides to tick eradication work. The mechanical side consists of building vats, making solutions and dipping cattle, and if there is no opposition to the dipping everything goes along smoothly and satisfactorily. However, where opposition arises, there is need of action of some sort. The first impulse is to resort to the law and make the objector dip. Some inspectors have a motto of "dip or affidavit", but that is not the wisest plan to follow in any instance. An inspector who cannot differentiate between the ob-stinate anti-dipper and the one who merely lacks knowledge of the benefits and necessity of dipping will not prove a success as an in-spector. We must not forget the fact that none of us are infallible, and that the cattle owner has his own ideas, sometimes peculiar, no doubt, but he is entitled to an opinion, and it is up to the inspector to dislodge him from his false notions about not dipping. His opin-ion should be respected, but he should be told that in justice to him-self he should first recognize the facts as regards the ultimate aims of tick eradication and so leave his mind open to conviction before he comes to a final conclusion.

It must be remembered that not so very long ago the Southern plantation owner was practically a king on his own plantation, and that feeling in a measure is still present, consequently nothing is so obnoxious to the Southerner as to be told or made to feel that he must do certain things which he considers unnecessary. Compulsion grates on his nerves, so, as an inspector, it is wise diplomacy to get away from force as far as possible and to picture by alluring words the benefits of eradication of ticks, the upbuilding of the cattle in-dustries, increased prices and the cessation of dipping when the last

*Address delivered at the meeting of Inspectors on Tick Eradication at Shreveport, La., May 18, 1918.

tick is gone. Boil down the facts and present them in a simple, unbiased way. Gain the man's confidence, friendship and respect, but do not fight him.

If there is no hope of converting the objector to your way, then proceed in a businesslike manner to apply the forces of the law at your command without unnecessary fuss. Have your evidence clear and clean-cut; don't go off half-cocked and wonder why you didn't get a verdict. You must bear in mind you are a stranger in a strange land, that the man on trial is among his boyhood friends and that you, yourself, must stand well in the community before you can hope for success. The inspector's personal deportment in the community often has a great deal to do with the outcome of cases brought before a jury.

Inspectors sometimes unthinkingly make indiscreet remarks in conversations which are carried to all parts of the country like a wireless message. I know of a case where an inspector inadvertently made a remark in a certain county where everything was going well up to that time, but after that it was Sherman's application to war.

Nothing great was ever achieved without enthusiasm. A successful inspector must be enthusiastic, he must be level-headed, he must be energetic. The things that usually hold back tick eradication are the indifferent local inspector (the lazy man), the incompetent local inspecor (too old for any use), and the skeptical owner (the "personal liberty" man).

What is this personal liberty? It is the benighted idea of some anti-dippers who have a total disregard for law and order and consider that their "personal rights" should be the law of the land and not what the statutes provide. Such a person is commonly termed a knocker, who always imagines himself a crowd, and is usually found at meetings to ask such questions as "What's good for hollow horn?"

The answer to the personal rights man is that he has not only rights but plain duties to perform as well, and that the right sort of a man will pay more attention to his duties than he does to his rights.

I remember while making a trip in Marion County, Miss., I laid special stress on cooperation and copartnership in tick eradication. One very old gray-haired citizen opposed to dipping got up and said: "That reminds me of the story of two men who went into copartnership on a day's hunt. They were to divide what they got that day. Well, all they killed was a turkey and a buzzard. So, when the dividing time came, they argued about who should have the turkey, but you know, in the end, someone got that buzzard, and that's the way this tick eradication is going to turn out."

It was up to me to say something, so I said: "You didn't say who got the buzzard in your story, but I'll tell you in my story that the tick has been getting the turkey for years, and there's plenty of evidence that the buzzard is always hovering around the house of the cattle owner that harbors ticks."

Every inspector is a necessary cog in the wheel to the success of tick eradication—he may do much to mar the work, and he may be a powerful help in its prosecution. The greatest success of an inspector depends largely on the ability he shows in prosecuting the work and "handling the people". If he knows his business, there need be no fear of his gaining the confidence of the cattle owners, and thus his work will be considerably lightened.

———◆———

CLINICAL AND CASE REPORTS

REPORTS OF CASES OF HEMORRHAGIC SEPTICEMIA*

W. S. FERRAND

I have been asked to report two or three experiences with hemorrhagic septicemia which I have had in the last year and a half.

CASE No. 1. A bunch of steers a year and a half to two years old were shipped from Kansas City, and on arrival two of them were noted to have a bloody diarrhea with quite a high temperature. No positive diagnosis being made the owner did nothing for a few days until one or two of his cows showed symptoms, and one cow suddenly died. I called Dr. L. E. Willey from Ames in consultation. Dr. Willey came that evening, we made a post mortem examination, and upon microscopic examination found the hemorrhagic septicemia organism. Vaccination was advised and serum secured from Iowa State College. We took the temperatures of all the cattle and found four or five running quite high. Serum was used for those

———

*Presented at the 30th Annual Meeting of the Iowa Veterinary Association, Iowa State College, Ames, Iowa, January, 1918.

running a high temperature, and vaccine for those which were apparently healthy. None were lost after treatment. Three animals had been lost before treatment.

CASE No. 2. Sixty head of steers were shipped from St. Paul, originating somewhere in Canada. They were on the road quite a number of days before arrival here and whether they were infected through the stockyards at St. Paul or elsewhere I do not know. Upon arrival three showed a lagging gait and a little diarrhea. These three cases were running quite a high temperature, with labored breathing. Two of them had quite a diarrhea, one showed no diarrhea, but had a bloody discharge in the feces. I telephoned for serum and used serum on the three that were running a high temperature. The rest of the herd was treated with vaccine, with no further losses.

CASE No. 3. A herd consisting of 60 calves was shipped from Kansas City. They were unloaded, one was sick, and another had to be hauled home. The owner let them go about two days. Upon being called I made a diagnosis of hemorrhagic septicemia and immediately secured serum and vaccine from the college. When I took the temperature four or five of them were running a temperature, but showed no other clinical symptoms. These were given serum and the remainder the vaccine. They all came through in nice shape.

DISCUSSION

DR. W. A. HECK: I have not had a great deal of experience with hemorrhagic septicemia, but have had a few cases in cattle coming out of Omaha and Kansas City stock yards and shipped to our section of the country. I have had excellent results in the treatment of hemorrhagic septicemia with the bacterins furnished by the biological manufacturers. I have never used any of the serum. I have also had good results from the use of bacterins in cases in which the disease was considerably advanced. In these cases I administered the bacterins several days apart, say once a week, and the animals recovered. I do not know whether or not I would have had better results with the serum.

I have had some cases in horses which I thought were septicemia, and I had some correspondence with and sent some specimens to Dr. Chas. Murray of Ames and he verified the diagnosis. He was not sure it was the primary cause of the disease, but thought it was probably secondary. The lesions found on post mortem examination were characteristic, and the microscope verified the diagnosis.

In one case an insurance company had insisted, before paying the loss, that a post mortem examination be made to ascertain the cause of death. Post mortem examination disclosed hemorrhagic septicemia. I sent a specimen to Dr. Chas. Murray for examination, and the diagnosis was confirmed.

DR. W. S. FERRAND: I would like to ask any of the members whether they have seen hemorrhagic septicemia in hogs. This fall I was called to see some hogs which were shipped in vaccinated. Thirty days after vaccination two hogs in one herd died suddenly, and I was called to make a post mortem examination. These hogs had been eating regularly and were apparently in good health but on going out to look at them in the afternoon two were found dead. On post mortem examination I found hemorrhages all through the intestines and in practically all the organs. I would like to know whether any of the members have found hemorrhagic septicemia in hogs.

DR. F. A. HINES: I would like to ask Dr. Ferrand if he found any lesions in the lungs.

DR. W. S. FERRAND: We did not find any marked lesions of the lungs.

DR. H. B. TREMAN: I would like to hear from Dr. Chas. Murray or from any other member in regard to the length of immunity that is conferred by the use of bacterins in hemorrhagic septicemia.

DR. CHAS. MURRAY: The immunity is of short duration. We have had cases of recurrence of the disease twelve to fifteen days after treatment where we had no reason to believe that infection existed in these animals at the time of treatment. In experimental animals immunity will hold as long as seven months. We have immunized rabbits with the simultaneous treatment, giving a live culture and protecting this with serum at the same time, and conferred immunity for seven months, and then used them in the ordinary course of work in the laboratory; in cattle the immunity is apparently of short duration.

DR. W. P. BOSSENBERGER: In speaking of hemorrhagic septicemia in hogs, we have had considerable to deal with in our neighborhood, and I have tried various methods of treatment. I have tried hog cholera anti-serum upon them and it did not give any results: I tried various antiseptic medicines, and they did not give any result. A bunch of hogs, immunized in the summer, came down with severe hemorrhagic enteritis. I gave these hogs a dose of serum and rectal injections of normal salt solution, with two drams of iodine to the quart. They seemed to improve for two or three weeks, then began to get worse.

I had some literature on the subject of bacterins in hemorrhagic septicemia in hogs, and thought I would try them out. I sent for some of these bacterins and tried them. Most of the hogs recovered.

I may say also that in hogs, among the various lesions found was an ulcerated condition of the bowels, sometimes just a necrotic sort of pus lesion, and scrapings from these ulcers when examined were found to contain many bacteria. They can be demonstrated in the blood in acute cases. In most of these cases where they died suddenly I found myocarditis. I have used serum in horses and bacterins in cattle and in hogs and have had good results in the number of animals I have treated.

DR. G. P. STATTER: Will some one discuss the possibility of transmitting infection to hogs devouring cattle that have died from hemorrhagic septicemia?

DR. H. B. TREMAN: I might cite an experience I was unfortunate enough to have with hemorrhagic septicemia. The client had lost several head of cattle before a diagnosis was made. The symptoms were so unusual that we were very slow in making a diagnosis. Four or five dead cattle were eaten by the hogs, with no bad results whatever. I know of several other cases where the first animal that died was eaten by hogs. I have knowledge of no case where there was transmission of the infection.

In order to make a positive diagnosis in this outbreak, after consulting several veterinarians, we called Dr. L. E. Willey from Iowa State College. He made a microscopic examination and confirmed our diagnosis. I ordered bacterins which were given; the man had lost about 12 head, but did not lose any more following the use of the bacterins. Since that time I have had 14 or 15 different cases of hemorrhagic septicemia, and in most cases have used the bacterins with very good results. There have been some cases where there has been the loss of one or two or three animals after the administration of the bacterin. I recall one case in which one animal died a week or ten days afterwards. During the period of two years of observation of this number of cases the disease has not recurred on the same farm except in one case, and that was just a week ago Friday. I was called back to the place where they had the disease last summer and had shipped in some cattle from Sioux City recently, or sometime during the winter, and have had a recurrence of the disease at that place. The first animal that died was one of those that were shipped in, and the next two were from those that had had the vaccine about six months before, so that it is apparent that the immunity was not carried longer than six months in that case. Outside of that, immunity has either been carried or they have not been reinfected. But in most cases young calves have come into the place since then without any trouble at all.

There is another point to which I desire to call attention. It seems rather curious to me and interesting in a way, and that is the fact in some cases the infection is quite virulent, and is transmitted rapidly from one animal to another in the same herd, but I have had no evidence of the disease apparently traveling from one farm to another. I have known one or two other cases, where the disease apparently was so well marked as to leave no doubt about the diagnosis, and of three animals sick in the herd one died. Yet nothing was done whatever, and no additional deaths occurred.

A MEMBER: When you give the bacterins, do you give more than one dose?

DR. H. B. TREMAN: I never have. I would say, however, I believe that if sick animals could have repeated doses of the bacterins at two to five day intervals, they would have a marked curative effect. I have treated a few cases medicinally which have recovered either from the treatment or in spite of it, I don't know which. I really believe that repeated doses of bacterins are indicated where it is convenient to give them.

DR. W. P. BOSSENBERGER: I find that to be the case in hogs. Hogs do not respond to less than two treatments, and often it is necessary to give the treatments from three to five days apart. In cattle I have given but one dose and they seemed to do very well. In hogs I find it necessary to give three or four doses.

DR. F. J. NEIMAN: I would like to ask Dr. Treman how long these cattle with hemorrhagic septicemia lived.

DR. H. B. TREMAN: Some of them lived 30 minutes, and others lived four or five days. Some of them apparently were sick for a week or ten days and got well.

DR. F. J. NEIMAN: I have not had any die in less than 30 to 46 hours.

DR. H. B. TREMAN: In 14 or 15 different herds I have seen hemorrhagic septicemia, and I believe that many different clinical symptoms are manifested. Sometimes there will be two or three symptoms shown in different animals in the same herd, but I do not hesitate to say that I have seen at least a dozen different clinical symptoms manifested in animals with this disease. There was one case that was especially interesting to me. I was called to see a young steer in a fair condition. He had been running on clover and the owner found him down about 6 o'clock in the evening. He had not been down very long. He showed evidence of brain lesions, being partially comatose at times, and again excitable, although paralyzed and unable to get up. He soon died. I had made a diagnosis of hemorrhagic septicemia before he died. On post mortem after careful observation I found absolutely nothing abnormal except the kidneys. They were normal in size and appearance, but showed blotches the size of the finger nail. There were no small petechial hemorrhages, but those brownish spots, hardly black, but a little bit darker than the normal appearance of the kidney. I simply did not know what it was. I didn't feel after we posted this animal that the condition looked like hemorrhagic septicemia, so I didn't advise the vaccination of the other animals. I sent a specimen to the laboratory for examination and bipolar staining organisms were found, and while the specimen was not in good condition the lesions were reported those of septicemia. There were a few evidences of putrefaction, but there were quite a number of bipolar staining organisms of the septicemic type found. The client did not lose any more and there was nothing done.

Dr. J. D. Cline: I quite agree with Dr. Treman when he says that hemorrhagic septicemia is a very peculiar disease, and I believe we are just beginning to learn a little about it.

I have had cases this year which I have diagnosed as hemorrhagic septicemia in cattle, and I believe we have hemorrhagic septicemia in horses. Before this time I have had some cases that died without any diagnosis.

As to vaccination and the results from it in cattle, I am still at a loss to know how much benefit is derived from vaccines. I have treated herds of cattle with the vaccine and also with the serum, and have had apparently good results. I remember one case where a man had lost a steer and a diagnosis of hemorrhagic septicemia was made. I advised vaccination. However, this man waited and no more of the animals became sick. Some animals recover without any treatment at all, with no more loss in the herd and when we compare those that have not been treated with the cases we had treated, I would like to know why we have a right to say the vaccines have been beneficial. We have apparently the same results with or without treatment. However, I want to say that after vaccination I have never had a loss in a herd. I have had the acute and chronic types of hemorrhagic septicemia to deal with. I believe this disease comes in very many different forms, and I also feel that it is a disease secondary in its nature. I do not believe that hemorrhagic septicemia in itself is a very deadly or fatal disease in the primary form, but I believe the disease comes on in secondary form. For instance, in most of my cases the cattle were shipped in, and I take it, were weakened by being in a different climate. In some cases, it is possibly due to the feed they are getting. In the cases I have had where a diagnosis of hemorrhagic septicemia was made there was gastro-enteritis as a symptom of the disease.

I differ with the gentleman who states that there is no benefit from the use of serum in hogs. I have never had a case in hogs that did not apparently show better results after serum was given. I am a little doubtful in my mind if in these cases there was not hog cholera mixed up with hemorrhagic septicemia. Hog cholera is becoming a more complex problem all the time. I am at a loss to know whether bacterins are beneficial or not, but with the results I have had I feel that they are beneficial, and I have only given one treatment. I have never had any loss after treatment, and have had recovery in herds without any treatment at all. I am in the dark about hemorrhagic septicemia and the use of vaccines.

Dr. Chas. Murray: I would like to ask Dr. Cline what he means by hemorrhagic septicemia not being a primary infection, when speaking of the predisposing causes of bad housing, change of climate, etc.

Dr. J. D. CLINE: I believe the shipping, change of climate, etc., weaken the animals so that infection sets in. It may really be the cause of the disease. At any rate, there is that weakened condition of the animals. We all know that we carry the pneumonia organism in our lungs, but we are not infected with pneumonia until we become devitalized. That is what I had in mind. In all cases I have had there seems to have been some cause back of the disease. As to hogs shipped in, I do not know. I have had no case where hogs infected with this disease were raised in the locality. I have had it in both cattle and hogs that were shipped in. In native animals I do not think I have had cases except in one or two animals which were probably first affected with some gastroenteritis or some condition where the tissues were devitalized, and that is why I speak of it as a secondary infection more than a primary cause. I may be wrong. I am bringing that point out for discussion.

Dr. W. P. BOSSENBERGER: In the last three years I could cite a dozen outbreaks of hemorrhagic septicemia in cattle fed low, and in them the disease may have been secondary rather than primary.

Dr. J. D. CLINE: Any animal that is fed low is out of the ordinary condition.

Dr. W. E. MACKLIN: In most of the cases I have seen, the outbreaks of the disease were in cattle that were shipped in. I received the report of an outbreak in October. In an hour's time one cow was dead. The owner looked over his herd and found another one that was isolated from the herd. Within the course of two hours this animal went down, struggled and died. An autopsy was made and we sent to Ames for vaccine, and vaccinated the rest the next day. The next day a neighbor lost two animals as suddenly with the same symptoms. The following day, three miles east, there were two deaths in another herd. No cattle had been shipped into that community. They were right out on the blue grass pasture. Post mortem examination disclosed no evidence of any other infection than hemorrhagic septicemia. We could find no other condition in the animals that would be predisposing to the disease. Ten days after the first herd was vaccinated a pure bred bull about three years old died.

Dr. L. A. WHITE: About two years ago I had an outbreak of hemorrhagic septicemia. The owner had lost one calf, and after a second one died he decided it was time to find out what was wrong. I made a post mortem examination on this animal and found typical lesions of hemorrhagic septicemia. I secured vaccine from Ames to treat the herd. Two in the herd were sick at the time, but there were no further fatalities. Since then I have had experience with twelve or fifteen different outbreaks of hemorrhagic septicemia, with no more than one loss on the place. I have advised vaccinating in each case, but for various reasons, financial being the principal one, vaccination was not resorted to, and no further losses occurred.

The carcasses of these animals in 50 per cent of the cases were fed to the hogs.

This fall I had an interesting case. The client called me out on Monday, after having lost two calves, and had one more sick. When I arrived at the place I found that he had dragged the carcasses of the dead animals into the hog lot, and they were frozen. All the organs I was able to tell anything about were the lungs and heart. The lesions in the lungs and heart were not sufficient to pronounce the disease hemorrhagic septicemia, although I told him my suspicions. In the meantime, I do not know whether he had lost confidence in my ability or not, however, he called in another veterinarian. We went out the next day and found that the calf sick the day previous had died. We posted the calf and found the typical lesions of hemorrhagic septicemia. I at once sent to Kansas City for vaccine. It was delayed in arriving. I think it arrived on Friday. I went out to the place to vaccinate and by that time the man had changed his mind. The two that were sick had recovered. He thought there was little or no virtue in vaccination. We did not vaccinate, and he has had no further fatalities. The hogs did not get sick, and the two animals that were sick recovered.

A MEMBER: I would like to ask Dr. Murray if he finds the same organism in cattle, hogs and sheep, and whether the lesions are the same.

DR. CHAS. MURRAY: Experimentally we have never been able to have the disease transmitted from one species of animal to another. We do have reports of septicemia, chicken cholera, hemorrhagic septicemia in cattle and maybe of sheep on the same farm, but there is no connection between the causative organism in one class of animals and another. I hesitate to say what I am about to say because I always recommend that carcasses of animals be disposed of otherwise than by feeding; but last fall there were 37 head of cattle that died from hemorrhagic septicemia in one herd. All of these were fed to hogs and no bad results from feeding ensued. We never have succeeded in producing hemorrhagic septicemia in pigs experimentally by feeding the carcasses of cattle that died of hemorrhagic septicemia. I am strongly of the belief that the disease is not readily transmissible.

A MEMBER: If animals are exposed and have been weakened in any way previously I can readily see how that may have something to do with susceptibility to infection. Most of these herds before being exposed may have been weakened physically. As to being a secondary infection, hemorrhagic septicemia may be a secondary infection, but it may be a primary infection as well.

DR. J. W. GRIFFITH: I have seen hemorrhagic septicemia in all forms, last summer in particular. I have often wondered if we are justified in using serums and vaccines in this disease. In some cases where I have telegraphed for it and have not gotten it in time, the

animals have apparently got along without it. I am of the opinion
that we are imposing an unnecessary expense on the farmer. I
have seen deaths after the use of the serum, and I have seen them
live where it was not used. So I raise the question, are we warranted in using serum and vaccine in these cases?

DR. D. H. MILLER: I have noticed this disease for many years.
We used to call it cornstalk disease. I have found more of it in
cattle that were shipped in. A client near Council Bluffs called me
last fall stating that he had lost a steer out of a herd of 40 or 50
two-year-olds that he had shipped in the week before. I made a diagnosis of hemorrhagic septicemia and advised vaccination, but he
didn't think he would have it done. The following morning he had
two or three more dead. He said that I had better get some vaccine.
I sent to Kansas City for vaccines and the next morning was ready
to do the work. I went out and found three more dead and another
one ready to die. The evening before we had looked at the cattle
quite late and everything seemed to be favorable. The animals appeared to be in perfect health. I used the vaccines and he did not
have any more deaths. I have wondered since whether the vaccines
did the business or whether the animals recovered in spite of their
use. I have had that occur many a time before.

DR. K. W. STOUDER: I had an outbreak the past fall, the man
having lost seven head. These cattle were all in the same field. In
a half dozen acres or so there were about 40 cattle, 90 head of hogs
and 15 or 20 horses. They were fed one hayrack load of green fodder a day. They changed the feed and surroundings and there was
no more loss. The cattle were eaten by the hogs, with no deaths of
the hogs, and nothing more was heard from them until this winter.
They telephoned me the other day saying they had lost one more
and wanted advice. I told them to change them around the same as
they did the other time. This was done, and there has been no further loss.

DR. S. K. HAZLETT: I have come to the conclusion that it is
not an easy matter to differentiate between hog cholera and hemorrhagic septicemia. My experience has not been as extensive as that
of many others. I wish to relate one case I had where a man that
owned a farm in Minnesota shipped cattle into St. Paul, sold a number of them, the others being tested for tuberculosis and shipped to
a farm in Iowa. Two animals had died when I was called and there
were four more sick. I made a diagnosis of hemorrhagic septicemia,
procured serum as quick as I could and treated them. There were
six deaths altogether. The treatment given the sick ones was eumen-
thol with sulphocarbolate internally. Some of the very sick ones
recovered, and some of them did not. This treatment was very satisfactory to me and to the owner. If there are any other outbreaks
in his immediate vicinity, I am quite satisfied they will call for vaccination. Here was another peculiar thing in this case: the cow that

first died was one that was shipped in, and the other five that died were those on the farm. None of the others that were shipped in died. That is rather peculiar.

We have been talking about feeding these carcasses to hogs. I do not advise feeding these carcasses to hogs, but the point was mentioned in regard to whether the carcass could be cooked. I can see no objections to the farmer cooking this meat and feeding it to his hogs. This was done with the last one that died. Some of the animals were buried. The two first ones that died were buried, and the rest were cooked and fed to hogs.

I think we should discuss the question whether or not these carcasses should be fed to hogs as this question the veterinarian must decide. As a rule, I do not advise it. However, I can see no objection if the carcasses are cooked.

I have heard no one say whether or not hides from these animals are given any treatment before being shipped. It seems to me, it is a proper thing to disinfect the hides before they are shipped.

DR. ORR: I have noticed that some outbreaks of hemorrhagic septicemia are quite virulent and believe there is some predisposing factor as a rule. I do not believe the disease is contagious in the same sense that hog cholera is. We do find in some of these cases a mixed infection. I think shipped in cattle are more predisposed to the disease than cattle under normal conditions. Cattle under normal conditions do not usually contract the disease.

DR. L. E. WILLEY: I would like to ask an explanation of this fact. Assuming cattle have been shipped in and are placed on a farm with cattle or calves that are perfectly normal as far as one is able to tell and running in pasture, and you have the appearance of the disease in the shipped in cattle, why then do you so often have loss in the domestic cattle which have not been weakened or predisposed through shipment?

DR. F. J. NEIMAN: One thing seems extraordinary to me regarding hemorrhagic septicemia in cattle that are shipped in. My experience has not been similar to that of some of the preceding speakers. I have never seen hemorrhagic septicemia develop in cattle recently shipped in. It has happened with us among the cattle raised in the locality, that have been there for a long time. We get cattle from Kansas City and Sioux City, but I have yet to see the first case of hemorrhagic septicemia in cattle that have been shipped in.

DR. W. S. FERRAND: In the first case I cited, the man had a herd of 40 head of steers shipped in. One was sick when the herd arrived, and the second case that developed was one of his own best milch cows, and both died. The steer that was sick on arrival died several days afterward.

Another point I want to bring out is this: I would like to ask any of the veterinarians present if they have ever used serum on the sick ones and vaccine on the well ones. I attribute my success to this practice. In every case where I find animals showing infection or clinical symptoms I have used serum, and vaccines on the well ones.

DR. J. D. CLINE: I would like to ask some one who is engaged in research work whether these organisms are found in the system of animals that have died of some other disease. It may become pathogenic from some cause. Is it normally found in the tissue? May not a great many cases we call hemorrhagic septicemia be some other disease? I believe we call many cases hemorrhagic septicemia when they are something else. I believe on microscopic examination the organism that causes hemorrhagic septicemia might possibly be found in the tissue of an animal dead of some other disease, and if anybody doing research work can answer that question, I would like to have them do so.

DR. CHAS. MURRAY: It is a common thing for the hemorrhagic septicemia organism to be a secondary invader. There are predisposing factors to disease, and there are primary and real causes of disease. Predisposing factors are important in putting the animal into a physical condition where the microorganisms are sufficiently virulent to produce disease.

As to the question of finding organisms in healthy animals, it is commonly known that they are found in healthy aimals, particularly in the nasal discharge. They are commonly found in the intestinal tract.

DR. S. A. DEMING: I wish to relate a little experience I had sometime ago. I believe I have learned to be guarded in my prognosis and my advice to my clients. About a year ago a client called and said one of his steers was crazy and wanted to know what the trouble was. The steer was dead when I arrived. I found in the dead steer what I thought were unmistakable evidences of hemorrhagic septicemia, and I told him what I considered the condition to be. He said his steers were ready for the market and he intended to ship them out Saturday. I agreed with him that this was the thing to do as my experience had been up to that time that when one died several would die. I said he was liable in a few days to lose a dozen or more of his steers. He said he was going to ship them Saturday, but failed to get his cars. The steers stayed in the yard two weeks, and there was no more septicemia, and he closed the incident by informing me that he thought I was a poor one from whom to seek advice. Perhaps some of the younger veterinarians will be a little more careful in offering a prognosis in hemorrhagic septicemia.

TEAT OPERATIONS*

THOS. H. FERGUSON, Lake Geneva, Wis.

The teat operations I am going to describe are a few simple operations that I have used for a long time in my practice with satisfactory results. My clients are satisfied with them, as indicated by their repeated calls for these operations. I will first take obstructions of the end of the teat, caused by injuries, frost bite, infection, etc., most commonly found in cows kept in the old fashioned wooden stanchion which favors injuries by treads, etc., from the adjacent cows much more than does the modern stanchion with pipe partitions.

The history of these cases are much alike. The owner or herdsman informs you that they were all right at the last milking, but milked with difficulty or not at all from the affected teat the next milking. Upon examination we find a hard swollen condition of the teat end with or without a wound or wounds. The quarter may be relieved of its milk by using a teat tube but these cases will terminate unfavorably if the use of the teat tube is persisted in. I have never yet found anyone able to lay down a rule whereby the layman could use a teat tube twice daily, for any length of time, without disastrous results to the quarter. The ordinary man considers a teat or tube clean if he is unable to see any dirt on them. I formerly used hard rubber teat bougies, or metal teat plugs, to dilate the affected duct, with unfavorable results; in fact, I have tried every apparently sane way of handling this condition, with very poor success until I began doing the operation I am about to describe.

It is absolutely essential in doing teat and udder operations to have the animal well restrained. First the teat is well cleaned, especially at the orifice, it is then dipped in etherized iodine. I carefully introduce a sterile teat bistoury, with the blade guarded into the orifice and up past the obstruction which is the inflamed swollen circular muscle that forms the valve. I then engage the cutting point of the blade to the superior or upper side of the muscle and put on enough pressure to divide the muscle, being careful not to punch through the skin or cut the mucous membrane at the

*Fifty-fourth Annual Meeting of the A. V. M. A. Clinic, Kansas City, Mo., August, 1917.

orifice of the teat. Repeat the procedure until the muscle has been divided three or four times at equal distances. The milk usually runs out in a stream until the quarter is one-fourth relieved when it is then necessary to empty the gland by milking. The after treatment consists of dipping the teat before and after milking in a 1/1000 solution of mercuric chloride and the milker's hands should be clean and dipped in the same solution before milking or handling the teat.

The next operation is for the fibrous growths that obstruct the duct of the teat, anywhere from the upper part of the lower third to the gland usually found at the upper part of the middle third. If a teat bistoury or curette is used on these cases the immediate results are good but in from three to ten days the trouble recurs. I find the best way to handle obstructions of this kind is to prepare the teat by washing with soap and water, rinsing with 1/1000 solution of mercuric chloride, dip in etherized iodine, inject a few drops of a 5% solution of cocaine into the field of incision; roll a rubber band up to the base of the teat to prevent bleeding, tense the teat by stretching, then with a sterile sharp scalpel make an incision down on to the fibrous growth, dilate the wound and dissect the growth out with a blunt pointed pair of scissors, apply etherized iodine to the wound. Leave the rubber band on two hours, then remove by cutting with scissors so as to not molest the wound.

AFTER TREATMENT. Apply etherized iodine and antiseptic powder twice daily for three days, then once daily. The milk will leak out sufficient to relieve the gland the first few days, then it will be necessary to strip it out by hand, with precautions against infecting the wound. If the wound does not become seriously infected this operation gives satisfactory results and will save a good many teat quarters that would be lost to other treatment.

Complete stenosis of the milk duct may occasionally be cured by slitting it completely from the base to and through the muscular valve at the apex of the teat, being careful not to cut through the mucous membrane at the orifice. Four incisions, equal distance apart, through its entire length are necessary.

Atresia of first calf heifers may be relieved in the same way after perforating the entire length of the teat with a large sterile probe. This condition is usually caused by being sucked by other calves while a calf.

In cases of severe wounds or other injuries to the teat ends, when the parts are beyond repair, complete ablation of the affected part is indicated and it is surprising how well some of these cases will terminate, providing the cow is on a good flow of milk when the operation is performed.

Blocking of the teat duct, with casein or blood clots, is best relieved by manipulation with the fingers. Every country practitioner should practice such manipulation until they become expert at it and by so doing save a good many teats and quarters.

Fistula of the teat is best operated when the cow is dry, preferably a month or more preceding parturition. Some object to casting a cow heavy with calf, but I have had no bad results from doing so.

The field of operation must be thoroughly cleansed with soap and water, thoroughly soaked in a 1/500 solution of mercuric chloride and the whole teat painted with tr. of iodine. The instruments, scalpel, tissue forceps, artery forceps, teat tube, scissors, needles, suturing material, sterilized by thorough boiling. Inject a few drops of 5% solution of cocaine into the field of incision and around the fistulous tract; introduce a long sterile, self-retaining teat tube into the teat, leaving it there for a guide, apply a clean rubber band to the base of the teat to prevent bleeding, grasp the fistulous tract with a pair of forceps and completely isolate it by an elliptical incision on each side of it down to the duct, make a clean dissection, removing all the skin leading down to the duct, then suture, using the mattress stitch, do all the operating and handling of the teat with sterile instruments, apply etherized iodine and collodion. If the operation has been done surgically clean the wound will heal by first intention and the teat will be o. k. when the cow freshens.

Removing supernumerary teats to improve the appearance of the udder is best done in heifers or when the cow is dry. Use the same restraint, remove the teat or teats close to the udder with a pair of sterile sharp scissors and cauterize the duct and wound with the small point of a thermo cautery at cherry red heat. No after treatment is necessary.

—Dr. J. E. Shillinger has removed to Little Rock, Ark., and will have charge of tick eradication in Miller County, Ark.

—Dr. James W. Murdoch has removed from Bismarck, N. D., to Omaha, Neb.

—Dr. Stephen L. Blount, Fort Worth, Texas, has been assigned to duty at National Stock Yards, Ill.

THE RELIEF OF LAMENESS*

L. G. W. HART, Chippewa Falls, Wis.

This paper is relative to the operation for relief of lameness in case of side-bones only.

HISTORY OF THE OPERATION. This operation was first brought to my notice in 1886 or 1887 when I was a student with James Hart, M.R.C.V.S., at that time in practice at Oldham,. England. Since my agreement to write this paper, I have endeavored to obtain all available information, relative to this operation, which I find rather limited. I have, through the kindness of Professor Joseph Hughes, been able to ascertain that this or a similar operation first came to his notice some twenty-five years or so ago. A description at that time appeared in some of the London veterinary magazines, recommended by Fred Smith of Bombay.

The description of the operation as given by Dr. Hughes is as follows: the quarter showing the side-bones is grooved from the coronary to the plantar border. The cutting through the horny wall extends through the dark crust lying over the layer, care being taken not to produce bleeding. The deeper part of the groove is then incised by a scalpel, so as to insure a separation of the area of horn, which it is intended to loosen. Having done this the grooves made through the wall are connected by cutting through the white line between the sole and the wall, a portion of the lower border of the detached portion is cut away, so that it may not reach the ground. The foot is now encased in a cotton pack, which is kept steadily saturated for several days. Following this, if any lameness is present, it is advised that a blister be applied at the seat of the side-bone.

The operation seems to have been lost sight of in America, at least, as near as I can find out, it has not been practiced to any extent in this country.

I will now describe the operation as performed by myself:

First clean the foot and surrounding area thoroughly and saturate the parts with a 1/500 solution of bichloride solution. Now, cocaine with a 4 or 5% solution of cocaine over the metacarpal

*Fifty-fourth Annual Meeting of the A. V. M. A. Clinic, Kansas City, Mo., August, 1917.

nerves. There are three important factors to take into consideration in doing this operation.

FIRST. Do not cut or injure the coronary band.

SECOND. Always make your cuts or incisions transverse to the fibres of the horny wall or crust, extending from the coronary to plantar border.

THIRD. Be sure to cut completely through the horny wall, leaving the section free.

I take the ordinary foot knife or gauge, and first groove out the horny wall at the superior part just inferior to the coronary band. These grooves are ⅜ of an inch wide and ½ to ¾ of an inch in length, and extend through the horny wall to the sensitive lamina. Beginning at a point where the side-bone is most prominent exteriorly or where the greatest tension is manifested on the coronary band, make two such grooves, the second midway between this part and the termination of the quarter of the hoof. I now take an ordinary stiff bladed saw, which has previously been rounded off in front, being sure there is plenty of set in the saw to allow free cutting. I now start my cuts at the plantar surface of the wall, make a few strokes with the saw to give same a foothold at this point; gradually raise the heel of the saw, to allow the rounded front end to cut its way down into the grooves. I have never exercised any particular precaution in not wound-ing the sensitive lamina. It looks to me as though it would be almost an impossibility to do this operation without bleed-ing. When the cutting is completed I insert some blunt instru-ment into the incisions, rotate same, to satisfy myself the sec-tions are free. I now insert two small wedges in each cut; a method adopted by myself, which may or may not be exercised. I leave same in for 24 hours to further insure complete separation of the sections. I have performed this operation during the past 20 years or so, whenever opportunity presented itself, with the very best of results, almost always putting the horse to work the following day. I have not made a practice of bandaging the foot but can see where same would be good treatment in some localities or under some con-ditions. Until the last few years I have not even used anti-tetanic serum. An operating table is indispensable.

AZOTURIA*

E. E. DOOLING, Syracuse, N. Y.

The reason I take Azoturia as a subject for my paper is because I have always been more or less of a crank on the subject; especially in regard to the drawing of the urine. During the month of April I had seven cases in six days so I was busy for a time. The first one was a gray horse, weight about 1550 pounds, that went down on the pavement. It was raining and he rolled around for about an hour before the ambulance came. From his general appearance I did not think he had any chance to live, so I thought I would experiment with him. I gave him two doses of sedatives but they did not do much good. I gave him 1½ pints of raw oil with 6ʒ of turpentine and after we got him home I left another 1½ pints of oil and 6ʒ of turpentine to be given every three hours, making 8 doses out of the one bottle. I continued the same treatment and nothing else for four days. He had 1½ pints of turpentine and 3 quarts of oil. I tried, after 48 hours, with the slings to see if he would stand but he could not. After 90 hours down he was able to stand with the help of the slings and the following day was able to get up and down alone. From his general appearance when I first saw him, I surely thought this horse would die. I did not draw his urine then, nor did I draw it at any time. Is it necessary that we should draw the urine in azoturia, unless it is done for the effect on our client, not the patient? After 4 days I used soda bicarbonate in tablespoonful doses, 3 doses in 24 hours. I fully realized that the doses of the turpentine were large. I had the experiment in mind for some time and when the opportunity presented itself I tried it and it was successful. I treated the six other cases in the same way and did not draw the urine in any case but one and that was for effect on the client.

*Presented at the meeting of the Central New York Veterinary Medical Association, Syracuse, N. Y., June, 1917.

—Dr. A. J. Dinse has removed from Hamilton to Moultrie, Ga.

—Dr. T. S. Hickman has removed from Kansas City, Mo., to N. Charleston, S. C.

ABSTRACTS FROM RECENT LITERATURE

THE PROPERTIES OF THE SERUM OF ANIMALS HYPERIMMUNIZED AGAINST GLANDERS, AND THE CHOICE OF ANIMALS FOR THE PREPARATION OF SUCH SERUM RICH IN SUITABLE ANTIBODIES. Bertetti, E., and Fuizi, G. *Atti della Reale Accademia dei Lincei, Rendiconti, Classe di scienze fisiche, matematiche e naturali*, Series 5, Vol. XXV, Part 5, pp. 131-135, Rome, September, 1917. Abstract in *Internat. Rev. of the Science and Practice of Agriculture.*—The writers have attempted to prepare anti-glanders sera rich in antibodies by using the following animals: the *ass*, which is very susceptible to glanders, and when infected naturally or experimentally, usually suffers from the acute form of the disease; the *mule*, in which the disease is usually very acute (though acute cases are fairly common in that animal and chronic cases are not rare); the *horse*, in which the disease is usually chronic; the *ox*, which is naturally quite immune.

The experiments were as follows:

Immunizing by using bacilli killed by chemical means. On August 30, 1916, a horse received an intravenous injection of a 7- to 8-day, half-culture on agar of glanders bacilli killed with a solution of bichloride of mercury. The following injections were made in decreasing doses: at the 12th injection 5 agar cultures were inoculated. The first injections were given close together; afterwards they were given every 5 days up to the end of January, 1917, when they were given every 12 or 13 days.

Immunity obtained by using bacilli killed by heat. On August 28, 1916, a horse, mule and an ass were treated like the horse mentioned above, with the difference that the bacilli were killed by heat.

Immunity obtained by means of bacilli killed by heat and by a malleinic toxin. Two horses and an ass were treated with bacilli killed by heat and by malleinic toxin obtained by a special process.

Immunity conferred on cattle by means of bacilli killed by heat and virulent bacilli. Two oxen were immunized subcutaneously; the first received injections of very virulent bacilli grown on agar; the second received cultures from the same stock, but killed by heat (1 to 6 abundant cultures in Petri dishes). The injections were made regularly every 5 days for about 8 months. The oxen supported the immunizing treatment very well.

RESULTS. In August, 1917, the subjects under treatment yielded serum having the following specific qualities: very energetic *precipitating* power; *agglutinizing* power very manifest, even at considerable dilutions, *e. g.*, of 1:10,000 to 1:20,000 (the heat test showed the specific nature of the agglutinins of these sera, in showing that they were such as would confer immunity); this serum has abundance of a specific *sensitizing* agent, easily recognizable either in presence of *Bacillus mallei,* or in presence of different bacillary extracts.

The animals under treatment did not all yield a serum of equal activity. Those inoculated with broth or agar cultures of *Bacillus mallei* and with mallein gave quite inactive serum.

If the *precipitating, agglutinizing* and *sensitizing* powers of the various sera obtained are classed by means of numbers from one to ten, the following scale is obtained: serum from oxen, 10; serum from horses, 8; serum from mules, 4; serum from asses, 1 to 2. The power of fixing alexins, precipitating malleinic poisons and agglutinizing the various races of *B. mallei* is perfectly proportional for all the sera.

CONCLUSIONS. 1. It is possible to obtain from the different animals (ox, horse, mule, ass) anti-glanders sera with strong precipitating powers in regard to various malleins and cultures of the bacillus obtained by filtration, of high agglutinizing power and containing specific sensitizing agents, easily recognizable in presence of the causal organism or its various extracts. 2. The existence of a more or less great individual disposition to glanders has an inversely proportional effect in the production of anti-glanders antibodies. In fact, these antibodies, which show the work performed by the organism in order to acquire immunity, are more abundant in ox-serum and diminish progressively through the horse, mule and ass. 3. According to the writers, the fact that oxen are immune to the disease should not be considered as being related to the lack of affinity between *B. mallei* and the cellular units of the organism, as these latter are certainly and actively affected by *B. mallei.* 4. It is inadvisable to treat the animals with agar or broth cultures of the glanders virus together with mallein, with the intention of producing a *complete* serum, for the soluble products of *B. mallei* contained in suspension in the broth cultures, or the crude mallein injected, possibly being modified only slowly, finally neutralize *in vivo* the antibodies produced by the bodies of the organisms, or else the haptophoric group of the precipitin absorbs and fixes the precipitin. 5. The precipitins contained in the anti-glanders sera prepared by the writers are thermolabile: temperatures between 55° and 60° C. destroy the functional, precipitogenous, and acting group of the precipitins, which are changed into precipitoids.

The work was carried out in the "Glanders Research Laboratory" of the 3rd Italian Army. The writers place their anti-glanders sera at the disposal of other workers. FISH.

MALE FERN EXTRACT FOR DISTOMIASIS. In the *Spanish Veterinary Review* for April, 1916, Dr. Maximilien Gonzales of Leon, Spain, reports excellent results from the use of five grams of ethereal extract of male fern mixed with 25 grams oil of almonds in the treatment of distomiasis in sheep. This dose was given in the morning on an empty stomach and repeated daily for four days. In some cases the medicine was administered through a stomach tube, but it was found more satisfactory to give it from a bottle with the usual precautions. The mixture should be thoroughly agitated before giving.

We believe this treatment was first introduced by Prof. Perroncito who demonstrated that male fern extract would kill most of the flukes, but he reported that there was serious tympanitis and anesthesia. Dr. Gonzales does not mention these conditions, but says that a number of sheep died during the treatment, but attributes death to the advanced state of the disease, as the sheep were not strong enough to stand the treatment. In one flock of ninety sheep, seventeen died by the time the third dose had been given. The treatment was discontinued and the remainder of the animals made a fine recovery. Dr. Gonzales concludes: first, that the cachexia in sheep, due to distomata, can be combated with male fern extract at all stages; second, the loss from treatment is directly in proportion to the advanced stages of the disease. N. S. M.

PYOTHERAPY IN THE TREATMENT OF HARNESS WOUNDS; SOME CONSIDERATIONS ON THE EFFICACY AND ABSOLUTE NON-SPECIFICITY OF ANTICRYPTOCOCCAL PYOTHERAPY ON THE HORSE. H. Velu. *Bulletin de la Société de Pathologie Exotique*, I, Vol. X, No. 10, pp. 901-903, Paris, December, 1917; II, Vol. XI, No. 1, pp. 12-17, Paris, January, 1918. Abstract in *Internat. Rev. Science and Practice of Agriculture.*—I. In the course of researches on the pyotherapy of epizootic lymphangitis the author has repeatedly found how efficacious is treatment with polyvalent vaccines (either anticryptococcal vaccine, or vaccine prepared from ordinary suppurations) for curing *non-specific* lesions, caused by harness.

During the negative phases, the periperal inflammatory reaction becomes intense; the separation furrow forms more quickly; the necrosis tissue is eliminated more easily, on account of the increased suppuration; surgical intervention becomes more easy, and the wound clears up without useless decay. During the positive phases, the wound cicatrizes almost without suppuration, with surprising regularity and quickness.

The author states that he has, by means of pyotherapy, rapidly cured arthritis and a severe traumatic synovitis, as well as obstinate bony fistulae. Lignières (Bacteriotherapy in the treatment of wounds, *Bulletin de la Société Centrale de Médecine Vétérinaire*, 1915, pp. 544-548) has already pointed out that specific organisms are not the only ones that give good results when injected into sick subjects. An anti-anthrax vaccination may stay the spread, in a herd, of a disease in no way connected with anthrax; wounds that won't heal may do so after injection of an organism unconnected with the disease, such as *B. coli*. On the other hand it is well known the injection of any antigen is followed by a hyperleucocytosis.

In conclusion, pyovaccine provides a very efficacious, simple and economic method within the reach of all practitioners, for reducing, in considerable proportions, the time lost in laying up for harness wounds.

II. The polyvalent anticryptococcal pyovaccine prepared at the Casablanca Laboratory has been used for treating pyogenous lesions of the horse due to pathogenic agents other than the cryptococcus. The results clearly showed the definite action of the pyovaccine.

In every case, the injections brought about decreased local inflammations, less pain, the diminution, then disappearance, of suppuration, and in certain cases, sterilization of the lesions. Their non-specific effect is undoubted, even when they do not bring about complete recovery.

The author quotes work of other experimenters on other vaccines, showing their non-specific action, and he concludes, speaking generally, that polyvalent, para-specific pyotherapy is a very simple and economical method which, whether by results already obtained, or those rightly expected, should take a prominent place in the practice of veterinary therapeutics.   FISH.

OAK POISONING OF LIVESTOCK. C. Dwight Marsh, A. B. Clawson and Hadleigh Marsh. Bureau of Animal Industry, United States Department of Agriculture.—The species *Quercus gambellii* in Utah and the shinnery oak or *Quercus havardi* in Texas and New Mexico are said to be the cause of oak poisoning in cattle. Sheep poisoning is unconfirmed. Horses are not reported to have been poisoned. The trouble occurs when cattle are driven to the summer range and there is little grass for them to eat. They do not eat the oak by preference.

The annual loss in the shinnery country is estimated at three per cent. Few of the cattle seem to suffer from their oak diet. If a small quantity of hay is fed daily no harm results from the oak. Under such conditions oak may be considered good forage.

There is extreme constipation. Feces are passed infrequently, are dark and hard, sometimes largely mucus, sometimes bloody. Constipation may be followed by diarrhea. External symptoms are gauntness, rough coat, nose dry and cracked, and head extended forward. There is extreme weakness with loss of appetite. Temperature and respiration are normal. The symptoms are noticed after feeding on the oak for about a week. Death may occur in two weeks or after an indefinite period.

Treatment consists of overcoming the constipation, keeping the cattle away from the ranges until the grass has a start, or seeing that the diet is not entirely oak. Three pounds of alfalfa hay daily with the oak will furnish a maintenance diet for a 2-year-old steer.   HAYDEN.

———◆———

TUBERCULOSIS IN CAMELS, IN EGYPT. F. E. Mason. *The Agricultural Journal of Egypt*, Vol. VII, pp. 6-11, Plates, Cairo, 1917. Abstract in *Internat. Rev. Science and Practice of Agriculture.*— Tuberculosis appears rarely to affect camels outside Egypt, but in that country it has long been known. In 1911, 1.63% of the camels slaughtered at the Cairo abattoir were found to be tuberculous, while for 1915 the percentage was 5.4. These figures are certainly higher than those for the entire infection in Egypt.

The author ascertained the cause of the disease by identifying the causal bacillus, controlled by inoculations in guinea pigs. The bacillus appears to be of the bovine type.

The author thinks that infection takes place primarily from cattle, the method being by inhalation. About 60% of the tuberculous camels are only affected in the lungs, bronchial and mediastinal glands. The disease is never found in camels from countries where they do not come in contact with cattle. The subcutaneous test with ordinary tuberculin can be successfully employed on suspected camels.   FISH.

---◆---

ARMY VETERINARY SERVICE

VETERINARY FORCE SUFFICIENT TO MEET ALL ARMY NEEDS NOW

The War Department has authorized the following statement from the office of the Surgeon General:

Examinations for commissions in the Veterinary Corps have been closed. There is available a force sufficient to meet all requirements of the Army for some time to come. In addition to the 1,700 officers and 10,000 enlisted men on active duty there is a waiting list of men who have passed the examinations and who will receive commissions when vacancies occur. As soon as the waiting list is exhausted a new examination will be held. Due notice will be published.

Veterinary graduates called under the selective service act will be taken into the service as privates. After a few months of service they will be allowed to take the examinations for veterinary officers. Should they pass, they will be given commissions as soon as practicable. Men over the draft age and under 40 years may enlist as privates and will have an equal chance with the selected men for commissions.

A training school for commissioned veterinary officers on active duty has been established at Camp Greenleaf, Chickamauga Park, Ga. One hundred men are graduated every month after having received a special two months' course.—*Official Bulletin,* June 27.

---◆---

The meat inspection service of the Veterinary Corps has expanded with the growth of the Army since the outbreak of the war. All meats and meat products purchased by the Depot Quartermaster in Chicago and the subsidiary depots in other large cities are carefully inspected for compliance with specifications. This covers practically all the refrigerated beef, canned meats, ham and bacon, which are sent to the overseas forces or issued to troops in this country. Veterinary meat inspectors remain in the packing houses and observe the processing from the selection of the meat to the sealing of the cans in which it is packed. Every step in the process receives a critical scrutiny in order that the Government may secure only meat from sound animals which has been properly prepared and preserved for transportation and issue.

The service in Chicago is supervised by Major George A. Lytle, V. C., N. A., assisted by 43 veterinary officers who are trained meat inspectors and 25 enlisted men. Meat inspectors who have been properly trained under the regulations of the Bureau of Animal Industry are the only ones engaged in this work and some difficulty is encountered in securing enough men for the enlisted force in particular. These enlisted men are not veterinary graduates but must have had at least one year's experience with packing house methods. Men of this class who are subject to the selective draft or who wish to enlist should communicate with the Surgeon General of the Army stating their qualifications.

A veterinary officer is attached to each division as meat inspector and to each cantonment is allowed a division or camp meat inspector with two enlisted assistants. Officers and men selected for this work are sent to Chicago for the course of instruction before assignment to stations.

———•———

—Majors D. S. White and R. J. Stanclift have received the rank of Lieutenant-Colonel. These gentlemen have been engaged in important administrative work since last autumn. Their many friends in the profession congratulate them on their promotion.

—Captain T. S. Hickman has removed from Kansas City, Mo., to the Animal Embarkation Depot, North Charleston, S. C.

—Lieut. G. L. Richards has been transferred from Camp Doniphan, Okla., to the American Expeditionary Forces, France.

—Lieut. L. J. Anderson has removed from Placerville, Calif., to 115th Field Signal Battalion, Camp Kearney, Calif.

—Lieut. L. N. Peterson has been transferred from Tallahassee, Fla., to the Animal Embarkation Depot, North Charleston, S. C.

—Lieut. Jesse L. Shahram of Hartford. S. D., is now stationed at Camp Greenleaf, Chicamauga Park, Ga.

—Captain G. A. Jarman has been transferred from the Remount Service, Kansas City, Mo., to the Medical Officers' Training Camp, Camp Greenleaf, Fort Oglethorpe, Ga.

—Lieut. A. A. Goodman, formerly at Falfurrias, Texas, has been transferred to Fort Bliss, El Paso, Texas.

—Lieut. S. K. Andreassen, formerly at Barnesville, Minn., is now stationed at Camp Lewis, American Lake, Wash.

—Lieut. Frederick Low has been transferred from Camp Dodge, Ia., to Camp Lee, Va.

—Dr. J. Hanrahan, formerly at Highwood, Mont., is now stationed at Camp Lewis, Wash.

—Dr. J. J. Kelly, formerly at Marshall, Minn., is now stationed at Fort Oglethorpe, Ga.

—Dr. H. E. Torgersen, formerly at Camp Cody, N. M., is now stationed at Camp Greenleaf, Chickamaugua Park, Ga.

—Dr. Maurice C. Hall of the Research Laboratories of Parke, Davis & Co. of Detroit, Mich., has received a commission as Second Lieutenant in the Veterinary Corps, and has been ordered to Fort Oglethorpe for duty.

—Lieut. Harve Frank, formerly at El Paso, Texas, is now stationed at Camp Funston, Kans.

—The marriage of Miss Edna Keeler and First Lieut. J. F. Jansen occurred at Ithaca, June 29. Lieut. Jansen has been stationed at Camp Beauregard, La., but has now been transferred to Chicago.

—Dr. W. R. McCall, formerly of Oklahoma City, Okla., is now with the 144th Field Artillery, Camp Kearney, Calif.

—Dr. R. T. Renwald, formerly at So. Omaha, Neb., is now stationed at Camp Lee, Va.

—Lieut. W. C. McConnell, formerly at Holdenville, Okla., is now stationed at Camp Greenleaf, Chickamauga Park, Ga.

—Lieut. C. J. Cook has been transferred from Camp Cody, N. M., to Chicago, Ill.

—Lieut. H. C. Pugh, formerly at Camp Devens, Mass., is with the American Expeditionary Forces.

—Major F. T. G. Hobday, formerly on the Flanders front, is now with the British Expeditionary Forces in Italy.

—Lieut. T. E. Wilke, formerly of Chicago, Ill., is with the Detroit Refrigerating Co., Detroit, Mich.

—Lieut. F. J. Reamsnyder, formerly of Elmhurst, N. Y., is stationed at Chicago, Ill.

—Lieut. R. O. Stott has been transferred from Fort Bliss, Texas, to 12th Cavalry, Columbus, N. M.

AMERICAN VETERINARY MEDICAL ASSOCIATION

THE A. V. M. A. MEETING, PHILADELPHIA,
AUGUST 19 TO 22, 1918

Arrangements have been practically completed for the 55th convention of the American Veterinary Medical Association which will be held at Philadelphia, August 19 to 22.

The local committees and officers of the association are much pleased with the interest manifested by members in all parts of the United States and Canada. A new feature of interest is the prominence which has been given this year's convention by the publications devoted to stock breeding and farming. A number of prominent breeders have signified their intention of attending the sessions for the purpose of establishing closer relationship with the veterinary profession. There seems to have been a general awakening to the necessity for conserving and promoting livestock interests to meet the demands of war and to anticipate the famine conditions for restocking which will occur after the war is over. The inquiries thus far received indicate a record-breaking attendance and the local committees are making every effort to provide a program replete with instructive and entertaining features. A tentative program, which is appended, has been assembled but is expected to be considerably enlarged dependent upon cooperation of Government Officials and Army Officers.

It is a matter of regret that special rates of travel could not be obtained, but it is suggested that persons coming from a distance purchase tickets to Atlantic City or other seashore resorts with stop-off privilege at Philadelphia.

The ladies' auxiliary of the entertainment committee has provided features which will keep their guests happy and contented, and leave pleasant memories of the 55th convention.

The headquarters of the convention will be at the Bellevue-Stratford Hotel where all sessions, except the clinic, will be held. The entire second floor of the hotel has been placed at the disposal of the association and there will be no confusion in locating the particular session in which one may be interested.

The Bellevue-Stratford is conveniently located at Broad and Walnut Streets in the heart of the city, being three blocks from Broad Street Station of the Pennsylvania Railroad and four blocks from the Terminal Station of the Philadelphia and Reading Railway.

The clinic on Thursday morning will be held at the Veterinary School of the University of Pennsylvania, 39th Street and Woodland Avenue.

Every member of the association should make special efforts to attend this annual meeting as matters of vital importance to the profession will be presented. Members of the veterinary profession who are not members of the association are cordially invited to attend and present their applications for membership.

PROGRAM*

MONDAY, AUGUST 19, 1918
9:30 A. M.

Meeting Called to Order by the President in the Ball Room.
Invocation.
Star Spangled Banner—one verse.
Canadian Anthem—one verse.
French Anthem—one verse.
Address of Welcome—Hon. E. T. Cattell for the Mayor of Philadelphia.
Response to the Address of Welcome—V. A. Moore.
President's Address.
Presentation and Adoption of Minutes of Last Meeting.
Report of Executive Board.
Secretary's Report.
Treasurer's Report.
Report of Committees.

1:30 P. M.

SECTION ON GENERAL PRACTICE
(Junior Cotillion Room)

Chairman's Address—T. H. Ferguson, Lake Geneva, Wis.
Secretary's Report.

LITERARY PROGRAM

The Chloramine Antiseptics and Disinfectants (Illustrated)—N. S. Mayo, Chicago.
Swine Practice—C. Courtney McLain, Meadville, Pa.
Certain Aspects of the Pathology of Spavin (Illustrated) S. A. Goldberg, Ithaca, N. Y.
Differential Diagnosis of the Diseases of the Pig—W. W. Dimock, Iowa State College.
Some Surgical Operations in Swine—T. H. Ferguson, Lake Geneva, Wis.
Election of Section Officers.

1:30 P. M. (Ball Room)

SECTION ON SANITARY SCIENCE AND POLICE

Chairman's Address—J. G. Wills, Albany, N. Y.
Secretary's Report—H. Preston Hoskins, Detroit, Mich.
Practical Methods of Prophylaxis Against Worm Infestations—B. H. Ransom, Zoologist, B. A. I., Washington, D. C.
Practical Methods of Treatment for Worm Infestations—M. C. Hall, 2d Lieut., V. O. R. C., Detroit, Mich.
Discussion of Papers on Parasites—E. L. Quitman, Chicago, and W. Horace Hoskins, New York.
Avian Tuberculosis in Swine—L. Enos Day, Chicago.
Practical Methods of Treatment and Prophylaxis for Arthropod Infestations—Seymour Hadwen, Pathologist, Dept. Agr., Ottawa, Canada.
Election of Section Officers.

*Subject to revision.

MONDAY, AUGUST 19, 1918
1:30 P. M. (Reed Room)

SECTION OF VETERINARY COLLEGES AND EXAMINING BOARDS

President's Address—M. Jacob, Nashville, Tenn.
Report of Secretary—C. D. Wall, Des Moines, Ia.
The Trend of Veterinary Education—W. Horace Hoskins, New York City.
Veterinary College Investigation—-E. A. A. Grange, Toronto, Ontario.
The Extension Veterinarian—Geo. M. Potter, Manhattan, Kans.
Fraternity—J. W. Sallade, Auburn, Pa.
Requirements for Enlistments for Veterinary Students in the Enlisted Medical
Reserve Corps—Capt. F. C. Waite, Sanitary Corps, N. A., Office of Surgeon General, Washington, D. C.
Animal Husbandry and Its Importance in a Modern Veterinary Course—H. H. Havner, State College, Pa.
Standardization and Cooperation of State Veterinary Medical Examining Boards—D. E. Westmoreland, Owensboro, Ky.
Election of Section Officers.

MONDAY, AUGUST 19, 1918
8:00 P. M.

President's Reception.

TUESDAY, AUGUST 20, 1918
9:30 A. M. (Ball Room)

WAR SESSION

Army Veterinary Matters—Major John P. Turner, V. C., N. A., Washington.
Bureau of Animal Industry as a War Auxiliary—John R. Mohler, Chief B. A. I., Washington, D. C.
Obscure Lameness and Some of Its Causes—George H. Berns, Brooklyn, N. Y.

Veterinary Corps

National Army Abroad—Major Louis A. Klein, Washington, D. C.
Veterinary Education—A. H. Baker, Chicago.
Discussion led by D. M. Campbell, Chicago, Ill.

TUESDAY, AUGUST 20, 1918
1:30 P. M. (Ball Room)

Miscellaneous Papers

The Veterinary Practitioner and the Control of Infectious Diseases—V. A. Moore, N. Y. State Veterinary College.
The Livestock Industry; Present and Prospective—J. J. Ferguson, Chicago, Ill.
Business.
Election of Officers.

TUESDAY, AUGUST 20, 1918
7:00 P. M.

Alumni and Class Meetings.

WEDNESDAY, AUGUST 21, 1918
9:30 A. M. (Ball Room)

JOINT SESSION

Hog Cholera in the East—Edward A. Cahill, Indianapolis, Ind. Formerly Director of Hog Cholera Control, Mass. Department of Animal Industry.
Tuberculosis Eradication—John A. Kiernan, B. A. I., Washington, D. C.
Standardization of Blackleg Vaccine—L. W. Goss, K. S. A. C., Manhattan, Kas.
Some Investigations on Sheep Diseases in Colorado—Geo. H. Glover, I. E. Newsom, and E. W. Alkire, Ft. Collins, Colo.
The Hog in Relation to Municipal Garbage—C. B. Palmer, Easton, Pa.
Subject Not Announced—E. L. Quitman, Chicago, Ill.

WEDNESDAY, AUGUST 21, 1918
1:30 P. M. (Ball Room)
JOINT SESSION
Symposium on Contagious Diseases
A Preliminary Report on the Value of Blood Tests in the Control of Contagious Abortion of Cattle—C. P. Fitch and W. A. Billings, University Farm, St. Paul, Minn.

The Bang Virus and Its Relation to Endo-metritis, Metritis, Abortion and Sterility—John F. DeVine, Goshen, N. Y.

Suggestions for Legal and Regulatory Measures Against Bovine Infectious Abortion—Ward Giltner, Mich. Agri. College, E. Lansing, Mich.

Discussion of Papers on Contagious Abortion—E. T. Hallman, Mich. Agri. College, E. Lansing, Mich.

TUESDAY, AUGUST 20, 1918
10:00 A. M.—Sight Seeing Auto Trip.
1:30 P. M.
2:30 P. M.—Theatre Party.
8:00 P. M.—Card Party.

10:00 A. M.—Auto Trip to Valley Forge.
1:30 P. M.
2:30 P. M.—Shopping Tour.
8:00 P. M.—Banquet at Bellevue-Stratford.

THURSDAY, AUGUST 22, 1918
9:30 A. M. (Ball Room)
BUSINESS SESSION
Stallion Enrollment—C. D. McGilvray, Winnipeg, Ont.

Subject Not Announced—Wm. M. Bell, Nashville, Tenn.

Hypertrophy of the Septum nasi of Horses and Mules—R. C. Moore, St. Joseph, Missouri.

THURSDAY, AUGUST 22, 1918
1:30 P. M.
Clinic, University of Pennsylvania Veterinary Department, 39th and Woodland Ave.

Visit to H. K. Mulford's at Glenolden.

3:30 P. M.
Boat Ride on Delaware River to Hog Island.
SOCIAL PROGRAM
(Mrs. H. B. Cox, Chairman)

MONDAY, AUGUST 19, 1918
10:00 A. M. (Ball Room)
Opening Exercises.
1:30 P. M.—Luncheon.
2:30 P. M.—Meeting Ladies' Auxiliary American Veterinary Association.
    Opening Prayer—Mrs. F. H. Schneider, Philadelphia.
    Address of Welcome—Mrs. H. B. Cox, Philadelphia.
    President's Report—Mrs. W. H. Hoskins, New York City.
    Reading and Adoption of Minutes of Previous Meeting.
    Reports of Various State Secretaries.
    Unfinished Business.
    New Business.
    Adjournment.
8:00 P. M.—President's Reception (Ball Room).

THURSDAY, AUGUST 22, 1918
10:00 A. M.—Visit to Girard College.
1:30 P. M.—Visit to H. K. Mulford Laboratories at Glenolden, Pa.
2:30 P. M.—Boat Ride on the Delaware River to Hog Island Ship Yards.

HOTELS FOR THE A. V. M. A. MEETING

Hotels Address	Distance from Headquarters	Rates			
		Single		Double	
		With Bath	Without Bath	With Bath	Without Bath
Adelphia—13th and Chestnut	2 blks	$3.00		$5.00	
Aldine—19th and Chestnut	6 blocks	3.00 up	$1.50 up	4.00 up	$2.50 up
Bellevue-Stratford—Broad and Walnut	Headquarters	3.50 up	2.50	5.00 up	4.00 up
Bingham—11th and Market	5 blks	2.50 up	1.50 up	4.00 up	3.00 up
Colonnade—15th and Chestnut	2 blocks	2.50 up	2.00	4.50 up	3.50 up
Continental—9th and Chestnut	6 blocks	2.00	1.50	3.00	2.50
Dooner's—10th above Chestnut	5 blocks	1.50 and 2.00	1.10 and 1.50	2.50 and 4.00	1.50 and 2.00
Green's—8th and Chestnut	7 blocks	2.50	2.00	3.50 and 4.00	2.00 up
Hanover—12th and Arch	5 blks	2.00 up	1.50 up	3.00 up	2.50 up
Stenton—Broad and Spruce	1 blk	3.00	2.00	5.00	4.00
Vendig—13th and Filbert	4 blocks	2.50 shower		4.00 shower	
Walton—Broad and Locust	1 block	2.50	2.00	3.50	3.00
Keystone—1528 Market St.	3 blocks	1.50	1.00	2.50	2.00
Little Wilmot—1410 S. Penn Sqr.	1½ blocks	1.50	1.25	3.00	2.50
St. James—13th and Walnut	1 block	3.00	2.50	4.00	3.50
Ritz-Carlton—Broad and Walnut	Opp. Headq'rs	5.00		7.00	
AMERICAN PLAN					
Aldine—19th and Chestnut	6 blocks	6.00	5.00	11.00	9.00
Windermere—224 S. Broad St.	½ block	3.00 up			

"AN ADVANCING PROFESSION"*

"Veterinarians are as essential to an army as surgeons are. They are preventing equine epidemics, saving the lame, wounded or over worked horses, keeping the army transport service in condition to feed the men and supply them with means of defense. The profession of veterinary medicine is justly recognized in modern armies as of equal importance with other professions. In civil life the profession is gaining by a clearer understanding of its usefulness as well as by the high standard which it has set for itself, a standard not below that of any other profession. When the world needs food and when a large part of its animal population has had to go to slaughter on account of war, it is of the utmost importance that epidemics be prevented and that all possible animals be saved for food or the work necessary to produce food. A profession with such notable achievements to its credit as the eradication of foot-and-mouth disease, the steady but sure reduction of Texas fever areas, the control of hog cholera and other epidemic diseases is entitled to the respect of stockmen and of the country. Everywhere relations between veterinarians and farmers are becoming closer as these things are better understood. The veterinarians are doing their part toward a better understanding of the aims, purposes and approved practices of their profession. For instance we are now asked to extend to all stockmen an invitation to attend and participate in the discussions of the American Veterinary Medical Association, which meets at Philadelphia, August 19th-23d. We cheerfully do it for the good of all concerned. Let us welcome the passing of the quack, a progress of veterinary science and the general appreciation of it."

*Extracted from the *National Stockman and Farmer*, Pittsburgh, issue of June 29, 1918.

—At the meeting of the Illinois Veterinary Medical Association, July 9-11, at Urbana, a resolution was offered urging the legislature to make an appropriation to establish a veterinary college under the control of the State University for the training of veterinarians, not only in medicine and surgery, but along all lines that shall promote, develop and protect the livestock industry of the State.

ASSOCIATION MEETINGS

TIPPECANOE VETERINARY MEDICAL ASSOCIATION

The Tippecanoe Veterinary Medical Association held its bimonthly meeting Wednesday, June 12th, commencing at 2 o'clock, at the Veterinary Building of Purdue University. The association had the pleasure and privilege of listening to Doctor J. E. Gibson and Doctor Clark H. Hays, government inspectors in charge of animal disease control in Indiana, and also Doctor L. E. Northrup, State Veterinarian, who favored us with a timely talk on vaccination of stock hogs to be returned to farms for feeding purposes.

Doctor J. E. Gibson explained the method by which the government hopes to be able to build many accredited tubercular free herds in the various states in which they are operating. Doctor Gibson eliminated many false notions in the minds of the practicing veterinarians relative to the government interfering with their business. He asked for their cooperation and showed the future possibilities by such team work.

Doctor Northrup pointed out in his talk how pork has been increased in Indiana by returning feeding hogs to Indiana farms from the public stock yards after vaccination. The past year's work has been very gratifying. Out of fifty thousand head of hogs shipped out of one public stock yard only one break was reported.

Doctor Clark H. Hays emphasized the necessity of cooperation by all forces within the State in order to do effective work.

An evening program was arranged at one of the local hotels. Dinner was served at 6 o'clock with thirty-five present. After dinner Mr. E. J. Llewelyn from New Castle, Ind., representing the State Council of Defense, gave a forceful and instructive talk on "The Danger Within". He pointed out the additional service the veterinary profession could render to the country at this particular time by refuting German propaganda that is being constantly floated over the country that would do unlimited harm in the remote districts unless some one counteracted such statements and give such communities real facts. Mr. Llewelyn stated that he could always count on a meeting of this kind bringing forth good results.

The election of officers for the ensuing year took place with the following result:

Honorary president, Lieut.. R. B. Whitesell (France) ; president, Dr. G. M. Funkhouser; vice president, Dr. J. E. Kixmiller; secretary-treasurer, Dr. L. C. Kigin.

U. S. BUREAU OF ANIMAL INDUSTRY VETERINARY ASSOCIATION, BUFFALO, N. Y.

At a meeting of Bureau of Animal Industry veterinarians held in Buffalo, N. Y., Thursday evening, June 20th, the U. S. Bureau of Animal Industry Veterinary Association was organized. The meeting was called by Dr. E. T. Faulder, who has advocated such a move for some time. The meeting was well attended; every veterinarian becoming a member. The objects of the association are to affiliate with the American Veterinary Medical Association, advance the interests of the Bureau veterinarians and make the Service more attractive.

The following officers were elected: Dr. J. M. Chase, president; Dr. W. C. Wooton, vice president; Dr. E. T. Faulder, secretary; Dr. E. R. Jackson, treasurer.

CENTRAL NEW YORK VETERINARY MEDICAL ASSOCIATION

The ninth annual meeting of the Central New York Veterinary Medical Association, held in Syracuse on Thursday, June 27th, 1918, opened at 10:00 a. m., with a clinic at the infirmary of Dr. H. A. Turner, now located at 1238 South State Street. The following cases were presented:

1. Spaying of cat; Dr. E. E. Dooling's case; surgeons: Dr. H. J. Milks and Dr. Dooling.

2. Bay gelding; quittor; Dr. J. A. Pendergast's case; surgeons: Dr. J. N. Frost and Dr. Pendergast.

3. Bay gelding; quittor; Dr. E. E. Dooling's case; surgeons: Dr. Frost, Dr. Dooling and Dr. H. A. Turner.

4. Gray gelding; roarer; Dr. H. A. Turner's case; surgeons: Dr. Frost and Dr. Turner.

5. Gray gelding; quittor; Dr. J. A. Pendergast's case; surgeons: Dr. J. A. Pendergast and Dr. W. M. Pendergast.

6. Demonstration of use of violet rays in case of mange on gray mare, by Dr. W. L. Clark.

7. Gray mare; quittor; Dr. W. M. Pendergast's case; surgeons: Dr. J. A. Pendergast and Dr. W. M. Pendergast.

8. Black gelding; quittor; Dr. E. E. Dooling's case; surgeons: Dr. J. M. Currie and Dr. Dooling.

The business session was opened at the St. Cloud Hotel at 2:30 p. m., with the following present: active members, Dr. H. A. Turner, Dr. W. B. Switzer, Dr. F. E. York, Dr. J. A. Pendergast, Dr. J. M. Currie, Dr. E. E. Cole, Dr. E. E. Dooling, Dr. Wilson Huff, Dr. Frank Morrow, Dr. W. L. Clark, Dr. C. R. Baldwin, Dr. W. M. Pendergast, Dr. R. C. Hurlbert, Dr. A. H. Ide, Dr. J. C. Stevens, Dr. J. V. Townsend, Dr. J. K. Bosshart, Dr. M. W. Sullivan, Dr. A. L. Danforth, Dr. O. P. Jones, Dr. J. H. Stack; honorary member Dr. V. A. Moore; guests, Dr. P. A. Fish, Dr. Otto Faust, Dr. J. N. Frost, Dr. H. J. Milks, Dr. O. B. Webber, Prof. Asmus.

Dr. W. M. Long of Baldwinsville was elected to active membership in the association and Dr. Otto Faust of Poughkeepsie to honorary membership. Dr. J. H. Stack was elected censor to succeed Dr. W. L. Clark. Dr. J. M. Currie was elected president; Dr. W. L. Clark, vice president; and Dr. W. B. Switzer, secretary and treasurer, all for the ensuing year.

A very interesting and profitable program of addresses and papers was furnished by members, as follows:

Address by Dr. W. M. Pendergast, retiring president.

Address by Dr. J. M. Currie, president.

Paper: Azoturia—My Late Experience With It—Dr. E. E. Dooling.

Paper: The Use of Violet Rays in Practice—Dr. W. L. Clark.

Address: The Veterinary Practitioner and the War—Dr. V. A. Moore.

Paper: Some Facts About the Tuberculin Test—Dr. W. M. Pendergast.

Paper: Report of Experience in Treatment of Sheep—Dr. J. C. Stevens.

The subjects presented called forth thorough discussion.

Adjournment was taken at 6:30 p. m., which closed one of the best meetings yet held.

The society has always been particularly fortunate in its friendships outside of the membership. At this meeting no less than five members of the faculty of the State College at Ithaca, in addition to Dr. Moore, Dean of that school, who is an honorary member, were present and their interest is appreciated.

W. B. Switzer, Secretary.

CAMP DODGE VETERINARY ASSOCIATION, MAY 28, 1918

Meeting called to order at 6:45 p. m., by the president, Major Gould.

As there was no new or unfinished business the program was opened.

Lieut. Leon M. Getz presented an excellent paper on Army Horseshoeing.

After being discussed by Lieuts. Mosher, Tillie and Major Gould, the rest of the members took Lieut. Getz in hand and quizzed him upon various phases of shoeing, the normal foot and of the treatment and proper mode of shoeing to remedy the various pathological conditions found in the foot.

Major Gould illustrated his method of treating contracted heels.

Lieut. Lester L. Jones presented a paper on Lice Among Army Animals, which was discussed by Lieuts. Smith, Parrish and Dawson.

Motion made and seconded to hold the next meeting Tuesday, June 4th, 1918, carried.

Motion to adjourn carried.

June 4, 1918.

Meeting called to order at 6:45 p. m., by the president, Major Gould. Sixteen members present.

Lieut. George Moon presented a paper on Army Horse Boards. This was ably discussed by Captain Edward J. O'Harra, Lieuts. MacNamara, Middleton, Underwood and Major Gould.

Lieut. J. F. Derivan delivered an excellent paper on Army Meat Inspection. It was discussed by Lieuts. Moon, Mosher, Moye, Elson and Smith.

Motion made and seconded to hold the next meeting Tuesday, June 11th, 1918; carried.

Motion to adjourn carried.

June 11, 1918.

Meeting called to order at 6:45 p. m., by the president, Major Gould.

Minutes of previous meetings read and accepted.

Paper presented by Lieut. R. G. Moore upon Cryptorchids and Their Castration. Discussed by Lieuts. Moon and Tesdell and other members of the association.

Captain Edward J. O'Harra presented a paper upon the Remount Depot, dealing with its personnel, purpose, etc. It was discussed by Lieuts. Moore and Nelson.

Motion to hold the next meeting Tuesday, June 18th, 1918, carried.

Motion to adjourn carried.

June 18, 1918.

Meeting called to order at 6:45 by the president. Minutes of the previous meeting read and approved.

Lieut. Wilbur Smith read an excellent paper upon Influenza, Its Complications and Treatment. It was discussed by Lieuts. Nelson, Moore and Dawson. A good many points in regard to the treatment, prevention, complications, etc., were brought out in the discussion.

Lieut. Underwood read a paper upon Swelling and Stocking of Legs; Cause and Treatment. The causes of this condition being so numerous it brought out a very good discussion which was led by Lieuts. Middleton, Tillie and MacNamara. Some rather pertinent suggestions in regard to chronic conditions of this kind were brought out in this discussion.

Motion to adjourn carried.

LIEUT. ROBERT C. MOORE, Secretary.

WESTERN NEW YORK VETERINARY MEDICAL ASSOCIATION

• The Western New York Veterinary Medical Association held its fifth annual meeting Friday, June 28th, at Buffalo, N. Y.

The meeting opened with a clinic which consisted of cases for observation, diagnosis and operation on both large and small animals.

At the business session which followed the following officers were elected for the ensuing year:

President, Dr. J. L. Wilder, Akron, N. Y.; vice president, Dr. W. E. Frink, Batavia, N. Y.; secretary-treasurer, Dr. F. F. Fehr, Buffalo, N. Y.

From 6:30 to 8 p. m., a banquet was held at the Teck Cafe, after which the meeting reconvened at the S. P. C. A. Hall, where the addresses and papers were given.

Dean W. Horace Hoskins of New York City addressed the association on the timely topic of conservation and preservation of

food, and pointed out among numerous other things the great
waste that was going on while thousands upon thousands were
slowly starving.

Dr. C. E. Gibbs of Fredonia gave an interesting paper on Hog
Cholera and Mixed Infection in Garbage Fed Hogs.

Dr. Geo. R. Chase of Attica read a very practical paper on
Dystocia in Cattle, citing numerous cases he has met in daily work.

The association voted the sum of twenty-five dollars to the
Red Star Animal Relief, through the local director of the S. P. C.
A., Mr. Preston.

Meeting then adjourned to the second week in December, 1918.

At a recent meeting of the Western New York Veterinary
Medical Association the following resolutions were recommended
and adopted :

Whereas, The present great need for more food products in
our country is becoming more apparent and pressing each day; and

Whereas, We as veterinarians are brought in close contact
with the breeders of livestock and the producers of dairy products;
therefore, be it

Resolved, That as a society of veterinarians and as individual
practitioners we use our influence among breeders and dairymen
to take better care of their stock and encourage the breeding and
raising of more food and milk producing animals; and, be it
further

Resolved, That the price of milk as fixed by the Federal Food
Administrator to the producer and to the distributor be more
evenly divided, the latter selling his supply at 48 cents per gallon
whereas the producer is only allowed 19 cents per gallon, thereby
permitting an excess profit by the middleman. Such acts do not
tend to stimulate increased production; and, be it further

Resolved, That the number of food producing animals is not
large enough to provide for the needs of our people and leave a
surplus to be shipped to our allies, thereby necessitating frequent
"meatless days"; and

Whereas, The cost to the consumer of pork, beef and mutton
is almost prohibitive, resulting in under-nourishment to the families of the poor; and

Whereas, The flesh of equine animals furnishes a wholesome
nourishing substitute and would be largely used in the place of
other meats if made available; therefore, be it

Resolved, That the Western New York Veterinary Medical Association in convention assembled advocate the use of horse meat as a substitute for beef and respectfully asks that an appropriation be made by Congress to provide for the Federal inspection of horses for food and that the sale of horse meat be legalized under proper restrictions; and, be it further

Resolved, that each practitioner take it upon himself while at his regular work to encourage such increase of food and food production; and, be it further

Resolved, That we pledge ourselves to cooperate in similar lines of work offered by the local Farm Bureaus, Grangers, State and National Authorities; and be it further

Resolved, That copies of these resolutions be sent to the Federal and State Food Administrators and to the veterinary journals.

Signed, J. L. Wilder, Edw. Rafter, Anderson Crowforth, E. L. Volgenau.

F. F. FEHR, Secretary.

COMMUNICATIONS

BRITISH APPRECIATION OF DR. LIAUTARD

Editor Journal of the American Veterinary Medical Association, Ithaca, N. Y.:

DEAR SIR:

Dr. Liautard's death will be much felt by members of the Veterinary profession in every part of the world, as he was indeed the Father of the Profession. I am publishing his photograph in the next issue of the VETERINARY JOURNAL, together with a biography which does not, however, express one-half of the esteem in which I and all my English colleagues have always held the name of Liautard. America is one of the strongest links in the chain which binds the veterinary allies together at the present time.

Please express through your columns the fact that we of the profession in England greatly deplore the fact that it is inevitable that such men are ever allowed to die, but that we consider the life he led and the results he attained must ever shine as a brilliant example for all other members (whether young or old) of the profession to follow.

Yours sincerely,

FREDERICK HOBDAY, Major.

A VETERINARY POET

Editor Journal of the American Veterinary Medical Association:
Ithaca, N. Y.

We have never suspected our old—excuse us, we mean our *long time* (for we are both still on the active list)—friend, Major Gerald E. Griffin, U. S. Army Veterinary Service, of being a poet. We have eaten and —— (deleted by the Censor) with him in this and other countries, and enjoyed his wit and blarney for lo these many years. We always thought a poet wore long hair. We are sure the Major is shy on this point, but external appearances are likely to be misleading.

"Ballads of the Regiment"* is a song of the old army and the frontier post, the camp and trail by one who knows them from long years of experience. We can see the troopers as they swing away over the buffalo grass and hear the rhythmic beat of hoofs, the creak of saddle leather, and can smell the sweating horses. After a long day's ride and "chow" while the cool night shadows are gathering we will light our pipes and sit by the camp-fire out of the wood smoke, and listen.

INSPECTED AND CONDEMNED

"Here's your horse," cried the auctioneer,
  (A trooper led him in)
"He's strong and sound, a worker, too,
  . Clean as a new-made pin.
What am I bid to start him off?
  (The crowd jeered where it sat.)
Twelve dollars bid! Twelve twenty-five!
  Who'll make it thirteen flat?"

A dark brown gelding, fifteen two,
  Just rising eighteen year.
A star and snip, the right hind white;
  Wire scar behind the ear.
U. S. I. C. burnt on near arm;
  C. 5 upon near thigh,
A bullet's mark across the breast,
  Received in years gone by.

I choke, my thoughts fly through the years,
  To days of long ago,
With "C" troop camping near the streams
  Fed by the mountain snow,
The carbine's crack. The savage yell.
  To horse! The troopers cheer.
The flying "clouts". The saber's flash.
  I charge on "Carbineer".

*The Geo. U. Harvey Publishing Co., New York. Price $1.00.

'Tis but a horse, a small brown horse,
Why should I grieve or care?
He served with me for twelve long years
That flag you see up there.
Companion of the camp and trail,
True friend who knew no fear;
To save him from an unkind hand
I'd die for "Carbineer".

Major, we are not going to violate these new fangled army regulations by asking you to "nominate yer pizen", so we'll simply say, may you live long, write many more ballads, and prosper. Here's How! MAYO.

NECROLOGY

GEORGE H. DUNN

Dr. George H. Dunn, a graduate of the Ontario Veterinary College of the class of 1894, died at Pittsburgh, Pa., July 2, 1918, of sarcomatosis of the intestines, at the age of 53. He formerly enjoyed a large horse practice, but of late years had specialized in canine and feline practice.

MISCELLANEOUS

—Dr. Frank C. McCurdy has removed from Buffalo, N. Y., to Baltimore, Md., in the federal meat inspection service.

—Dr. Howard S. Miller has left Buffalo and joined the federal force at Richmond, Va., in the eradication of tuberculosis.

—Dr. Otto E. Jung has transferred to Little Rock, Ark., to engage in hog cholera control work conducted by the B. A. I. in co-operation with the State of Arkansas.

—Dr. Sid Galt has been assigned to tick eradication work at Fort Worth, Texas, as assistant to the inspector in charge.

—Veterinary Inspector D. S. Otey has been transferred from meat inspection at Waterloo, Ia., to field work in hog cholera control with the force of Dr. J. P. O'Connor at Poteau, Okla.

—Dr. F. L. Cusack has removed from Carrington to Wimbledon, North Dakota.

—Dr. W. R. Lee, formerly at Chicago, Ill., is now at Columbus, Nebraska.

—Dr. C. L. Moles, formerly with the B. A. I. at Cedar Rapids, Ia., is now located for practice at Central City, Ia.

—Dr. J. F. Shigley, formerly at Kenmare, N. D., is now with the Beebe Laboratories at St. Paul, Minn.

—Instructions have been issued by the Bureau of Animal Industry for the transfer, effective August 1, 1918, of Dr. A. W. Swedberg from Omaha, Neb., to Denver, Colo.

—Dr. John W. Hermann has transferred to Grove City, Pa., where he will engage in tuberculosis eradication under direction of the B. A. I.

—Dr. William Grimes of Paterson, N. J., has exchanged places in the federal meat inspection service with Dr. George N. Suits of New York City.

—In a recent hearing relative to unsatisfactory meat sold the Government by Wilson & Co., Dr. A. Eichhorn of Pearl River, N. Y., appeared as one of the witnesses for the defense. Dr. Eichhorn explained the meaning of "stale" meat and "moldy" meat. "Mold"—a vegetable growth—did not mean that meat upon which it appeared was unfit for consumption. It may easily be removed with a mixture of vinegar and water, and did not spoil the meat. "Stale" meat was not so "lively" as fresh meat, but was in no way inferior, the nutritive value being unaffected, thus it was good for human consumption. Dr. Eichhorn did not change his testimony under cross examination by the Government's counsel.

—Dr. Archibald R. Ward, late of the Bureau of Animal Industry stationed at Washington, has severed his connections with the Maryland State College of Agriculture at College Park, Md., to assume the duties of Director of the Veterinary Biological Laboratories of the H. K. Mulford Co., at Glenolden, Pa.

—Dr. W. L. Williams of the N. Y. State Veterinary College at Cornell University, visited British Columbia in June to initiate treatment of cattle at the Provincial Government Farm in connection with contagious abortion. He also met the members of the B. C. Veterinary Association, conducted a clinic and gave a lecture upon the cause and treatment of the disease. Dr. Carl Cozier Bellingham, Wash., secretary of the Washington State Association, was also in attendance. A banquet was given by the B. C. Veterinary Association in honor of Dr. Williams at the Hotel Vancouver with President S. F. Tolmie, M. P., in the chair. Appropriate toasts were made and responded to and Dr. Tolmie outlined the nature of the proposed Veterinary Advisory Board for Canada. The members freely expressed their thanks to Dr. Williams for the services he had rendered.

—Among the names for promotion and appointments in the Most Distinguished Order of Saint Michael and Saint George for services rendered in connection with the war, on the occasion of his Majesty's Birthday, is the name of Major Frederick Hobday to be an Additional Member of the Third Class, or Companion of the said Most Distinguished Order.

—Dr. G. E. Koch has removed from Toronto, Ont., to Ardenode, Alberta.

—Dr. L. F. Ross, formerly of Belpre, O., is at Nashville, Tenn., on influenza control work with Army horses.

—The U. S. Civil Service Commission announces a competitive examination for veterinarians, men only, on Aug. 21. Vacancies in the Bureau of Animal Industry, at an entrance salary of $1500 per year, will be filled from this examination.

—Dr. H. M. Martin, formerly of York, Pa., is now associated with the Animal Pathology and Hygiene Department, University of Nebraska, Lincoln, Neb.

—CHANGE IN ARMOUR & CO.'S BRANCH HOUSE ORGANIZATION. A number of important changes have been made in the branch house organization, affecting the territories with headquarters at New York City, Jacksonville, Fla., Little Rock, Ark., Dallas, Tex., Spokane, Wash., and San Francisco, Calif. The changes came in the nature of promotions to the various men affected. Mr. U. P. Adams leaves the superintendency of the outlying district of New York to assume the superintendency of the Jacksonville, Fla., territory. Mr. Adams is succeeded by Mr. F. A. Benson, formerly superintendent of the Little Rock district. Mr. Benson will be succeeded by Mr. J. S. Livesay, formerly assistant district superin- tendent of the Lynchburg, Va., territory.

On the Pacific coast, Mr. Sommer, superintendent of the Spokane territory, has been transferred to San Francisco. Mr. W. B. Spinks will succeed Mr. Sommer at Spokane. Mr. J. E. Hoban, who has been Mr. Spinks' assistant, succeeds Mr. Spinks in the superintendency of the Dallas territory.

—To Prevent the Introduction and Spread of Communicable Diseases Among Livestock in Tennessee. It has been determined by the Commissioner of Agriculture and the State Veterinarian that enormous losses among horses and mules are incurred every year as the result of infections from influenza, strangles and their complications, which are highly infectious and contagious diseases. Since these losses affect our horse and mule industry to the extent of lessening our State and National efficiency along agricultural and commercial lines, it is therefore ordered by H. K. Bryson, Commissioner of Agriculture, and M. Jacob, State Veterinarian:

Section 1. That all public stock yards and stables operated for the sale, assembling, feeding and distributing of horses and mules in Tennessee be maintained under sanitary conditions at the expense of the owner, as provided in the following sections:

Section 2. That all portions of public stock yards and stables used for the handling of horses and mules, as set forth in Section 1, be subjected to thorough cleaning and disinfection at least once every week, or oftener if considered necessary by the Federal or authorized State inspectors. The cleaning and disinfection to be conducted as follows:

(a) The original cleaning shall consist in the removal of all manure and litter.

(b) All mangers, watering troughs, racks, etc., shall be properly cleaned before each disinfection.

(c) After the original cleaning and disinfection, the manure in horse and mule pens need not be removed more often than once a month, provided there is applied once a day a new or fresh layer of straw, shavings, sawdust or other acceptable fresh bedding.

(d) The disinfection shall include watering troughs, mangers, buckets, halters, floors, partitions, walls, etc.

(e) The disinfection shall consist in the use of 3 per cent solution Liquor Cresolis Compound or any other recognized disinfectant.

Section 3. That all horses and mules showing symptoms of influenza, strangles or any other infectious and contagious disease shall be immediately isolated to premises or quarters not occupied by healthy horses and mules.

Section 4. That the operation and enforcement of this order shall be under the immediate supervision of the inspectors of the United States Bureau of Animal Industry, the War Department, and the State Department of Agriculture.

H. K. Bryson, Commissioner of Agriculture.

M. Jacob, State Veterinarian.

—C. W. Clark has removed from Park Falls, Wis., to Ashland, Wis., 117 Front St. W.

AN ACTION TO ENJOIN THE LIVE STOCK SANITARY BOARD FROM DESTROYING CERTAIN MARES INFECTED WITH DOURINE AS DETERMINED BY THE COMPLEMENT-FIXATION TEST. SUPREME COURT OF NORTH DAKOTA.

Syllabus: (1) The court cannot enjoin the carrying out of an order of the Live Stock Sanitary Board for the killing of a mare under the provisions of Section 2686 of the Compiled Laws of 1913, which gives to that board the power "to quarantine any domestic animal which is infected with any such (contagious or infectious) disease or which has been exposed to infection therefrom, and to kill any animal so infected", where no appeal has been taken or review of the decision of the board demanded under the provisions of Section 2686 of the Compiled Laws of 1913, which provides that, "within twenty-four hours thereafter (the notification of the board) its owner or keeper, may file a protest—whereupon an examination of the animal involved shall be made by three experts, etc."

(2) The 5th and 14th amendments of the Federal Constitution and their counterparts in the Constitution of the several states gave no new rights but merely guaranteed the permanence of these already existing.

(3) What is and what is not due process of law depends upon the circumstances and the constitutional provisions which provides for a preliminary court procedure are often held to have no application to statutes which are passed in the exercise of the so-called police power of the state.

(4) Sometimes summary proceedings are necessary and summary abatement of nuisances without judicial procedure was well known to the common law prior to the adoption of the State and Federal Constitutions.

(5) There is no property right in that which is a nuisance and no right of liberty in that which is harmful to the public weal.

(6) The state may interfere with private industry whenever the public welfare demands and in this particular a large measure of discretion is necessarily vested in the legislature to determine not only what the interests of the public require but what measures are necessary for the protection of these interests.

(7) The state may delegate to an administrative board the power to adopt reasonable regulations and to adopt what tests it deems necessary in order to ascertain the existence of a disease. This is not a delegation of legislative power. It merely relates to a procedure in the law's execution.

(8) The finding or adjudication of a Board of Health cannot generally be made conclusive upon the owner as to the fact and existence of the nuisance, or that it comes within the terms of the statute prohibiting it, so as to deny the owner the right to a trial by jury and the recovery of damages, if the property so destroyed

is not, in fact, a nuisance, or does not, in fact, come within the terms of the statute. Summary proceedings, however, may be authorized by the legislature against the thing declared to be a nuisance, and such property may be destroyed without a hearing before a jury provided that the right to the action for damages remains. Due process of law is not violated by such procedure.

(9) Where the statute provides for the destruction of infected animals in the discretion of a live stock sanitary board, but provides that before such destruction the owner may appeal to a board of experts, and the owner neglects to take any such an appeal he cannot in an injunctional proceeding to restrain the destruction of the stock, question the determination of the board as to the fact and existence of the disease.

(10) Where a statute authorizes a public board to quarantine or kill disease infected animals, the determination of which of the two remedies shall be adopted lies within the discretion of the board and cannot in the absence of fraud be controlled by the courts. In all of such matters the only question in which the courts or the juries are concerned is the ultimate question whether the animal was diseased or not, or came within the provisions of the statute.

(11) The so-called complement-fixation test for the detection of the disease known as dourine appears to meet with the approval of the scientists of both the United States and Canada, and the courts will not interfere with the discretion of the Live Stock Sanitary Board in adopting the same, and in ordering horses to be killed, which react thereto, even though it is a chemical test merely and the horses show no physical symptoms of the disease.

(12) Section 2686 of the Compiled Laws of 1913, leaves it to the discretion of the Live Stock Sanitary Board whether horses which are infected with the disease known as dourine shall be killed or isolated, and the courts will not interfere with or seek to control such discretion.

(13) The fact that the disease known as dourine can only be communicated in the act of breeding and that the owners of diseased mares offer to isolate the same and give bonds that they shall not be bred does not prevent the Live Stock Sanitary Board from ordering their destruction.

—Malcolm J. Harkins has removed from Glenolden, Pa., to Conshohocken, Pa.

—Dr. H. M. Hamilton of Paris, Ky., has reported for service in the Veterinary Reserve Corps at Camp Greenleaf, Ga. Upon his departure from Paris a banquet was given in his behalf at which a gold wrist watch was presented to him.

JOURNAL

OF THE

American Veterinary Medical Association

Formerly American Veterinary Review

(Original Official Organ U. S. Vet. Med. Ass'n)

PIERRE A. FISH, Editor   ' ITHACA, N. Y.

The American Veterinary Medical Association is not responsible for views or statements published in the JOURNAL, outside of its own authorized actions. Reprints should be ordered in advance. A circular of prices will be sent upon application.

VOL. LIII., N. S. VOL. VI.   SEPTEMBER, 1918.   NO. 6.

Communications relating to membership and matters pertaining to the American Veterinary Medical Association should be addressed to Acting Secretary L. Enos Day, 1827 S. Wabash Ave., Chicago, Ill. Matters pertaining to the Journal should be sent to Ithaca, N. Y.

ANNOUNCEMENT

"The pen is mightier than the sword," but we have resigned the pen to enter the military service. At this writing we are unable to announce definitely who our successor will be; but we bespeak for him the kind indulgence and hearty cooperation that has been accorded us.

In changing the office of publication and transferring the equipment, there is likely to be some delay in the date of publication. For this delay, under the circumstances unavoidable, further indulgence must be asked.

It has been our aim to make the JOURNAL the organ of the veterinary profession as well as the organ of the American Veterinary Medical Association. For whatever measure of success we have attained, we wish to render our due appreciation and thanks to the members of the profession and association, through whose cooperation success has been possible.   P. A. F.

THE FIFTY-FIFTH ANNUAL MEETING OF THE A. V. M. A.

The choice of the place for the fifty-fifth annual meeting of the association was very fitting. In these days when, in addition to the purpose to benefit from the program of such a meeting, it is desired to keep up the spirit of patriotism among our members no other place than Philadelphia could have been better chosen. The birth place of our Liberty holds much that is dear to the mind of Americans. Independence Hall, the "Betsy Ross" house, and many other places of historical interest take on special significance in these times. The veterinarians and their friends who visited Philadelphia could not help but take away a deeper consecration to the cause that holds the minds and hearts of all liberty loving mankind. As one of the centers of veterinary learning and things that pertain to veterinary medicine the place of meeting was a happy choice. Meetings in connection with the business of the association began as early as Saturday. The executive board, by early sessions, cleared the way to handling the great mass of business to be brought before the members. On Sunday afternoon the Association of State and Provincial Veterinary Colleges met in the "Red" room of the Bellevue-Stratford. The attendance at this meeting was good and the interest in the numerous reports and papers was of high order. Following the president's and secretary's reports there were committee reports and papers on such subjects as entrance requirements, curriculum, faculty, teaching, histology, physiology, diagnosis, parasitology, pathology and bacteriology, therapeutics. Major Fish introduced Captain F. C. Waite of the Surgeon General's office, who talked upon the subject of entrance requirements. Captain Waite added much to the general program on Monday by his discussion on "Requirements for Enlistments for Veterinary Students in the Enlisted Medical Reserve Corps". Most of the discussion in this section centered upon entrance requirements, teaching the fundamentals such as histology and the knowledge and skill of the teachers. It is to be inferred from the general discussion that the section work is too general and that not enough in the way of specific recommendation has been given.

The fifty-fifth annual meeting of the American Veterinary Medical Association was called to order by the president, F. Torrance, in the ball room of the Bellevue-Stratford. After the invocation the members sang one verse of the Star-Spangled Banner, the Canadian National Anthem, and the French National Anthem. The Hon. E. J. Cattell gave the address of welcome for the Mayor of Philadelphia. Dr. V. A. Moore, for the association, gave a pleasing response to Mr. Cattell. Part of the report of the executive board was given at this session and was amplified in later sessions.

The program for Monday afternoon was divided into three sections. One was almost a symposium on swine diseases, another section was a symposium on parasitic diseases, and the third section dealt entirely with matters of veterinary education. The rest of the program was in joint session. Tuesday morning was given over to army veterinary relationships. Major Turner and Dr. Mohler were the only men scheduled who were able to appear in this session. The papers given by these two men were of great value to the association. Dr. V. A. Moore and Mr. J. J. Ferguson gave the papers of the afternoon. These two men completed the literary part of Tuesday's program. The rest of the day was given over to business and the election of officers. Wednesday furnished its quota of good papers. The afternoon session, which was a symposium on contagious abortion, showed a lack of agreement in the association upon the subject and the president was authorized to appoint a committee to report at the next annual meeting. Only two papers were read on Thursday morning. The rest were read by title. Business and the clinic in the afternoon completed the work of the association. The association made it hard to conform to the constitutional limitations as applied to papers and discussions. More might be accomplished in the meetings if these limitations were lived up to.

It was voted to add another district to the jurisdiction of the executive board. About 1000 new members were elected to membership. Of this large list a very large number came from the B. A. I. and the Veterinary Corps of the Army. It was deemed wise to form a section in the association to be known as the B. A. I. section. A large sum of money was set aside to be invested in equal proportions in war bonds of Canada and the United States. The sum of $2500 was appropriated from the funds of the Allied Veterinary Relief Fund to be sent to Prof. Vallée of Alfort, France, and to be used for the relief of indigent veterinarians in

the allied armies. A little over $5000 was reported in this fund
by Dr. T. E. Smith, the treasurer, It was voted that a committee
be appointed to establish a Liautard Memorial. The resignation
of Major P. A. Fish as editor of the JOURNAL OF THE A. V. M. A.
having been accepted Dr. Dalrymple of Louisiana was elected in
his stead. An amendment to the constitution was offered by Dr. N.
S. Mayo which would combine the office of secretary and the editorship. Dr. W. H. Dalrymple of Louisiana invited the association to
New Orleans for the meeting in 1919. This was referred to the executive committee with the recommendation that the invitation be
accepted.

Dr. V. A. Moore of the New York State Veterinary College at
Cornell University was chosen as the next president. Dr. N. S.
Mayo was elected secretary and Dr. M. Jacob was elected treasurer.
$1000 was appropriated for the use of the legislative committee
during the coming year..

An impressive ceremony in the course of the meeting was the
presentation by Dr. Eagle of the portraits of Dr. Salmon, Dr.
Melvin, and Dr. Mohler to be hung in the art gallery of the Saddle
and Sirloin Club, space having been set aside in that gallery for
the portraits of veterinarians who have given valued service to
the livestock industry. It was voted on behalf of the association to
accept the portraits and that they be presented to the club at the
December meeting of the Live Stock Sanitary Association.

Mr. E. S. Bayard, editor *National Stockman and Farmer,* and
Mr. J. J. Ferguson were elected by unanimous vote to honorary
membership in the A. V. M. A.

The stay of the society in Philadelphia was not entirely given
over to business. Monday evening we had the pleasure of attending
the president's reception in the ball room of the Bellevue-Stratford.
Tuesday evening there were alumni and class meetings. Wednes-
day evening the annual banquet was held in the ball room of the
Bellevue-Stratford. Major P. A. Fish acted as toastmaster. The
speakers were Mrs. A. T. Kinsley for the ladies, Hon. E. J. Cattell,
Mr. E. C. Bayard, Mr. W. Freeland Kendrick, and Dr. V. A. Moore.
On Thursday afternoon there was a boat ride on the Delaware to
Wilmington. Of especial interest on this trip was the great Hog
Island shipyard. To Mulford's is due a vote of thanks for the
splendid trip and also the opportunity that many of the members
availed themselves of to visit the Mulford plant at Glenolden.

C. E. HAYDEN, Ithaca, N. Y.

DISEASES INTERFERING WITH REPRODUCTION IN CATTLE AND THEIR SIGNIFICANCE TO THE STATE*

W. L. WILLIAMS, Ithaca, N. Y.

Some three years ago, I estimated that the infection responsible for contagious abortion in cattle was causing an annual loss in the State of New York of ten million dollars. In 1916, the Secretary of Agriculture estimated the losses from contagious abortion in the United States at twenty millions, just below the losses from tuberculosis, estimated at twenty-five millions. It is evident that either there was a great divergence of opinion in the two estimates or New York had a grossly unjust share of the losses—one-half the total in the nation. The cattle of New York are as healthy as any group of dairy cattle of equal concentration and under similar climatic conditions to be found in America or in the world.

Statistics regarding chronic infectious diseases are inevitably inexact. If an acute disease, as hog cholera, breaks out in a herd of one hundred swine, and fifty die, the owner knows he has lost fifty per cent by death and has incurred further loss in the condition of the recovered animals and in other ways. He can compute his losses upon quite a secure basis. In a chronic disease, the owner does not know when it began, cannot diagnose the disease in all the affected animals, and does not know when or how the disease will end.

Among all chronic diseases, estimates and statistics upon the contagious abortion of cattle are most subject to error and most liable to mislead. The fundamental difficulty is that there is no generally accepted definition. The original, and unquestionably still the most popular conception of contagious abortion in cattle is the observed disaster of the expulsion of a dead fetus. Careful researches seem to indicate that approximately one-half the embryos and dead fetuses are expelled unobserved. Many calves also are born prematurely or at full term which are more or less seriously involved in the same infection, and they too are excluded from the statistics upon contagious abortion.

My conception of contagious abortion of cattle differs radically

---

*Presented at the N. Y. State Agricultural Society, Albany, N. Y., Jan. 16, 1918.

from that commonly prevailing. I have defined contagious abortion as a virtually universal infection of the genital and other organs of cattle which, under favorable conditions, induces no recognizable disease, but when virulent may induce sterility, abortion, premature birth, and, with these or with birth at full term, a metritis or inflammation of the uterus or womb, frequently complicated with retained afterbirth. Further, the infection within the uterus underlying these disasters, if it does not kill the fetus, nevertheless invades it, and frequently induces, before or shortly after birth, such diseases, or rather symptoms of disease, as calf scours, pneumonia, etc. This radical difference in the conception of contagious abortion is the probable explanation for the wide divergence between the estimated losses from contagious abortion made by the Secretary of Agriculture and by me.

Whatever conception of contagious abortion is held, it is well-nigh impossible to secure accurate data upon which to base estimates of losses. If it is attempted to base estimates of losses upon the number of observed abortions, the foundation is insecure. The ordinary farmer or dairyman remembers an abortion for only an astonishingly short time. The majority of farmers having dairy herds of ten cows, in which one cow aborts every two years for ten years, will not recall many of the abortions at the close of the ten-year period. Yet he has lost by abortion five per cent of his calf crop. Records are not ordinarily kept in grade herds. In pure-bred herds, the records of living calves at age for registration is essential. Many breeders make notes of abortion, and some of retained afterbirth. Incidentally, the number of calves registered in the official herd book might indicate the practical reproductive efficiency, if it were known how many females of breeding age were in the herd, but this is only rarely known, and, so far as I have observed, never publicly stated.

There are in the United States, in connection with agricultural schools and colleges and experiment stations, a great number of dairy herds kept for research and teaching. The authorities report frequently the records made by individual cows, the average milk and butter yield in a given time for all cows in milk in the herd, the amount and cost of foods used in producing such records, etc., but the management of no public herd, so far as I have discovered, has ever recorded any data to indicate the reproductive efficiency. Apparently, if one cow in such a herd makes thirty pounds of butter in a week, the management considers that success, even though one of her associates aborts and yields essentially no milk, another has retained afterbirth and dies, and a fourth is sterile for the year or forever. The yield of thirty pounds of butter by one of the four cows does not save the group from bankruptcy.

For obvious reasons, private owners of registered cattle do not report the vital statistics of their herds. The breeding efficiency in all large herds is such that accurate vital statistics, if published, would place the herd at a disadvantage with all other herds whose owners rest their case upon the general statement that they have no sterility, abortion, premature birth, retained afterbirth, calf scours, or calf pneumonia. Viewed from the standpoint of observed abortions alone, among the few herds from which I have been able to secure reasonably accurate data over a period of years, the abortion rate has ranged as high as seventeen per cent and has not fallen below ten per cent. The abortions have always been highest in heifers—usually in first, though sometimes in second pregnancy. In those herds where heifer calves are regularly grown in considerable numbers and enter the breeding herd at the rate of ten or more annually, the abortion rate in first pregnancy over a series of years frequently reaches thirty to fifty per cent, and has not fallen below twenty per cent in any herd from which I have been able to obtain data over a period of eight to ten years.

In smaller herds, especially where but few heifers are grown, the abortion rate is apparently much lower. The average rate of abortion in dairy cows certainly exceeds five per cent. If the dairy cows of New York number 1,500,000, and five per cent are known to abort annually, the total abortions in the state number 75,000. In many localities, dairymen can sell a large new-born calf for five dollars, to be grown for veal. Calves of the smaller breeds are not so valuable for veal, but high-grade heifer calves are much more valuable and the values of pedigreed calves of either sex mount into thousands. It would appear very conservative to place the loss of the aborted calves alone at an average of five dollars each— a total of $375,000 per annum.

It is reasonable, according to my observations, to say that two per cent of aborting cows die—a total of 1500 animals, which, at $75.00 each, amounts to $112,500.

Not less than ten per cent of observed aborters become permanently sterile and have to be sent to the butcher, at an average loss of probably thirty dollars each—a total of $225,000.

I have estimated that two per cent of aborters die. The dairying efficiency of the remaining ninety-eight per cent, or 73,500 cows, which abort is probably reduced fifty per cent for the prospective lactation period. In order to be safe, let the estimated loss be thirty per cent of the milk flow, considering the normal lactation as twenty-five pounds per day for three hundred days, or a total of seven thousand five hundred pounds.

The cow which aborts loses thirty per cent—2250 pounds—of milk, worth two cents per pound, or $45 for each aborting cow—a total loss in value of milk of $3,307,500.

Those cows which do not die or become permanently sterile do not breed promptly. High dairying efficiency demands that a cow calve once every twelve months. Every month that a cow exceeds this period between calves is, on the average, a total loss to the dairyman. On the average cows which abort and breed again probably run over at least two months, or there is a period of fourteen months between two calvings, and if a cow's keep is estimated at five dollars per month, or ten dollars for the two months in the one year, there is a further total loss of $735,000.

These various items total $4,755,000, as the estimated annual losses caused by observed abortions in New York. Upon this basis, my figures are still far in excess of those of the Secretary of Agriculture, who estimates the total for the United States at $20,000,000. New York possesses about seven per cent of the dairying cattle of the nation. Consequently, her pro rata of the loss should be $1,400,000, instead of $4,755,000.

If the common conception is accepted of limiting the term "contagious abortion" to those losses due to observed abortions in cows and the immediate consequences, my estimate of ten millions annually for New York is apparently too high. If my conception of what constitutes the infection of contagious abortion is accepted, the estimate becomes entirely too low. Under the broader conception, most of the losses from sterility in cows not observed to abort must be added. The data I have been able to obtain indicate that five per cent of heifers fail to conceive, or conceive and abort unseen and are sold to the butcher as sterile, and that approximately as high a percentage of sterility prevails among cows of all ages. In other words, approximately five per cent of the cows and heifers of breeding age go to the butcher each year because of permanent sterility. Retained afterbirth plays a conspicuous part in causing sterility, whether the cow has aborted, calved prematurely, or calved at full term. Retained afterbirth causes many deaths, and when at all severe either seriously injures or wholly ruins the milk production during the involved lactation period.

One of the most stupendous and very largely unrecognized losses of dairymen is temporary sterility, or delay in conception. It has been stated that the highest dairy efficiency calls for healthy calving once in each twelve months. Pursuant to this plan, the dairyman or breeder ordinarily breeds a cow at the first opportunity between fifty and eighty days after calving. If she fails to become pregnant within ninety days after calving and must be bred several times, if she is an average cow, it means that she must run dry for an undesirably long period, or her milk yield must be extremely low over a long period. Besides, and especially in registered cows, there is a diminution in the number of calves. The cost of this delay, falling singly, cow by cow, attracts little attention; studied carefully, the losses are staggering. If estimates are based upon one calving each twelve months and each cow is expected to be dry two months, a cow is actually at remunerative efficiency eighty-three per cent of the time. If conception is delayed one month, the efficient milking period is reduced to seventy-seven per cent of the time—a reduction of six per cent. It is probably safe to say that upon the average dairy cows calve once in thirteen months, instead of once in twelve months, and must be kept one unprofitable month in excess of the two dry months estimated as judicious before calving. If it is assumed that keeping a dry cow costs five dollars a month, and that each of the one and one-half million dairy cows are fed for one useless month for each lactation period, the item is one of $7,500,000 for the state.

It is slowly becoming recognized by veterinarians and breeders that the infection within the uterus, which may cause sterility, abortion, retained afterbirth, and other disasters to the cow, frequently passes from the uterus to the fetus prior to birth. Immediately after birth, the infection from the uterus of the diseased cow may flow down along the tail, thighs, and udder to the teats and be taken with the milk by the calf, to constitute the fundamental cause of scours and pneumonia. These cause the death or serious deterioration of a vast number of calves. In the largest herds of the best breeding cattle, the losses are frequently total for months at a time, and losses of thirty to forty per cent for sev-

eral years in succession are by no means rare. Therefore, the
deaths are most keenly felt in valuable calves which it is desired to
grow for breeding and dairying purposes. In the State of New
York, the deaths of calves from this disease probably exceed 100,-
000 annually. Considering that a large proportion of them are
highly bred and valuable for breeding purposes, it is safe to estimate the losses from this cause at more than one million dollars.

If this broader conception of contagious abortion—or whatever it may be called—is accepted, but brief study is required to
show that the estimate I have made of $10,000,000 annual losses is
none too high. Such estimates dictate also a reversal of position between tuberculosis and abortion, with regard to the monetary losses
caused by each. Abortion is unquestionably the more expensive
disease, by far, and it is an open question which of them is the
greater menace to human health.

What do these losses signify to the State? A careful study of
this disease, or group of diseases, shows that it involves by far the
most seriously the large herds of highly pedigreed cattle. From
these the most cows are sent to the butcher for sterility; here the
most is expended in keeping a sterile cow for months or years, in
the hope, not always realized, of ultimately having her breed; here
retained afterbirth is commonest; and here also scours and pneumonia take the most frightful toll in the death of calves.

The losses fall primarily upon the cattle owners. In many instances they are men of independent weath, who take up the breeding of highly pedigreed cattle as a sport or for idealistic reasons
and have ample incomes from other sources to maintain the herd,
regardless of its essential bankruptcy. Ultimately the State must
meet the losses. The great breeding herds are the logical source of
supply of valuable breeding stock for the improvement of the common cattle. Without such sources where scientific breeding is
nurtured, the common cattle cannot keep up that constant advance
in efficiency ever demanded by the State. Each year the cost of
cattle food and of labor advances, and just as surely the efficiency
of dairy cows must keep pace, or the owner must fail. The world
war has found the dairies of America inefficient, just as it has
found many, if not all our industries. Few industries are being
more sorely tried. The embarrassments are numerous and serious.
Complaints regarding the industry are heard on all sides. The
consumer complains of the high cost, the producer complains of the

ruinous costs of food and labor, and health boards criticise the high bacterial count in the milk and the unsanitary conditions in the dairy. The official veterinary service kills, quarantines, and otherwise interferes with the movements and uses of cattle by their owners. Dairymen complain that dairying does not and cannot pay, and are said to be dispersing their herds; breeders of purebred cattle complain even more seriously, and are dispersing and scattering to the winds great herds of vast economic possibilities to the State. Public-spirited men are busying themselves in efforts to check the scattering and destruction of valuable cattle, but are not wholly successful. The fact is that the world war is testing both cattle and men. We all hear that thousands of valuable dairy cattle are being sent to the shambles. Personally, I have seen no accurate data upon the point. Unquestionably, great numbers of dairy cows are being slaughtered, but just how efficient they are in the dairy is not revealed. How many cows free from tuberculosis and yielding thirty pounds of milk with 4.5 per cent of butter fat daily are being sent to the shambles? I doubt that many such cows are being sold. I have examined thousands of dairy cows in abattoirs, but am not accustomed to seeing there highly efficient dairy cows in full flow of milk.

Possibly the reports mean rather that cows which have a high potential dairying value are being slaughtered. This is doubtless true, and in this field many lamentable errors are made—and made in both directions. I recall a highly valuable cow which had been bred many times, but was apparently incurably sterile. Being dry, she was butchered, and was found pregnant. Evidently this was not so much a want of prudence as of knowledge. The opposite error is equally common. A notable cow in the State of New York made a world's butter-fat record and was sold for $10,000. At once she became sterile. After four years of effort, she became pregnant and dropped a fine bull calf potentially worth the cost of the cow. The calf died when a few days old from scours, and the cow is again sterile. There has been a very considerable expense added to the original cost of the cow. In each of these cases, there has been serious loss to the owners. However, the loss is not limited to the owner. The $10,000 cow, with a butter record of more than forty pounds per week, was quite as much an asset of the State as of the owner. The progeny of such a cow is needed for breeding up less efficient cattle. Her failure to reproduce living young, and her failure to yield milk, is a State loss. The ten thousand dollars lost through this cow are paid ultimately by the users of dairy products, veal, and beef.

A serious financial burden falls upon the small dairyman when he goes to the great breeding herds for purebred sires for grading up his stock. Each high-producing cow which aborts, and each calf from a high-producing dam which dies of scours or pneumonia, adds to the price of the bull he must buy. If each thirty-pound cow would produce a healthy calf annually, the market price of calves from thirty-pound cows would drop. If the breeding powers of each thirty-pound cow could be preserved to eighteen years of age or over, and she would produce sixteen calves, such highly efficient cattle would multiply rapidly. In herds from which I have been able to secure reasonably good data, the cows have produced upon an average about three live calves each. In small herds, the average is perhaps a trifle higher, but does not exceed, so far as I can determine, an average of four calves per cow. That is, the average dairy cow does not live to six years of age and produce a calf each year beginning at two years. The average dairy cow fails to reach the prime of dairy life, but dies or is sold before six years old because of inefficiency. Part of such inefficiency is clearly fundamental, and the animal fails in the dairy in spite of good health. Far more heifers and young cows are discarded owing to disease which greatly lowers or wholly destroys their efficiency.

In another respect, it is a serious matter for the small dairyman to go to a large herd for breeding stock of either sex to introduce into his dairy. The abortion group of diseases has become so intense and widespread that the dairyman must incur a severe risk of introducing a more intense type of infection into his herd than that which already exists. Careful observations indicate very strongly that animals procured for breeding purposes from extremely badly infected herds may be followed by a trail of disaster wherever they go. The complaint from this standpoint is growing as we learn more and more of the nature of these diseases, and it is becoming of greater importance each year that the large breeder shall be more vigorous and more careful to preserve the soundness of his herd. The small dairyman can make very scant progress by going to the breeder of valuable cattle and securing a sire which is so badly infected that he will cause serious losses in the herd.

Neither can the small diaryman well afford to breed his cows to a valuable sire in a neighboring herd which is virulently infected.

In another respect the question of this group of diseases is highly important. Whenever a cow aborts, calves prematurely, or calves at full term and has retained afterbirth, there occurs for a longer or shorter period a voluminous and highly repulsive discharge from her genital organs. Part of this, flowing down along the tail, thighs, and udder, eventually gets into the milk. No definite disease of the human family has been traced to this source, but grave apprehensions are being aroused that this filth may interfere very seriously, in a variety of ways, with human health. The belief cannot be avoided that these discharges are injurious to human health, though to what extent and in what manner we do not know at present. The malignant sore throat of man is attributed wholly to contaminated milk, though in just what manner this contamination occurs is not known. Various writers on human medicine have suspected that diseases of the tonsils and adenoids are due to milk infection, and some writers suspect that infection from the use of cow's milk may play a part in the production of abortion and other diseases of the genital organs of woman.

The State is especially interested in the fact that the diseases of the genital organs of cattle, by lowering enormously the reproductive and dairying efficiency, increase correspondingly the cost of milk and of veal and beef. Every pound of milk produced pays a toll to disease. The cost of cattle diseases is rarely fully recognized. In order of importance, the average dairying expenses are food, labor, and disease, with disease crowding labor closely and not infrequently taking precedence. The State is also intensely interested in these diseases from the standpoint of human health.

The State Agricultural Society has a special interest in this great problem. Agriculture needs cattle—and especially dairy cows—for maintaining the fertility of the soil. The climatic and soil conditions of the State of New York render this problem of supreme importance. The decrease in the number of dairy cows in the State which is now going on is a serious blow to the productiveness of the soil. Therefore, if for no other reason, agriculturists should do everything in their power, as a body, to maintain and increase the number of dairy cows.

Throughout the history of our race, cow's milk has contributed the chief food of children, and milk and other dairy products have

constituted a leading food of adults and of the aged. Dairy products excel among all human foods, in economy, efficiency as nutri-
ents, and healthfulness, when procured from healthy cows and
kept under sanitary conditions. The human race has subsisted for
so long largely upon dairy products as a staple food that it is impossible to turn from them. The growth of our cities is constantly
demanding more and more milk. The metropolis is reaching out
for hundreds of miles—about as far as milk can be economically or
safely transported—in order to get an adequate milk supply. In
spite of this, the number of dairy cows decreases, and now in the
world war every dairy herd is being severely tried, and wherever
a cow is inefficient she must be sacrificed for economic reasons.
Unfortunately, many of these cows are not fundamentally inefficient, but are inefficient because of preventable disease. This
makes the present rapid decrease in dairy cows all the more de-
plorable. No one can seriously blame a dairyman for selling a dry
cow which was not efficient because of retained afterbirth during her last lactation period and will not calve for several months.
He knows too well that she may abort or again have retained afterbirth after she has cost a large sum for food.

War conditions demand efficiency in every walk in life. This
is just as true of dairying as it is of the making of ammunitions or
of any other industry. If a cow fails, she must go, even though
the failure is due to ignorance or carelessness on the part of the
owner. It is the failure—not the potential worth of the cow—
which must decide the question. Possibly the present conditions
may lead to great good by thoroughly awakening the dairyman and
the State to the condition of affairs and leading to some efficient
measures for overcoming the evil.

Up to the present, there has been great confusion regarding
the conditions necessary for the control of this disease. Generally,
dairymen and breeders have taken the matter very lightly except
when a storm breaks in their herds and a large per cent of their
cows abort or nearly all their calves die, and the milk production
is reduced alarmingly. Then they suddenly take alarm and appeal
for some rapid and cheap aid. Consequently they resort to various
patent medicines—some quack cure-all—in an effort to overcome a
chronic infection which has existed in their herds for years and has
only recently become visible to them by a great increase in its virulence. When the storm has swept by, they again lapse into forget-

fulness and fancied security until the infection again gathers force and they again have very serious losses.

One of the greatest difficulties in the situation is to have the dairyman and breeder recognize the scope of the disease as it has been outlined. The average man insists upon regarding abortion as one disease, sterility as another, retained afterbirth as a third, and calf scours and pneumonia as a fourth and fifth: they refuse to consider them as the varying symptoms of one great infection. If they could but once come to a realization of the relationship existing between them, a great step in advance would be made. They would recognize the fact that the infection exists in essentially all herds: that some herds are so slightly infected that no recognizable harm is produced, and that other herds are so severely infected that there is appalling destruction. Still more important, they should recognize that, with the knowledge now available, they may by proper measures reduce the losses very greatly, within economic bounds.

The breeders of purebred cattle should especially be brought to recognize the fact that their herds are the great centers for the nurturing and distribution of chronic diseases. From the large purebred herd, stock for breeding purposes radiates out in every direction. If diseased, these animals are capable of carrying such infections and disseminating them widely. It should be recognized as a moral crime for a breeder to sell knowingly highly infected animals to go into other herds. According to the views expressed, he cannot sell animals absolutely free from this infection, so far as known, nor, if he could do so, could they go into smaller dairy herds which are free. It is possible, however, for him to sell animals so nearly free from the infection that the degree of infection will compare favorably with that in the herds to which they are to go, and breeding may go forward without visible disease.

It has been suggested by numerous veterinarians and others that contagious abortion should be named among the contagious diseases of cattle coming under the control of the State Veterinarian or other veterinary police authority, so that animals so infected may be subjected to quarantine or other restrictions. Such laws have been enacted in a few countries. So far as known, they have accomplished no good. Such attempts at control are exceedingly imprudent, and unfortunate for the State, as well as for the dairyman and breeder. Too little is known of the disease for it to be handled equitably and safely by legal restrictions. However, there are constant mutterings regarding such restrictions, and it would be well indeed to take note of these complaints and try to control the infection in a herd as far as the present knowledge of the disease will permit.

The State should do its utmost to increase the sum of the knowledge of the disease and to transmit that knowledge to veterinarians, breeders, and dairymen. It cannot be hoped that dairymen or breeders, working upon their own initiative, will materially advance our knowledge of the disease. The study of the disease has been considered entirely too much the business of the owner of the dairy or breeding herd. Individual dairymen can do little to learn the true character of the disease and the means of prevention. The work must be done through co-operation, and the co-operation must be had through the agency of the State. The State is capable of improving the situation in a variety of ways:

(1) By educating and distributing throughout the State an adequate number of competent veterinarians, thoroughly versed in the latest knowledge regarding the diseases of cattle and ready to aid the dairymen and breeders with advice wherever necessary.

(2) By research work, through adequate veterinary organization, making careful and exhaustive studies of these diseases.

(3) By issuing reports, bulletins, or other publications, which may be distributed among veterinarians, dairymen, and breeders, advising them as far as may be practicable what they may do to control the disease.

In the first respect—educating veterinarians—the State of New York has taken a high place in America. The State has founded and equipped a commodious veterinary college, which, however, is not yet complete. Up to the present time, the State of New York has expended about one-third as much on the buildings and equipment of her veterinary school as the little country of Belgium expended upon her veterinary school a few years prior to the world war. When the New York State Veterinary College at Cornell University is compared with other veterinary schools in America, however, there is little complaint to be made. With better facilities, more and better instruction could be given. The agriculturists of New York should have a keen interest in veterinary education and see that their school is brought up to the highest state of efficiency for the needs of the State. There is need for better, rather than more veterinarians, in the dairying regions of the State. The college is graduating a sufficient number of veterinarians to furnish an adequate supply in every part of the State. Whatever dearth of veterinarians there may be can be largely corrected in time, if the breeders and dairymen will take a greater interest in veterinary science and let it be known that they need and are ready to support a good veterinarian in their community.

Until recently, American veterinarians have known little of the diseases of cattle. Almost all the veterinary schools of America have been located in great cities and conducted primarily for gain by their private owners. The members of their faculties have not had experience with the diseases of cattle, and there are no clinical facilities for teaching regarding these. Fortunately for the State of New York, when its state veterinary college was founded in 1896 it was located at Ithaca, under the management of Cornell University, in the midst of an extensive dairying district. The clinic in the college at Cornell University has afforded large numbers of cattle for research and observation by the teaching staff, in order that they may be more able to teach students regarding the diseases of dairy animals. Of equal importance, the clinical facilities with dairy cattle furnish necessary material for illustrating to students the nature of these diseases, and methods of handling. The college has—and long has had—the largest cattle clinic on the American continent.

The college has not been unmindful of the interests of dairymen and breeders with reference to research work. Much time has been given to research upon the various diseases of cattle prevalent in the State of New York—especially upon the ruinous group of diseases to which contagious abortion belongs. The study of these diseases was undertaken almost as soon as the college was founded, and the research work has grown constantly, until two years ago a special department was founded for this work, with a professor and an assistant giving their entire time to research upon the diseases of breeding cattle. In this respect, it is unique among the colleges of America.

Two years ago the legislature was asked for a special appropriation of $15,000 for erecting, equipping, and maintaining buildings and for procuring cattle for special researches in connection with contagious abortion. The hearty and vigorous support of numerous cattle breeders in the State enabled the appropriation bill to be passed. The building has been completed, with accommodations for thirty animals. Before it was fully completed, it was filled with cattle. While there is an opportunity for much interesting work with the room and the number of animals available, the equipment is still inadequate. The amount appropriated for the building, equipment, and cattle—$15,000—represents about one and one half per cent of the estimated annual loss to dairymen and breeders from this one disease in the State of New York.

For several years, the college has issued annually an extensive report, in which the account of the investigations of this disease has occupied a prominent place. The report has been comparatively technical, and only a limited number have been printed by the order of the legislature. These have been distributed as widely as possible to those breeders who were presumably most deeply interested. In addition to these reports, the Department of Research in the Diseases of Breeding Cattle has issued popular bulletins which have been distributed as widely as possible among breeders and dairymen. It is hoped that in the future still more will be done and a larger audience reached.

—Dr. E. A. A. Grange, for many years Principal of the Ontario Veterinary College, has retired from that position and been made Principal Emeritus. He has been one of the leading veterinarians of the country, has held many important positions in veterinary service and is well known to the members of the American Veterinary Medical Association.

Dr. C. D. McGilvray, V.S., M.D.V., of Winnipeg will succeed Dr. Grange as Principal on the first of September. Dr. McGilvray has been for many years the chief veterinary officer in the Province of Manitoba where he has done excellent work in the control of glanders and other contagious diseases. He has published an important paper on the suppression glanders in that Province. He also was the first to bring to the attention of the American Veterinary Medical Association garbage feeding as a source of hog cholera.

—Dr. S. H. Burnett, formerly of the New York State Veterinary College at Ithaca, N. Y., is now located at Laramie, Wyo., in connection with the Agricultural Experiment Station.

MYSTERIOUS LOSSES AMONG CATTLE IN THE PACIFIC NORTHWEST*

A Clinical Study

Dr. C. H. Schultz, Seattle, Wash.

During the last three years, losses among livestock in our states have been severe. Every month newspaper notices appear, stating that a great number of animals had perished under mysterious circumstances; investigations have been conducted, to be sure, but the problem has evidently not yet been solved. Several diseases should be considered, some at least, of bacterial origin; isolated instances where poison was used with criminal intention may have caused some losses; plant and forage poisoning have been blamed in several localities, without obtaining definite proof, however. In every number of our veterinary publications articles appear, discussing destructive outbreaks among cattle; without being able to announce a definite diagnosis. Hemorrhagic septicemia is usually mentioned in connection with these outbreaks, but investigators have found it exceedingly difficult to demonstrate and isolate *Bacterium bovisepticus*. Drs. Mack and Record presented a paper at the annual meeting of the A.. V. M. A., in Kansas City, under the title "Studies of an obscure cattle disease in Western Nevada". It brought forth a most interesting discussion; although several veterinarians expressed their views in a liberal manner, a definite diagnosis has not been established.

In Washington, we have similar outbreaks and have had them for years. It is possible that true hemorrhagic septicemia in violent form occurs, but in several instances consideration of history and clinical appearances supported by careful bacterial studies failed to demonstrate the presence of pathogenic bipolar organisms. Dr. A. U. Simpson, M.D., our city bacteriologist, a most conscientious investigator, was not able to demonstrate *Bacterium bovisepticus* in specimen from three different localities, although the lesions and appearance of tissues would be accepted as characteristic of hemorrhagic septicemia.

After many observations and as careful a study as circumstances would permit, I diagnosed what is commonly known as

---

*Presented at the Oregon-Washington State Veterinary Meeting at Portland, Ore., June 14th, 1918.

"red dysentery" of cattle as the cause of a great part of these
losses. The purpose of this article is to call your attention to this
disease, to explain some of its peculiarities and destroy as much
as possible the shroud of mystery that has always surrounded it,
not only during its appearance here, but wherever it has been observed.

The cause of red dysentery in cattle was first recognized and
described in connection with the disease by Dr. F. A. Zurn, in
Leipzig, Germany, in 1878. The material which he examined was
obtained from calves which died from the disease while pasturing
on moist land. Since then the malady has been recognized from
time to time and descriptions have appeared, especially in European
journals. From 1885 to 1891, it destroyed many animals in Switzerland, where it was identified by Dr. Zschokke (veterinary college Zurich) and Drs. Guillebeau and Hess (veterinary college
Bern). Their articles were published in 1892 and 1893, and are
used as references in our textbooks today. Another article on the
same subject from the pen of Dr. Zublein appeared in a Swiss
veterinary journal in 1908. In 1905, an outbreak of a mysterious
disease destroyed a great number of cattle in Tunis (Africa) ; at
first anthrax, blackleg or piroplasmosis was accepted as the cause,
but M. E. Ducloux identified it as red dysentery, a disease which
had not been recognized in that part of Northern Africa before.
During the last decade its distribution on all continents, with the
possible exception of Australia, and on many islands has been reported.

The specific cause of the scourge is a protozoan, a minute organism that belongs to the primitive, unicellular forms of the animal kingdom. The bacteria, on the other hand, belong to the simplest, smallest forms of the vegetable kingdom. The organism under discussion passes through a complicated life-cycle and has a
peculiar ability to adapt itself to marked changes of environment.
Some of its forms are very resistant and can dry out or freeze for
months and begin to multiply when moisture and temperatures become favorable. The organism in question is known as coccidium
oviforme or coccidium zurni. It belongs to the

   Phylum Protozoa,
    Subphylum Plasmodroma
     Class Sporozoa (Leukart)
      Subclass Telosporidia (Schaudinn)

which is divided into different orders by different authorities:

1. Order, Gregarinidae,
2. Order, Coccididae,
3. Order, Haemosporidiae.

Systematic Zoology shows that coccidia are closely related to the haemosporidia, which multiply in and are especially destructive to the red blood-cells of their host. The malaria parasites belong to the haemosporidia; their life cycle resembles that of the coccidia in many ways, but it is still more complicated, because they require a change of hosts to complete it.

The close relationship of these two groups of destructive parasites has not received due consideration and should be remembered when symptoms of the early stages, with high temperatures are considered.

In Neumann-MacQueen's work on "Parasites and Parasitic Diseases of Domestic Animals", II edition, an interesting list of tissues and organs in which coccidia have been demonstrated by different investigators will be found; it shows that nearly every organ has been invaded by these destructive protozoa. Several authorities (Balbiani, Novy) have also found them in the blood-stream. These facts have often been overlooked, but should be duly considered because they may help to explain the serious and often mysterious disturbances produced by coccidia.

In "A treatise on Zoology", second fascicle, 1903, by E. Ray Lankester, on page 206, the statement is made, that:

"Coccidia are chiefly parasites of epithelial cells, and since the infection of the host appears to take place in all cases by way of the digestive tract, it is the epithelium of the gut or its appendages, such as the liver, that is most often the seat of the parasite. In a considerable number of cases, however, the parasitic germs, after entering the system by way of the gut, go further afield before settling down. Passing through the gut wall the parasites are transported, probably by the circulation of the blood or lymph, to their specific habitat."

All classes of animals may be attacked by this type of protozoa. They have been found in centipedes, insects, clams, crayfish, fish, frogs; they often cause fatal diseases among rabbits, mice, moles, sheep, goats, cattle, swine, many kinds of wild animals, but especially among the different species of birds, from house-sparrows to wild swans. Even the human family has been attacked—several cases of coccidian diarrhea in man have been observed and reported. Another peculiarity of coccidia is that they do not always attack the same organs. They are mostly cell-parasites, that means that they bore into a cell of the lining of the intestines, for example, and enlarge and multiply in it. This destroys the cell, the young attack new cells and in course of a few hours serious injury to the attacked tissue results. Some of these protozoa multiply in the intestines; this occurs commonly in cattle, sheep and chickens; other kinds prefer the kidneys, as in mice and frogs; in rabbits they invade the intestines, the liver and gall ducts, the lungs, nose and eyes; in swine often the lungs; in birds usually the intestines, but they may be found in the chest, on the lungs, on the ribs, on the liver, in the kidneys, the nose and even the eyes. Young animals of all species are most frequently attacked. Protozoa as a class are far more destructive to the young than to older hosts; if an animal passes through an attack of a disease, it acquires a certain degree of resistancy against a subsequent attack. This may, to some extent, explain why not so many older, full grown animals are afflicted. Another peculiarity may here be mentioned in connection with protozoan diseases; it is that the processes which produce so-called "immunity", or to be correct, "resistancy", are very complicated and not well understood. An animal may have a certain amount of resistancy when in good health, but if weakened by overwork, hunger, or another disease, this resistancy is lessened or may be entirely destroyed. This explains why animals are "more or less resistant". When an animal takes up from some source or other a certain amount of virulent material, it becomes sick if the organisms are able to multiply rapidly; but if they cannot multiply, it remains apparently healthy. This happens when the resistant power is high, and the parasite can multiply only slowly or not at all. Such an animal becomes therefore a "carrier" of that disease; itself resistant, immune, it carries the cause of disease and disseminates it, maybe not always, but periodically, at least.

This is one of the peculiarities of protozoan diseases. If all the animals that come in contact with a carrier are resistant, no outbreak occurs. But if such a carrier goes into a neighborhood where susceptible animals are, the disease reappears (no one can tell from where) and, conditions being favorable, a sudden outbreak occurs, assigned to a mysterious cause.

It is also necessary to consider, that coccidia pass through a very complicated life-cycle. This phase has received especial attention from the German scientist, Dr. Fritz Schaudinn, whose classical studies of malaria are world-famous. He worked out the life-cycle of coccidia in the centipede and mole; since then investigators have studied it on rabbits, chickens and other small animals.

. In the Twenty-seventh Annual Report of the Bureau of Animal Industry, 1910, U. S. Department of Agriculture, a short sketch of diseases caused by protozoan parasites appears. Several pages are devoted to the subject of coccidia; their complicated life-cycle is explained by a full page illustration and comprehensive text.

About 1905, a fatal disease that destroyed the grouse on the moors in Scotland became so virulent that nearly all the young birds died. A special commission was appointed to investigate it. The results of this investigation were published in the "Proceedings of the Zoological Society of London" during 1909 and 1910. In a most interesting series of articles, Dr. H. B. Fantham states that the cause of the plague was a coccidium; and gives an exceedingly useful and interesting account of the mode of multiplication of the parasite, which resembles that causing the disease in cattle.

Dr. E. Montgomery, pathologist in Nairobi, British East Africa, identified and described the disease in young cattle during 1911 and 1912. Another interesting article from the pen of Dr. Walter Jowett, pathologist of the Department of Agriculture of Cape Colony, in Capetown, South Africa, was published in 1911.

Red dysentery in cattle is caused by coccidium oviforme (egg-shaped coccidium). Under the microscope it appears as an oval, body about 30 microns long, half as thick, with a well defined double outline; its protoplasma may appear quite clear, with a large nucleus. Young forms show faint outline; they are protected by surrounding cells and under favorable conditions multiply rapidly by simple division.

Sometimes one protozoa divides into a great number of daughter-cells and the process is repeated for many generations. It is this primitive but rapid division that destroys the host. Whenever these rapid division forms are found in great numbers, the disease exists in a dangerous form. After a certain time this quick asexual method of multiplication stops. The minute protozoa become differentiated into male and female forms; fertilization then takes place and better developed but still unicellular organisms with a well marked double outline, a resistant tough capsule, are formed. Into the larger of these the male forms penetrate at a certain point and soon there appear in the roundish or egg-shaped, transparent parasite four small oblong bodies, spores. These are also surrounded by firm membranes; each one divides again into two small organisms, so that a fertilized female cell eventually produces eight minute offsprings, sporozoites. These forms are all very resistant; they can stand drying out, freezing, and may lay dormant for a long time. Whenever conditions are favorable for further development, they emerge from their protective capsules. These resistant forms may be lodged on grass, or in the dried condition on hay, oats, corn; or they may be found in contaminated waterholes. As soon as they are taken into the intestinal tract of suitable animals, their capsules are dissolved and the motile minute parasites bore into suitable cells and begin the rapid, simple process of agamic multiplication.

These different phases of development provide material. for most interesting studies and are even today not definitely known. They are very important, because if they were fully understood it would help us to devise protective measures. We know, for example, that these protozoa can only attain full development in the presence of oxygen; certain temperatures are more favorable than others. Moisture is necessary. Other important points, on the other hand, are still in dispute. Many observers say that they are obligatory parasites, others say that they are only facultative parasites. This point is very important, because an obligatory parasite can only develop within its host, but a facultative parasite is able to live or even develop and multiply outside of the host.

Here, then, is an important question that needs most careful investigation, and, since these organisms are so primitive and therefore often very difficult to recognize it will require careful observations.

Dr. Eckhardt, in an article on intestinal coccidiosis in poultry, published on pages 177-180 of No. 11, March 12th, 1903, of the *Berliner Tierarzliche Wochenschrift,* makes the statement that "coccidia are only facultative parasites which multiply rapidly in moist garden soil on hot sultry summer days especially in decaying or putrid substances. When taken up by animals in water or food the disease appears. Some birds die suddenly without visible symptoms."

Guillebeau in 1892, reported that coccidia were able to divide and multiply in different manner when subject to different temperatures—this is important when we consider that animals become infected because they eat contaminated hay—dried during hot summer weather on irrigated fields, where the temperature would correspond to 104°-110° F., as against temperatures of 70°-75° F., or lower, which are often found on moist pasture lands in the western part of our state.

The disease is commonly caused by the ingestion of coccidia on grass, hay or water. The early symptoms may vary, depending upon susceptibility of the animal and amount of virulent material taken up. Some cases terminate fatally in two or three days. The owner observes that animals are humped up, look distressed, and finds them dead on the next day—often with good pasture all around them. Other animals in the same pasture are not affected; several may appear sick later on; when examined they show more or less discharge, water or slimy, at times streaked with blood, from the nose; they may show slight inflammation of the eyes. Some animals eat, others do not. Usually cattle appear dull, seem subject to chill, stand humped up, coat is staring, rumination is suspended, they grind their teeth; drooling is quite noticeable, defecation is usually very scanty. The abdomen is markedly tucked up and they drink a great deal of water if not too far away. Evidently moving about causes pain and they will lay down or stand quietly if not disturbed. During these early stages a raise of temperature to 104° or even 107° F. will be registered on the thermometer. Constipation is the ever-present important symptom. The attack may cause death in a few days, even before diarrhea sets in. In other cases the period of constipation, during which feces, formed into hard pellets or dislike masses, covered with mucous, sometimes streaked with blood, are passed—is followed by well marked diarrhea. The feces become watery and show remnants of imperfectly digested food. The discharge soon becomes offensive, because the bile is not secreted properly and its antiseptic property is lacking. The secretory glands of large parts of the intestines are involved, croupous casts are passed out in large massés; often they show bloody streaks. If discharge from nose becomes cream-like and yellowish, the upper air passages and even the lungs may be involved. In severe cases, all these processes are rapidly progressive; emaciation, weakness and general debility, due to the destructive processes in the intestines and the inability to absorb nourishment causes death in a few days.

On the other hand, some animals will pass through a mild attack without marked symptoms. They may stand about humped up; milk cows give less milk; are drowsy, show constipation and scant, hard, rather dry feces, invariably covered with a thick layer of mucus, at times streaked with blood. After a period of constipation extending over several days, diarrhea sets in. The last part that passes out is quite thin and contains a mass of pale yellow or clear mucous. It may have an offensive odor and show bloody streaks. This stage may only last during an evening and the animal appear all right the next day. Similar periods re-occur from time to time.

These are chronic cases of coccidiosis; in other words, a mild form of red dysentery of cattle. The animal that is afflicted is resistant—because it has become accustomed to the parasite. Therefore the coccidia for reasons which are not well understood, multiply only in a more or less limited part of the intestines (usually the last part of the colon and the rectum), cause a chronic moderate inflammation and small defects in the lining of the gut, but nothing more serious. This process may involve only part of the rectum, or it may affect the gut from the cecum (blind gut) to the anus; it may also be more or less severe. In dairy cows that were slaughtered for other causes, the parasites could often be observed on the folds of the fourth stomach, which appears to present conditions especially favorable for the development of coccidia.

In very mild attacks, practically no disturbance will be observed. In the more severe cases of this chronic form, the constant drain on the host is severe. Animals produce less milk, drop calves too soon, show a ravenous appetite and instead of being well nourished and good producers lose flesh, so that they must be discarded. The mucous that such animals pass in their feces is produced by the intestinal cells as a result of constant irritation; it requires nitrogenous material, albumen, for its production and costs a good deal to produce. I wonder if the remarkably low per cent of milk solids which have been reported in some of our dairy herds must not be charged up to this cause. Observations, which extend over several years, from April, 1915, until now, convince me that this disease in its chronic form is very common among our dairy cattle. It can be observed in all the dairies that feed alfalfa hay obtained from irrigated districts in Eastern Washington. Evidently the alfalfa fields in irrigated districts are infested and supply contaminated hay.

The beginning and course of the chronic form is usually so insidious that it has been overlooked. Stock owners call their veterinarian only when animals are in great distress. This type of disease requires careful consideration of history, clinical symptoms and microscopic examination of feces, not only once, but during different periods, because as already stated, the parasite goes through a well defined cycle of development and cannot always be recognized.

An important factor in the dissemination of coccidia is the number of chronic carriers, animals that have the disease in a mild form. .

The fertile, encapsulated forms that alone can infect pastures or cause the disease in susceptible animals are not formed in animals that perish, but in those that recover. These resistant forms are passed out in feces and usually develop on the pastures if temperature and other conditions are favorable. After they have reached full development, they are very resistant and may remain dormant for a long time, certainly for several months. Their existence outside the body is still an obscure chapter. In Switzerland, several cases of red dysentery have been observed, the disease being caused by feeding contaminated hay in winter. In other cases it appeared among young stock in summer on pastures which were frozen and covered with snow during several months.

It goes without saying, that the disease can and is further distributed by animals that are shipped from one part of the country to another. Especially would this be important if it is demonstrated beyond a doubt that coccidia are only facultative parasites; that is, that they can multiply and exist in waterholes or on carcasses of dead animals or on miscellaneous matter, such as decaying fruit or roots, manure or slime in ditches. A carrier would drop them on a pasture, the weather being favorable (hot) and the ground moist, the protozoa would multiply and dry up. Some weeks afterward young stock is driven into the same field and after a few days animals begin to die, others have diarrhea and become thin and weak. Not very mysterious, after all!

A severe outbreak among young cattle running on the range, near Alder, Pierce County, Washington, a town on the Tacoma and

Eastern Railroad, and one in a large dairy herd near Seattle, were traceable to such causes.

In regard to the cause of death, we again find it difficult to arrive at definite conclusions. In some cases where animals have been afflicted for several days with fever and constipation, followed by diarrhea and gradual loss of flesh and increasing weakness, the lesions in the intestines were insignificant, certainly not severe enough to cause death. We ascribe death in such cases to the absorption of poisonous substances and the inability of the body to get rid of them. In severely acute cases, the escape of blood through the intestinal mucosa and intense diarrhea cause death. In peracute cases, die suddenly or in severe cases lasting but a few days, showing great distress, dyspnea and high temperatures, the blood will be found to be very dark, coagulating poorly or not at all, evidently unable to carry oxygen; hemolysis may be more or less pronounced, all characteristic of a septicemia.

Whenever the disease has appeared in chronic form, many unthrifty, poorly developed, cachectic animals will be observed. Young animals fail to grow, show great weakness and emaciation, although they eat, chew their cud, and appear hungry. These often develop progressive anemia and pronounced cachexia. On post mortem, but slight lesions can be found. The condition is due to inability to digest and faulty absorption. Others are chronic cases; they improve but have frequent recurrent attacks of severe diarrhea; systematic examinations will demonstrate that they distribute periodically great numbers of zygotes; hence they are carriers of the protozoa—never very sick, resistant against the mild infection, they scatter the protozoa wherever they go.

The difficult part, therefore, is to recognize the trouble early. We cannot eradicate it, but we should be able to guard against the sudden destructive outbreaks, where the mortality has at times reached 60%. The severe outbreaks among young stock, where animals die very suddenly, must be controlled by preventive measures, sanitation, and as far as possible by protective serum or vaccines. These can only be developed along rational, satisfactory lines if we understand the ways and means of attack of the hidden, mysterious enemy. The losses caused by red dysentery among all classes of domestic animals have often been very serious. In some parts of Africa (Tunis and Cape Colony), in Asia and many European countries, thousands of cattle have perished. The economic losses in the western part of our state are considerable, among pure bred as well as grades. Three years ago, after the identity of the disease was established, I began to make trips to localities where animals died from mysterious causes. Wherever cattle died suddenly, the owners were convinced that their stock had been poisoned.

Mr. Albert Jacobson, our city chemist, has carefully analyzed stomach contents from many such cases, without being able to demonstrate poisons. Professor Johnson of the University of Washington has had similar experiences. Examinations of tissues and blood for bacteria, especially *Bacterium bovisepticus,* anthrax symptomatic anthrax, malignant oedema, and other pathogenic organisms, have been carefully carried out in the laboratories of the Public Health Service, the State Board of Health and the Department of Health and Sanitation. Dr. A. U. Simpson, M.D., our city bacteriologist, an exceedingly conscientious investigator, took great interest in these problems—but has seldom been able to demonstrate pathogenic bacteria.

A few miles south of Seattle, near Allentown, is a large wet pasture. It is not fenced and cattle of all kinds use it for a common feeding ground. Several open ditches meander through it and furnish contaminated surface water. The land is usually covered with water during the rainy season and is therefore washed off. As soon as the weather is warm, mild cases of red dysentery can be observed. In calves, attacks often assume a severe and fatal form; owners claim that the animals are poisoned, because they do well as long as they are fed in their yards. It is my supply field for infested material which can be found in one form or another throughout the year.

On September 22, 1915, Mr. A. W., who owns a small dairy on the hill near Bryn Mawr, three miles from Renton, brought to Mr. Jacobson's laboratory the omasum and abomasum of two young cows that died in the morning without having shown symptoms of disease. He requested careful chemical analysis of stomach contents for a series of poisons. The mucosa of the fourth stomach of one animal was rather pale, no evidence of corrosive poisons could be detected; a great number of minute, pearly gray, translucent nodules, arranged in groups, were readily seen upon careful examination. They protruded slightly above the mucosa and appeared to extend to the fundus of the crypts; they corresponded nicely to the description of coccidia as found in Hutyra and Marek.

The other stomach showed but few of these, but many very small, deep ulcers, where blood escaped, were found. Evidently the fine pellicle which covered them had broken open and the parasites escaped, leaving a minute but deep defect reaching at least to the basement membrane of the crypts.

Careful analysis for several poisons which might have been used gave negative results. An investigation of the premises showed that six other cows were afflicted with offensive slimy diarrhea. The owner stated that a nice Guernsey grade which appeared languid and thin, had not been doing well all summer. The calves were kept in a small pen, they were unthrifty, languid, sunken eyed; had diarrhea, two showing slight whitish secretion in the lid sacks and marked slimy discharge from the nose. The microscope demonstrated masses of schizonts in the mucous from cows and calves.

Mr. W. F. B., near Clifton, Washington, whose ranch is located at the head of Hood's Canal, lost several valuable Guernsey grade heifers during the year 1915. The losses were attributed to poison—six animals were found to have died suddenly at one time in one pasture. Stomach contents were analyzed by Professor Johnson in the laboratories of the University of Washington in Seattle, with negative results. The case was tried in the courts in Shelton, and is therefore of record; accused party was discharged. Several trips were made to this ranch and owner stated that cattle began to die the year after alfalfa hay from the irrigated districts in Eastern Washington had been fed, during the winter months. On July 9th, 1916, several animals on the place were afflicted with quite severe chronic diarrhea; one heifer showed marked slimy discharge from the nose and was certainly not doing well. Microscope showed schizonts and epithelial cells in great numbers in slimy mucous.

On December 9th, 1916, a nice heifer was found dead, apparently from the same cause which killed the animals on other occasions. Careful post mortem examination and study of collected specimens left no doubt—an acute attack of red dysentery.

On ranches located nearby, calves and colts begin to suffer from severe diarrhea and dysentery late in the summer when pastured in low bottoms, but usually recover when driven into the hills. Several die every year; others are stunted because they are chronic cases. On this place rational prophylactic measures have stopped the losses, no further outbreaks have been reported.

An interesting outbreak occurred on upland pastures a few miles southwest of Redmond, Washington, during May, 1917. Mr. C. drove 23 large healthy grade Holstein heifers from Kent to his pasture about the middle of May. The animals were turned loose in the south forty acres, where a small stream and springs provided good drinking water; a clearing, an old orchard and some old buildings surrounded by alder and small timber made it an ideal place; grass was abundant, so that the animals prospered. When pasture became short, the herd was driven across the road into the north forty acres. The land had been cleared with stump pullers, the logs burnt and the ground seeded to clover. The soil was clay, impervious to water. A small stream in one corner supplied running water. The weather was dry and quite hot, the whole herd had to go to the creek to drink, no other supply being available. The heifers were doing well. A week later rains set in; the large stump holes acted as catch-basins for surface water. After a few rainy days, the weather became hot and sultry; the animals remained on the hill and drank water from the stump holes. In a very few days the caretaker reported to Dr. J. P. Johnson, at the time veterinarian in general practice in Redmond, that some of the heifers were very sick, acted as if they had pneumonia and suffered from severe offensive diarrhea. Several appeared drowsy, thermometers registered temperatures of 105° to 107.4°; respiration was labored and rapid; marked discharge from nose was slightly streaked with blood; some were frothing at the mouth and grinding their teeth; abdomen was drawn up and they appeared to be in great pain and distress. Pulse weak and rapid, often almost imperceptible. Scanty defecation was followed by severe, offensive diarrhea. Most animals were sick 6 to 8 days; 13 died out of the 23. Post mortem examinations were made by several veterinarians, wihout definite results, however.

Dr. Johnson found all the organs in a state of severe congestion. In the abdominal cavity, the serous layers were dry and rough; peritoneum was severely inflamed; the liver was brownish, very friable; stomach empty; in several places the intestinal mucosa was separated from its basement membrane, permitting the dark, tarry blood to escape into the lumen of the bowel. The rectum and part of the colon were filled with a mass of dark, poorly clotted blood. Tinged slimy mucous escaped from the nose. In some cases dark blood escaped into the subcutaneous tissues and caused deeply tinged blotches. The bladder was filled with darkly tinged urine. Most remarkable conditions, when we consider that the animal was destroyed and the post mortem held at once. Blood when kept in a bottle remained dark, it did not coagulate. Liver and spleen were sent to laboratories in Seattle. No cultures of pathogenic bacteria could be demonstrated. Cultures resembling *Bacterium anthracis* were obtained from one specimen, they proved to be non-pathogenic to laboratory animals. In this connection it is well to remember that Dr. V. A. Moore described in his Microbiology twenty organisms which resemble *Bact. anthracis.*

After remaining several days on the infected pastures, the herd was driven into another corral where good water was available, several afflicted heifers improved rapidly and made good recoveries. Some of the animals that ate eagerly of baled alfalfa hay about 8 o'clock one evening were found dead next morning. If the history had been unknown, such cases would surely have been designated as poisoning, especially in range countries. After the herd was removed to the corral, animals which showed no symptoms registered temperatures around 105°, proving that high temperatures are to be expected in the early stages. Treatment consisted in stimulants and as good care as circumstances would permit.

On June 16th, I made a trip to the infected pasture and waterholes. From slime and sediment oocytes showing spore formation were obtained by washing and sedimentation methods. The remaining ten heifers were again running in the north pasture; doing well. Two weak animals were still afflicted with slimy diarrhea. In mucous which they passed, a great number of epithelial cells, a number of schizonts and well developed macrogametes could readily be demonstrated. In this instance it has been demonstrated beyond a doubt, that the outbreak was due to a common source of infection, the infected water-holes, that the disease was not only occasionally directly transmittable, and that a period of dry hot weather, followed by warm rains and hot sultry summer days permitted rapid multiplication of the destructive organisms. It was unfortunate that it was not possible to leave the pasture with the infected water-holes and turn a number of susceptible Whidby Island yearlings loose in the same field, so as to observe the earliest symptoms and undertake a comprehensive study of the protozoan and its development in the drinking water or on the grass. The dangerous but interesting conditions can be reproduced artificially in hothouses or on favorably located fields in summer time. It would be quite worth while and I hope to find such an opportunity sooner or later.

When in July, 1917, a notice in our daily papers stated that range animals valued at $150,000 had perished in a few days near Klamath Falls, Oregon, I decided to make a trip to that locality. Arriving in the Oregon city on August 2nd, it was found impracticable to go to Malin, where the losses were so numerous and sudden, the animals having been removed to other pastures. I am greatly indebted to Mr. J. F. Kimball of the Weyerhauser Timber Company, and Dr. G. C. Mitchell for rapid transportation and a great deal of really useful information. Although several diseased animals were located, observed and studied, nothing even approaching poisoning could be identified. On the other hand, cattle observed on dairy farms, as well as on the range, showed infection identical in every way to the cases found near Seattle. Evidently losses in the State of Oregon are due to the same cause as those in Washington. We can readily see what occurs around watering places where cattle congregate as soon as the dry season has set in. The holes become contaminated from droppings, which remain moist and warm so that protozoan or bacteria can develop and multiply. Drying out for weeks has no deleterious effect on encysted coccidia, it represents simply a suitable resting period. This phase of the coccidian life cycle has not yet been investigated as it should be, and presents a most interesting subject for systematic investigation.

When warm showers dissolve the miscellaneous matter in which the parasites are, they begin to float around the waterholes. Whenever susceptible animals take them up on feed or in the drinking water, outbreaks occur. This assertion is borne out by numerous observations—contaminated material, a period of dry hot weather, warm rains to liberate the contagion and then susceptible animals make an ideal combination for an outbreak. This was well illustrated in the outbreak near Redmond and on LaConner Flats.

Cattle run on alfalfa pastures which become contaminated from the manure; when moisture and warmth are supplied the organisms multiply and are carried on to the stems of the plants where they encapsulate and dry out during hot summer weather or when the hay is cured. Fed to our dairy cattle in Seattle, it has not infrequently caused severe outbreaks of diarrhea, affecting a great number of animals in some herds. Three such instances are described in my notebook.

Dairymen in Seattle know that cattle bought on Whidby Island—mostly Guernsey grades—often become sick when first fed alfalfa hay. One well known firm lost eight animals from this cause during the late summer and fall of 1916.

Having obtained assignment to slaughterhouse inspection last summer, cattle from many parts of the country could be observed soon after arrival. Stomachs and intestines could be examined and studied soon after slaughter in a systematic manner. During the dry hot season, it was not unusual to find steers afflicted with intermittent diarrhea. Cattle from Toppenish Flats, Washington, steers from Myrtle Point, Oregon, others from the vicinity of Roseburg, were all quite heavily infected. About three weeks after the heavy rains flushed out the water-holes and stagnant creeks, these chronic carriers cleared up. No doubt can therefore exist as to the dissemination of this group of parasites and the enormous losses which red dysentery causes to our livestock industry. Investigations along this line have not received the attention which they deserve and special efforts should be made definitely to establish the identity of the causes of the many mysterious outbreaks which have ravaged the stock raising districts in Oklahoma, Texas (Ward County), California, Oregon, Montana, Idaho and Washington.

In July, 1916, Dr. C. E. Richards, M.D., from Des Moines, Wash., brought specimen of tissues to the city laboratories and stated that cattle near Des Moines died from acute attack of coccidiosis. The doctor had studied the disease in Iowa and was probably one of the first to recognize and diagnose it in cattle in our state. Losses around that settlement were quite severe during the summer of 1916.

Dr. Julian Howard, veterinarian, located in Stanwood, Washington, has also recognized the disease and found the coccidia in feces of afflicted cattle and sheep.

In the fall of 1915, Dr. H. Welch, veterinarian at the experiment station in Bozeman, Montana, reported that he had identified acute coccidiosis and demonstrated the parasites in the intestines of pure bred Holstein calves which died from rather obscure causes.

While the technique of examinations for coccidia is not difficult, it is not given in our text books. No satisfactory method of
making permanent mounts for future reference and comparative
studies is taught in our laboratory courses, and even text books on
microscopic methods do not give us much help. We are taught
that it is necessary to section tissues to demonstrate the parasites.
When I made the statement in Oakland, California, before the A.
V. M. Association, that examination of feces gave us a safe and
quick method to diagnose this disease in its early stages, I was
challenged at once and severely criticized. In Dr. Law's text book
of veterinary medicine, II edition, 1905, Vol. 2, page 265, we find
the terse statement that "Diagnosis can always be made by microscopic examination of fresh warm feces"!

In "Bacteriankunde und pathologische Mikroskopic" by Dr.
Med th. Kitt, IV edition, 1903, the suggestion is given, to examine
feces, fragments of mucosa, mucous or croupous membranes because coccidia in great numbers would be found. The author
states that 50 to 100 parasites may be found in one field under the
microscope.

Illustrations in the numerous short articles published and
accessible cannot be considered satisfactory. They leave the impression that coccidium oviforme is an obligatory cell parasite and
lay great stress on the presence of the encapsulated forms of the
zygote and spore-formation. These forms occur only in animals
where the rapidly destructive asexual division (schizogony) of the
parasites has reached its limit. In all severe cases, especially in
those that end fatally in a few days, the schizont alone may be
found in immense numbers—in masses, and this rapidly multiplying asexual (agamic) division form should be studied, so that it
can be recognized. The position of the parasite in the cell is frequently very useful to identify it. This is what pathologists look
for. Since it would be very useful to be able to stain and mount in
a simple but permanent manner mucous containing these parasites,
a practical method which has been found to be acceptable and
which has given satisfactory results will be described in detail.

Dr. Ph. B. Hadley of the Rhode Island Experiment Station has
devoted a great deal of time to the study of this group of diseases,
especially among fowls and birds. He found it difficult to distinguish and identify coccidia among intestinal contents but over-
came the difficulty by bringing out a differential staining method.

The article, "Regarding the value of the Van Giesen and Roman-
owsky malarial stains for the detection of coccidia" is found on
page 147, No. 1, Vol. 52, originale Abth. I, *Centralblatt fur Bacte-
rien kunde*. The article is written in English and contains very
useful information. My efforts along this line did not produce
satisfactory results and it was only when Rosanilin violet, which
Dr. Hadley kindly sent me, was used that marked differentiation
was obtained. These stains are not permanent, however.

The greatest stumbling block apparently has been the attempts
to subject such material to bacteriological methods, especially that
of dehydration with heat or alcohol.

The parasites are of appreciable dimensions, although schizonts
in early stages of rapid development may only be 3 μ and appear
round or oval, somewhat resembling small lymphocytes or baso-
phile leucocytes. Unstained or when flooded with weak Loeffer's
meth. blue sol., they show a delicate fine outline and a denser
faintly variegated nucleus. Schizonts stain with difficulty and always unevenly. Merozoites are mobile, and can be distinguished
by the peculiar grouping and method of division as seen in the
fully developed trophozoite. Epithelial cells of certain types may
be mistaken for merozoites. All these forms are soft, jelly-like
masses and may become markedly distorted by the manipulations
on the slide or undue pressure of the coverglass.

In "Principles of Microbiology", by Dr. V. A. Moore, Ithaca,
N. Y., 1912 Edition, chapter on protozoa, page 429, the author
states that:

"The coccidia in the liver show themselves in two principal
forms. The free coccidia, schizonts, merozoites or young macrogametes are most frequently spherical or elongated, 12 to 14 microns broad and 17 to 22 microns long. Some are almost homogeneous and very refrangent, with darker central point; they resemble cells undergoing fatty degeneration. Their volume varies
from 6 to 8 to 30 microns. They are often included in epithelial
cells and solitary or grouped in small masses in the same cell. The
encysted coccidia (oocyst) may also exist in the interior of a cell
and like the preceding, they are sometimes lodged in large giant
cells.

It is not rare to find white particles floating in the bile, similar
to the contents of tumors and almost exclusively formed of coccidia.

: Rivolta once found numerous encysted coccidia in the epithelium of a dilated gall bladder.''

Many hundreds of examinations have been made and prove that as a result of the irritation caused by these parasites an unusual amount of mucous is secreted by the goblet cells. During the early diarrheatic period, mucous is produced copiously, forming casts or false membranes; later on, in flake or shreds, finally, when the intestinal mucosa has been severely attacked and became exhausted, in minute particles only.

Coccidia are usually found in these mucous masses and flakes. They may be present in immense numbers without cells or tissue fragments. Feces containing mucous are washed in large amounts of cold water until the water runs off clear. Large particles can then be fished out, small ones aspirated with suitable pipette: large amounts are best washed over fine sieves or on a double layer of gauze. In case of very offensive diarrhea, decomposition must be arrested by adding to the collected material as soon as possible an equal amount of Kaiserling No. 1 solution; slimy discharges are easier to manipulate when this is done.

The rinsed mucous and tissue shreds when collected are kept in equal parts of water and Kaiserling solution No. 1, which leaves the mucous nicely transparent, inhibits growth of all but few miscellaneous bacteria and fungi and is easily obtained. Certain resistant fungi, however, have produced marked mycelia and even gonidia in specimen bottles containing 50% Kaiserling solution No. 1. Tissues fragments and especially epithelial cells show good fixation, so that cell inclusions and nuclei remain well preserved. If Kaiserling's solution No. 1 cannot be obtained, preserve washed specimens in 10 to 20% formalin solution; specimen kept preserved for years stain well.

When ready to examine for parasites, fish out a reasonable amount and wash carefully in several changes of water to remove preservatives. Place selected particles on a slide, cover with cover glass and examine while wet under the microscope with low power lens. Once familiar with the parasites, they will be recognized without difficulty. A drop of Loefflers' blue (dilute) should be added and produces a transparent specimen. It may be necessary to tease the mucous particles apart to form a thin layer.

For permanent slides, the best results are obtained when the water in the mucous and tissue fragments is gradually replaced by glycerine. This process toughens the mucous flakes, does not injure cells or parasites and makes the specimen beautifully transparent.

Mucous does not always give the same reaction. A large mass, the size of an egg, produced in a competent, well nourished intestine, free from blood, is quite different from the minute particles found in diarrheatic evacuations of an animal which will die in twelve hours. The latter is rather difficult to wash, stain and examine. Stains must therefore often be selected by trial. Usually it is best to fix material, rinse well and then stain it. Sometimes it was found of advantage to stain before fixing because penetration was better.

Large and firm mucous masses, such as cylindrical casts or ribbon-like false membranes for example, must be cut up into thin pieces to permit the stains to penetrate.

When characteristic forms have been found in mucous that is reasonably free from miscellaneous detritus, so as to be suitable for permanent slides, the mucous is carefully carried through suitable staining processes, rinsed in water and dehydrated and clarified by being gradually carried through 30% to 60%, and then into pure glycerine. The last steps must be carried out slowly, requiring two or three days to obtain the best results. Only stains which contain but little alcohol and which are not soluble in glycerine will be found satisfactory.

Mayer's hemalum or Mayer's acid hemalum, which will show a reddish tinge, produced very satisfactory results. Length of time and degree of dilution required to obtain good nuclear differentiation varies and must be ascertained when staining. It is best to use the stain diluted 1 to 3 of water and stain 24 to 36 hours. Rinse thoroughly and wash in tap water for twelve hours.

Old Delafields hematoxylin penetrates well, but does not give so neat a nuclear differentiation.

Alum-Carmine is one of the best stains, usually it gives well marked differentiations of nuclear structures and clarifies nicely in glycerin.

As counterstain, Bismark brown (vesuvin) has proven to be acceptable, especially when followed by picric acid solution, which acts as a mordant and intensifies it.

1 gram Bismark brown dissolved in 300 ccm. of 3% carbolic acid solution by heat, then filtered makes a serviceable, penetrating

stain which brings out bacteria as well as miscellaneous vegetable structures. Dilute as required and stain 12 to 36 hours. To demonstrate bacteria the stronger solutions are best; for cells and other material, weaker solutions are to be preferred. Trials are necessary. Rinse stained mass lightly and place into aqueous solution of Picric acid, 1 gram in 300 ccm. of water. This bath will intensify the stain and give better definition. After mucous has been stained and rinsed, it is finally mounted in glycerin as stated above. Changes should not be made too rapidly to avoid shrinking and distortion of the protozoa.

It is of advantage to carry material stained in Bismark brown solution through glycerin slightly acidulated with Picric acid.

Eosin soluble in water will also give satisfactory contrasts for hematoxylin stains.

A good quality of cement should be used to paint over the edges of the coverglasses. Oxide of zinc well rubbed up in good fishrod (marine) varnish, which is easily obtained, makes tough dense rings, insoluble in alcohol, but soluble in xylol.

A collection of slides prepared in this manner will keep well and permit a demonstration of these dangerous parasites at any time. The zygotes and fully developed cysts are protected by dense capsule—which forms soon after fertilization of the macrogamete—are easily recognized when found, but they occur usually (there are exceptions) only in animals that recover. Whenever the microscope demonstrates the presence of macrogametes and zygotes, forms which are constant in their appearance and can therefore be identified beyond all doubt, and schizonts become less numerous, a favorable prognosis can be given, because the dangerous agamonous multiplication of the parasites, which is so injurious to the host has reached its limits. The improvement of the animals at this stage of the disease in twenty-four hours is most remarkable and unless toxemia is very severe or injury to the intestinal mucosa has caused serious defects, recovery will be quite rapid. In severe lengthy cases the search for agamonous division forms of the coccidia is tedious and difficult, because the parasites are small, multiplying rapidly, are poorly developed, probably only immature trophozoites or schizonts being present, which are very difficult to stain and identify. In such cases several animals should be examined and better developed forms will surely be found.

Diseases of this class require careful observations and consid-

eration of the clinical symptoms during their entire course, as well
as numerous microscopic examinations of blood, excreta, nasal discharges, discharge from sores, urine, etc., before a definite diagnosis
can be established. It is also necessary that clinical findings shall
be compared—checked up—with examinations of organs and tissues from animals that died. Specimens must be secured during
the early as well as during the late stages of the disease, so as to
permit a comparative study of the injuries to the tissues and enable
us to find the point of attack, study the progress and demonstrate
the cause of death. Our present knowledge of the distribution and
importance of this parasitic disease of cattle and other animals is
entirely inadequate.

A careful, systematic survey of the entire situation should be
made, so as to identify and study the different diseases which
cause these severe losses among cattle. When the identity of a
disease has been established, an outline for a campaign against it
can be laid down and measures to prevent its spread can be adopted.
Sometimes successful treatment can be inaugurated. The success
of such an investigation often depends upon the cooperation and
support which the stock owners extend to those that are entrusted
with the study and solution of the problem.

(The different stages of development of coccidium oviforme
were demonstrated on a series of slides prepared from material
collected during the outbreaks near Redmond, Washington, from
dairy cattle near Seattle and from Big Soda Springs on Keane
Creek, near Pinehurst, Oregon.

Zygotes and oocysts showing spore formation, macrogametes
in different stages of development on some slides, while the schizogonous cycle: rapidly dividing schizonts, trophozoites and merozoites were to be seen on others.)

—Dr. L. A. Maze, formerly with Parke, Davis & Co. at Rochester, Mich., has purchased the practice formerly conducted by Dr.
O. E. Parker at Pontiac, Mich. Dr. Parker is now at Fort Oglethorpe, Ga.

—Dr. A. W. Swedberg of the B. A. I., who has been at Omaha,
Neb., since January, 1917, on Tuberculin Testing, has been transferred to Denver, Colo.

A PHYSALOPTERA FROM THE DOG, WITH A NOTE ON THE NEMATODE PARASITES OF THE DOG IN NORTH AMERICA

MAURICE C. HALL, PH.D., D.V.M., AND MEYER WIGDOR, M.A.
Reseach Laboratory, Parke, Davis & Company, Detroit, Mich.

In a series of over 300 dogs examined post mortem at Detroit, we found a single female specimen of *Physaloptera* in one dog, No. 300, an incidence of about 0.3 per cent. The head of the worm was so deeply and firmly imbedded in the duodenum about an inch below the pylorus, that we were unable to remove the parasite by what we regarded as a reasonable amount of traction without danger of breaking it. The worm and the tissue to which it was attached were, therefore, placed in normal saline solution for a time, and in the course of an hour the worm relinquished its hold and separated from the intestinal wall.

The description of a new species of nematode on a single female specimen is not a wholly satisfactory proceeding from the standpoint of those who describe such species or those who must consider their descriptions later. On the other hand, if it is desirable to describe the rare parasites of dogs, which parasites have considerable bearing on the subject of the dog as a carrier of parasites usually occurring in other hosts, then it is desirable that we have some name by which these parasites may be discussed. It simplifies discussion, and it is no serious matter that a parasite may be found to bear more than one name and that all but one of its names must be rated as synonyms.

On these grounds we are describing the nematode found by us in the dog as a new species. It is entirely improbable that this is a customary or even common parasite of the dog. It is probable, though not certain, that it is a parasite of some wild mammal, but it might even be a parasite of a bird or reptile, temporarily present in the dog after the dog had eaten the infested animal. In any case it is quite apt to be a species heretofore undescribed, as there has been but little study of the genus *Physaloptera* on this continent.

Species *Physaloptera rara* Hall and Wigdor, 1918.

SPECIFIC DIAGNOSIS.—*Physaloptera*: Anterior extremity of the body somewhat attenuated. Cuticle strongly annulated (in the

female at intervals of 50 to 200 μ), the first annulation behind the
head forming a sort of collar, with the head somewhat sunk in the
depression formed by this collar. Mouth with 2 large lateral lips
(Figs. 1 and 2), each of which is prolonged anteriorly by 3 prominent teeth in a row, a somewhat smaller tooth being external to the
middle tooth of the three. Each lip bears a pair of conspicuous
papillae, one of the pair being situated near each end of the lip
and toward its base, and a third papilla near the middle of the lip
base. The esophagus length is 4.8 per cent of the total body length.

MALE unknown.

FEMALE 24 mm. long, with a maximum diameter of 1.34 mm.
The head is 90 μ long and 200 μ wide at the base. The collar in
which the head is set is 324 μ wide. The teeth on the lips are about
12 μ long and about 10 μ wide at the base. The collar-like depres-

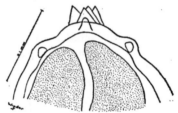

FIGURE 1. *Physaloptera rara.* Head. Lateral view.

sion about the head is formed by the cuticle delimited by the first
transverse striation. The third pseudo-annulus thus formed breaks
on one side and runs obliquely back; this may be accidental (Fig.
3). The esophagus is 1.16 mm. long, the muscular portion being
526 μ long; the maximum width of the esophagus is 102 μ. The
nerve ring surrounds the muscular esophagus at a point near its
union with the glandular portion. The inconspicuous vulva is in
the anterior portion of the body, 3.63 mm. from the anterior end.
The vestibule of the ovejector (Fig. 4) proceeds inward a short distance and then turns toward the anterior end of the worm for a
distance of about 0.6 mm., when it turns back past the vulva, the
remainder of the genitalia lying in the posterior body between the
vulva and the anus. The vestibule is 880 μ long. The succeeding
portion, the unpaired portion of what Seurat calls the "trompe",
which is the distal portion of the ovejector, is 2.16 mm. long and is
directed posteriorly throughout. This bifurcates and the 2 branches
form a loop and meet the corresponding portions of the uterus.

The most posterior ovarian loops (Fig 5) are in the vicinity of the anal region. The anal aperture appears to be set deep in a depression formed by a fold of cuticle (Fig. 6). The external aperture of this cuticular depression is 420 μ from the posterior extremity of the body. The posterior extremity is comparatively blunt. This was the only specimen present, so there were no fertilized eggs in the worm.

Host.—*Canis familiaris.*

Location.—Duodenum.

Locality.—Detroit, Michigan.

Seurat (1917) divides the species of *Physaloptera* from mammals into 2 groups; in one group, such worms as *Ph. clausa,* the

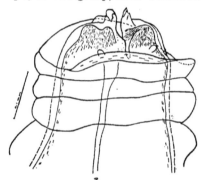

Figure 2. *Physaloptera rara.* Head. Dorso-ventral view.

external tooth of the lip is approximately as large as the internal teeth, the latter forming a 3-pronged fork; in the other group, such worms as *Ph. abbreviata,* the external tooth is very large and the internal teeth are small and set at intervals. *Ph. rara* evidently belongs in the first group. The surprisingly short glandular esophagus distinguishes this species from the other species with which we have compared it wherever this feature is described for other species. It is unfortunate that we have for study only a single specimen of the worm, as this feature is rather widely different from the corresponding condition in other species.

We take this occasion to summarize what is known in a general way of the nematode parasites of dogs in North America, thereby completing a series of papers on the parasites of dogs in North America. The other papers, published in recent issues of this journal, dealt with protozoan, cestode, trematode, acanthocephalid and arthropod parasites. While these records are not exhaustive, they are the first comprehensive summary of our knowledge of the parasites of dogs on this continent.

NEMATODA. *Filaria osleri* was described from dogs in Canada by Osler (1877). It has since been found in Europe and has recently been reported again from this continent, after an interval of almost 40 years, by Milks (1916) at Ithaca, N. Y. The worm occurs in nodules in the trachea, bronchi and lungs.

Dirofilaria immitis was described from the heart blood of the dog in this country by Leidy (1856). The worm was subsequently

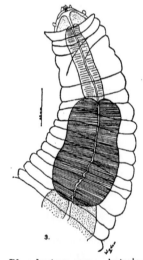

FIGURE 3. *Physaloptera rara.* Anterior extremity.

found to be widely distributed over the world. It has been reported a number of times from the United States, being collected by Curtice, Hassall, Wheeler and others. It does not appear to be uncommon in the South, but it is evidently uncommon in the northern United States. We have not found it in the post mortem examination of over 300 dogs at Detroit.

Spirocerca sanguinolenta (*Spiroptera sanguinolenta*) has been reported from a tumor of the esophagus in a dog at Washington by Sommer (1896). More recently, Haythorn and Ryan (1917) have reported 6 cases of the occurrence of this parasite in dogs at Mobile, Ala., and note that the U. S. Bureau of Animal Industry has specimens from one case at Atlanta, Ga., and from 2 cases at

Washington, one host said to be a lynx from the Zoological Park. (The other specimens at Washington are probably Sommer's.)

Trichuris depressiuscula, the whipworm, is a common parasite of dogs in the United States. We found it in 39.7 per cent of the first 300 dogs examined here by us, with an average of 21.4 worms per dog. The largest number present in a dog in this series was 677 and the next largest 299.

Trichinella spiralis has been experimentally developed by us in the dog here at Detroit.

Dioctophyme renale occurs in the kidney and abdominal cavity of the dog in the United States. The records of its occurrence in this country have been summarized by Riley (1916) and Hall (1916; 1917). Since the publication of these summaries, this para-

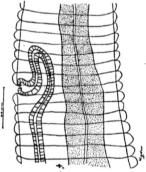

FIGURE 4. *Physaloptera rara.* Vulva region, showing loop of ovejector.

site has been reported from the dog at Tama, Iowa, by Maxfield (1917), and in a paper by MacNider (1917) on nephropathy of the dog, we find the following: "At autopsy the kidneys of 4 of the animals were found to be the seat of infections by a parasitic worm, with surrounding areas of lymphocytic infiltration and connective tissue hyperplasia." These last cases are from North Carolina, and we regard them as probably cases of *D. renale*.

The occurrence of *D. renale* was reported by Hall (1917) in 2 dogs out of 67 dogs examined post mortem at Detroit. In a continuation of that series of examinations, this parasite was subsequently found by us in Dog No. 242, a mongrel male with some characteristics of the rough-coated terriers, so that our percentage for the series of 300 is only 1 per cent. The worm found was a male and was located in a tough cyst in the pelvic cavity to the

right of the urinary bladder. This appears to be an unusual location, as the worm is usually free, rather than encysted, when it
occurs in the abdominal cavity.

Maxfield's case, MacNider's 4 cases and our case make a total
of 6 cases that should be added to the totals for the United States.
In addition, we note the following from a letter to one of us (Hall)
from Dr. Ralph W. Nauss of the California State Board of Health:
"I note what you say regarding the prevalence of *Dioctophyme
renale* among dogs in Chicago. This parasite was frequently found
in dogs during my student days—1902-5—at the Northwestern
University Medical College. On a later occasion, in 1911, when

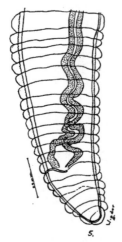

FIGURE 5. *Physaloptera rara*. Posterior extremity, showing ovarian loops.

doing experimental surgery on dogs at this same institution, one
case I remember distinctly of finding a female in the right kidney
and a male (quite small in comparison with the one contained in
the kidney) in the abdominal cavity beneath the liver." The new
cases listed here make it reasonably certain that this parasite has
been found in the United States in at least 50 cases and probably
in more than 50 cases. In a general way the distribution of the
cases follows the Atlantic sea-board and the Great Lakes region,
a distribution which is in accord with the supposition that the
parasite has an intermediate stage in fish.

Ancylostoma caninum, the common dog hookworm, is generally
distributed over the United States, though the available evidence

indicates that it is more common in the South, as might be expected. However, it might be noted in passing that very little has ever been published regarding the parasites of southern dogs. We found hookworms in 33.3 per cent of our series of 300 dogs, with an average of 15.2 worms per dog. The largest number present was 282, and the next largest number was 165.

Uncinaria stenocephala has only b,een reported once, by Muldoon (1916), from the dog in the United States. Muldoon reported it from Ithaca, N. Y.; from correspondence it appears that no specimens of the worm were preserved. This is unfortunate,

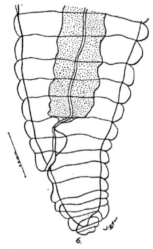

FIGURE 6. *Physaloptera rara.* Posterior extremity.

as the record was published without corroborative data and there is a possibility of misidentification.

Belascaris marginata is the roundworm which appears to be most common in dogs in the United States. We found ascarids (the majority of them *B. marginata*) in 53.3 per cent of our 300 dogs, over half of them, with an average of 25.2 worms per dog. The largest number present was 2054, and the next largest was 204. Without this extremely large number, 2054, the average per dog was 12.3.

Toxascaris limbata appears to be much less common in this country than the foregoing species. Ransom (1913) reports *Tox. ascaris* from the dog, apparently at Chicago. We recently found specimens of this species fairly common in our ascarid material from dogs.

Agamonematodum gaylordi was described from tubercles in the hyperplastic thyroids of experiment dogs at Craig Brook, Maine, by Ransom (1914).

HEAVY INFESTATIONS. Dog No. 170 had 2054 ascarids (*B. marginata*), most of them very small immature worms. Following anthelmintic treatment, 5 of these worms had been collected from the feces and 64 had been collected post mortem from the large intestine and cecum and credited to the efficacy of the anthelmintic. Of the remainder, 89 were found in the stomach and 1,896 in the small intestine. Some of the very small larvae might have been passed in the feces and escaped detection, so that there is a possibility that there were even more ascarids present than the large number accounted for.

This dog was much emaciated and had prominently enlarged thyroids. The animal received 2 anthelmintic treatments, the second 5 days after the first, and died the evening after the second treatment. Death was probably due to the cachectic condition of the animal, which in turn was apparently due to the gross infestation with ascarids, though the anthelmintic treatment in such a weakened animal may have hastened the end. Post mortem examination showed the following: The margin of the left lobes of the lung were congested; the external vessels of the heart seemed congested; the liver was cirrhotic; the spleen was dry and tough; the peripheral portion of the medulla of the kidneys was hyperemic; the bladder was distended; the gastric mucosa was gelatinous and showed some dark areas that apparently had been hemorrhagic; the jejunum showed locally inflamed areas and the ileum was inflamed and had some local hemorrhages; the colon was inflamed, the rectum hemorrhagic, and the glands of the rectum and cecum were very prominent.

Some of the young ascarids collected from this dog were put in Kronecker's solution (a slightly alkaline physiologic saline solution), where they lived for 64 hours with a room temperature of about 26° C. The adults of this dog ascarid were found by Hall (1917) to survive for 14 days in Kronecker's solution.

To get some information in regard to the developmental period of these ascarids, 30 young worms, none of them more than 1 cm. long, were put in gelatine capsules and fed to Dog. No. 173. The feces of this dog had been examined for the five-day period previous to the feeding and once 3 days before and no worm eggs of any sort had been found. Ascarid eggs first appeared in the feces 11 days after the feeding the worms to the dog, indicating that the female ascarid of the dog attains maturity and begins egg production within 11 days after reaching a length of about 1 cm. This dog was killed 48 days after these ascarids were fed to it. During that time the dog had vomited 3 ascarids on one occasion and 7 on another occasion. On post mortem examination the dog had 83 ascarids, which with the 10 worms vomited makes a total of 93 ascarids following the feeding of only 30 ascarids. We may assume that immature worms were present during the period when fecal examination showed the absence of eggs, or that the dog acquired the additional worms from eggs in the feces as a result of the experimental infestation, or that the dog acquired the additional worms from eggs present in the cage from previously infested dogs. Experiments noted below indicate that the second assumption is a possibility.

The experiment in infecting this dog with ascarids is of interest in connection with the work of Stewart (1916; 1917) and of Ransom and Foster (1917), on the life history of ascarids. Stewart demonstrated experimentally that when infective eggs from ascarids of man or of swine were fed to rats or mice, the embryos would escape from the eggs in the digestive tract and subsequently appear in the liver, spleen and lungs, later stages apparently migrating from the lungs up the trachea to the mouth and ultimately being swallowed in saliva and attaining the intestines, where they did not develop, but passed out in the feces. In view of the general failure which had followed most of the attempts to infect animals directly with infective eggs of suitable ascarids, Stewart concluded that rats and mice acted as intermediate hosts of ascarids, the infective larvae escaping in the saliva or feces of the rat and presumably attaining their definitive host in contaminated food or water. Ransom and Foster have stated that Stewart's conclusions do not necessarily follow from his findings, and we suspect that most helminthologists at present would agree with Ransom and Foster in this, even though inclined to give all due credit to Stewart for what is evidently a very interesting and valuable piece of work. Ransom and Foster have confirmed Stewart's work experimentally and have obtained similar results with guinea pigs. They further note one case where a young pig was fed ascarid eggs and died a week later; numerous ascarid larvae were found in the lungs, trachea and pharynx. They correlate this finding with Epstein's (1892) success in developing *Ascaris lumbricoides* of man by feeding eggs to young subjects, and state that age is an important factor in determining susceptibility to ascarid infestation.

In the case of Dog. No. 173, the animal was in a wire cage with a solid metal bottom and the cage was placed on top of some similar, but larger, cages which usually contained dogs. We consider this a location that would not be much disturbed by rats or mice which might infect the food or water of the dog in the cage, especially as the building is a concrete rat-proof structure with practically no place for rats or mice to hide except in the dog cages. The only food that might have come in contact with rodents is the stale bread, but this is furnished in entire loaves, free from rodent feces and, so far as we have noticed, apparently free from tooth marks that might indicate the presence of rodent saliva. The indications are that this dog acquired his infestation with worms in excess of the 30 originally fed to it, by contamination of food or water with eggs from the original worms.

In this connection it might be noted that Ransom and Foster call attention to the fact that heavy infestations of the lungs in rats and mice produce a serious pneumonia which is frequently fatal, and conclude that it is not improbable that ascarids are frequently responsible for lung troubles in children, pigs and other young animals. In the case of Dog No. 170, there was a congestion of the margins of one lung found post mortem, as noted, but it is difficult to correlate this with the ascariasis. The recent invasion of the lungs by about 2000 ascarids should theoretically give rise to a generalized pneumonic condition, if anything, rather than a congestion confined to the margin of the left lobes; still, inflammation might have occurred and subsided. We do not disagree with their conclusions and we regard the ascarid as a dangerous parasite, but in this case the presence of so many young ascarids in the intestine with a lack of the lung condition which might be expected suggests to us that the injury to the lung in the case of the rat and mouse fed with human or pig ascarids is partly due to the fact that these worms were in an unusual host, a condition which often leads to added injury. Thus in our experience trichinae in rats do not give the thermal and other clinical conditions found in man, the reaction in man, the unusual host, being much more severe. It is also true that the large clinical experience of the world in dealing with so common a parasite as the ascarid has credited it with the production of a wide range of symptoms in connection with the gastro-intestinal tract and the nervous system, but pneumonic conditions, except from the invasion of the lung by the wandering adult worm, do not seem to have been associated with it. Of course, clinical experience may be at fault here, as it has been in other instances.

In connection with the well-known wandering habits of the adult ascarid, it may be noted that this habit of entering the ducts of the pancreas and the liver and of traveling up the esophagus and leaving the pharynx by way of the nares, the trachea or the Eustachian tubes is apparently much more common in the case of the ascarids of man and swine than in the case of the ascarids of the dog. We have only seen one such case in the dog. This animal, a six-months-old pup, was found dead one morning with an ascarid projecting from one of the anterior nares. Behind it was another worm. On removing the head, another ascarid was found in the pharynx and posterior nares. Another worm was found in one bronchus. There were 19 worms in the intestine. Apparently death was due to these ascarids. The possibility of post mortem wandering cannot, of course, be absolutely excluded, but in our experience post mortem wandering of parasites in the dog must be a very rare thing, as we have almost no evidence of it.

We had one case of severe infestation with whipworms, a rough count showing approximately 677 worms, of which 421 were in the cecum and 253 in the colon and rectum to within 3 inches of the anus. In the cecum there was a mild hyperemia associated with the attachment of the worms.

MULTIPLE INFESTATIONS. Of our 300 dogs, 156 had only one kind of nematode worms, 91 had 2 kinds, 21 had 3 kinds, and none had more than 3 kinds.

CULTURE METHODS FOR EGGS. The culture method recommended for coccidia by Cole and Hadley (1910), the use of a 10 per cent potassium bichromate solution, gave us very good results in culturing ascarid and hookworm eggs. At room temperatures of 20° to 29° C. ascarid eggs would form the two-celled stage overnight. In 4 days embryos could be seen moving about in the eggs. Ascarid eggs kept under the same conditions, but in a solution of tap water, showed the two-celled stage in about half the eggs in 18 days, the other half being still in the one-celled stage.

Hookworm eggs in the potassium bichromate solution at room temperatures of 20° to 23° C. showed actively motile embryos within 36 hours.

BIBLIOGRAPHY

EPSTEIN, ALOIS. 1892. Ueber die Uebertragung des menschlichen Spulwurms (*Ascaris lumbricoides*). *Verhandl. Versamml. Gesell. Kinderh. Deut. Naturf. u. Aerzte*, v. 9, pp. 1-16.

HALL, MAURICE C. 1916. American records of *Dioctophyme renale*. *J. Am. Vet. Med. Assn.*, v. 3 (3), Dec., pp. 370-371.

HAYTHORN, S. R., AND A. H. RYAN. 1917. Aortic aneurisms in dogs with the report of six cases. *J. Med. Research*, v. 35 (3), Jan., pp. 411-423, pls. 28-29.

LEIDY, JOSEPH. 1850. Descriptions of three filariae. *Proc. Acad. Nat. Sci.*, Phila., v. 5 (6), Nov.-Dec., pp. 117-118.

MACNIDER, WM. DEB. 1916. A pathological study of the naturally acquired chronic nephropathy of the dog. Part 1. *J. Med. Research*, v. 34 (2), May; pp. 177-197, pls. 7-9.

MAXFIELD, FRED M. 1917. Common parasites of the digestive tract. *Am. J. Vet. Med.*, v. 12 (5), May, pp. 295-297; discussion on pp. 298-300, 314.

MILKS, H. J. 1916. A preliminary report on verminous bronchitis in dogs. *Rept. N. Y. St. Vet. Coll.* for yr. 1914-1915, pp. 129-135, 2 pls.

MULDOON, W. E. 1916. Uncinariasis in dogs. *Rept. N. Y. St. Vet. Coll.* for yr. 1914-1915, pp. 136-141.

OSLER, WILLIAM. 1877. Verminous bronchitis in dogs. *Veterinarian*, Lond., (594), v. 50, 4 s., (270), v. 23, June, pp. 387-397, 2 figs.

RANSOM, BRAYTON H. 1913. *Cysticercus ovis*, the cause of tapeworm cysts in mutton. *J. Agric. Research*, v. 1 (1), Oct. 10, pp. 15-58, pls. 2-4, 13 text figs.
1914. (*Agamonematodum gaylordi*). In *Bull. Bu. Fisheries*, Wash., Doc. 790, v. 32, Apr. 22, pp. 500-501, fig. 123.

RANSOM, BRAYTON H., and WINTHROP D. FOSTER. 1917. Life history of *Ascaris lumbricoides*. *J. Agric. Research*, v. 11 (8). Nov. 19, pp. 395-398.

RILEY, WILLIAM A. 1916. The occurrence of the giant nematode, *Dioctophyme renale* (*Eustrongylus*) in the United States and Canada. *J. Am. Vet. Med. Assn.*, v. 2 (6), Sept., pp. 801-809.

SEURAT, L. G. 1917. Physaloptères des mammifères du Nord-Africain. *Compt. Rend. Soc. d. Biol.*, Paris, v. 80 (4), pp. 210-218.

SOMMER, H. O. 1896. Results of an examination of fifty dogs, at Washington, D. C., for animal parasites. *Vet. Mag.*, v. 3 (8), Aug., pp. 483-487.

STEWART, F. H. 1916. On the life history of *Ascaris lumbricoïdes*. *Brit. Med. J.*, (2896), v. 2, pp. 5-7, 3 figs.
1916. The life history of *Ascaris lumbricoides*. *Brit. Med. J.*, (2809), v. 2, p. 474.
1916. Further experiments on *Ascaris* infection. *Brit. Med. J.*, (2910), v. 2, pp. 486-488.
1916. On the life history of *Ascaris lumbricoides*. *Brit. Med. J.*, (2918), v. 2, pp. 753-754.
1917. On the development of *Ascaris lumbricoides* Lin. and *Ascaris suilla* Duj. in the rat and mouse. *Parasitology*, v. 9 (2), pp. 213-227, 9 figs., 1 pl.

HISTORICAL FACTS CONCERNING THE PATHOLOGY OF SPAVIN*

S. A. GOLDBERG

Department of Comparative Pathology and Bacteriology, New York State Veterinary College at Cornell University, Ithaca, N. Y.

The term *spavin* apparently had its origin from the Latin *spavenius* used by Jordanus Ruffus in the middle of the 13th century. Originally it indicated various pathological processes in the neighborhood of the tarsal joint. Later the term became confined to disease processes occurring on the median side of the tarsus. Due to the different externally noticeable changes in the hock joint there are modifying terms used as prefixes to the term *spavin*, such as *bog, blood, moist, dry* or *bone, occult spavin*, etc.

There was at one time considerable confusion in the classification of spavin. DeSolleysel used the term *dry spavin* for lameness resembling spavin lameness but which did not originate from spavin. True spavin he named ox spavin. Saunier introduced the term *muddy spavin,* a form of spavin usually occurring in horses raised in damp, marshy localities. Gibson selected the term *bone spavin* because the swelling is of a hard consistency and also to distinguish it from a *soft blood spavin.* Bourgelat (1789) acknowledged only one form of spavin which he named *callous spavin.* By the term dry spavin he understood a form of lameness originating in the muscles and their nerves. He considered *ox spavin* as a swelling on the median side of the hock joint arising from stagnated lymph which is at first soft, later becoming hard as gypsum and very commonly occurring in oxen.

At the present time spavin is considered to begin by a rarefying ostitis in the subchondral bone, spreading to the joint to form erosions and ankylosis, and to the periosteum to form exostoses.

The knowledge of the pathology of spavin was, up to the beginning of the 19th century, very meagre. There were a large number of theories concerning the development of the thickening on the median surface of the hock joint. The basis of most of these theories is in harmony with the medical view of humoral pathology at that time.

---

*The publication of these notes was prompted by the fact that most of this literature is not available to the English speaking Veterinarians.

Thomas de Gray in 1639 wrote "A splint is, in the beginning, a very gristle. However, if it be long left alone, it will come to be a hard bone or excression. A ring bone begins first with a slimy humour which in time groweth to a hard gristle.   *   *   * A dry or bone spavin is a great hard crust as hard as a bone if it is let run, sticking or indeed growing to the bone."

Gibson (1754) places the origin of spavin in a soaking of the ligaments with moisture which condenses, forming a swelling composed of hardened glue which later grows like the callous of a fractured bone resembling a piece of flint without any visible pores, except the foramina for the passage of nerves and blood vessels such as are found in other bones that compose the skeleton.

According to vonSind (1770), strong muscular exertion produces an irritation in the vessels allowing the escape of the juices. These juices accumulate in the joint ligaments and on account of their corrosive nature act upon these parts producing a gradually hardening callous known as spavin.

Laffosse (1772), who places the cause and development of spavin in the same class as coronary ringbone, gives the changes as follows: "Following excessive work on heavily strained fibres, they lose their power of speed and cease to require the circulation of lymph. The latter stops, hardens, and causes a stiffness or tension which is at first of an inflammatory nature but soon becomes separated and a sort of horny growth results."

DeSolleysel (1775) thought that the bony swelling arises on the inner and lower part of the hock joint through a confluence of cold humours that gradually becomes bone hard by evaporation and dissolution of its delicate substances.

VonBusch (1788) wrote, "Spavin is indisputably no other than this lymph becoming thickened in many ways, and finally hardened. The ligaments, cartilage and tendons of the hind knee joint contain especially numerous circulatory vessels for the purpose of nourishment. The lymph contained in these vessels becomes tenacious by lengthy inactivity, sudden chilling, etc. It thickens and gradually accumulates. Thus, the spavin begins."

In 1800, Taplin wrote, "A splint is either an enlargement of the periosteum by an original rupture of small vessels, and the extravasated fluid collected and indurated by time or, it is a callosity originally formed upon the bone and becoming ossified, constitutes a bony substance, seeming a deformed part of the bone itself.

* * * A bone spavin is exactly in a greater degree behind what a splint is acknowledged to be before.''

Von Rohlwes (1801) treats spavin as follows: ''Violent stretching of the binding tendons of the hock joint excites an inflammation at the points of attachment. An inflammation invariably causes an afflux of juices which bring about a thickening of the bone itself. Every bone is covered by a strong membrane. Should this membrane become injured, the bone becomes free to enlarge. Hence, whenever the membrane is injured by an inflammation brought about by an afflux of juices, the bone becomes thickened.''

Havemann in 1805 was the first to show that in spavin the articular surfaces themselves are diseased. He says, ''The cause of the lameness lies always in the diseased articular surfaces. The lameness begins as soon as the articular surfaces of the flat bones become denuded of cartilage. This is followed by a sort of growing together of the bones.'' He distinguishes between the hard or bone spavin, the soft or moist spavin, and the occult or invisible spavin.

Von Arnim (1806) considers the cause of spavin similar to that of rheumatism, and a cure very difficult or impossible.

Von Hochstetter (1824) combines under the term spavin all harmful influences diminishing the strength or the flexibility of the hock joint. He considers forceful injury and swelling of the tibial flexor as the cause of bone spavin.

Dietrichs (1829) supports Havemann's view. He says that spavin is a local disease of the hock joint affecting the articular surfaces. He is of the opinion that the primary lesion is in one or more of the articular cartilages of the hock joint.

Regarding occult spavin he says, ''The swelling is, in many cases, unimportant. It is hardly visible, and yet the animal shows marked lameness. This is usually the case when the spavin is observed in the process of development, at the stage when the articular cartilages mainly, are affected and before the bones are grown together.''

According to E. F. Gurlt (1831) spavin is a disease of the horse characterized by exostoses on the median side of the hock joint associated by ankylosis of the articular surfaces and ossification of the ligaments. Like von Rohlwes, he considers that the bony outgrowth comes out of the bone itself following a disease of the periosteum. He says that too little is known about the changes in the cartilage to form an opinion. He asserts also that the growing together of the central with the third tarsus and the latter with the metatarsus usually occurs first.

Hering (1834) supports, in general, Havemann's ideas about spavin. He asserts, however, that not very seldom diseased articular cartilages are found which are not associated with lameness of the horse. Also that in *visible spavin* the articular surfaces are usually found unchanged.

Havemann's spavin theory is further supported by G. W. Schrader (1839). In his numerous investigations of diseased hock joints he found that, as a rule, the articular surfaces between the central and third tarsus are the first to suffer. This chondritis is followed by suppuration of the articular cartilages resulting in caries of the bones that are sooner or later united. According to his view the exostoses appear only after the articular surfaces are markedly diseased and the external border of the third tarsus has been affected by caries. He also points out the fact that many horses without exostoses show marked lameness, while others with exostoses show slight or no lameness.

Bartels (1843) claims that spavin originated with an inflammation of the tendinous attachment of the hock joint. In place of *visible* and *occult* spavin he uses the terms *tarsal* and *navicular spavin*. He used the former where the spavin is located in the upper part of the hock joint accompanied by long standing lameness. The latter, where the spavin is situated in the central and third tarsus not accompanied by lameness of the animal.

Bouley (1850) expressed his opinion that the affection of the articular surfaces is of marked importance in spavin. He says, "Spavin is not an external swelling situated at the articular margin of the flat tarsal bones alone. It is more than that. It is a constant expression of an internal lesion of the articulations of these bones as well."

According to Hertwig (1850) every bony outgrowth on the inner side of the hock joint should be considered as spavin. In very few cases this outgrowth begins as an acute inflammation of the ligaments and the bone, brought about by external injuries to the hock joint. It begins more often as a chronic inflammation, principally of the bone. In such a hock joint the bone is found redder, more vascular, and more porous than normal. The periosteum is slightly thickened and between the bone and periosteum there is found some coagulable liquid. Then the spavin outgrowth arises. In spavin without exostosis, the process begins in the articular surfaces or in the tissue of the bone itself. He holds that, besides strong exertions and kicks, rheumatism may be the cause of this affection. Later Hertwig said that the changes arising in the joint always follow a chronic arthritis.

According to Lawrence (1850) stiff joint or anchylosis arises from some accidental wound in the joint, in which case the synovia escapes outwards. This escape of the synovia occasions great irritation and inflammation, and if the orifice of the wound is not soon closed, the membranes begin to thicken, bony matter is thrown out from the heads of the bones, thereby uniting them in one mass, and the use of the joint is gone. * * * The inflammation from a wounded joint is very different from that which takes place in any muscular part. For as ligaments are not so vascular as muscles, they are consequently much slower in forming granulations, or, in other words, they possess not so perfectly the powers of regeneration.

E. Gurlt (1853) considers spavin a chronic arthritis affecting first the articulation between the central and third tarsus and later the ligaments that bind these bones and the periosteum. He remarks that the swelling and the ankylosing exostosis take place exclusively on the median side of the tarsus. The calcaneo-astragalar articulation as well as that between the astragalus and the central tarsus remain free when they are surrounded by bony outgrowths.

O. F. W. Schrader, Jr. (1860) examined many hock joints of horses that he treated for spavin during life. He considers spavin to be a chronic arthritis with the following possibilities: The process may begin in the cartilage due to strong and continued injurious influences such as pressure which causes a weakening and destruction of the cartilage followed by an affection of the bones. The synovial membrane may be primarily diseased. This causes a diminished amount of synovia or a diseased synovia which in turn affects the cartilage. Finally the subchondral bone may become primarily diseased by repeated jarring, pressure, etc. This causes a disturbed nutrition followed by necrosis of the cartilage.

Anacker (1864) claims that spavin is a chronic deforming and proliferating arthritis. He considers the changes in the cartilage as an amyloid process.

According to the researches of Stockfleth (1869) the inflammatory process in spavin may originate in the ligaments, or in the articular surfaces. In the former the symptom complex arises as a chronic inflammation of the capsular ligament. In the latter the seat of origin is in the median part of the articular surfaces whence it spreads slowly. The articular cartilage gradually disappears and the denuded ends of the bones may grow together.

According to Dieckerhoff (1875) spavin is a complicated chronic inflammatory process originating in the inner leaf of the bursa of the fanshaped muscular attachment of the tendon of the tibial flexor. From here it spreads to the capsular ligament and to the periosum of the lower part of the hock joint producing a chronic synovitis, a softening and dissolution of the articular cartilage, and an inflammation of the bone marrow.

Among the etiological factors he mentions a faulty histological setting in the structure of the hock joint as well as defective body structure, a peculiar temperament, and external influences, such as excessive exertions of the horse, especially excessive burdening of the posterior extremities.

In 1880, Gotti, after examining a large number of hock joints mostly from horses showing spavin symptoms during life, concluded that spavin originates in the bones of the hock joint. He found that the process usually begins with a very slow ostitis of the central and third tarsus and of the metatarsus. In the course of this ostitis there is a widening of the Haversian vessels causing a nutritive disturbance of the bony connective tissue. The latter is finally transformed into plastic marrow tissue which produces a decalcification of the bone. The ostitis later leads to a chondritis characterized by a slow and continued inflammation of the articular cartilage accompanied by active proliferation and destruction of the ground substance.

In the inflammatory process of the bone, Gotti recognized two stages. A destructive period, during which the newly formed marrow tends to spread slowly, and a regenerative period during which the newly formed marrow tends to be transformed into compact connective or bony tissue. Should the proliferating process reach the articular surfaces, it is possible for the marrow elements to be transformed into osseous tissue and lead to a true ankylosis.

He considered the formation of osteophytes as secondary, usually following the disorder of the joint, and developing at the time when the changes have reached the margin of the articular surfaces.

According to von Klemm (1887) the etiology of spavin is as follows: "In all cases where the heel is trimmed low the hock joint is excessively extended through the forward pressure on the joint by the tendon of the flexor pedis. This is the case when the thigh is loaded. In connection with this extension there is undoubtedly an excessive tension of both tibial flexors which, with their five tendinous heads must, in their turn, have an injurious effect on the points of insertion around the hock joint. Should the horse be cow hocked or the median side wall trimmed low, the injury occurs only on the median tendons thus bring about a spavin." He stated that in fifteen military horses whose heels were trimmed particularly low, nine showed spavin in from one to two months.

Bayer (1890) supported the views of Gotti.

Müller considers spavin as a *chronic deforming arthritis.*

According to Pflug (1892) the exostoses are the primary lesions of spavin. He considers them as arising from an inflammatory process, an *ossifying periarthritis* which is often complicated by an arthritis.

Hoffman (1892) at first supported Dieckerhoff's views of spavin. Later he declared that spavin is an inflammation of the bone, a hyperemia leading to a *rarefying ostitis* and finally to formation of lacunae.

Höhne considers spavin not as a primary disease of the hock joint but as a complication of gonitis.

Smith (1893) differentiates between an *articular* and a *nonarticular* form of spavin. He considers spavin to be a *chronic deforming arthritis.*

An interesting treatise of spavin appeared in 1893 by Aronsohn. He summarizes as follows:

1. Spavin begins with a periostitis brought about by an injury to the median terminal tendons of the tibialis anticus and by overstretching the long and short lateral ligaments. This periostitis leads to exostoses on the median surface of the hock joint.

2. The arthritis is mostly secondary and occurs only on both lower articulations of the hock joint.

3. The capsular ligament and the synovial membrane of this joint show only slight changes. An enlargement of the synovial villi is, macroscopically, not shown.

4. There is very little proliferation of the articular cartilage before degeneration takes place. Peripheral proliferation of the articular surfaces followed by ossification is never found. Eburnation of the denuded bone is likewise not seen.

5. Free bodies are never found in this joint.

6. Eventually, the disease process leads to a partial, rarely to a complete, osseous ankylosis of the articular ends. The latter is never found in the tarso-metatarsal articulation.

7. Atrophy of the tarsal bones is rare. When it occurs, it is hidden by the articular ends and by the ossifying periostitis. The endosteal changes consist of an osteoporosis and an osteosclerosis. They do not influence the periosteal formation of bone.

8. The affection of the tibio-astragalar joint consisting of a fibrous thickening of the capsular ligament and a proliferating inflammation of the synovial villi is a secondary complication of spavin.

He admits that an arthritis may cause a periarthritis and all the above described changes; but he claims never to have noticed, in spavin, diseased articular surfaces without any changes in the periosteum. He holds that those cases where there are erosions on the edge of the articular surface without any periarthritic changes, indicate nutritive or functional disturbances without any important significance. He thinks it unlikely that the small joints of the tarsus, on account of their rigid structure and naturally limited movement, should be primarily diseased.

According to Eberlein (1898) the process begins by a reddening and softening of the subchondral bone of the central and the third tarsus, at the anterior and median part of the joint and 2 or 3 mm. from the margin. This spreads towards the articular cartilages to form erosions, and towards the periosteum to form exostoses.

The synovia is diminished to but a few drops. It is alkaline in reaction and of normal appearance. In cases of ankylosis, it thickens and gradually disappears. He did not find any bacteria in the synovia, in the bone, or in the cartilage.

The cartilage is at first changed in color. It is bluish red instead of whitish, and dull instead of shiny. Later there begins a superficial fibrillation followed by deeper destruction of the cartilage. This becomes noticeable as punctiform erosions which later become confluent resulting in elongated erosions.

Microscopically the earliest change is an increased number of lymphoid marrow cells in the Haversian canals. These are at first lined along the walls of the canals. Later they are gradually increased in number until the canals are completely filled, and they appear as proliferating granulation tissue. At the same time there is a disappearance of the bony tissue, indicated by a widening of the canals. This widening takes place in various directions so that the Haversian canals become irregular in shape. The dissolution of the bone is accomplished by numerous giant cells, osteoclasts, that originate, according to Kölliker, from the osteoblasts. This process is known as *rarefying ostitis* or *inflammatory osteoporosis*.

Soon after this resorptive process there appears a regenerative process in which there is a new formation of bone, known as *osteosclerosis* or condensing ostitis. This process tends to counterbalance the damage done by the previous process so that finally the bone becomes even denser than the original bone.

The osteo-porosis spreads to the neighboring parts and causes therein a destructive process. In this manner it reaches the articular surfaces. Here, however, it is checked by the articular cartilage. The granulation tissue then spreads out beneath the cartilagenous surface causing a disturbed nutrition of the articular cartilage. This is followed by a fibrillation of the upper and a softening of the deeper layers of the cartilage. Together, they produce a splitting and a sinking of the articular cartilage. Usually, however, there occurs a true chondritis in the form of progressive and retrograde inflammatory processes. In this case the inflammation of the bone affects the cartilage directly producing a proliferation of the cartilage cells. The number of cells is increased and they lie together in groups. Between these groups of cells there are round or oblong, large multinucleated giant cells which produce a degeneration and resorption of the newly formed cells. This results in a loosening and fibrillation of the cartilage and in a destruction of the ground substance, and is eventually followed by a splitting of the cartilage. The proliferating granulation tissue very often simply penetrates the cartilage, i. e., it grows into the cartilage and dissolves it until it reaches the articular surface. Should the osteosclerosis now quickly follow, the chondritis may cease, and there may remain on the articular surface white punctiform elevations, the so-called *lime points*. In other cases the chondritis spreads rapidly and leads to a destruction of the articular cartilage.

There is often found ankylosis between individual bones, particularly between the central and the third tarsus. This growing together of the bones may be in the form of a pseudo-ankylosis produced by fingershaped hyperostoses gripping one another, or it may be in the form of osseous ankylosis arising from the articular surfaces. The latter does not take place over the entire articular surface but in parts of it, so that on section of the joint there are seen elongated fissures in ankylosed parts of the joint. There is, therefore, only partial ankylosis as a rule and rarely only complete ankylosis. Eberlein claims never to have seen a fibrous or cartilagenous ankylosis, so that he regards ankylosis in spavin as being exclusively of an osseous nature.

Etiologically, he holds that spavin is due to pressure on the smaller bones of the hock joint. The extrinsic causes for this pressure are overstraining of the hock joint due to too quick movements, jumping, heavy loads, improper shoeing, etc. The intrinsic cause consists of an internal anlage due to faulty conformation of the hock, to temperament, and to the age of the animal. Heavy musculature in the pelvic region predisposes to spavin, particularly when the hock joint is not built correspondingly strong. A long dorsum is also a predisposing factor. Horses with violent temperaments are more susceptible to spavin than phlegmatic horses. This is so because they attempt their work with greater exertion. Young horses are affected more often than older ones.

In affected joints the erosion is at first noticed 2 or 3 mm. from the margin. The reason for this lies, according to Eberlein, in the form of the articular surface. He claims that if pressure is exerted on a joint after it has been freed from its ligaments, it will be seen that the *closing border* is not at the margin of the joint, but a few mm. from it. On account of this fact, every mechanical lesion will exert itself more heavily on this closing border, so that the first inflammatory changes must occur on this part of the bone and cartilage.

This view of Eberlein that spavin begins in the subchondral bone is accepted today by most veterinarians. Hertwig (1850) was the first to point out this possibility and Gotti was the first to assert that it always begins in the subchondral bone. Williams claims that spavin is a local manifestation of a general disease.

Some French authors (Kitt) claim that diseases through which young animals pass predispose them to this condition.

BIBLIOGRAPHY

ABRAHAM, P. S. Arthritis Deformans in the horse. Dublin, 1884.

ARONSOHN. Beitrag zur Kenntniss der pathologischen Anatomie des Spates beim Pferde. *Inaug. Diss.*, Giessen, 1893.

BARTELS. Der Spat und die Heilung desselben ohne brennen. *Viehzucht u. Thierheilk*, I Jahrg. Helmstedt, 1843 (cited by Aronsohn).

BUCHE, KARL. Über die Histologie u. Pathologie der periarticulären Krongelenkschals. *Inaug. Diss.*, Hanover, 1912.

DIECKERHOFF. Die Pathologie und Therapie des Spates der Pferde. Berlin, 1875.

EBERLEIN. Der Spat der Pferde. *Monatsh. f. prakt. Tierheilk*, IX Bd. (1898), 49.

ENGEL, HANS. Über Kongenitale Ankylosen an den Gelenken der Hände und Füsse. *Inaug. Diss.*, Berlin, 1902.

FISCHER, C. W., and UDALL, D. H. Etiology and Pathology of the Spavin group of lameness. *Thesis*, 1901.

FRÖHNER. Compendium der spezielle Chirurgie für Tierärzte. 1905, p. 256.

GIBSON, WM. A. A new treatise on the Diseases of Horses. Vol. II, London, 1754, p. 252.

GOLDBERG, S. A. A Case of Erosive Osteo-Arthritis in a calf. *Cornell Veterinarian*, Vol. V, No. 2 (July, 1915), p. 90; *Am. Vet. Rev.*, Vol. XLVII, No. 6 (Sept., 1915), p. 735.

GOLDBERG, S. A. The Structural Changes that Occur in Certain Non-Specific Inflammation of Joints. *Report of the N. Y. State Vet. College at Cornell University for the Year* 1914-15, p. 142. Abstracted in the *Cornell Veterinarian*, Vol. VI, No. 1 (1916), p. 57.

GOTTI. Ricerche Sopra un lento Processo arthritis al Tarso del Cavalo. Bologna, 1880.

GRAY DE THOMAS. The complete Horseman and expert Farrier. London, 1639, p. 324.

HAMILTON, J. W. Synovitis. A clinical lecture. *Ohio Med. and Surg. Jour.* Columbus, 1860.

HARGER, S. J. J. Anatomo-pathologic study of ringbone and spavin as indicated by examination of pathological specimens. *Am. Vet. Rev.*, Vol. XXV (1901), p. 992.

HERTWIG, F. Practisches Handbuch der Chirurgie für Thierärzte. Berlin, 1850 (cited by Eberlein).

HOCHSTETTER, V. Theoretisch-praktisches Handbuch der Pferdekenntniss und Pferdewartung. Bern, 1824 (cited by Eberlein).

KARNBACH. Die Omarthritis chronica deformans des Pferdes. *Monatsh. f. prakt. Tierheilk.* Bd XIV, p. 97.

KARNBACH. Die Hufgelenkschale des Pferdes. *Monatshefte f. prakt. Tierheilk.* XI Bd. (1900), p. 516.

KITT, TH. Lehrbuch der pathologischen Anatomie der Haustiere. 4 Aufl. I Bd. Stuttgart. 1910.

KRUEGER. Die chronische Arthritis u. Periarthritis Carpi des Pferdes. *Archiv. f. Tierheilk.* (1905), p. 295.

LAWRENCE, RICHARD. The Complete Farrier. London, 1850, p. 77.

NICHOLS, E. H., and RICHARDSON, F. L. Arthritis Deformans. *Jour. Med. Res.*, Vol. XXI (1909), p. 149.

PFLUG. Spat. Encyklop. der gesammt. Thierheilk. u. Viehz. IX Bd. Wien u. Leipzig (1892), (cited by Eberlein).

RVINI, CARLO. Delle Infirmitadi De'cavalli. Venetia. 1602, p. 314.

SCHRADER, G. W. Verzeichniss menier Sammlung krankhafter Knöschen vom Splunggelenk des Pferdes. Bemerkungen in Bezug anf spat. *Mag. f. d. gesammte, Tierheilk.* V. Jahrg. Berlin (1839), p. 95.

SCHRADER, JR., O. F. W. Ueber dis chronischen Gelenkkrankheiten des Pferdes. *Magaz. f. d. gesammte Thierheilk.* XXVI Jahrg. Berlin (1860), p. 1.

SMITH, F. Some Joint Diseases of the Horse. *Jour. Comp. Path. and Therap.*, Vol. VI. Edinburg (1893), pp. 1, 149, 195.

STOKFLETH. Ueber Spatbehandlung. *Tidsskr. f. Veterin.* 1868, *nach. Report d. Thierheilk.* XXX Jahr. (1869), (cited by Eberlein).

TAPLIN, WM. Modern System of Farriery. London, 1789, p. 55; Philadelphia, 1794, p. 32.

PRAEGER. Beitrag zu den Ansichten uber den Spat. *Magaz. f. d. gesammte Thierheilk.* V. Jahrgang. Berlin (1839), p. 205.

URDISKIE. Die Pathologische Anatomie der Krongelenkschale des Pferdes *Monatshefte f. prakt. Tierheilk.* XI Bd. (1900), p. 337.

WILLIAMS, W. L., FISCHER, C. W., and UDALL, D. H. Spavin Group of Lameness. *Proc. Am. Vet. Med. Asso.* 42 (1905), p. 283.

ZALEWSKY. Die Gonitis chronica deformans des Pferdes. *Monatshefte f. prakt. Thierheilk.* XII Bd. (1901), p. 481.

JUSTIN MORGAN—THE MAN AND THE HORSE*

MAJOR C. A. BENTON, New York, N. Y.

The Morgan Horse was at his top notch when Hale's Green Mountain Morgan, in 1851, swept the country from Vermont to Massachusetts, as perhaps the most sensational animal that had ever appeared in America.

For twenty years the Morgans held their popularity. It was only after the Civil War that their decadence began, when the *craze for speed,* started by the wonderful career of Dexter, caused everyone to turn his attention to the long striding trotters, represented by the descendants of Rysdyk's Hambletonian.

Those were the years when Hambletonian stallions began to be taken to Vermont and bred on Morgan mares, hoping to produce fast trotters. The result was disastrous. Environment was against the violent cross. The breeders failed to get what they expected, and spoiled what they had.

Not until about 1890 did the supreme folly of the experiment thoroughly impress those who had known the excellence of the original Morgan stock, either from personal experience or the statements of those who had owned and driven them.

At about that period classes began to be made for ''Morgans conforming most nearly to the original type''. It was discovered that very few were left, and they were to be found only in those parts of Vermont, such as Caledonia County, in the neighborhood of St. Johnsbury, where the hills were so steep, and the roads so

---

*Presented at the February meeting of the Massachusetts Veterinary Medical Association.

ill adapted to extreme speed, that none but the old fashioned type, with their short sharp trotting gait, with no sign of straddle behind, no inclination to pace, built low to the ground and substantial in form, could live.

Ethan Allen 3rd, a much inbred descendant of Hale's Green Mountain Morgan, was one of the first to command recognition as the true type of Morgan horse. He was bought and taken west the second year after he showed up a winner. Fortunately, after 16 or 17 years' absence, when 24 years old, his limited offspring attracted attention and he was brought back to Caledonia County, where he lived his last 3 or 4 years, leaving possibly about 100 descendants in Vermont and adjoining states.

Ethan Allen 3rd was a son of Ethan Allen 2nd, and strongly inbred to Peter's Vermont, and other blood which had been kept untainted by the men of the Peter's family, the Orcutts, and the Ides, who stand as sponsors for sound Morgan breeding just as the Booths and the Bates families have in the history of English Short Horn cattle.

Other sons of Ethan Allen 3rd were Mcginnis' Comet and Ethan Allen 4th (both dead), Bob Morgan, Rob Roy, Croydon Prince, Morgan Falcon, Delvyn. These are the horses that have helped to uphold the lines of Hale's Green Mountain Morgan in the home state.

Many excellent mares, bred in these lines, were taken West, some to western New York, Ohio, Illinois, others to Virginia, and some even as far west as the State of Washington. Their names and location were made a study by Mr. Henry S. Wardner, the first president of the Morgan Horse Club, in which work he was aided by the cooperation of Dr. A. H. Hinman of Dundee, Ill.

Another branch of the Morgan family, one of the very best, is that starting with Billy Root, an impressive sire, whose prepotency carries to our own day. Billy Roberts, of late years, was the most typical scion of that branch of the Morgan family, Lyndon, and Reynard, own brothers, in two of the most conspicuous Morgan breeding studs of Vermont, still hold up the Billy Root end. Some of the best Morgan brood mares are recognized as from the Billy Root blood.

A combination of these strains has been brought back to Vermont, in Jerome, an aged stallion; thus, it appears that there still exists a few representatives of the original Morgan strain.

Justin Morgan, the horse, was foaled in 1789 and died in 1821; Sherman Morgan foaled in 1808, died 1835. From that time up to 1848 Bulrush Morgan, Woodbury Morgan, Royal Morgan, Gifford Morgan and Vermont Morgan were the prominent descendants. After that Billie Root, Black Hawk, Hale's Green Mountain Morgan, Morrill, Flying Morgan, the Streeter Horse, and Stockbridge Chief were recognized as the best examples of Morgan blood. Just subsequent to this, Ethan Allen, Peter's Vermont Morgan, Goldust, and Gen. Knox were quite famous.

Later on, the breeding of Morgan stallions are susceptible of verification, in which connection comes the thought that it is to be regretted that equine history is not written when it is made.

Reverting to Justin Morgan, there has been and exists today, a well definited uncertainty as to his true breeding. On conformation and type, anyone who has been a keen and interested observer, would be inclined to think that the theory that he was a Dutch horse correct. There must be something in the old saying that "like begets like" while on the other hand such authorities as Linsley and Joseph Battell published pedigrees of Justin Morgan that clearly indicate his descent from Byerly Turk and Godolphin Arabian, and his dam by Diamond son of Wildair. Take your choice.

Whatever the truth may be, nothing is more certain than that the Morgan horse was, and is a good one and that it is difficult to indicate any service for which he is not useful. The records made by the breed on the track, in cavalry service during the Civil War, and his nature in rugged New England country are an open book. He is without question one of the most useful horses known and the preservation of the breed, as a breed, is to my mind of paramount importance. The breeding should be perpetuated under conditions that will not include what some people call, an improved type. Hale's Green Mountain, son of Gifford, has been wisely adopted by the Morgan Horse Club as the model type. Is it not good enough?

Man developed civilization, but not alone; side by side, prospering and suffering together has been his best ally, the horse. As the Pony Express, at the plough, or hitched to the crude stone boat he has drawn sap through the New England sugar bush, and carried the country doctors and circuit riders on their errands of mercy; why shouldn't we talk about him? Nowadays our lives, yes, even our thoughts, have become so artificial that it is far cry

from early New England days when the ties that bound our fore-
fathers to their horses were closely interwoven.

In 1837 the 1st Dragoon Guards from England were mounted
on Morgans from Vermont and pronounced by their officers as fully
the equal of the best English troop horses.

Twenty-four years later the 1st Vermont Cavalry went to
southern battlefields mounted on Morgan horses and records prove
them to be the best and most efficient cavalry regiment in the Federal Army.

It makes but little difference as to a verified ancestry. Justin
Morgan must have been well bred to accomplish what he did, en-
dowing his offspring with the power of perpetuating his good
qualities through generations from his to the present one. As the
Morgan Horse Club say, "for all practical purposes of the Morgan
horse breeder of today, Justin Morgan may be regarded as "Adam".

With this introduction let us go somewhat in detail as to both
Justin Morgan, the man, and Justin Morgan, the horse, in which
connection I desire to thank Mr. Wm. H. Gocher of Hartford,
Conn., for most of the valuable information upon which it is based.
Mr. Gocher, as secretary of the National Trotting Association, has
given the subject most careful investigation and his opinion is
recognized as worthy of most serious consideration.

Within a radius of fifty miles of the grounds of the Vermont
State Agricultural Society, there was laid between 1795 and 1821,
the foundation of a breed of horses which have carried the name
of Vermont over the world. It established a type which became
the trademark of the first great American family of horses and it
is so distinct and different from all others that when an Australian,
a South American or an Englishman refers to a horse as a "Vermont Morgan" an idea of his general appearance is conveyed as
lucidly to the residents of these countries as it would be if addressed
to a New Englander.

As is well known, Ethan Allen won his honors as a trotter.
He was the champion four-year-old stallion of his time, and when
Magna Charta, Fearnaught and Lady Maud acquired champion-
ship honors, those who were breeding utility Morgans made an
effort to produce trotters. This was an error which the Morgan
Horse Club has done more than any other organization to point
out, as the compact form of Morgan is not what can be looked for
in the champion trotter of today, although a dash of the blood adds

finish to many of the plainer families, as is well illustrated in Uhlan, the fastest trotter that the world has seen. This blending with other lines, however, has in a measure shown good results as on account of it, strains of Morgan blood can be found in the pedigree of many of the greatest trotters, and show ring winners both in harness and saddle classes.

For the first few generations, the Morgan was a male line family. The breeding of the dams of all the early stallions of note is either unknown or when known traces to horses that did not possess in a marked degree any of the qualities which made their descendants famous. The germ of merit came from the sire, and notwithstanding this method of breeding, the original type for a time increased in size and was reproduced so uniformly that it became fixed in New England.

The breed which passed into history as the Morgan horse bears the name of the man who brought the tap root to Vermont in 1795, and while he was always in humble circumstances, and died in debt under the roof of a friend who had adopted two of his children, his fame will endure beyond the advent of the much heralded, but evidently remote, horseless age.

Justin Morgan, the man, was born in 1747, in or near Springfield, Mass. Upon arriving at the age of twenty, he developed tubercular symptoms and as he was unfitted for heavy work on a farm, he took up school teaching, giving singing lessons, standing other people's stallions for public service and finally keeping a tavern for a living. Up to 1788 he was located at West Springfield, Mass., and at that time owned two-thirds of an acre of land on which there was a house and barn. While there among other horses, he had in 1784, one from East Hartford, Conn., named True Briton. He was also known as Beautiful Bay and later as Traveller, and had been standing for service at several places in Massachusetts for a number of years. At the beginning of his stud career, so far as public announcements show, True Briton was simply a stallion, "to fame unknown," but later in life, he was represented as an English horse, or what would not be termed a thoroughbred, and finally he had a story tacked on to him in which it was set forth with great particularity that prior to the Revolution, he was one of Colonel DeLancey's race horses, and was stolen from him during the war, ridden into the American lines at White Plains, New York, and ultimately sold by one Smith to Joseph

Ward of Hartford, Conn., and he in turn sold him to Selah Horton, who lived on the other side of the Connecticut River in East Hartford. He was the owner of the horse when Justin Morgan stood him at West Springfield.

In 1788, Justin Morgan, possibly on account of his health, sold his home in West Springfield for thirty-three pounds, seven shillings and sixpence and removed to Randolph, Vermont, with his wife and daughter Emily, born in 1784, and son Justin, born in 1786. After his departure, John Morgan, a distant relative, secured True Briton and stood him during the seasons of 1788 and 1789. He removed to Lima, New York, his departure from West Springfield dating from 1790, and he never returned.

While travelling about Vermont teaching, Justin Morgan saw that there was an opportunity to make a little money with a good stock horse, so he communicated with some one in Hartford, possibly Selah Horton, the owner of True Briton, and procured a horse named Figure which he advertised for service in the Windsor, Vermont, *Journal* in 1793 as the "famous horse Figure, from Hartford". Justin Morgan also stood Figure in 1794, and in 1795, he again advised his patrons by an advertisement in the Rutland *Herald* that "Figure sprang from a curious horse owned by Colonel DeLancey of New York" and by that announcement an effort has been made to show that Figure was the horse afterwards known as Justin Morgan and that Justin Morgan bred him while he lived in West Springfield, notwithstanding the fact that Linsley and others, including Justin Morgan's son, fixed the date of this horse's birth at 1793, beyond a shadow of doubt.

But three years of life remained for Justin Morgan. As yet he had done nothing to carry his name beyond the boundaries of Randolph. He had no home ties and his health bad. In the summer of 1795, after making a season with Figure, he told his friends that he was going down the Connecticut River to Springfield to collect money that was due him, possibly on the house and lot which he had sold in 1788. He rode away and nothing more was heard of him until he returned to Randolph in the early fall, leading a three-year-old gelding and followed by a little nubbin of a two-year-old colt. At a later date, he told his friends that he took the pair in payment of the debt, and that the colt was a Dutch horse. This was the horse that made Vermont famous, and those who today discuss the merits of the family should stop for a moment

to recall that dusty, travel worn figure coming back to Randolph
with a three-year-old gelding and a two-year-old colt, neither of
which could at that age bring him in any revenue.

For the time being, fame and fortune passed him by, but his
home coming in 1795 meant much to Vermont as he was followed
by a horse that made the Green Mountain State and those bordering on it, the headquarters of a famous type of horses, and now,
after a lapse of over a century, would not the citizens of Vermont
be honoring themselves if they erected in Randolph or some appropriate place, a monument in memory of this man and his horse?
As for the horse, no one knows who bred him and the only suggestion that can be made is that it was the man who was in Justin
Morgan's debt. That man, in all probability, was Abner Morgan.
No one has ever taken the trouble to learn who he was, what he did
for a living, what he owned, or what became of him. He is the
missing link in the story of the horse Justin Morgan.

The only statement in existence in regard to this horse from
anyone who knew Justin Morgan appeared in a letter written by
his son to the Albany *Cultivator* in 1842. It was also the first
statement, and at the time it was written he was not guided by the
memories or suggestions of others. He said the colt was a two-
year-old when his father brought him to Randolph in 1795, and
that his father called him a Dutch horse. That is all. The writer
of this letter was twelve years old when his father died, and the
only accurate knowledge in connection with the origin of the horse
Justin Morgan begins and ends with it. At a later date, John
Morgan, still living at that date at Lima, New York, introduced
the True Briton story and ultimately supplied Justin Morgan with
a dam, while the facts are that John Morgan never saw the man
Justin Morgan after he left West Springfield in 1788, and it is self
evident that he never had any correspondence with him in regard
to this horse or he would have mentioned it when he wrote the
Albany *Cultivator*. Half a century later, John H. Wallace loomed
up with his iconoclastic hammer and knocked every peg from under
the True Briton end of the pedigree by showing that the horse did
not stand for service at West Springfield the year Justin Morgan
was got, even if he was bred there, which is a point that has never
been determined.

But before going any further with the Morgan family, it
might be well to stop and look up the Dutch horse. It was intro-

duced in America by the founders of New Amsterdam, the New York of today. Some of them were brought from Holland as early as 1625. By 1650 they were very numerous and used for all kinds of work.

In 1665, after New Amsterdam was surrendered by the Dutch to the English, Governor Nicholls established a race course at Hempstead Plains on Long Island, and offered prizes for races. These events were no doubt contested under saddle as there were no vehicles suitable for harness races in existence then. It was probably the former as the racing was continued for many years and trotting under saddle did not come into vogue on Long Island until early in the nineteenth century, when the descendants of Imported Messenger began to appear on the road in New York, New Jersey and Pennsylvania.

It will therefore be seen that racing was established among the Dutch in New York before the English race horse was considered a separate breed, in fact, it was only being started under the patronage of Charles II, who, after the Restoration in 1660, revived all kinds of sports in England, and especially horse racing. He also kept a number of running horses and frequently rode them in their races at Newmarket. It is therefore safe to presume that the horses which raced on Hempstead Plains in 1665 and for many subsequent years, were Dutch horses, tracing direct to those which were imported from Holland. Dutch horses were also sent to other ports than New Amsterdam, as there has been found at Salem, Mass., an entry in 1635, setting forth the fact that in that year two Dutch sloops landed twenty-seven mares and three stallions. The mares were valued at thirty-four pounds, while the English horse of that period cost six pounds, and ten for freight. The difference in value can in all probability be attributed to the size of the English horse, between thirteen and fourteen hands, while the Dutch horses were between fourteen and fifteen hands, and by the date of the Revolution, this had been increased so that the average horse was fifteen hands.

Dutch horses were plentiful in New York State and especially in the valley of the Hudson River, where the wealthy burghers had large estates and that they were also bred in New England is evidenced by the fact that one of them named Young Bulrock stood for service at Springfield, Mass., in 1792, the year that Justin Morgan was got. He was described in an advertisement as a "horse

of Dutch breed, of large size and a bright bay color''. Was this
the sire of Justin Morgan? Certainly there are better grounds for
claiming it than that he was by True Briton, a horse that is not
known to have been there that year, and which was advertised in
the *Connecticut Courant* to stand in East Hartford, Conn., although the announcement was afterwards withdrawn.

At this point, it would also be well to stop and compare the gait,
form and style of the Dutch horse, with Linsley's description of
Justin Morgan, which is as follows:

"The original, or Justin Morgan, was about fourteen hands
high, and weighed about nine hundred and fifty pounds. His color
was dark bay with black legs, mane and tail. He had no white
hairs on him. His mane and tail were coarse and heavy, but not so
massive as has been sometimes described; the hair of both was
straight, and not inclined to curl. His head was good, not extremely small, but lean and bony, the face straight, forehead broad,
ears small and very fine, but set rather wide apart. His eyes were
medium size, very dark and prominent, with a spirited but pleasant
expression, and showed no white round the edge of the lid. His
nostrils were very large, the muzzle small, and the lips close and
firm. His back and legs were perhaps his most noticeable points.
The former was very short; the shoulder blades and hip being very
long and oblique and the loins exceedingly broad and muscular.
His body was rather long, round and deep, close ribbed up, chest
deep and wide, with the breast bone projecting a good deal in
front. His legs were short, close jointed, thin, but very wide, hard
and free from meat, with muscles that were remarkably large for a
horse of this size, and this superabundance of muscle exhibited itself
at every step. His hair was short, and at almost all seasons soft
and glossy. He had a little long hair about the fetlocks and for two
or three inches above the fetlocks on the back side of the legs; the
rest of the limbs were entirely free from it. His feet were small
but well shaped, and he was in every respect perfectly sound and
free from any sort of blemish. He was a very fast walker."

When the above and the accepted picture of the horse is compared with the type of English thoroughbred of that period, they
will be found as far apart as it is possible to be among horses of
about the same weight. On the other hand, an English writer describes the Dutch Hartdraver, that is, a fast trotter, as follows:

"These horses run from fourteen to sixteen hands; the head

small, the shoulders well laid back; the haunches prominent, the croup short and broad, and the limbs muscular and clean, but often fringed with longish hair up the sinew above pastern joints.'' This is taken from a book that was published in London in 1845 and would almost fit the Morgan of today.

Also, in order to show that the trotting speed of the Dutch horse is not of the mythical kind that was attributed to the Narragansett pacer, it is only necessary to refer to the history of the Orloff trotter. This breed was originated by Count Alexis Orloff. He began with an Arabian horse named Smetanka which he bred to a Danish mare. She produced Bolkan. He was larger than his sire and was in turn bred to a Dutch mare which breed at that time had a reputation for its trotting qualities. This Dutch mare, in 1784, nine years before Justin Morgan was foaled, produced Barss, to whom all of the Orloff trotters trace, and there are now over 18,000 of them with records of 2:30 or better, through his sons Dobry, Lebed, and Lubezny.

In Russia, the Dutch mare gave the Orloff horse the trotting step. Did young Bulrock do the same thing in America for the Morgans? He came from a family that was noted for that quality and the results in Russia show that he had the power to transmit it. True Briton, if any of the stories told about him can be believed, came from a family noted for its running qualities, and the ability to transmit it and the turf test in America, proves conclusively that thoroughbred sires have never succeeded in siring trotters in either the first, second or any other generation, except in the line through Messenger, to which all of the Hambletonians and Mambrinos trace.

There is, therefore, nothing left but to add that Justin Morgan, so far as an established pedigree is concerned, is a ''Topsy''. He simply grew. That he had a sire and dam, we must admit, but their breeding, if they had any of merit, is unknown. The name of his breeder is unknown, and the chances are that it always will be. The only clue is supplied by Justin Morgan's son, who, as before stated, said that his father called the colt a Dutch horse. It is the only testimony that should be accepted. It was the first impression on the subject placed on the memory of a boy and all of us know that they are lasting. It is also unfortunate that Linsley and other early writers on the Morgan horse did not look up the Dutch horse. The fact that Linsley ignored it entirely shows that he never gave it a thought.

SERUM OR INULA AND ECHINACEA IN THE TREATMENT OF CANINE DISTEMPER*

A. SLAWSON, New York City

The purpose of this paper is to discuss briefly the relative merits of two kinds of biologics used in the treatment of canine distemper. A few similar products will be mentioned to bring out more clearly the meaning of what I am endeavoring to place before you. The etiology and symptomatology of canine distemper are so well known that no attention will be given them in this article. It is my aim rather to deal with two points only, viz., the method of treatment and the action of the therapeutic agents in question which in this case are anti-canine distemper serum and inula and echinacea, also to compare these with similar biologics.

METHOD OF TREATMENT. Anti-canine distemper serum is injected subcutaneously, three injections of 4 to 7 c.c. being the rule. This article referring to canines only. It may be stated that subcutaneous injections of this serum cause little pain, no edema and no lameness. This is also true of normal serum, leucocyte extract or nuclein.

Inula and echinacea, a proprietary compound composed of echinacea augustifolia and inula helenium, is injected intramuscularly, six injections of from 2 to 5 c.c. being the usual number. This injection causes considerable pain, lameness for a day or two, and often a transitory cellulitis or serous infiltration with its consequent pain and swelling at the point of the injected material.

Viewing the method of injection of these substances from the standpoint of the comfort of the patient and the impression on its owner, not forgetting the satisfaction we derive as a profession in being able to administer our treatment humanely, the balance in favor of either a subcutaneous or intramuscular injection inclines strongly toward the subcutaneous method.

ACTION OF THERAPEUTIC AGENT. Anti-canine distemper serum acts as an anti-toxin and sets free in the system specific anti-bodies. These act quickly upon *B. bronchisepticus*, especially in the early stages of the disease, besides increasing the leucocytosis already present, thus giving the serum additional bactericidal power.

*Presented at the April, 1918, meeting of the New York City Veterinary Medical Society.

Inula and echinacea causes leucocytosis with a rise in opsonic index but with no specific action upon *B. bronchisepticus*. Plain serum, leucocyte extract, and nuclein possess similar properties to inula and echinacea, the two former products being of animal, the latter of plant origin.

Inula and echinacea has been spoken of as a curative agent in distemper but in cases treated by me it has been necessary to resort to anti-canine distemper serum to effect a final cure. I have found the action of inula and echinacea in repeated injections no different from the action of nuclein, leucocyte extract or plain serum, all of which I used before the advent of the specific serum. I have had three cases treated repeatedly with inula and echinacea by others, and pronounced cured, which two weeks later were brought to me for further treatment. To me the inula and echinacea treatment in dogs is not satisfactory because it is given via the intramuscular route, and because it is not specific.

It is not my desire to go more deeply into the serum treatment of canine distemper because this was gone into fully in my paper on this subject entitled "Serum Treatment of Canine Distemper" read at Kansas City last summer. This paper was published in the JOURNAL OF THE A. V. M. A. in the July, 1918, number.

CLINICAL AND CASE REPORTS

TREATMENT OF SUPPURATING CORNS IN HORSES, WITH A CASE

R. W. SHUFELDT, M.D.
Major, Medical Corps, U. S. A. Army Medical Museum.

The patient here referred to and described is a gray gelding, about ten years of age, that was treated at the veterinary hospital of Dr. Harry Bosley of Washington, D. C. Mr. Roy Reeve, Photographer of the Army Medical Museum of the Surgeon General's Office, made the two photographs, from which the cuts illustrating the article were made—the former having been taken direct from the patient, and each shows the conditions described below. It will be noted that the disease is in the right fore-foot (Fig. 1), and it resulted from the animal having worked on the asphalt streets of Washington for a period extending over four years. Both the whole of the sole of the hoof and the wall from heel to quarter have been removed.

This condition is quite common, as we would naturally suppose, for the reason that it arises from the horse having been used on cobbled or asphalted streets for too long a time; or, as sometimes happens, from having been quartered in stalls with concreted floors, or other material of an equally hard nature.

Shoes that have remained on too long will also give rise to these suppurating corns, for the heel of the shoe becomes imbedded

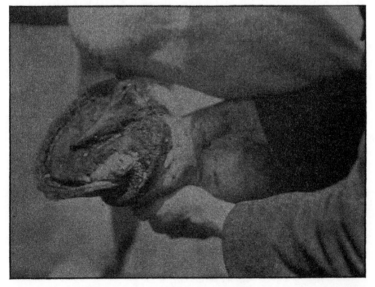

FIGURE 1—Gray gelding about ten years old exhibiting a suppurating corn on sole of right fore-foot.

in the sole of the hoof at its heel, and this, in time, causes sufficient irritation to start the inflammation at the point of greatest pressure.

Flat-footed horses are more subject to this disease than those with more shapely hoofs, and this is especially true should the victims be heavily built animals. Generally, the corn makes its appearance on the inside of the hoof of a fore-foot, while the one in the present instance is on the outside.

The premonitory symptom consists in a slight lameness, and

this gradually increases from day to day, particularly should the cause of it be persisted in, or kept up. Local fever soon makes its appearance on the hoof-wall where the corn or suppuration will eventually appear. Should one tap on the hoof at this point the patient will flinch and exhibit other evidences of local tenderness accompanied with pain.

We should now promptly remove the shoe and pare away the sole of the hoof at the heel, and this when skilfully done will soon

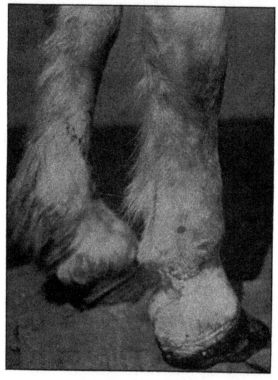

FIGURE 2—The same animal showing feet with whole of sole removed and the disease shown in Figure 1 cured. Dr. Harry Bosley, operator, Washington, D.C.

expose the cause of the trouble. First, a red spot or area is exposed, and by continued paring the center will be arrived at, and we may look for the escape of a small quantity of pus. This is all due to the usual tissue and capillary changes that take place at the seat of an acute, or later, a chronic inflammation. Eventually, this inflammation will extend up the hoof wall and the discharges make their appearance at the coronary band. At this stage, the horse is quite unable to walk, or even put the foot to the ground, and evidently is at no time free from more or less severe pain.

Doctor Bosley, who kindly furnished the notes for this case, informs me that the condition here described lasted about a fortnight, that is, prior to the taking of the photographs—while at the stage shown in the pictures the animal was regaining the flesh that it had lost, and was improving in other respects. As resolution became established, both pain and suppuration subsided, flesh and appetite were regained, and the case gradually passed into recovery.

At the time the photographs were made, here reproduced in Figures 1 and 2, this horse had a slight limp, and it will be fully seven or eight months before the hoof will assume, through growth, its normal size and appearance again.

This growth is already inaugurated as will be noted by observing in the figure the ridge at the coronary band. It is more extensive than the original, for an effort is being made on the part of the new hoof tissue to accommodate itself to the enlarged and changed conditions.

TREATMENT. Doctor Bosley informs me that he has treated many of these cases and is usually successful along the following line, which can also be used in the case of vicious nail punctures.

First of all, the diseased foot should at once be kept in a tub of cold antiseptic solution—night and day—until the acute inflammation subsides or entirely disappears. Usually this is done in a soak stall, using a small tub, and changing the solution frequently. As soon as indications are favorable the hoof wall should be punctured in order to release the accumulated pus. This, if satisfactory, should immediately be followed by the removal of all dead hoof tissues in the diseased parts of the sole and hoof wall, which procedure should promptly relieve the pressure.

When pain and sloughing have both sufficiently subsided, the new hoof growth should be stimulated by the use of mild applications at the coronary band, in the hair above it. In connection with this, mild antiseptic astringents may be applied to the exposed soft tissues, to promote healing and to maintain their healthy state.

The animal here shown passed on to complete recovery under

this mode of treatment, and I am informed by Doctor Bosley that horses, even in these days, are only too often shot when suffering from this condition, the malady being considered incurable by most veterinarians, whereas many animals might be entirely cured were the above treatment carefully followed.

SOME FACTS ABOUT THE TUBERCULIN TEST*

Walter M. Pendergast, Syracuse, N. Y.

In this paper I am not going to give you a history of the tuberculin test as that part is familiar to most of us, but to give you a few of the experiences which I have met with in tuberculin testing. I have had occasion to do considerable tuberculin testing under State supervision and have had many opportunities to perform post mortems on the reactors, thus checking up the results of the tests as to the reliability of the tuberculin test. I will say from my experience that when an animal gives a typical reaction you can be almost absolutely sure that it has tuberculosis in some form. In the past four years I have injected 1420 animals with tuberculin. Some of the animals have been testing yearly. Out of these tests we had one hundred twenty reactions or about 8½%. Of these one hundred twenty reactors I have made sixty-seven post mortems, sixty-five of which showed positive lesions of tuberculosis. One of the two not showing lesions gave a very uncertain reaction, she being the only reactor in a herd of over forty animals. I was very doubtful of her being tuberculous before her slaughter. I think oftentimes, when we fail to find a lesion in a typical reactor, that we have overlooked a small lesion in a gland, or other organ, which may easily occur. The past winter I had occasion to perform post mortems on 12 reactors in a herd of eighteen animals. In one animal that had given a low reaction, I had not found any lesion but after the carcass had been split and hung on the hook I discovered a very small infected lymph gland near the brisket that had been incised when the butcher split the carcass and in the center of this gland was a perfect tubercle.

Now as to the unreliability of the test, I will cite the case of a cow tested by me on May 15-16, 1916, and on July 20-21, 1917, and

*Presented at the meeting of the Central New York Veterinary Medical Association, Syracuse, N. Y., June, 1917.

showing no reaction. Previous to May, 1916, I had tested this cow twice with no reaction, but have not a record of those two tests. This cow was originally in a very badly infected herd about 70% tubercular. This cow was always in fine physical condition until the early fall of 1917 when she injured one of her hind feet. This injury developed into a fistula of the heel and was about three months in healing. She, being very lame, lost a great deal of flesh but we did not suspect anything at this time. On the annual test of this herd the past winter we found four reacting cows, one heifer, and five young bulls. We had not had a reaction in this large herd for nearly three years and was unable to discover the source of infection.

This cow about this time was observed to be coughing some and in quite poor flesh. I took it upon myself to examine her physically and discovered her lungs to be in bad condition. She being a very valuable cow and about seven months pregnant the owner wished to save the calf if possible.

She was segregated but died about one month later. Post mortem showed a very bad generalized case of tuberculosis of both lungs and pleura. We then discovered that two of the reactors had been in a small pasture with her last fall, the reacting heifer had been in an adjoining box stall for about a month, and the five reacting bulls had been watered in the same pail that she drank from. This evidence cleared up the source of infection. On her test of May 16, 1916, you will notice that she gave a temperature of 102 at 6 p. m. and it is possible if the test had been carried further that she might have shown a reaction. Below are her two tests:

JULY 20-21, 1917

9 a.m.	2 p.m.	4 p.m.	12 a.m.	2 a.m.	4 a.m.	6 a.m.	8 a.m.	10 a.m.	12 m.
100.8	101.7	101.8	101.3	101.3	101.5	101.3	101.6	101.3	101.7

MAY 15-16, 1916

11 a.m.	4 p.m.	10 p.m.	6 a.m.	8 a.m.	10 a.m.	12 m.	2 p.m.	4 p.m.	6 p.m.
101.1	101.3	101.9	101.1	100.9	101.6	100.9	101.3	101.8	102.

Here is a case of a cow 13 years old that passed the test Jan. 18-19, 1918. She was in a herd of ten animals, five of which reacted, two being generalized on post mortem.

Retested, this cow May 13-14, 1918, injecting 7 c.c. tuberculin. She gave a typical reaction, and at post mortem showed two calcified lesions in one lung that seemed to me to be of quite long standing. I think the extra 2 c.c. tuberculin caused this cow to react.

We ought to be very careful in regard to passing cows that give suspicious elevations of temperature, especially in herds with a considerable number of positive reactors. Below are temperatures of two reactors. In this herd we had twelve reactors in a herd of eighteen animals.

Age	9 a.m.	11:30 a.m.	3:30 p.m.
2½ yrs.	102.	101.5	101.8
8 yrs.	101.9	102.1	102.6

Age	12 a.m.	2 a.m.	4 a.m.	6 a.m.	8 a.m.	10 a.m.	12 p.m.	2 p.m.
2½ yrs.	101.8	102.	102.	103.1	103.7	103.4	102.	102.6
8 yrs.	101.3	101.9	101.9	102.7	103.3	102.9	103.2	102.6

These two animals proved tubercular on post mortem, but lesions were slight. Many cows have been passed as free from tuberculosis on just such temperatures as these and it behooves us to be more careful.

In regard to testing pregnant animals that are very near parturition, it has been my experience that if an animal is free from tuberculosis, the tuberculin does not have any effect on the animal, although I do not advise testing an animal with a high preliminary temperature.

Below is the temperature of a cow due to calf four days from date of test:

MARCH 2, 1917

Age	1 p.m.	3 p.m.	8 p.m.
6½ yrs.	103.2	102.2	103.

MARCH 3, 1917

Age	4 a.m.	6 a.m.	8 a.m.	10 a.m.	12 m.	2 p.m.	4 p.m.
6½ yrs.	102.7	103.	104.4	104.2	104.8	103.4	103.6

The owner insisted on testing her as she was consigned to a sale. Under the circumstances I marked her suspicious and held her for retest. About two months later owner called me up and told me this cow had suffered from tympany several times and wanted advise in the matter. I advised him to have her slaughtered as I suspected enlarged tubercular glands between lungs. Held post mortem on her on May 23, 1917, and found an enlarged mediastinal gland about seven inches in diameter. This enlarged gland pressing on the oesophagus caused her to bloat.

In regard to the examination of the lymph glands on post mortem, I wish to call attention to the prescapular lymph gland in front of the shoulder. I remember one reactor in which the only lesion was located in one of the prescapular lymph glands. These glands are not very often infected, but should be always examined for lesions may be found there.

In conclusion I would urge the need of more careful observation during tuberculin tests. Be sure and give dosage enough, especially in old animals. Also be careful in passing animals that give low suspicious temperatures. I consider the physical examination very important, especially in herds that show a considerable number of reactors. Mistakes will occur in tuberculin testing, even when the greatest care is taken, but that is all the more reason why we should be as thorough as possible in our tuberculin testing.

THE VIOLET RAY IN VETERINARY MEDICINE

W. L. Clark, Seneca Falls, N. Y.

Electricity is a force in nature which scientists have, as yet, been unable to define. Some have said that electricity is life. We know that our bodies are charged with it and in the continuous struggle of the body against disease, electricity is always fighting on the side of health. It always operates toward the normal and against the abnormal and thus supernormal as well as subnormal conditions excite its antagonism. It is the great equilibrator.

Undefinable as is this force, it is unquestionably the most rational and logical therapeutic agent that man has at his command.

One of our quaint humorists has said: "If I were a doctor, I'd treat the patient and fergit the disease." This states the extreme metaphysician's view, but the physicist is also liable to go to extremes by dealing only with inanimate things and ignoring the patient's mental attitude. Electricity is the one remedy that both can use because it treats both the patient and the disease. That electricity by the high frequency violet ray method does invoke favorable mental forces is natural because its application is pleasant to the patient and quick in its manifestations. But that it will accomplish results independent of this is shown by the fact that the long list of its successes in the treatment of many ills and diseases has been established largely by results incidental to a result sought for, as, for instance, in the discovery that it has restored gray hair to its natural color, when it was being applied for another purpose and when no such outcome was anticipated.

Nothing in the science of therapeutics has proven so valuable to the physician and suffering humanity as the development of high frequency electricity. As this marvelous force is so efficient and convenient and economical I believe more veterinarians will use it in their practice.

The tendency of electricity to restore and maintain the natural equilibrium has long been understood, but to apply the treatment in an agreeable form and without injurious effects has been the problem, but it has now been solved by the use of the Violet Ray High Frequency Generator. In this we mean the voltage in electricity which means force. Amperage means the volume, and frequency means the vibrations per second.

Scientific research has determined that the body does not require a large volume of electricity to yield up its ills, but a strong force which will seek out and rescue every cell from the ailment with which it is struggling. This must be done in such a way as to prevent pain or muscular contraction. These objects have been perfectly accomplished by the violet ray high frequency generator through the following processes:

1st. Beginning with the ordinary illuminating voltage (110) the generator intensifies it until it mounts into hundreds of thousands while at the same time consuming only about one-quarter of the current required in a 16 candle power lamp. This gives the desired force.

2nd. The amperage (volume) is reduced from one-half to an infinitesimal fraction. This reduces the quantity to the proper degree.

3rd. The frequency is increased from 120 oscillations in alternating current (no oscillations in direct current) to hundreds of thousands per second from either direct or alternating current. This eliminates pain and muscular contraction.

The reason that the sensory nerves do not comprehend the electric current under the high frequency principle is the same that makes it impossible for the eye to see very rapid motion, or the ear to distinguish high sound vibrations.

I will now quote from the work of one of the foremost electro therapeutists in the country the following statements of effects resulting from the application of high frequency currents:

1. Increase of blood supply to the objective point.
2. General increase in ovidation and local nutrition.
3. Increase oxygen in blood.
4. Increase absorption of oxygen.

5. Increase in expulsion of carbon dioxide.

6. Increase secretions.

7. Increase elimination of waste products.

8. Injection of ozone through lungs and tissues.

9. Locally germicidal.

10. Increase in bodily heat without increase in temperature.

11. Soothing or stimulating according to character and length of treatment.

12. Caustic when strong sparks are applied.

13. Arterial tension increased by spinal spark application.

14. Absorption of plastic exudates promoted.

These effects are mainly local, yet apply to a lesser degree to the entire system as the current traverses the whole body. It may be seen from the above what a wide range of uses high frequency has. In fact it still remains for its limits to be established. It may be briefly stated as a cellular massage. The study of high frequency is endless as each day brings new revelations, but simple tests will quickly establish its merits.

Pain can be promptly relieved or greatly alleviated.

The air is quickly purified and the ozone is very perceptible. Water may be purified by a moment's contact. Warts, moles, etc., may be promptly and effectively removed.

It can be stated with assurance that high frequency is absolutely indispensable to the veterinarians, for which no cure-all claims are asserted to excite prejudice. It may be safely declared that this modality is a help-all and cure-much. It may be applied independently or in connection with medicinal dosage because it prepares the body to receive the help which the medicine offers, and it may be applied to force surface applications.

In my general practice I have used it on all animals, large and small, and have had very good success. My first case was that of a dog which was a case of paralysis following distemper. When he entered the hospital he could not use any of his limbs at all. I applied the violet ray after exhausting the pharmacopea and in two weeks had the animal moving all four limbs. Two weeks more showed improvement to such a marked degree that I was very agreeably surprised as now he would sit on his hind limbs like a kangaroo. I used the surface electrode and applied it about fifteen minutes, in all three times daily, then as symptoms improved applied it twice daily until he began to place weight on the front legs, then treated only once daily.

In all the treatment was of eight weeks' duration, until the patient was able to go about. I kept the patient two weeks longer as I wished to see if the results were permanent, which they were, and animal now is in fine condition.

CASE No. 2. Pustulus skin eruptions on arm was treated by surface electrode 15 minutes three times daily and in ten days the patches began to heal and in a month they were all healed. Applications of sannax oil was used then for the restoration of hair.

CASE No. 3. Sow with paresis of hind parts occurring after farrowing. In one week patient was able to walk about and treatment was discontinued. Treatment consisted of surface electrode 3 times daily.

CASE No. 4. Sow with paresis of hind parts same as above. Treatment same. Duration two weeks.

CASES NOS. 5, 6 and 7. Azoturia in horses. Surface electrode 15 minutes' duration, 6 hour intervals. First patient able to stand alone in 24 hours. Second case, patient able to stand alone in 48 hours. Third case, patient showed symptoms in one limb. In 24 hours improvement noticed and in 3 days discharged.

INGUINAL HYSTEROCELE

W. J. CROCKER
Laboratories of Pathology and Bacteriology, University of Pennsylvania, Veterinary School

A five-year-old bull bitch presented a firm swelling the size of a human fist, which had existed for a period of several months in the right posterior mammary gland. The condition was diagnosed as a neoplasm of the mammary gland and the owner sent the animal in to be destroyed. At autopsy the cadaver was placed in the dorsal position, an incision made through the skin from the chin to the pubis and the skin together with the mammary gland separated from the abdominal wall and laid back. Opposite and anterior to the external ring of the right inguinal canal the greater portion of the right horn and round ligament of the uterus and part of the omentum protruded from the canal and flattened, thinned and bulged the mammary gland outward producing an enlargement the size of a fist. When opened the right inguinal canal disclosed the remainder of the right uterine horn together with the mammary vessels and nerves.

The bitch is more predisposed to inguinal hysterocele than the females of other domesticated animals because the round ligament of the uterus of the bitch is well developed (unstriated muscle and fat) and extends from the extremity of the uterine horn through the distinct inguinal canal to the ramus of the os pubis and tends to direct the uterine horn into the canal. In the females of other domesticated animals the internal inguinal ring tends to close at an early age, contains spermatic vessels and nerves but does *not* contain the round ligament of the uterus. On external examination inguinal hysterocele may be confused with tumors of the mammary gland of the bitch.

ABSTRACTS FROM RECENT LITERATURE

MARASMUS OF ARMY HORSES. M. Urbain, Vétérinaire, Infirmary, C.V. Belgian Army. *Revue Generale de Médecin Vétérinaire*, June, 1918.—On our arrival at the Central Veterinary Infirmary of Belgium we were struck with the increasing number of horses evacuated for "marasmus".

The autopsies of these marasmatic horses reveal two worms: a cylicostome and the Strongylus equinus (caecum, colon). These parasites were constant in the cases of marasmus in those of our observations that were followed by autopsies. We frequently noted the co-existence of gastrophilis (stomach), ascaris (duodenum), Anoplocephala mamillana (fecal matter) and the Filaria equina (peritoneal cavity).

This is not the first time that the cylicostome has made its appearance in veterinary pathology. Cuillé, Marotel and Roquet observed them in horses appearing to be in good health, eating ravenously and still growing thinner and thinner until they died of marasmus.

The mucous membranes were pale and the pulse and temperature normal.

In Brazil we contributed largely to the proof that osteomalacia of the horse is due to a cylicostome. (I. *A osteomalacia ou a cara inchada. O. Dia Mai 1914—Contribuicao para o estudo da cara inchada. A. Estancia juillet 1915.*)

With us there is no doubt that horses affected with a state of marasmus should be suspected of having a large number of parasites in the intestines. They exert a triply pathogenic action by despoiling the animal through the number of parasites, the irritation of the mucous membrane by their presence or by the traumatisms they produce or by diverting extremely active toxins into the organism as has been shown is the case with other nematodes, especially the Ascaris megalocephala.

It will not be denied that the various intestinal parasites found alone or concurrently in horses occur in all conditions of health or in deaths in no way associated with a state of marasmus. The objection is not without value. However, one must not lose sight of the very great part played, as much with external as internal parasitic diseases, by the soil, while seeming at least equal but otherwise preponderating to that of the parasite itself. In the one of which we speak, advanced age, cold, acclimation, more or less bad alimentation, concomittant diseases such as mange has truthfully exercised this preparing influence on the "soil". Further, we can see no other causes that can explain the chain of symptoms and lesions observed, no fever, persistance of the appetite, deficient nutrition and no infectious lesions.

SYMPTOMATOLOGY. 1. Healthy appearance.

2. Progressive loss of flesh.

3. A voracious appetite: inconstant pica.

4. Absence of fever and febrile symptoms.

The animals eat ravenously all that comes before their teeth, oats, straw manure, and the ingestion of sand may cause recurrent colics and death.

We have often observed the ingestion of non-alimentary material in the diseases causing general malnutrition, such as hookworm of humans, bovine piroplasmosis, equine osteoporosis, canine rickets, etc.

In the last stages of the disease the patient becomes enfeebled to the point of being unable to rise alone after lying down but still continues to eat all it can reach during its decumbency. Placed on its feet the patient is normal again. The mucous membranes are rather pale.

The temperature oscillates between 36° and 38° C. Cases of hypothermia are not rare but hyperthermia is constantly absent. The pulse is normal or sometimes small and the heartbeats are strong as in dilatations. The respirations are normal in rhythm and number.

The feces are quite moist and permeated with grains of oats and coarse forage. Digestion is impaired.

The patients stand sometimes on all four, sometimes on the two fore legs and at other times on the two hind legs.

Microscopic examination of the feces reveals ova of strongyli.

LESIONS. The lesions are those of verminous cachexia. The muscles are emaciated, the connective tissue shows points of serous infiltration, and there is a transudation of sero-fibrinous liquid in the peritoneal, pleural and pericardial cavities. The parenchymatous organs are not "infectious". In the lumen of the intestines (colon and caecum) there are found numerous adult worms and larvae of the cylicostome and strongyle (sclerostome). The intestinal walls are not changed in color except occasionally they may show a slight enteritis. The mucous membrane when ridden of the alimentary matter exhibits small cysts caused by the presence of embryos, which after penetrating the mucous membrane becomes enveloped by the inflammatory reaction of the environs. The cystic cavities end by opening into the intestines where the parasites develop into perfect worms. These facts have already been established in parasitology. Verminous granulations are often seen in the liver and lungs. These are white or yellow, spherical, calcified nodules varying from the size of a millet seed to that of a bean, that is easily enucleated. They are distributed over the serous membranes and in the depth of the organs and are constituted of a central caseocalcareous mass with a fibrous shell. Microscopic examination reveals in the contents a nematode larva that is always altered and sometimes difficult to identify. The heart is dilated.

ETIOLOGY. The best understood cylicostome is the *Cylicostomum tetracanthum*. According to Neveau-Lemaire it is a nematode belonging to the family *Strongylidae* and sub-family *Strongylinae*. The male is 8 to 17 millimeters long and the female 10 to 24 millimeters long. The mouth is encircled by a projecting cuticular fold carrying six papillae. The buccal cavity is armed with a crown of triangular denticles. The caudal pouch has two lateral lobes united by an anterior and a posterior lobe more or less elongated. There are two spiculae curved at each extremity.

We have pointed out the following species: Cylicostomum tetracanthum, labratum, labiatum, coronatum, bicoronatum, poculatum, calicatum, alveatum, catinatum, nassatum, radiatum, elongatum and auriculatum.

According to our observations the ova segment as soon as laid like those of the Strongylus equinus, but they are always longer and thinner. The longitudinal diameter is more than double that of the transverse. The cylicostome lives in the colon and caecum.

We think it is useful to draw the attention of those who seek to find them post mortem, to the difficulty of finding them because of their obscurity. To be sure that they exist the colon and caecum must be well stretched out and incised with a bistoury. The alimentary mass thus exposed is examined closely without disturbing it. Very thin white threads, through the action of cold, are seen to wiggle about in the most liquid parts. These are gathered with the point of the bistoury stretched out on the blade and placed on some container to carry them for the microscopic examination.

The Strongylus equinus or Sclerastomum equinum, better understood than the preceding and being larger is, according to Neveau-Lemaire, a nematode 18 to 35 millimeters (male) and 20 to 55 millimeters (female) long.

The mouth is distended by concentric, chitinous rings, the most external ones of which present six papillae while the internal ones are armed with denticles. The buccal cavity is supported by a single longitudinal dorsal rib and at the bottom is provided with two rounded sharp plaques. The caudal pouch of the male is almost trilobate. The tail of the female is blunt and the vulva is located toward the posterior third of the body. The ovum is ellipsoid and is slightly bulged in the middle. It measures 92 μ long by 52 μ thick.

It should be stated in passing that the agamic strongyli can lodge in the arteries (colic and mesenteric) and produce verminous aneurisms which disengage emboli and cause grave intestinal congestions and fatal colics. It might also be said that strongylosis is seen especially in aged horses. Nearly all of the marasmatic subjects we have seen were aged.

EVOLUTION. Coupling as much with the sclerostome as with the cylicostome occurs in the colon and caecum. The ova already segmented at the time of laying are expelled with the excrement. They develop in water and damp grounds at a temperature of 15 to 20° and after a time varying from two days to twenty days give birth to the embryos which, ingested by a horse, becomes encysted in the mucous membrane of the large intestines where its evolution continues. As horses are infested by the drinking water or by wet pastures it is of great interest to avoid in the future the purchase of horses infested before importation by knowing the regions whence they originated.

DURATION, COURSE AND TERMINATION. Cylicostomo-strongylosis is a chronic disease. It is only after some months (six or seven) that the infested animal shows signs of malnutrition. The patient once well enfeebled lies down and dies from infection of the wounds of decubitus. Sand colics or pica can, however, bring a fatal termination more rapidly.

DIAGNOSIS. The epizootic character of the affection, absence of fever, progressive loss of flesh, and abnormal appetite constitute the principal elements of the diagnosis. The microscope, by revealing the ova of the cylicostomes and of the strongyli, removes all doubt.

PROGNOSIS. The prognosis is unfavorable as cylicostomo-strongylosis is a grave disease. The beginning is so insidious that it passes unperceived and thus does not permit of effectual intervention.

TREATMENT. The treatment is curative and preventive. The curative consists of eliminating the intestinal parasites and of toning up the system. If the expulsion of the worms inhabiting the lumen of the intestines is theoretically easy the destruction of those fixed in the intestinal walls and the encysted larvae presents great difficulties. To expel the worms thymol should be employed (Giles and Theobald), or santonin, calomel, terebinthinae, creolin, or picric acid. As the parasites live in the large intestines it would perhaps be an advantage to inject the vermicide with a trocar and cannula. To attack the encysted larvae intravenous injections of atoxyl or cacodylate of sodium should be tried. The system is toned up with good alimentation (green food), special hygienic care and the administration of such tonics as arrhenal, atoxyl, cacodylate of sodium, etc.

As noticed above, the worms hatch in damp grounds at temperatures of 15 to 20°, there is danger of purchasing animals and forage from infected regions. It should also be desirable that the manure from infected animals is not accumulated near stables nor spread upon pastures. It should be sold for use on tilled land. The manure could be sprinkled with lime water and the contaminated pastures could be treated with sulphur.   L. A. MERILLAT.

REACTION PRODUCED BY THE INTRA-PALPEBRAL INJECTION OF MALLEIN. Lanfranchi, A., in *Il Moderno Zooiatro,* Series V, Year VI, No. 9, pp. 197-202, fig. 1. Bologna, September 30, 1917. Abstract in *Internat. Review of the Science and Practice of Agri.*— The diagnosis of glanders by means of the reaction produced by the intrapalpebral injection, proposed by the author in 1914, has been widely used, having been officially adopted for use in the Allied armies. As the author has applied it to a considerable number of cases, he has been able to make many observations, which have led him to the conclusions given below.

If, on account of numerous reactions produced by intra-palpebral injections or for other causes, sclerosis of the conjunctive tissue is observed in the lower eyelids, the mallein should be injected into the upper eyelid.

In the case of a negative intrapalpebral reaction in subjects already tested several times by this method, and for which the period of the last intrapalpebral reaction is unknown, a minimum period of 15 days should be allowed to pass before repeating the injection. If this precaution is not taken, a subject still infected with the living organism may be thought to be free from glanders.

FISH.

———◆———

COCCIDIOSIS IN YOUNG CALVES. Theobald Smith and H. W. Graybill. *The Journal of Experimental Medicine,* Vol. XXVIII, No. 1, July 1, 1918.—"Discharges of blood per rectum, associated with oocysts of coccidia, were observed occurring in young calves during the warmer season of the year. In a small percentage of cases death was probably due directly to the coccidiosis. Although the disease, known as red dysentery in Switzerland, may have existed in this country for some time, there seems to have been no knowledge of its existence and no reports of it have thus far been published. The coccidia have been artificially cultivated and shown to produce four spores. Two oocysts of quite different dimensions and having minor differential characters were encountered in the same animal in several instances.

The invasion of the epithelium of the small intestine was slight. The chief seat of the parasitism was the large intestine. The lesions following the loss of epithelium were superficial hemorrhages and filling up of the denuded tubules with polymorphonuclear leukocytes." HAYDEN.

THE INTRA-PALPEBRAL REACTION IN THE DIAGNOSIS OF EPI-
ZOOTIC LYMPHANGITIS. (1). Lanfranchi, A., in *Il Moderno Zooia-
ro*, Series V, Year VI, No. 10, pp. 217-225, fig. 5. Bologna, Oct.
31, 1917. Abstract in *Internat. Review of the Science and Practice of Agriculture.*—The clinical diagnosis of epizootic lymphangitis, although generally fairly easy, is, however, not always possible, and under practical conditions the microscope is not always
available for identifying the characteristic *Rivolta cryptococcus.*
For this reason, the writer has sought a sure method for diagnosing this infection, based on the so-called "allergic" local reaction,
i. e., on a special state of specific hypersensibility of the affected
subjects.

The test materials are prepared in the following manner: to
1 part of pus, collected aseptically and known to be free from
other microorganisms 2 parts of ether are added; shake well, then
leave to stand for 24 hours; the ether is then evaporated off on the
water bath; make up to the original volume with distilled water
and leave to stand for 24 hours; then heat at 80° C. on the water
bath for 15 to 20 minutes and allow to cool; centrifuge for 20 to 30
minutes at 2000 to 3000 revolutions per minute; decant off the
liquid part, which constitutes the vaccine to be used for inoculating
in 2.5 to 3 c.c. doses, according to the number of cryptococci used.

The injection into the eyelid is carried out in the usual way.

In healthy animals, or those infected with a disease other than
epizootic lymphangitis, the injection gives rise to an edema localized at the points of injection, or which at the most extends to the
lower eyelid only. This edema is produced in 1 or 2 hours after
inoculation, attains its maximum between the 8th and 9th hours,
then being slowly reabsorbed, and disappearing entirely after 20-
24 hours. On the other hand, in animals infected with epizootic
lymphangitis, the local reaction, which commences 2 to 4 hours
after the injection, already extends, between the 4th and 6th hour,
over all the lower eyelid, sensibly reducing the palpebral opening;
the edema spreads gradually and, after 24 to 49 hours, reaches the
lower border of the zygomatic crest, passes it a little in front while
progressing backwards towards the lower mandibular arch, which
it may even reach. This local reaction lasts several hours, then
slowly diminishes up to the 3rd, 4th or 5th day. The purulent
conjunctivitis occurs 4 hours after inoculation and increases in
24-48 hours.

One test for the intra-palpebral reaction has no influence on successive tests. The most intense and lasting effects of the reaction are shown by animals in which lesions have already commenced.

The use of this method of diagnosis, combined with treatment by arsivan, which was tested by Favero (*Moderno Zooiatro*, Scientific Part, 1917, No. 6, p. 129), who suggested its use, would, thinks the author, cause the disappearance of the centres of infection from which the disease spreads.   FISH.

PRELIMINARY REPORT ON THE VIRULENCE OF CERTAIN BODY ORGANS IN RINDERPEST. W. H. Boynton. *Philippine Journal of Science,* Vol. XIII, Sec. B, No. 3, May, 1918.—The virus of rinderpest attacks primarily the involuntary muscles, the endothelial lining of the capillary vascular system, and the parenchymatous tissue. The virus does not have its source of development in the blood stream. The tissue cells seem to be its real source.

Extracts were prepared from liver, spleen, lymph glands, heart, intestines, thymus, skeletal muscle, larynx, pharynx and back of tongue of animals having been bled for virulent blood or having died after the regular course of rinderpest. Extracts were kept as sterile as possible and for the purpose of the experiment were injected into animals highly susceptible to the disease. In the work it developed that the tissues best adapted to the production of virus were the liver, spleen, lymph glands, heart, fourth stomach, caecum and colon. In a 0.5 per cent phenol extract of liver, spleen, and lymph glands the virus persisted in a virulent form from eight to fifty-five days. The best extract is one in 0.75 phenol and not over 15 days old. It seems to be plausible that similar or even better results may be obtained with the virus of hog cholera along the same lines.   HAYDEN.

NOTE ON THE USE OF ORGAN EXTRACTS IN PLACE OF VIRULENT BLOOD IN IMMUNIZATION AND HYPERIMMUNIZATION AGAINST RINDERPEST. W. H. Boynton. *Philippine Journal of Science,* Vol. XIII, Sec. B, No. 3, May, 1918.—The virulent blood and the organ extracts from a Batanes bull furnished 20 liters of virulent material. Since the virulent blood produced was 9000 c.c. the whole amount of virulent material was over twice that produced by the ordinary methods. The amount might have been tripled if the animal had been handled by the "Martoglio" method. Both simultaneous immunization and hyperimmunization were accomplished with tissue extracts in the provinces and at the laboratory. The extracts were just as potent as virulent blood when used in simultaneous immunization work. Kept at 15° C. 2000 c.c. doses were used with safety for hyperimmunization. Such a dose should not be given after having been exposed for a period of eighteen hours to the climatic conditions of the tropics. The extracts are easily produced and could be used at any immunization station. The method should be applicable to hog cholera, reducing the enormous cost of the virus.   HAYDEN.

THE INSUFFICIENCY OF MAIZE AS A SOURCE OF PROTEIN AND ASH FOR GROWING ANIMALS. Hogan, Albert G. (Dept. of Chem., Kas. State Agri. Exp. Station, Manhattan, Kas.) in the *Journal of Biol. Chem.*, Vol. XXIX, No. 3, pp. 485-493, 3 diag., Baltimore, April, 1917. Abstract in *Internat. Rev. of the Science and Practice of Agri.*—Agriculturists have known for a long time that maize kernel does not suffice as a diet for growing animals. Experiments on young rats have shown the first limiting factor for growth to be a lack of certain inorganic constituents. When the mineral deficiencies were corrected, normal growth was not obtained, even after the addition of considerable quantities of purified protein, thus proving a lack of suitable growth accessories. According to McCollum, and his collaborators, maize kernel is lacking an accessory called by them "fat-soluble A". The author's previous experiments show that mineral deficiencies in maize are tolerated much better by swine, and protein deficiencies are tolerated better by rats. Assuming that maize is poor in one or more of the growth accessories, swine are much less affected by it than are rats.

The author has continued his earlier work in order to determine specifically what inorganic elements in the ash, and what amino-acids in the proteins are deficient in quantity, thus constituting limiting factors. It was first shown that the addition of tryptophane and lysin improved the proteins of maize, and later, that tryptophane is the first limiting factor in the proteins of the maize kernel, and that lysine is the second. The most important mineral deficiency of maize is calcium.   FISH.

WHITE SNAKEROOT OR RICHWEED (EUPATORIUM URTICAEFOLIUM) AS A STOCK-POISONING PLANT. C. Dwight Marsh and A. B. Clawson. *United States Department of Agriculture, Bureau of*

Animal Industry, Circular 26, Feb. 28, 1918.—White Snakeroot is among the suggested causes of the disease milk sickness, trembles, slous, tires, etc. Whether or not it is the cause of the disease its importance as a stock-poisoning plant has received little recognition. Trembling is one of the most noticeable symptoms of its poisonous nature. Marked depression and inactivity may be the first symptom noticed. Constipation is the rule and sometimes the feces are bloody. Nausea and vomiting are not uncommon. Respiration is normal except on exertion when it may become labored and quickened. On the average there is no significant change in temperature. Weakness is very pronounced. Animals may live several days after the first symptoms. Symptoms in general are typical of milk sickness. No animals seem to be immune to the toxic principle of the plant.

There seems to be very little difference between toxic and lethal doses. The toxic substance is eliminated slowly and thus there is a distinct cumulative effect. The plant is most poisonous in a fresh state. Poisoning is produced by a poisonous principle in the plant.

Most cases of so-called milk sickness occur in localities where the plant grows. Many if not most cases of the disease are caused by the plant. Some cases may be bacterial in origin. Trembling seems to be characteristic of eupatorium poisoning while a subnormal temperature is distinctive of the bacterial disease.

Most cases of poisoning by the plant occur when there is a shortage of other foods. Purgatives, such as epsom salts and laxative foods are well indicated. Since the toxic substance is eliminated slowly recovery is slow and rather prolonged attention should be given the animal. Clearing the land will act as a preventive measure. Animals should not graze where eupatorium is abundant. Losses should be avoided by prevention rather than by reliance on remedies.   HAYDEN.

—Dr. Wm. C. Woodward has resigned as Health Officer of the District of Columbia and is now Commissioner of Health, Boston, Mass. Dr. Wm. C. Fowler has succeeded him in Washington.

—Dr. R. H. Fessler has removed from Elmhurst, Long Island, to 225 N. High Street, Harrisonburg, Va.

ARMY VETERINARY SERVICE

INFORMATION RELATING TO APPOINTMENTS IN THE VETERINARY RESERVE CORPS OF THE ARMY

Examinations for commission in the veterinary section of the Officers' Reserve Corps are open for veterinarians in civil life. All appointments will be in the grade of second lieutenant and future promotions based entirely on the qualifications of the officer.

The officers of the Veterinary Reserve Corps are appointed and commissioned by the President, after having been found upon examination prescribed by him, physically, mentally and morally qualified to hold such commissions. Commissions are issued for periods of five years, at the end of which time the officers may be recommissioned subject to such further examinations and qualifications as the President may prescribe. They are subject to call for duty in time of actual or threatened hostilities only. While on active duty under such call they are entitled to the pay and allowances (including quarters, fuel and light) of their grade. They are entitled also to pension for disability incurred in the line of duty and while in active service. They are not entitled to pay or allowances except when in active service, nor to retirement or retired pay.

Appointees must be citizens of the United States, between 22 and 55 years of age, must be graduates of recognized veterinary colleges or universities, and must at the time of appointment be in the active practice of their profession in the States in which they reside.

The examination is physical and professional. It is conducted by boards consisting in each case of one medical and two veterinary officers of the army, designated by the War Department.

The examination as to physical qualifications conforms to the standard required of recruits for the United States Army. Defects of vision resulting from errors of refraction which are not excessive, and which may be entirely corrected by glasses, do not disqualify unless they are due to or are accompanied by organic disease. Minor physical deficiencies may be waived.

The professional examination may be oral. If the applicant fails therein, he may if he desires have a written examination. An average of 75 per cent is required to qualify in the examination. The examination comprises the following subjects:

1. General anatomy.
2. General pathology, therapeutics and surgery.
3. General bacteriology and parasitology.
4. Hygiene, including feeding and watering, stabling, heat and light, and ventilation.

Applications for appointment in the Veterinary Reserve Corps must be made in writing, upon the prescribed blank form, to the Surgeon General of the Army, Washington, D. C., who will supply the blank upon request. This blank may also be obtained from the examining board. The correctness of the statements made in the application must be sworn to by the applicant before a notary public or other official authorized by law to administer oaths. It must be accompanied by testimonials based upon personal acquaintance, from at least two reputable persons, as to the applicant's citizenship, character, and habits, and by his personal history given in full upon the blank form furnished him for the purpose.

A veterinary examining board has been appointed at the following places:

ALABAMA

Anniston, The Camp Veterinarian, Camp McClellan.

ARKANSAS

Little Rock, The Camp Veterinarian, Camp Pike.

CALIFORNIA

Linda Vista, The Veterinarian, Aux. Remount Depot, Camp Kearney.

San Francisco, The Veterinarian, The Presidio of.

DISTRICT OF COLUMBIA

Major Joseph N. Hornbaker, V.C.N.A., S.G.O., Unit F, 7th and B Streets, N. W.

FLORIDA

Jacksonville, The Veterinarian, Aux. Remount Depot, Camp Joseph E. Johnston.

GEORGIA

Atlanta, The Veterinarian, Aux. Remount Depot, Camp Gordon.
Chickamauga Park, The Senior Veterinary Instructor, Medical Officers' Training Camp, Camp Greenleaf.

ILLINOIS

Chicago, Major Geo. A. Lytle, V. C., N. A., 3615 Iron Street.

IOWA

Des Moines, The Veterinarian, Aux. Remount Depot, Camp Dodge.

KANSAS

Fort Leavenworth, The Post Veterinarian.

Fort Riley, The Senior Veterinary Instructor, Mounted Service School.

KENTUCKY

Louisville, The Camp Veterinarian, Camp Zachary Taylor.

LOUISIANA

Alexandria, The Veterinarian, Aux. Remount Depot, Camp Beauregard.

MASSACHUSETTS

Ayer, The Veterinarian, Aux. Remount Depot, Camp Devens.

MICHIGAN

Battle Creek, The Veterinarian, Aux. Remount Depot, Camp Custer.

MINNESOTA

Fort Snelling, The Post Veterinarian.

MISSOURI

St. Louis, Major C. W. Greenlee, V. C., N. A., Medical Supply Depot.

MONTANA

Fort Keogh, The Purchasing Zone Veterinarian.

NEW MEXICO

Deming, The Veterinarian, Aux. Remount Depot, Camp Cody.

NEW YORK

Fort Jay, The Veterinarian.

OHIO

Chillicothe, The Veterinarian, Aux. Remount Depot, Camp Sherman.

OKLAHOMA

Fort Sill, The Veterinarian.

PENNSYLVANIA

Philadelphia, Major Samuel H. Gilliland, V. C., N. A., Veterinary Laboratory, 39th and Woodland Avenue.

SOUTH CAROLINA

Columbia, The Veterinarian, Aux. Remount Depot, Camp Jackson.

TEXAS

Fort Worth, The Veterinarian, Aux. Remount Depot, Camp Bowie.

Houston, The Veterinarian, Aux. Remount Depot, Camp Logan.

Fort Sam Houston, The Veterinarian, Aux. Remount Depot, Camp Travis.

VIRGINIA

Newport News, The Supervising Veterinarian, Port of Embarkation.

Petersburg, The Senior Veterinary Instructor, Veterinary Training School, Camp Lee.

WASHINGTON

American Lake, The Veterinarian, Aux. Remount Depot, Camp Lewis.

WYOMING

Fort D. A. Russell, The Veterinarian.

The applicant should proceed to the most accessible point in the foregoing list and report to the board. He will be required to defray all travel or other expenses incurred in going to the point of examination, while there, and in returning to his home.

The applicant should take with him to be submitted to the board (a) the application blank, completely filled out and sworn to before a notary public, (b) testimonials based upon personal acquaintance from at least two reputable persons and (c) a certificate from the proper official that the applicant is duly registered to practice veterinary medicine in the State in which he resides. The application (a) can be filled out after arrival at the place of examination but time will be saved if it is prepared at home beforehand.

Successful applicants who are commissioned in the Veterinary Reserve Corps are placed on a waiting list and called to active duty as their services may be required. No assurance can be given any person as to when he may be called, but the present chances for active duty at an early date are good. Officers receiving commissions should, therefore, continue their civil occupations until such time as they receive instructions from the War Department.

—Major H. E. Bemis of Ames, Iowa, is now with the American Expeditionary Forces in France.

—Major John H. Gould, Captain Joseph F. Derivan, Lieut. Geo. W. Moon, Lieut. Lester L. Jones, Lieut. Roy H. Tesdell, Lieut. Jean R. Underwood, Lieut. Spencer K. Nelson, Lieut. Guy M. Parrish, Lieut. Orrin H. Crossland, Lieut. Ralph A. Parsons and Lieut. James B. McNamara, who have been stationed at Camp Dodge, Des Moines, Iowa, have all been transferred to the 88th

Division and are with the American Expeditionary Forces, overseas.

—Major John H. Gould and Captain Joseph F. Derivan spent a few days at Camp Upton, L. I., and Hoboken, N. J., on their way overseas.

—Capt. Lawrence A. Mosher, V. C., N. A., was married to Miss Arlye Fuller of Hillsdale, Mich., at the First Episcopal Church, Jersey City, N. J., July 31, 1918. Capt. Russell E. Elson, V. C., N. A., Camp Upton, L. I., attended him as best man.

—Captain Ross A. Greenwood, V. C., N. A., has been transferred from Hdqs. Army Artillery to Hdqs. 77th Division, American Expeditionary Forces, as Division Veterinarian.

—Captain Jos. F. Crosby, formerly at Fort Sill, Okla., is now Camp Veterinarian at Camp Dodge, Des Moines, Iowa.

—2nd Lieut. Harrold L. Campbell, V. R. C., reported for duty with Depot Brigade No. 152, Camp Upton, L. I., Aug. 9. Lieut. Campbell has been at the Veterinary Officers' Training School at Camp Greenleaf, Ga.

—2nd Lieut. Spencer K. Nelson, V. C., U. S. A., received his promotion to 1st Lieutenant August 3, 1918.

—Lieut. R. O. Stott has been transferred from the 12th Cavalry, Columbus, N. M., to the Remount Depot, Fort Bliss, Texas.

—Dr. R. S. Whitney of Jersey City, N. J., has entered the service and is stationed at Camp Sevier, Greenville, S. C.

—Dr. H. P. Bonnikson, formerly of Berkeley, Calif., is now in the service as Lieutenant in the Veterinary Reserve Corps. He is located at 4130 Drexel Blvd., Chicago, Ill.

—Dr. M. V. Wilmot has transferred from Fort Riley, Kas., to Veterinary Reserve Corps No. 1, Camp Greenleaf, Chickamauga Park, Ga.

—Lieut. J. G. Nash, who has been stationed at Fort Riley, Kas., is now with the American Expeditionary Forces, overseas.

—Dr. Chas. M. Stull, formerly Lieutenant with the 1st Cavalry, Douglas, Ariz., has been promoted to a Captaincy and is now Camp Veterinarian at Camp Bowie, Fort Worth, Texas.

—Lieut. S. C. Dildine has been transferred from Louisville, Ky., to 557 N. 13th Street, St. Louis, Mo.

—Lieut. L. J. Anderson, who has been located with the 115th Field Signal Battalion at Camp Kearney, is now with that Battalion with the American Expeditionary Forces, overseas.

—Dr. Ray Gaskill, formerly at the Remount Depot at Camp Kearney, Calif., is now a Lieutenant in the Veterinary Corps, National Army, and is stationed at Kelly Field, San Antonio, Texas.

—Dr. Simeon Yetter of Far Rockaway, N. J., is now a Lieutenant in the Army Veterinary Service and is stationed at Camp McClellan, Ala.

—Lieut. Samuel M. Langford has been transferred from Camp Sevier, S. C., to the 14th F. A., Fort Sill, Okla.

—Lieut. John J. Martien, Camp Funston, Kas., is now with the American Expeditionary Forces, overseas.

—Dr. Walter G. White of Lansdowne, Pa., is now a 1st Lieutenant with Major McKillip's Veterinary Hospital, No. 6, Somewhere in France.

—Dr. H. M. Cameron, who has been stationed with the 24th Engineers, Newport News, Va., is now with the American Expeditionary Forces.

—Dr. N. L. Nelson of the 55th Field Artillery Brigade, formerly at Camp Sevier, S. C., is now with the American Expeditionary Forces.

—Dr. G. W. Rawson of Norfolk, Va., is now a Lieutenant in the Veterinary Officers' Reserve Corps stationed at Camp Wadsworth, Spartanburg, S. C.

—Lieut. John J. Handley, formerly at Camp Hill, Va., is now with the First Division, American Expeditionary Forces, France.

—Dr. M. L. Walter of Napoleonville, La., is now in the service as Lieutenant with the 7th Battalion, Camp Greenleaf, Ga.

—Dr. W. E. Simonson, Cherokee, Iowa; Dr. Roy E. Onderkirk, Reynolds, Ill.; Dr. W. M. Lynn, Pittsburgh, Pa.; Dr. Will D. James, Martinsville, Ill., and Dr. D. E. Reece, Rossville, Ill., have entered the Medical Officers' Training Camp at Camp Greenleaf, Chickamauga Park, Ga.

—Dr. R. C. Dunn has removed from College Station, Texas, to 263 West Market Street, Tiffin, Ohio.

—Dr. A. Berdan has removed from Miles City to Great Falls, Montana.

AMERICAN VETERINARY MEDICAL ASSOCIATION

PRESIDENT'S ADDRESS

F. Torrance, Ottawa, Can.

It has been customary, on occasions of this kind, for your president to indulge in some remarks, laudatory of the veterinary profession, and also at times to criticize its short comings, and frequently to give it the benefit of his advice. These are tasks for which I am but little fitted by ability or inclination, and I must ask your indulgence for a few remarks of a more or less rambling nature.

First, I would say a word as to the war, and on our part in it as a profession. Both American and Canadian veterinarians take a just pride in the prompt alacrity with which the profession responded to the call to arms. The veterinary corps of our countries were rapidly recruited, not merely with the young and inexperienced, desirous of the excitement and change of army life, but with many of the best men in the profession, men who gave up important positions in our colleges, responsible posts in the Government service, and sacrificed lucrative practices to serve their country. We honor them for what they are doing, and experience a lively satisfaction when one and another are singled out for promotion or the award of some honor or distinction.

It was fortunate that previous to the entry of the United States into the war, the army veterinarian, through the efforts of this association, had received the rank to which he was entitled, and equally fortunate that the work of a past president of this association, C. J. Marshall, now Lieut.-Col. Marshall, and others had gathered information respecting the organization of Army Veterinary Service.

The war found our profession in America unprepared. There were extremely few veterinarians experienced in military work, and these few had gained their experience in the Spanish American War, on the Mexican frontier, or, in the case of Canada, in the Boer campaign. These were but small affairs in comparison with the present war, and the experience gained from them extremely limited. Our civil veterinarians had to learn the business of war from the foundation up, learning and building at the same time— learning to obey the discipline of the army and building on the foundation of a knowledge of veterinary science the substantial edifice of army veterinary service.

The many phases of army veterinary work have called for extensive and varied accomplishments; the selection and purchase of remounts, the care of these in transit and in depots, their transport over seas, their maintenance in health while in active service, and lastly, their protection from disease, and the treatment of the wounded. These varied activities of the army veterinarian require the exercise of his professional knowledge to a high degree and often put to the test his courage and powers of endurance.

We may well be proud that the veterinary corps of our armies have done their work more efficiently than ever before. They are indispensable to the success of an army in the field. The motor transport ends with the end of the road, and from the end of the road to the guns and to the men in the trenches, supplies must be taken by horses or by human carriers. Horses, mules or donkeys are used for this work as much as possible, and are exposed not only to the casualties of shell fire, but must undergo the hardships inseparable from war, exposure to all kinds of weather, often without shelter, and while doing the hardest kind of work in most unfavorable conditions. Under these circumstances, it is surprising to learn that the mortality of horses in the British Army is less than 10% and compares favorably with the average losses of horses engaged in industrial work in our cities.

War has demonstrated the value of the veterinary profession to the nation and increased its importance as a necessary cog in the machinery of modern life. This leads to improvement in the profession itself. The demand for well educated veterinarians, not only for war, but to care for the enormously valuable livestock of the country, now and hereafter, will increase the attendance at our veterinary colleges, will render it easier for these to obtain the financial support necessary to their success, and render possible a high standard of education and efficiency.

An indication of how the importance of veterinary knowledge has been impressed upon the British is found in the recent establishment of a Veterinary Research Laboratory for the Army. This is at Aldershot, England, and is called "The Research Laboratory, Army Veterinary Services". The director is Colonel Watkins-Pitchford, who worked with Theiler in South Africa for many years, and the staff consists of a bacteriologist, a chemist, an entomologist, and a pathologist. The investigation of the newer diseases, brought to light during the war, is to be its chief function. Those in authority must appreciate the value of scientific research.

One cannot leave the subject of the veterinarian and the war without referring to another aspect of the situation, the veterinarian at home in war time. The privilege and honor of serving our countries in the army is enjoyed by many, but denied to others whose age, infirmities or circumstances keep them at home. To them have come increased responsibilities. The man who has joined the army and left his practice to his fellow practitioner should not find on his return that his trust was misplaced, and his business taken from him in his absence. The home fires must be kept burning, a welcome ready for these men when they return, and every opportunity afforded for them to resume their former life. Should any fail to come back, and there will be some who have given their lives for freedom just as much as though they fought, their families and dependents must not suffer. It should be our sacred duty to look after them, and that this may be done systematically and carefully, I commend to you that we all continue and increase our contributions to the Veterinary Relief Fund of this association.

There is still another duty of the veterinarian at home. That is, the conservation of our livestock not only to prevent and cure the diseases from which they may suffer but also to encourage and advise our breeders so that they may increase their flocks and herds. The losses of livestock from preventable diseases amount to millions of dollars annually. It is our duty to reduce this loss to a minimum. It can be done by the methods now in use and through the education of the farmer by the broad dissemination of knowledge of livestock sanitation. The country practitioner has a great opportunity to help his country if he will advise his clients not only as to the treatment of diseases, but will interest himself in the farmers' problems regarding feeding, breeding and rearing livestock. There is too much careless and happy-go-lucky breeding of mongrel livestock, too much loss of young animals from ignorance how to care for them, too much waste of feed through ill-balanced rations. These are all matters where a word in time from a well informed practitioner will do a world of good. The veterinarian and especially the country practitioner should be a good stockman as well, and, in my opinion, our veterinary colleges should give their students instruction in livestock judging, breeding, and management.

This naturally brings me to the subject of veterinary education, a topic of perennial interest and of great importance to this association. The committee on intelligence and education will report on the condition of the colleges and I have no desire to forestall their work. I might, however, refer to one or two features of the present situation.

War has made unforseen demands upon the profession. Men who received a training at college to fit them for general practice were suddenly called upon to perform duties for which they had no previous experience and about which their college teaching had said little or nothing. The future should find the profession better prepared for such emergencies and our veterinary colleges might include in their curricula courses on the management and sanitation of horses, etc., in remount depots, on transport by land or sea, protection against contagious diseases, and the treatment of large numbers of animals affected by such diseases as mange, ringworm, etc. When the war is over, there will be available many men well qualified to teach these subjects from personal experience.

Veterinary education has made great progress, and this association can take credit to itself as one of the most important factors in causing the improvement. Stricter matriculation examination has raised the student to a higher plane, longer terms have increased and broadened his course of study, and laboratory facilities have given him the opportunity to become skillful in handling the test tube and the microscope. In a word, our colleges are now turning out scientific veterinarians, but are they also turning out practical veterinary surgeons?

As the profession rises in the educational scale it attracts men from higher walks in life. The recruits which formerly joined the profession from the blacksmith's forge, and the livery stable, are kept out by the matriculation examination. The farm and the city are now the chief sources of the raw material of the veterinary surgeon. An increasing proportion of the students reach college without previous knowledge of the practical handling of animals. That intimate acquaintance with the habits and customs of horses, for instance, which is common knowledge to the boy on the farm, or to the man who works in livery stable or blacksmith shop, is quite unknown to the city youth. If the college does not give him the opportunity of acquiring this practical knowledge of animals, he will find himself badly handicapped when he begins to practice.

There is an art, as well as a science of veterinary medicine. To be a good practitioner one must be trained in both the art and the science, and to my mind there is danger at the present time of developing the scientific side of veterinary education to the neglect of that training of hand and eye which lies at the foundation of the veterinary art.

The passing of the Kansas City Veterinary College, which has transfered its students and its records to a State institution, is a sign of the times. This was one of the most successful of the private schools and its closing indicates the growing difficulty of competition with the State colleges. The increasing curriculum, lengthening terms, and expensive laboratories incidental to modern veterinary education, have rendered it more and more expensive to provide, and lessened the profits of private institutions. We may expect in future that veterinary education will become more and more a function of the State, accepting it as a public duty to provide efficient veterinarians to safeguard the health of the immensely valuable livestock of the country.

It may be appropriate on this occasion to refer to the more important discoveries of the year in veterinary science or in other fields which influence our own. In surgery the increasing use of Dakin's solution is reducing the time required for the healing of wounds, and probably, if we may argue from its effects on humans, is greatly lessening the pain suffered by the wounded animal. Fistula and quittor have received much attention and their surgical treatment has been improved. Our secretary, Dr. Merillat, has published a book on this subject of much interest and value to the practitioner.

In medicine, an important aid to the diagnosis of diseases of the viscera has been contributed by a French veterinarian, Dr. J. A. Roger, in an article entitled "Le clavier équin". He advances the theory that pain or disease in a definite part of the abdominal organs has its effect upon some corresponding area on the surface of the body. Pain in the colon, for instance, strikes a sympathetic cord in a limited area on the side of the body, and renders it hypersensitive. The surface of the body becomes a sort of key board, on which one can experiment until the sensitive area is detected. By patient observation and experience, these areas can be mapped out, and a very definite diagnosis of the seat of the trouble reached. Dr. Roger himself has located many of these areas in reference to the corresponding internal organs and claims to be able to locate with accuracy such lesions as intestinal calculi, ruptures, volvulus, and intussusception.

The anatomy of the nervous system, and the connection between the sympathetic and the spinal nerves in the dorsal and lumbar regions, makes it quite probable that this close relationship between the internal organs and the surface of the body is a fact which has hitherto been overlooked.

In *control work*, the application of modern methods of diagnosis and sanitation are producing gratifying results in diminishing the annual losses from glanders, hog cholera and other diseases. Through the extensive use of mallein, the horses in the field have suffered little from glanders. It is interesting to note, however, that mange has given more trouble in the field than anything else. In ordinary peace times, horse mange is of little importance; in the present campaign in France it has been a veritable plague. The usual remedies, such as dipping, have given only a partial success in its treatment, and now the horses are being "gassed" in air tight chambers filled with the hot fumes of burning sulphur. Much success is claimed for this method.

Some years ago Dr. Leonard Pearson pointed out the clinical similarity between meat poisoning in man and forage poisoning in animals. This suggestion received the attention of Mohler, Buckley and Shippers of the B. A. I., who found that *B. botulinus* is capable of producing fatal results in horses and mules. A very interesting study of botulism was made by Robert Graham, A. L. Bruckner and R. S. Pontius, who have demonstrated the relationship of an organism resembling *B. botulinus* in actual cases of forage poisoning in Kentucky.

Toxicology has received important contributions. One of the most interesting is the discovery of the cause of the disease popularly known as "milk sickness". At one time this was supposed to be due to a bacterium, the *B. lactimorbi.* Investigators in the Bureau of Animal Industry have established the fact that it is the result of plant poisoning by white snake root (*Eupatorium urticaefolium*). Cattle and sheep are affected by this plant, which causes what is commonly known as "trembles", while the milk of affected cows produces in human beings "milk sickness".

Bracken poisoning in horses has been proved by the officers of my department to cause "staggers", and in England, Sir Stewart Stockman shows that it may cause a fatal disease of cattle.

Bovine haematuria is probably a result of a kind of plant poisoning. Hadwen has shown it in British Columbia to be closely related to oxaluria and in all likelihood caused by eating plants containing oxalic acid. Moussu, the great French authority, is favorably inclined to this theory, and Kalkus in Washington has lately written a bulletin in its support.

The shortage of fodder in Western Europe has led to the eating of plants not generally considered good forage, hence Stockman reports poisoning from rag-wort (senecio jacobaea). This disease was known in Nova Scotia for many years as Pictou cattle disease, from the locality in which it was prevalent. The weed had been introduced from Scotland and spread over a considerable area. Now that the cause of Pictou cattle disease is understood, there is little heard of it.

There is one feature in connection with plant poisoning that it not often emphasized. That is, that in many cases, no effects are seen until considerable quantities of the poisonous plant have been consumed and the animal has been under its influence for some time. During periods of drought, when ordinary forage plants are scarce, animals are driven by hunger to eat plants they usually refuse. Under such circumstances are observed cases of plant poisoning not seen at all in times of plenty. Bracken, snake root and ragwort are good examples of these slow poisons.

Parasitology is assuming greater importance to our profession than ever and some recent discoveries indicate an attractive and promising field for the explorer. The life history of that common parasite, ascaris lumbricoides, has recently been worked out by Ransom and Foster in America and Stewart in India. They prove that after the mature eggs are swallowed, the larvae do not remain in the intestinal tract during their development into the adult worm, but migrate through the tissues until they reach the lung. Here they may cause such an amount of irritation as to bring on pneumonia resulting in the death of an animal. The large mortality of young pigs is partly caused by this and has heretofore been wrongly ascribed to other causes, such as swine plague. After undergoing a certain amount of development in the lung, the young worms are coughed up, swallowed and complete their career in the site where they are usually seen.

Important contributions in parasitology have come from Prof. Railliet on the life history of the oxyuris, from Van Es and Scha1k on parasitic anaphylaxis, from W. E. Dove in the United States on bots, and by Hadwen and Cameron in Canada, and by Rouband in France on the same subject.

Rouband has exploded an old idea concerning the manner in which the bot larvae reach the stomach of the horse. Formerly it was thought that when the horse licked them off his legs, he swallowed them with his saliva. It is now proved that the young larva sticks to the tongue and burrows beneath its mucous membrane, whence it journeys beneath the surface of the pharynx and oesophagus till it emerges and attaches itself to the wall of the stomach. The migration of these larvae may produce serious lesions in the region of the throat.

Strongyli in horses have been receiving attention and I note with some regret that two parasites well known to me under the familiar names, *S. armatus* and *S. tetracanthum,* have disappeared, and can only be recognized with some difficulty among a crowd of worms rejoicing in brand new names such as *Cylicostomum, Oesophagodontus, Triodontophorus* and *Gyalocephalus.* The new nomenclature is doubtless scientific and probably necessary, but the modern parasitologist is adding much to the white man's burden, especially of those veterinarians not freshly graduated.

The life history of animal parasites is most interesting and strange facts are frequently brought to light. A recent discovery shows that one of the bot flies of South America (*Dermatobia*) catches blood sucking flies and lays its eggs upon them, so that they may be carried on to the host they wish to infect. Recently much good work has been done on parasites, not only of horses and cattle, but also of swine, sheep and dogs. Hall of Detroit deserves mention for excellent progress on dog parasites.

The observers I have mentioned and other workers in this field have lifted a corner of the veil with which nature has so long concealed the mysteries of parasitic life. The prospect thus open to our view is offering a tempting field for the investigator and promises a rich reward to the diligent and patient worker, and valuable results in the protection of our livestock. Parasites exact a heavy toll every year, the damage running into millions of dollars, so that the value of these efforts to control their ravages can hardly be overestimated.

The past year has cost us the lives of several distinguished men, and it is fitting that we should here refer to some of them and offer a tribute to their memory. Dr. Melvin, the Chief of the Bureau of Animal Industry, was taken from us last December, after a long and plucky fight against a slow and relentless disease. As a public man and the head of a large and important department of the public service, Melvin showed himself capable of dealing successfully with the immense work of the Bureau, a work which grew and developed enormously under his care. During his administration, the present system of federal meat inspection was begun, and has grown tremendously in size and importance. He had also to deal with more than one outbreak of foot-and-mouth disease, the last, occurring in 1914, the most serious in the history of the country. Not a little of the success of the Bureau in dealing with this was due to his wisdom. The efficiency of the Bureau service today is a tribute to his skill as an administrator, as well as to that of his able successor, Dr. Mohler.

While the country, as a whole, may well mourn the loss of this able and efficient public officer, his personal friends, and they are many, well remember him affectionately for his sincere friendliness, and the unfailing courtesy and interest that characterized his intercourse with others. Melvin was a man to be both admired and loved. Admired for his work and loved for his genial personality. May his memory be kept green.

The death of Liautard marks an epoch in the history of the veterinary profession in America. Liautard was one of the makers of that history, and by his teaching, by his example, and by his untiring industry has done more than any other American to place our profession where it is today. As one of the organizers of the United States Veterinary Medical Association he helped to lay the foundation of this great organization, which is now the largest veterinary society in the world. As editor of the *American Veterinary Review* he exercised an influence over the whole profession in America, and always used that influence for progress and improvement. As an author, his contributions to our literature placed many useful text books in the hands of the student. These were a few of his activities, and in all of them he attained pre-eminence. But it is on his reputation as an educationist that his fame chiefly rests. For many years Liautard was the moving spirit in veterinary education in New York, and as Dean of the New York

College of Veterinary Surgeons, and later as Principal of the American Veterinary College, he set the pace in veterinary education. His standing as a graduate of that great veterinary school at Alfort, France, his unique personality and his great skill as a teacher, combined to give him great influence over his students. There are doubtless many in this audience who could give testimony to the great affection with which he was regarded by his students, and to the value his influence and example have been to them in their lives. Their loss is a personal one. A great teacher and friend has been taken from them. But from the rest of us, the veterinary profession as a whole, there has gone one of our great men, full of years and of honors. One of those gifted few who, rising above the common level, see clearly the distant goal, and point our steps in the right direction. The profession owes much to Liautard and in recognition of that debt we should, I think, take steps to honor his memory in some more tangible way than by a resolution. I would suggest that a committee be appointed to formulate a plan for this purpose, and to report before the close of this meeting.

I cannot let this occasion pass without also referring to the death of Sesco Stewart. He was president of this association many years ago, when I first joined it, and has always taken a most active interest in it. Those who attended the meeting in Kansas City last year will remember his untiring efforts to ensure the success of the meeting, and to make us feel at home in the fine building his industry and success had provided for the Kansas City Veterinary College. He was a skillful and persistent pleader of the cause of the private schools whenever he felt that the association was going too fast in raising the standard of veterinary education. But when a standard was once adopted, he was loyal to the association in carrying it out. His college was marvellously successful, and the facilities it afforded for teaching, and for the well being of the students were a surprise to those that saw it for the first time. It was a monument to his energy, sagacity and industry. His place in this association will be hard to fill, and we will long miss his regular attendance, his interest in every important question, and especially in the welfare and progress of the profession.

The work of the association during the year has felt the influence of the great war. Several of our officials, including our secretary, Dr. Merillat, are actively engaged in military affairs, and it became necessary to appoint others in their places to carry on. Through the kindness of Dr. Mohler, Dr. Day was permitted to undertake the duties of secretary, with the assistance of Dr. Kroner, Dr. Merillat's assistant. I trust you will find that in spite of these changes, the work of the association has not suffered.

But I have already detained you too long. You must be eager to attack the excellent program which has been provided for you, and I gladly give the signal to go "over the top".

ASSOCIATION MEETINGS

REPORT OF THE 25TH ANNUAL MEETING OF THE MISSOURI VALLEY VETERINARY ASSOCIATION HELD AT OMAHA, NEBRASKA

The 25th annual meeting of the Missouri Valley Veterinary Association, held at Omaha, Nebraska, July 15, 16 and 17, was marked by a good attendance, and a very keen interest in the various problems under consideration.

The program was opened by an exhaustive report on a few of the common drugs, by the committee on therapeutics, presented by Dr. W. E. Stone, chairman of the committee. Reports of other standing committees were not as complete as might be desired, due to their recent appointment and detention from attendance by other pressing duties.

Among the highly commendable papers rendered, were the following: "Some Complications Following Influenza" by Dr. W. P. Bossenberger, Williams, Iowa; "Hog Cholera, Its Control and Eradication" by Dr. C. F. Harrington, Denver, Colorado; "Interesting Cases in Connection with Hog Cholera Control Work in Iowa" by Dr. J. S. Koen, Des Moines, Iowa; "The Control of Some Important Infectious Diseases in the Conservation of our Livestock" by Dr. A. Eichhorn, Pearl River, New York; "The Conservation of Edible and Inedible Fats" by Dr. J. I. Gibson, Des Moines, Iowa.

The author of the latter paper pointed out the enormous waste in animal by-products resulting from lack of suitable methods and regulations for collecting and extracting these products from dead animals. A special resolution covering this problem was adopted by the association, which it is hoped may serve as a stimulus to the entire country to take up this important and timely work.

Dr. Eichhorn discussed the pressing need of conserving the animal food supply by the application of sanitary rules and biologic therapy for reducing the enormous losses brought on by the spread of our great animal scourges. Among the points emphasized, should be mentioned the dissemination of anthrax infection through the innundation of land by streams polluted with the remains of carcasses of dead animals, and by tanneries handling hides of diseased animals. He recommended the active cooperation of veterinarians with the sanitary authorities, to suppress those dangerous diseases which constitute so great a menace to the present welfare of our country.

Dr. Bossenberger's paper showed evidence of careful and painstaking study of the many complications following attacks of influenza in horses. Among these complications he mentioned pneumonia, pleurisy, myocarditis, arthritis, conjunctivitis, in various forms and combinations, recommending rational means of treatment and prevention.

Dr. Harrington discussed the plan practiced by the B. A. I. in the control of hog cholera and related infections. An interesting discussion was elicited, tending toward careful differentiation of porcine diseases, satisfactory treatment depending so largely upon a proper comprehension of the disease or combination of diseases present in a herd. Considerable progress seems to have been made in the control of hemorrhagic septicemia or swine plague by the use of killed cultures, either alone, or in conjunction with hog cholera serum, where protection from both diseases must be sought. Necrotic enteritis and stomatitis of pigs were generally conceded to be the most troublesome of the complicating diseases. Treatment by the employment of copper sulphate or permanganate of potash in the drinking water, has met with success in the hands of many.

Dr. J. S. Koen gave a number of interesting observations made during several years' control work in the State of Iowa. Generally speaking, the hog cholera situation in the Missouri Valley is highly satisfactory. Serum producers, however, are finding their laboratory facilities insufficient to take care of the calls made upon them for anti-hog cholera serum.

A paper of unusual merit and interest by Dr. L. Van Es, who

has recently taken the chair of Veterinary Pathology at the University of Nebraska, dealt with the possibilities and limitations of the State diagnostic laboratory in conducting laboratory investigations to assist the practitioner. He placed especial emphasis upon the necessity for both the practitioner and upon the laboratory men acquiring a comprehension of the nature of each other's work, in order that their cooperation may prove of greatest value. The practitioner in need of laboratory assistance was given specific directions as to preparing material for shipment, and was impressed with the necessity of supplying all available data relative to the case in hand in order that the laboratory might work more intelligently.

Dr. A. W. French, Cheyenne, Wyoming, related his experience with the intradermal tuberculin test. During the past year his department has applied the test to approximately 12,000 cattle, all reactors being later tested and in all cases confirmed by the thermal test given from four to seven days later. He prefers the intradermal test, particularly on range animals, on account of the convenience in handling, and the possibilities for doing a large amount of work with a small expenditure of time and labor. To date, the intradermal test seems to have proved fully as satisfactory as the thermal. He recommends the two tests in conjunction, for beginners, until a knowledge of the character of the reaction from the intradermal test is acquired by experience with those reacting.

Dr. G. H. Glover handled, in a very sane and commendable manner, the problem of "The county agent in relation to the veterinary practitioner". He pointed out that the field of each is distinct; that it is possible for them to aid each other materially, by getting together and discussing their problems in a thoroughly friendly manner, and the futility of creating ill feeling by injudicious statements and actions. He made a strong plea for the settlement of any differences which may arise, first through personal and friendly contact with the agent himself; failing in this, that the matter be taken up through the director of the veterinary department at the State college, who has authority to pass upon all projects dealing with veterinary matters, which are undertaken by such agents. The complaint may be carried to the director of extension, the president of the college, and still higher, when necessary.

Other papers of note were read by Dr. C. E. Salsbery, Kansas

City, Missouri, on "Observations on the Use of Biological Products"; Dr. D. M. Campbell, on "The Duties of Veterinarians during the War Period"; and "Sunstroke in Horses" by Dr. W. S. Nichols.

The social program was somewhat modified to conform to war conditions, a patriotic program consisting of an illustrated talk by I. C. Brenner, vocal solos by Dr. J. I. Gibson, and a community singing of patriotic airs, being substituted for a banquet. Dr. W. H. Hoskins gave an inspiring address.

The officers for the ensuing year are as follows:

President, C. C. Hall, Omaha, Neb.; vice president, J. W. Chenoweth, Albany, Mo.; secretary-treasurer, R. F. Bourne, Ft. Collins, Colo.; directors, L. U. Shipley, Sheldon, Iowa; A. T. Kinsley, Kansas City, Mo.; B. W. Murphy, Topeka, Kans.; P. L. Cady, Arlington, Neb.; G. H. Glover, Ft. Collins, Colo.

In each case, the officer elected was the only nominee presented. Twenty-eight additional members were added to the rolls, and as a mark of appreciation for conspicuous service rendered to the veterinary profession, Drs. W. Horace Hoskins and A. Eichhorn were elected honorary members.

A motion to remit the dues of all members in active service with the army was passed by unanimous vote. Two veteran members, Drs. James Vincent of Shenandoah, Iowa, and J. T. Burns, Walnut, Kansas, were reported as having died during the past year, and appropriate resolutions extending the sympathy of the association to their families were adopted. Approval of a higher salary standard for employees of the Bureau of Animal Industry, as a means of securing adequate and competent veterinary service in this Bureau was covered in a special resolution.

About forty ladies were in attendance, and a program of entertainment for which they are most grateful and appreciative, was arranged by the wives of the local members. All in attendance felt that the meeting was highly satisfactory, and at no time were meetings of its character more necessary to the profession, the livestock interests of the nation, and the concerted action of the profession toward the assistance of the Government than at the present time.

The following resolutions of general interest were adopted:

ANIMAL BY-PRODUCTS

WHEREAS, The present method of disposal of the carcasses of

dead animals by burial is not only unsanitary but wasteful of valuable animal products; therefore, be it

Resolved, By the Missouri Valley Veterinary Association that the various States take such action as will provide for the disposition of animal carcasses in a manner that will conform to modern sanitary requirements and make available various valuable animal products so essential to agricultural interests and the successful prosecution of the war; and be it further

Resolved, That copies of this resolution be sent to the Secretary of War, the Secretary of Agriculture and the livestock sanitary authorities of the various States.

THE USE OF HORSEFLESH

WHEREAS, Horseflesh is a nutritious and wholesome food and not objectionable to many people in this and other countries; therefore, be it

Resolved, By the Missouri Valley Veterinary Association that the Federal Government and the various States make available this valuable meat, and that they promulgate such rules and regulations as will safeguard its use; and we further

Resolve, That copies of these resolutions be sent to the Secretary of Agriculture and the livestock and pure food authorities of the various States.

INSPECTION OF IMPORTED HIDES

WHEREAS, The war demand has caused a great increase in the importation of hides and other animal products from countries without adequate livestock sanitary service; and

WHEREAS, Such importations are a constant and serious menace to the livestock industry and the public health of the United States because of the danger of transmitting serious diseases; therefore, be it

Resolved, By the Missouri Valley Veterinary Association that the federal authorities provide that proper veterinary supervision shall be maintained at ports from which such shipments originate, and that copies of this resolution be sent to the Secretary of the Treasury and the Secretary of Agriculture.

PAY OF BUREAU VETERINARIANS

WHEREAS, There is an immediate and growing need for competent and thoroughly trained veterinarians for the federal service; and

WHERAS, The recent increase by the Secretary of Agriculture

is appreciated, yet such important service has not advanced in proportion to the educational requirements and the increased cost of living; therefore, be it

Resolved, By the Missouri Valley Veterinary Association that we recommend that such changes be made in the laws that will provide for the proper remuneration of the veterinarians in the federal service and to this end we pledge our support.

PLEDGE OF LOYALTY

WHEREAS, The exigencies of war demand the best efforts of all patriotic citizens, individually and collectively; and

WHEREAS, We as official and practising veterinarians are the direct conservers of the health of food-producing animals of the nation; be it

Resolved, That we pledge our best efforts and personal service to the President of the United States and to all persons responsible for the successful prosecution of the war.

APPRECIATION TO LOCAL ORGANIZATIONS

Resolved, By the Missouri Valley Veterinary Association that we extend our sincere thanks to the local committee on arrangement, the Chamber of Commerce, the Ak-Sar-Ben and the management of the Hotel Rome for their many and splendid endeavors that have made this meeting so successful and enjoyable.

R. F. BOURNE, Secretary.

THE SOUTHWESTERN MICHIGAN VETERINARY MEDICAL ASSOCIATION

The midsummer meeting of the Southwestern Michigan Veterinary Medical Association was held at Lake of the Woods, Decatur, Mich., Thursday, Aug. 1. Except for a few minor changes the following program was carried out to the letter:

The meeting was called to order by President Hosbein at 10:00 A. M. After the president's address and routine business, two unusual and interesting case reports were presented by Dr. J. W. Randall and Dr. James M. Miller. A paper on "Death by Asphyxia in Horses from Auto Gas" was presented by Dr. E. C. Goodrich, St. Joseph, Mich.

At the afternoon session the following papers were presented: "The Accredited Herd and Its Importance to Livestock Breeders," W. R. Harper, Secretary State Livestock Sanitary Commission.

"Many veterinarians have gone to get the 'Huns'; large districts are left without veterinary service while other territories are overcrowded with veterinarians. How can we overcome the situation for the period of the war?" Answer by Dr. Geo. Dunphy, Lansing, Mich., State Veterinarian.

"Cholera Immune Herds," County Agricultural Agent Wickard of Van Buren County.

"Let's Get Together and Keep Together and Help Win the War," Harry Lurkins, County Agent.

After the presentation of papers the free clinic was held, in charge of Dr. John Neville, assisted by Drs. Howard, Japink, Krieger, Magrane, Clemo, Graham, Bowman, McMichael and Winter.

The ladies were entertained with a boat ride and music while the members held the afternoon session.

This was the best attended meeting ever held. Seven new members were taken into the association.

The next meeting will be held in January, date and place to be decided at a later date.

E. C. GOODRICH, Secretary and Treasurer.

NEW YORK STATE VETERINARY MEDICAL SOCIETY

The twenty-eighth annual meeting of the society was to have been held in Brooklyn in the summer of 1917. Due to the uncertain status of affairs it was voted by the members to dispense with the usual meeting in order that the veterinarians would be in a better condition to meet the demands of the country upon them. As time progressed and it was better known just what our profession could do it was deemed unwise not to hold a meeting this summer. The executive committee accordingly at a meeting held in January decided to submit the proposition to a vote of the members. A canvass was made and a large majority of those voting chose Ithaca as the place for the meeting. Later the committee fixed on July 24, 25 and 26 as the time.

The meeting convened at 10:00 A. M., July 24, at the New York State Veterinary College at Cornell University. In place of President J. G. Schurman, who is absent on leave for Y. M. C. A. work abroad, Prof. D. S. Kimball welcomed the society to the University. Prof. Kimball is acting president while Dr. Schurman is absent. Attorney Fitch Stephens gave an address of welcome on behalf of the City of Ithaca. Dr. W. B. Switzer did great credit to the society in his response to these two excellent speakers. The most of the first morning was taken up by the addresses of welcome and the usual order of business of the association. The paper on "Calf Scours" by Dr. W. A. Hagan and Dr. C. M. Carpenter was given at this session.

The afternoon was taken up with the literary program. Dr. John McCartney gave a paper on "Some Present Day Problems in Milk Sanitation"; Dr. W. L. Williams on "Abortion and Sterility", and Dr. Leo Price on "A Preliminary Report on the Intrapalpebral Mallein Test". These papers were all excellent and elicited a great deal of valuable discussion.

In the evening the members and visitors enjoyed a good dinner at the Clinton House. The after dinner speakers were S. Bruce Wilson, Y. M. C. A. representative with the U. S. Aviation and Vocational schools at Ithaca, and Captain W. E. Muldoon of the V. T. S., Camp Lee, Va. Mr. Wilson was formerly at Camp Dix and was well able to talk on his subject "How Our Army Is Made". Captain Muldoon said that he didn't know what he was going to talk about when he started and didn't know what he had said when he was through. With all this handicap he gave a most interesting and instructive talk on the men in the V. T. S. Dr. Way, who was our impromptu toast-master, called on Dr. Wills, Dr. V. A. Moore, and Dr. W. H. Hoskins for short talks.

The program for the second day of the meeting was varied and highly instructive. Dr. Cassius Way and Dr. A. G. Hall gave a paper on "The Tuberculin Test and the Seven-Day Re-Test", Dr. A. Slawson on "Serum Treatment of Canine Distemper—Results During the Present Year", Dr. H. S. Beebe on "A Few Remarks in Reference to Recent Veterinary Legislation", Dr. G. A. Knapp on "Some Recent Experiences with Hemorrhagic Septicemia in Cattle", Dr. R. W. Gannett on "Clinical Observations on Foot Diseases of the Horse", Dr. H. B. Leonard on "Accredited Herds", Dr. S. A. Goldberg on "Microscopic Foreign Bodies in the Tissues", and Dr. E. Sunderville read the paper prepared by Dr. G. S. Hopkins on "Facial Sinuses of the Sheep". Clinic was held throughout the morning of the third day in the operating rooms of the college.

On the evening of the second day Dr. and Mrs. V. A. Moore

entertained the society at a Lawn Party at their home at 914 East State Street. Refreshments were served. Music and readings helped to entertain their guests throughout the evening. This evening was one of the best parts of the program. For the visiting ladies a lunch at the University Club, a motor ride about the city, "Retreat" at the field of the Aviation School, a boat ride on Lake Cayuga, lunch at the Cafeteria of the Home Economics Building of the University, an organ recital by Prof. J. T. Quarles, a theatre party and the evening entertainments furnished a very pleasant ime.

Dr. Geo. A. Knapp of Millbrook was elected president for the ensuing year, Dr. H. S. Beebe of Albion vice president, Dr. C. E. Hayden of Ithaca secretary-treasurer, and Dr. H. J. Milks of Ithaca librarian. Sixteen new members were recommended by the board of censors and were duly elected to membership. The seventeenth application was received on the last day of the meeting and since the applicant is one of the profession most highly eligible he will be elected at the next annual meeting. Dr. James Law and Dr. Wilson Huff were elected to be honorary members of the society.

There has never been held a better meeting of the New York State Veterinary Medical Society than the twenty-eighth annual meeting. Attendance, excellency of scientific papers and entertainment were all above par. However, the meeting at Brooklyn next year is to be better than the one just closed. ·

C. E. HAYDEN, Secretary-Treasurer.

OREGON AND WASHINGTON VETERINARY MEDICAL ASSOCIATIONS

The Oregon and Washington Veterinary Medical Associations held a joint meeting at the Imperial Hotel, Portland, Oregon, June 13, 14 and 15, 1918. More than seventy veterinarians were present. This is a much larger number of veterinarians than has ever before been assembled for any meeting in the Northwest. The two state presidents, Doctor L. C. Pelton of Washington and Doctor S. M. Reagan of Oregon had Doctor S. B. Nelson, Dean of Veterinary College of Washington State College, preside at the meeting.

With Doctor Nelson in the chair, the meeting was called to order Thursday morning June 13 and an address of welcome was given by Mr. C. C. Colt, President of the Union Meat Company of Portland. Doctor Pelton responded. The first paper was by Doctor C. W. Lassen of Pendleton on "The Intrapalpebral Mallein Test". Lieut. E. B. Osborne of Camp Lewis led in a discussion of this paper. Lieut. Osborne has tested some 3000 horses with this test in the past three years during which time he has acted as Assistant State Veterinarian of Oregon or as Veterinarian in the Army. All veterinarians present who have used this test were enthusiastic in its praise.

The next paper was by Doctor W. H. Lytle, State Veterinarian of Oregon, on "The So-Called Walking Disease of Horses". Discussion was led by Doctors Nelson and Simms. This peculiar and baffling disease has appeared in the wheat belt of Oregon and Washington from time to time during the last ten or fifteen years. Losses have been very heavy at some periods. Doctor Lytle seemed to believe that the trouble is quite possibly of parasitic origin.

Doctor J. W. Cook of Brownsville read a paper on "Diarrhea in Horses". He reported that this trouble was very common in his section of Oregon during the past winter. Some seventy-five to eighty cases occurred in a very small area. It was recalled that the past winter had been a very mild one with a great deal of moisture. The possibility of a mold that grew on the hay as being the causative agent was suggested. Doctor Cook reported that practically all cases yielded to treatment very nicely. Several other veterinarians practicing in the Willamette Valley reported that this disturbance was more or less common in their neighborhood during the winter months.

Doctor E. C. Joss, Federal Inspector in charge of Western Division, read a paper on "New Zealand and Australian Meat Inspection System and the Possible Adoption of this System in the Pacific Northwestern States". The discussion of this paper was led by Doctor E. E. Chase, Chief City Meat Inspector of Portland, Oregon. Two papers on tuberculosis were read, one by Doctor Sam B. Foster, veterinarian in charge of tuberculosis eradication in Oregon and Washington, and the other on Avian tuberculosis by Doctor Peter Hanson, Veterinary Inspector of the City of Portland. Doctor Foster reported some very interesting results obtained in eradicating tuberculosis in the pure-bred herds of the Northwest. Doctor Hanson exhibited a tubercular fowl, showing the disease in the advanced stage. He reported that Avian tuberculosis is very common in the Pacific Northwest and that large numbers of tubercular fowls are slaughtered at Portland.

There were three papers on hog cholera. The first was by Mr. W. F. Richter of Portland, Oregon, a representative of the Cutter Laboratories of Berkeley, California. The second was by Doctor Beattie of the Union Stock Yards of Portland, Oregon. The third was by Doctor W. W. Sullivan of Twin Falls, Idaho. Doctor Sullivan is the Federal Inspector in charge of hog cholera control in the Twin Falls district. It seemed to be the opinion of the veterinarians present that the serum alone method of vaccination is advisable in the major portion of the Northwest. Practicing veterinarians reported that hog cholera is not at all prevalent in the Northwest at the present time. The State Veterinarians of both Oregon and Washington advise that very few outbreaks of this disease are being reported and that they are being controlled quite nicely through the use of serum alone. Doctor Sullivan emphasized the fact that vaccinating to prevent hog cholera is not a hit or miss method but that it is a scientific procedure requiring the careful work of a scientific man if the proper results are to be obtained.

A paper on anthrax was read by Doctor C. A. Jones of Sedro Woolley, Washington. Doctor Jones gave some of his experiences in recent outbreaks of this disease.

A paper entitled ''Diagnosis of Diseases of Sheep'', prepared by Doctor E. T. Baker of Moscow, Idaho, was read by the secretary of the Washington association. This was followed by very interesting discussions. A case report by Doctor H. Nunn of Corvallis regarding tetanus in a mare with a suckling foal was read by the secretary of the Oregon association.

Doctor C. H. Schultz of the Department of Health and Sanitation of Seattle, Washington, read a paper entitled ''Mysterious Losses Among Cattle in the Pacific Northwest''. This paper reported the results of several years' investigations of diseases of cattle in this section of the country. Doctor Schultz brought out the fact·that coccidia are found in many outbreaks of a so-called mysterious disease among cattle. He exhibited slides showing beautiful specimens of coccidia in all of their various stages. These organisms were obtained upon the feces of animals suffering from the disease. Nearly every veterinarian present reported that cattle losses in his district had been quite common in the past and that symptoms had been very similar to those described by Doctor Schultz.

A portion of Friday, June 14, was spent at the packing plant of the Union Meat Company, Portland, Oregon. A most delightful luncheon was served to the veterinarians by the Meat Company. During the afternoon of the same day the veterinarians visited the slaughter house at which horses are killed for the Portland market. Doctor E. E. Chase, Meat Inspector of the city, slaughtered a tubercular cow and demonstrated the method of examining slaughtered animals for tuberculosis.

On the night of Friday, June 14, a most delightful banquet was served at the Imperial Hotel.

Election of officers for the two associations resulted as follows: For the Washington association—Doctor L. C. Pelton of Seattle, president; Doctor W. Ferguson of Spokane, vice president; Doctor Carl Cozier of Bellingham, treasurer. For Oregon—Doctor F. E. Eames of The Dalles, president; Doctor Roy Smith of Eugene, first vice president; Doctor B. E. Nevel of Prineville, second vice president; Doctor Peter Hanson of Portland, fourth vice president; Doctor B. T. Simms of Corvallis, secretary and treasurer. It was voted to hold another joint meeting in 1920, electing Portland as the meeting place two years hence.

On Saturday morning, a polyclinic was held at the hospital of Doctor G. H. Huthman. On Saturday afternoon the veterinarians made an automobile trip up the famous Columbia River Highway. This is considered one of the most scenic highways in America. Even Doctor C. H. Schultz of Seattle admitted that this was the equal of the famous scenery of Switzerland, saying that the trip made him homesick for his Swiss mountains.

Thanks are especially due to Doctor E. E. Chase of Portland who, as chairman on the committee of local arrangements, made the joint meeting a most successful one.   B. T. Simms.

VIRGINIA VETERINARY MEDICAL ASSOCIATION

After the business transactions of the association and the President's address the following program was carried through:

Some Phases of the Work of the Bureau of Animal Industry in Its Relation to the War—J. R. Mohler, Chief of the B. A. I., Washington, D. C.

Antibodies (tissue reacting products) in Their Fight Against Infection—G. A. Roberts, Raleigh, N. C.

Thoracic Choke Due to Abnormal Trachea—L. O. Price, Blacksburg, Va.

Parturient Apoplexy—W. G. Chrisman, Blacksburg, Va.

Lieut.-Colonel C. J. Marshall, Assistant Director of Veterinary Service, Washington, D. C., was unable to be present to give his paper on Some Phases of Army Veterinary Activities.

On July 12, at 1 o'clock, luncheon was served to sixty members and guests. The guests of honor were Governor Westmoreland Davis; President J. D. Eggleston of the Virginia Agricultural College; Hon. J. Thompson Brown, Chairman of the Virginia Livestock Sanitary Board; Dr. G. A. Roberts, Professor of Veterinary Science of the A. & M. College, Raleigh, N. C.; Major Gill, Veterinarian in Charge of the U. S. Embarkation Station at Newport News, Va.; Captain Gregg, in charge of the British Remount Station, Newport News, Va., and Lieut. Glover, his assistant; Captain Dunn, Lieuts. White, Mickle, Kelsey and Naylor.

After adjournment many of the veterinarians visited Camp Hill to see the largest veterinary hospital in the world.

The next meeting of the association will be at Richmond, Va., Jan. 16 and 17, 1919.   W. G. Chrisman, Secretary.

———◆———

COLORADO VETERINARY MEDICAL ASSOCIATION

By far the most interesting meeting which the Colorado Veterinary Medical Association has ever held was their semi-annual gathering at Ft. Collins on June 27 and 28. The attendance was large considering the small size of the association and the interest was very intense. The most important items of business were amendments to the by-laws providing for raising the dues from $2 to $3 per year and striking out the requirement that applicants for membership should hold a license to practice within the State. This latter change resulted immediately in veterinarians from both Wyoming and New Mexico joining the association, there being no organization in either one of these states. Six new members were elected.

Entertainment consisted in an automobile ride for the ladies some thirty miles up the Poudre Canon, followed by a picnic lunch near the river for all members and their ladies. The noon luncheon was taken at the mess hall with the two hundred and six soldiers who are located at the college for special training in the Mechanic Arts.

Drs. A. T. Kinsley and H. Jensen of Kansas City were present to add to the interest taken in the program. The president's address dealt largely with our duties and obligations as veterinarians in the present war. Some cases of probable mistaken diagnosis were detailed by D. C. Patterson, one of them particularly being a question as to diagnosis where hogs were dying of what was variously diagnosed as cholera and necrobacillosis.

Hemorrhagic septicemia in sheep was considered more formally by A. A. Hermann and I. E. Newsom, the former giving his experience in treating large numbers of these animals by means of bacterins and the latter offering a detailed account of some experiments which seem to show that the disease is quite prevalent in the State. Later the discussion became general and nearly every one took part.

Dr. A. W. French, State Veterinarian of Wyoming, read a paper on the "Intradermal Test for Bovine Tuberculosis", giving his experience on many thousands of animals in the State where the testing was conducted from the State Veterinarian's office. He had no hesitancy in saying that for the conditions as they exist in Wyoming the intradermal test is much to be preferred over the subcutaneous.

The high point of the meeting, however, came in the discussion of hog cholera. Dr. E. E. Tobin discussed what constituted a proper fee for the use of biologics. This resulted in the appointment of a committee to report on the question. Dr. A. G. Wadleigh, who is veterinarian to the Monte Vista Hog Growers' Association, gave some suggestions on vaccinating hogs as the result of his experience. Dr. C. F. Harrington, B. A. I. hog cholera specialist, working in the State Veterinarian's office, gave a paper on "Cholera, Its Control and Eradication". Dr. A. T. Kinsley discussed very clearly and concisely the differential features of the various diseases which may be confused with hog cholera. His address brought out a great deal of discussion regarding the indication of the various symptoms and lesions which have formerly been considered as being associated with this disease. On the following day, Drs. Kinsley, Harrington and Thrower conducted a post mortem examination on two pigs that were affected with a disease that simulated hog cholera. On these animals they exemplified what had been brought out in the discussion the day previously.

In fact, it was the concensus of opinion that this demonstration was the most helpful single event that occurred during the meeting.

A round table discussion on "The Relation of the Veterinarian to the County Agent" was led by Dr. G. H. Glover and participated in by Drs. E. H. Lehnert of the University of Wyoming, G. W. Dickey of Colorado Springs and H. T. French, Director of the Extension Department in Colorado.

The clinic lasted all day Friday and was replete with interesting operations and cases. A demonstration of hog cholera vaccination was given by Dr. H. E. Kingman of the Colorado Agricultural College and Dr. J. D. Thrower of the Denver Hog Ranch Company. Each demonstrated his own technique. After the members had gone many clinic cases remained untouched for want of time.

I. E. NEWSOM, Secretary.

NATIONAL ASSOCIATION OF BUREAU OF ANIMAL INDUSTRY VETERINARIANS

At the annual meeting of the association the following temporary officers were elected:

President, Dr. J. S. Koen, Des Moines, Iowa; secretary, Dr. S. J. Walkley, Milwaukee, Wis.; treasurer, Dr. L. Enos Day, Chicago, Ill.; vice president-at-large, Dr. F. P. St. Clair, Omaha, Neb.; vice president eastern zone, Dr. Leland D. Ives, New York City; vice president central zone, Dr. M. Guillaume, Chicago, Ill.; vice president southern zone, Dr. J. S. Grove, Oklahoma City, Okla.; vice president western zone, Dr. B. W. Murphy, Topeka, Kansas.   S. J. WALKLEY, Temporary Secretary.

SOUTHERN TIER VETERINARY MEDICAL ASSOCIATION

The fourth annual meeting of the Southern Tier Veterinary Medical Association was held at Binghamton, N. Y., on July 5, 1918. Thirty-four veterinarians were present.

During the morning a clinic was held at the hospital of Dr. A. W. Baker, who had provided ample material. The following cases were handled: Roarer, examined by Dr. P. J. Axtell and pronounced inoperable; repulsion of lower molar, Dr. R. R. Bolton and Dr. D. W. Clark; sterile cow, Dr. R. R. Birch; cryptorchid, Dr. P. J. Axtell; tumor, dog, Dr. H. J. Milks.

Following luncheon at Hotel Bennett the meeting was called to order by President Battin, and a short business session was held, during which nine new applicants were admitted to membership. Dr. H. J. Milks was elected president; Dr. P. J. Axtell, vice president, and Dr. R. R. Birch was reelected secretary-treasurer.

Dr. Leonard of the Bureau of Animal Industry, Tuberculosis Eradication Division, read a very concise and interesting paper entitled "Accredited Herds" in which he explained the aims and methods of the system followed by the Bureau, with respect to placing herds on the accredited list.

This paper was discussed by Dr. V. A. Moore and Dr. J. G. Wills. Dr. Moore directed special attention to the dangers incident to accrediting herds without the most searching methods of establishing clean bills of health, and to the consequent discredit which might fall on an otherwise excellent system. He stated further that in districts where herds are badly infected, it is especially dangerous to place too much confidence in the health of animals that fail to react to tuberculin.

Dr. Wills brought out the point that in cleaning up herds preparatory to placing them on the accredited list, the practicing veterinarian has an important part to play, and that it is only through intelligent and sympathetic understanding between herd owner and veterinarian that any progress worth while can be expected.

Dr. R. R. Bolton read a carefully prepared and well received paper on "The Examination of the Eye". This is a phase of veterinary medicine that receives too little attention, and Dr. Bolton's paper covered the subject thoroughly.

In the enforced absence of Dr. E. F. Vorhis, who was to read a paper entitled "The Business Side of a Country Practice", Dr. P. J. Axtell discussed the subject extemporaneously, calling attention to the business and professional aspects of veterinary practice. He regarded professional ability as most important, but asserted that it should be supplemented by business ability and business methods, as people have no confidence in one who is unbusinesslike.

Dr. J. W. Ardell discussed the subject from the standpoint of the young practitioner, just establishing a practice. His remarks might be summed up thus: "Be at your place of business and do not permit that place of business to be a livery stable, unless you are manager."

After voting fifty dollars to the relief fund for Belgian and French veterinarians the meeting adjourned.

R. R. BIRCH, Secretary.

REVIEW

THE CORNELL VETERINARIAN—SHEEP NUMBER

Vol. VIII, No. 3, July, 1918

From time to time and as conditions have warranted, it has been the policy of the *Cornell Veterinarian* to publish special numbers or to use single issues for opportune subjects. The regular July issue is devoted to sheep. The editor, Dr. E. M. Pickens, and Dr. V. A. Moore each have editorials that are succinct. The part that the veterinarian may and should play in giving aid in the revival of the sheep industry as an important national industry is very aptly shown in the editorial by Dean Moore.

Following the editorial pages there are nine leading articles. "Farm Flock Husbandry" is presented by M. J. Smith, Department of Animal Husbandry, Cornell University. Dr. G. S. Hopkins has an illustrated and instructive article on "The Paranasal or Facial Sinuses of Sheep". The knowledge of these sinuses is essential to the veterinarian should it become necessary to remove the larvae of oestrus ovis from them. Dr. E. Sunderville has written on the "Anatomy of the Digestive Tract of Sheep", and C. E. Hayden on "Digestion in the Sheep". "The Veterinarian and Sheep Practice: Especially as It Relates to Intestinal Parasites", delivered before the students of the New York State Veterinary College at Cornell University by Dr. Cooper Curtice of the Bureau of Animal Industry, is extremely practical and helpful. Dr. James Law has written a thorough discussion on "Digestive Disorders (colic) in Sheep". This article is followed by one from the pen of Dr. V. A. Moore on "Infectious Diseases of Sheep". The discussion is the usual clear, scientific presentation for which the author is noted. "Obstetrics of Sheep" should and does receive consideration at the hands of Dr. W. L. Williams. The readers of the number are fortunate to have these three articles from the men of all the profession most competent to write them. Dr. J. N. Frost and Dr. F. B. Hopper have a short but helpful paper on "Docking and Castration of the Young Lamb". There are six case reports, all of which are written from sheep practice. The extraneous matter in the number is very little. Practically all of it is given over to the sheep industry. As one reads the issue it cannot but be felt that its purpose to stimulate the interest and knowledge of both breeders and veterinarians in the revival of the sheep industry will be fulfilled.   C. E. HAYDEN.

MISCELLANEOUS

EDITOR DALRYMPLE

As the last form is closing, word has reached us that Dr. W. H. Dalrymple of the Louisiana State University at Baton Rouge, La., has accepted the editorship of the JOURNAL OF THE AMERICAN VETERINARY MEDICAL ASSOCIATION. Doctor Dalrymple is too well known in the American veterinary profession to require an eulogy from us. His broad experience, his high-mindedness upon all ethical questions, his staunch patriotism and his cosmopolitanism, are guarantees of the future success of the JOURNAL. We ask for him complete and loyal cooperation.

With the publication of this number, which completes the sixth volume of the New Series, we retire in favor of Doctor Dalrymple, to whom all JOURNAL communications should be addressed in the future.   P. A. F.

—Dr. E. P. Caldwell, formerly at Caldwell, Idaho, is now at 323 Federal Bldg., Salt Lake, Utah.

—Dr. L. B. Fox has removed from Bartlesville to 215 Exchange Bldg., Oklahoma City, Okla.

—Dr. B. L. Cook has removed from Farmington, Minn., to Red Wing, Minn.

—The annual meeting of the Eastern Iowa Veterinary Association will be held Oct. 16 and 17, 1918, at Cedar Rapids, Iowa. The meeting will probably be held at the Montrose Hotel, which will be the headquarters for the committee for registration of members.

—366,392 WAR ANIMALS PURCHASED FOR THE ARMY. The War Department authorizes the following:

The number of animals purchased by the Remount Division of the Quartermaster Corps from the beginning of the war. April 6, 1917, to July 15, 1918, is as follows:

United States:	Horses	Mules	Total
Mature	174,676	123,640	298,316
Young	4,238	......	4,238
France	58,093	5,745	63,838
Total	237,007	129,385	366,392

—HORSE MEAT IN FRANCE. The people of France are eating two thousand donkeys and mules and three hundred horses a day. The average weight of those slaughtered for meat is 500 pounds. Last year about 70,000 horses were utilized as meat. The British Army furnishes 200 horses a day. The best cuts sell at about 36 cents a pound. By utilizing horse meat as human food, France has relieved the meat shortage to a great extent. Wounded horses which are not fit for war service are sold at prices ranging, in our money, from about $14 to $128. There is said to be an abundant supply.

—A mysterious cattle disease resembling paralysis is causing large losses to Transvaal farmers. The disease is believed to be connected in some way with an outbreak of infantile paralysis or poliomyelitis among human beings in the same districts.

—Denmark's stock of swine, which amounted to about 2,500,000 head at the outbreak of the war, has now dropped to 400,000, according to latest estimates. Further serious inroads on this stock are being compelled by the impossibility of importing fodder, principally corn. In 1913 Denmark's total exports of pork were nearly 250,000 tons, of which just under one-half went to England. All exports have now been stopped, and the outlook for supplying the domestic consumption's requirements will be dark if the war continues much longer.

—TRIBUTE TO THE HORSE. Says a writer: "God bless the noble animal, he is everywhere when wanted, doing everything required of him. Charging in the face of fire and like a perfectly drilled battalion, carrying cavalry riders across plains, down deep ravines or up rugged steeps, failing only when either nature becomes exhausted or the bullet from a foeman's gun lays him low. There is no load too heavy for him to draw, no surface so dangerous as to cause him to refuse to strain every ounce of strength, no quagmire too deep or broad but what he bends nobly, resolutely to the task which has been given him. Ever and always he is at his master's call.

—The 11th annual meeting of the American Association of Pharmaceutical Chemists was held at Cedar Point, Ohio, June 17-20. It is reported to be the most successful meeting in the history of the association. Professor Kremers described his work as head of the Wisconsin Pharmaceutical Experiment Station, the only institution of its kind in the country. He asked for cooperation and assistance in arousing Congress to the need for appropriating the necessary funds for the experimental culture of medicinal plants on a large scale. Their cultivation is of national importance in the promotion of the self reliance of the United States in the production of medicines.

—CATTLE DIPPING BREAKS RECORDS. Reports to the Bureau of Animal Industry disclose that May set a new record in the work of eradicating the cattle-fever tick. In that month the number of cattle dipped was 5,468,600, the largest number reported in any one month since the campaign began actively in 1906. The big figures are believed to indicate the unanimity with which southern livestock raisers have joined in the fight to free the South from the tick by 1921. The number of dipping vats available in May was 25,911 and 338 Federal inspectors, 284 State inspectors, and 1,426 county inspectors supervised the work.

—PROMPT VETERINARY TREATMENT. Not long ago a farmer of the old school experimented for a couple of weeks on his sick hogs. He fed a hog tonic and various concoctions the knowledge of which he inherited from ancestral swine breeders, but a few more hogs got sick each day and they began to die faster and faster. He winced under the strain as hog after hog went under the sod. He thought it might be cholera, but he did not know. Finally his wife persuaded him to call a graduate veterinarian and to agree to follow his suggestions. She thus virtually secured a promise that her husband would vaccinate his remaining hogs and stop the loss. A post mortem revealed unmistakable cholera lesions and all the hogs on the place, big and little, were given the serum and virus, with the exception of a few very young litters. Over 150 head were treated and thirty of them were noticeably sick. Only seventeen of these died and all of the others were saved. He paid $137 for the treatment—the value of four of the fifteen hogs that he had buried during his trial of home doctoring.

After recounting this experience and the outcome, this gray-haired man declared that the burial of $450 worth of hogs had taught him that prompt veterinary advice and treatment is the best investment a farmer can make when an animal is seriously sick and he does not know what will cure it. He regretted that he had not called the veterinarian sooner, but he thanked his lucky stars—and his wife—that he called the doctor when he did.

The high value on livestock will doubtless serve to teach many others that the money paid for needed veterinary services is well invested. The moment an owner admits to himself that he does not quite know what is wrong or what will cure an ailing animal, it is time for him to call the veterinarian. A few dollars spent for such service during the year will save a few hogs or calves, a cow or a horse. It is a better interest-paying investment than Liberty Bonds and just as necessary for the feeding of the national army.— *Breeders' Gazette.*

—AIDS IN FURNISHING ARMY REMOUNTS. The United States Department of Agriculture is cooperating with the War Department in producing horses for the Army. G. A. Bell of the Department of Agriculture has recently returned from Virginia, Vermont, and New Hampshire, where, with a representative from the War Department, 135 horses were purchased. These horses were 3-year-olds and were purchased from farmers who bred their mares to stallions owned by the Department of Agriculture. Through an agreement made by farmers and the Government, the Government agrees to pay $150 for each colt sired by Government-owned stallions, provided it passes the requirements of the War Department, or the farmer, by paying the service fee, can keep the colt for his own use.

WOMEN'S AUXILIARY TO THE A. V. M. A.

At a meeting held at Philadelphia, Aug. 19, 1918, the following officers were elected:

Mrs. W. H. Hoskins, president; Mrs. H. Jensen, Kansas City, Mo., vice president; Mrs. Chas. E. Cotton, Minneapolis, Minn., recording secretary; Mrs. Lockhart, Kansas City, Mo., corresponding secretary.

The following Constitution and By-Laws were adopted:

WOMEN'S AUXILIARY
ARTICLE I
SECTION 1. This organization shall be known as WOMEN'S AUXILIARY TO THE AMERICAN VETERINARY MEDICAL ASSOCIATION.

ARTICLE II
SECTION 1. The object of this association is to give necessary financial assistance to the family of any veterinarian engaged in war work if his life has been forfeited in pursuance of such work, or if he has been temporarily or permanently disabled.

ARTICLE III
SECTION 1. The sisters or sister, wife, daughter or daughters and mother of a veterinarian who is eligible to A. V. M. A. membership shall be eligible to membership. Contributing members may be carried from year to year when contributions are made by others than those eligible to regular membership.

ARTICLE IV
SECTION 1. Meetings shall be regular and special.
Sec. 2. Regular meetings shall be held annually at the time of the meet-

ing of the A. V. M. A. The exact date to be chosen by the hostesses and president.

Sec. 3. Special meetings may be called by the president or on written request signed by fifty members. No other business shall be transacted except what is stated in the call for the same.

ARTICLE V

SECTION 1. The officers of the association shall consist of a president, 1st, 2nd, 3rd vice presidents, secretary, corresponding secretary, treasurer, and an auditing committee of three appointed by the president.

Sec. .2. The officers and chairmen of permanent committees shall constitute an executive board.

Sec. 3. The officers shall be elected at a regular annual meeting and hold office for two years from the date of their election. Vacancies in the office of the secretary or treasurer shall be filled by appointment for the unexpired term by the president.

Sec. 4. The chairman of the permanent committee shall be appointed by the president.

Sec. 5. The treasurer shall pay out money on vouchers countersigned by the president and secretary.

Sec. 6. The treasurer shall account to the association for all moneys received. She shall give bond to the association in the sum of $1000.00, acceptable to the executive board. At the expiration of her term of office she shall account for and turn over to her successor in office all moneys, vouchers and account books belonging to the association.

BY-LAWS
ARTICLE I

SECTION 1. Twenty-five per cent of the women registered at any meeting shall constitute a quorum for the transaction of business.

ARTICLE II

SECTION 1. There shall be an initiation fee of fifty cents. The annual dues shall be fifty cents payable in advance on or before date of annual meeting. Any member two years in arrears for dues shall be automatically dropped from the roll of membership. Reinstatement on payment of arrearages and approval of the committee on membership or executive committee.

ARTICLE III

SECTION 1. Nominations for office shall be made orally, not more than three nominees for each office. A majority of all the votes cast shall be necessary to elect.

Sec. 2. The officers shall assume their duties at the close of the annual meeting at which they are elected.

THE HORSE TO HIS MASTER

I am a Horse! You are a Man:
I've been your slave since I began.
And though I'm strong enough to shake
My shackles off and make a break
For freedom that would lift the lid,
You've noticed that I never did.
By day and night I've worked for you

And done the best that I could do;
And though I may not always like
Your methods, yet I never strike;
In heat or cold, in wet or dry
I'm always ready—Glad to try
To do the very most I can
To satisfy my master, man.
Therefore, my master, if you please,
Considering such facts as these,
Say, don't you think it ought to be
Your pleasure to look out for me,
If for no other reason than
My greater usefulness to man?
Of course, you might be worse, I know
You sometimes treat your own kind so, but I'm a Horse,
And truer than the man-slave to his master, man,
And furthermore, my nature is
Much more dependent than is his.
And as I trust you, Sir, you should
Do all you can to make it good. Nor do I ask a lot, I guess,
To be a fairly fair success—Good food, good shelter and good care,
I think it just about my share, no other pay I ask—
No touch I make, but this.—Is that too much?

—W. J. LAMPTON.

—The use of horseflesh for human consumption in France has
greatly increased. Last year more than 70,000 horses were killed
for food in Paris.